Gastrointestinal Surgery: Advanced Techniques

Gastrointestinal Surgery: Advanced Techniques

Edited by Diana Pollard

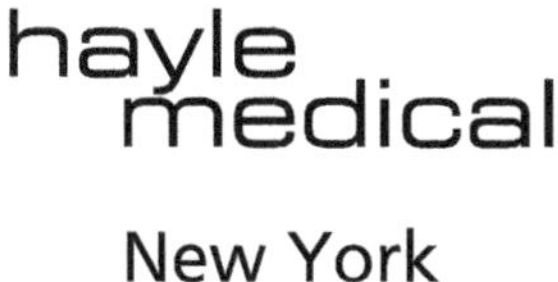

New York

Hayle Medical,
750 Third Avenue, 9th Floor,
New York, NY 10017, USA

Visit us on the World Wide Web at:
www.haylemedical.com

ISBN: 978-1-63241-609-4

Cataloging-in-Publication Data

Gastrointestinal surgery : advanced techniques / edited by Diana Pollard.
p. cm.
Includes bibliographical references and index.
ISBN 978-1-63241-609-4
1. Gastrointestinal system--Surgery. 2. Digestive organs--Surgery.
3. Surgical technology. I. Pollard, Diana.

RD540 .G37 2019
617.4--dc23

Table of Contents

Preface

The gastrointestinal tract is responsible for the assimilation of food and expulsion of wastes in the form of feces. Various organs are responsible for these functions, including mouth, the esophagus, stomach and intestines. Gastrointestinal surgery can be classified into two parts, i.e., upper gastrointestinal surgery and lower gastrointestinal surgery. Upper gastrointestinal surgery is the practice of surgery which focuses on the upper parts of the gastrointestinal tract. Lower gastrointestinal surgery is the type of surgery which is concerned with colorectal surgery and the surgery of the small intestine. This book unravels the recent studies in the field of gastrointestinal surgery. It will also provide interesting topics for research which interested readers can take up. Researchers, doctors and students in the field of gastroenterology will be assisted by this book.

All of the data presented henceforth, was collaborated in the wake of recent advancements in the field. The aim of this book is to present the diversified developments from across the globe in a comprehensible manner. The opinions expressed in each chapter belong solely to the contributing authors. Their interpretations of the topics are the integral part of this book, which I have carefully compiled for a better understanding of the readers.

At the end, I would like to thank all those who dedicated their time and efforts for the successful completion of this book. I also wish to convey my gratitude towards my friends and family who supported me at every step.

Editor

1

Laparoscopic gastric pouch and remnant resection: a novel approach to refractory anastomotic ulcers after Roux-en-Y Gastric Bypass: Case report

Daniel C Steinemann[1,2], Marc Schiesser[1], Pierre-Alain Clavien[1] and Antonio Nocito[1*]

Abstract

Background: Anastomotic or marginal ulcers occur in 0.6 to 16% of patients after laparoscopic Roux-en-Y-Gastric Bypass. Initial therapy aims at eliminating known risk factors including smoking, Helicobacter pylori infection, use of non-steroidal anti-inflammatory drugs and inhibition of gastric acid secretion. While this approach is successful in 68 to 88% of the cases, up to one third of patients need a subsequent surgical revision. However, marginal ulcers still recur in up to 10% of cases after revisional surgery, thus constituting a serious challenge for bariatric surgeons.

Case presentation: We herein report a case of an insidious marginal ulcer refractory to both medical therapy with high-dosed proton pump inhibitors and sucralfate as well as surgical therapy consisting of the lengthening of a short alimentary limb and later resection of the gastroenterostomy and construction of a new tension-free anastomosis. Only after gastrectomy by laparoscopic en-bloc resection of the gastrojejunostomy, the gastric pouch and resection of the gastric remnant with reconstruction by esophagojejunostomy the patient remained free of symptoms.

Conclusion: By laparoscopic resection of the entire gastric pouch and the gastric remnant the risk to leave a suboptimally vascularised or even ischemic pouch in situ was avoided. The esophagojejunostomy was then created in healthy, good vascularised tissue. In our case this novel approach was effective in the management of a refractory anastomotic ulcer and might represent a rescue option when simple revision of the gastrojejunostomy fails.

Keywords: Roux-en-Y-Gastric Bypass, bariatric surgery, anastomotic ulcer, marginal ulcer, obesity

Background

A specific complication after laparoscopic Roux-en-Y-Gastric-Bypass (LRYGB) is a marginal or anastomotic ulcer (AU) occurring at the gastrojejunal anastomosis. While AU can remain asymptomatic in 62-92% of the cases [1-4], they can frequently cause disabling pain or complications such as perforation and bleeding [5,6]. The incidence of AU varies from 0.6% to 16% in endoscopic studies [1-4].

* Correspondence: antonio.nocito@usz.ch
[1]Department of Visceral and Transplantation Surgery, University Hospital Zurich, Raemistrasse 100, 8091 Zurich, Switzerland
Full list of author information is available at the end of the article

The etiology of AU is unclear. Two classes of risk factors have been suggested: operative and patient related factors. Although large gastric pouch, vertically oriented pouch [7], gastro-gastric fistula [8], local tissue ischemia due to anastomotic tension [9] or presence of foreign bodies in the ulcer ground (e.g. nonabsorbable sutures) [10] have been previously discussed, there is still a lack of high level of evidence demonstrating these factors to be significant. In contrast, better data exist for patient related factors, showing that smoking (odds ratio (OR) 30.6), use of nonsteroidal anti-inflammatory drugs (OR 11.5) and lack of proton pump inhibitor (PPI) prophylaxis (OR 3) represent significant risk factors [11].

Therefore, ulcer therapy starts with elimination of patient related risk factors and inhibition of gastric acid secretion. While this approach is successful in 68 to 88%, up to one third of the patients need a subsequent surgical revision [8,12]. Although revision surgery is successful in most cases, AU recur in up to 8% [8], thus leading to a distressing situation for both patients and bariatric surgeons.

We herein report a case of an insidious AU refractory medical and surgical therapy, which finally required an aggressive approach consisting of laparoscopic gastric pouch and gastric remnant resection.

Case presentation

In a 50 year male patient with a BMI of 45 kg/m^2 an antecolic, antegastric LRYGB with a 100 cm alimentary and a 60 cm biliary limb was performed. The gastrojejunostomy was constructed using a 25 mm circular stapler (EEA 2535, 3.5 mm Staples, Covidien®). Simultaneously, a 6 cm silastic (Fobi) ring was placed around the gastrojejunostomy. A few weeks after discharge, the patient, who continued smoking after surgery, presented with strong epigastric pain, postprandial regurgitation and vomiting. He was unable to eat solid food and to attend work. Endoscopy revealed two AU at the gastrojejunostomy. Oral PPI therapy (esomeprazole, 80 mg/die) was initiated and, since it was thought to be partly responsible for the symptoms, the silastic ring was removed. Intravenous high-dose PPI (esomeprazole, 240 mg/die) led to healing of the AU. However, epigastric pain and regurgitation did not ameliorate. A 99 m Tc-mebrofenin scintigraphy revealed severe biliary reflux. Seven months after LRYGB the patient was referred to our department.

At the initial consultation the patient was taking up to 600 mg/day esomeprazole and 200 mg/day tilidin orally. As an AU could not be detected further diagnostic investigations were performed:

- Upper gastrointestinal (GI) contrast series revealing a small gastric pouch without signs of a gastric fistula and normal passage.
- Double balloon push enteroscopy demonstrating a short (40 cm) alimentary limb.
- High-resolution esophageal manometry revealing a normotensive propulsive peristalsis and a normotense lower esophageal sphincter.
- 24 h-impedance pH-metry - performed under antacid medication - showing no pathological acid or non-acid reflux.
- MRI in Sellink technique showing no obstruction of the small bowel.

Apart from the biliary reflux diagnosed by scintigraphy consistent with a very short Roux-limb by push-enteroscopy, no other reason for the epigastric pain was detected. We performed a laparoscopic lengthening of the Roux limb by additional 120 cm resulting in a new alimentary limb of 160 cm. Oral PPI therapy (80 mg/day) was continued and sucralfate (4 g/d) was added.

After a short period without pain and regurgitation, symptoms recurred two weeks after Roux limb lengthening. Despite PPI therapy endoscopy revealed a recurrent AU at the gastrojejunostomy (Figure 1). Therefore a laparoscopic resection of the gastrojejunostomy was performed followed by a construction of a new, tension-free anastomosis using a 25 mm circular stapler (EEA 2535, 3.5 mm Staples, Covidien®). PPI therapy and sucralfate were continued. Again the patient was discharged free of symptoms on postoperative day five.

One month later and one year after initial LRYGB surgery, the patient was again not free of epigastric pain. Gastroscopy showed again a large AU at the gastroenterostomy. Meanwhile, the patient was finally motivated enough to quit smoking and was enrolled in a stop-smoking program. Since gastrin level was not elevated (111 ng/l) an underlying gastrinoma could be excluded. Furthermore, Helicobacter pylori and hyperparathyroidism as additional potential causes for anastomotic ulcers were also ruled out. Nevertheless, epigastric pain and the AU persisted.

At this point an aggressive approach was decided consisting of a gastrectomy by laparoscopic en-bloc resection of the gastrojejunostomy and the gastric pouch with transsection 2 cm proximal to the angle of His and resection of the gastric remnant (Figure 2). The gastrointestinal continuity was re-established by the construction of an esophagojejunostomy using a 25 mm circular stapler (Figure 3). Two days after surgery an upper GI contrast series showed no leakage or stenosis at the level of the esophagojejunostomy. The patient was

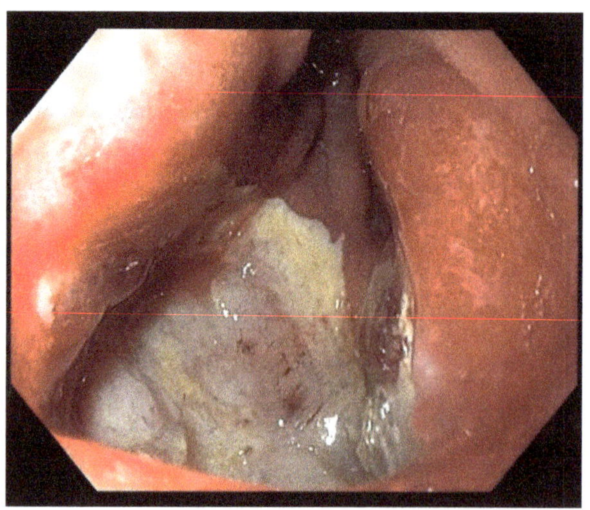

Figure 1 Recurrent anastomotic ulcer in the intestinal part of the gastrojejunostomy.

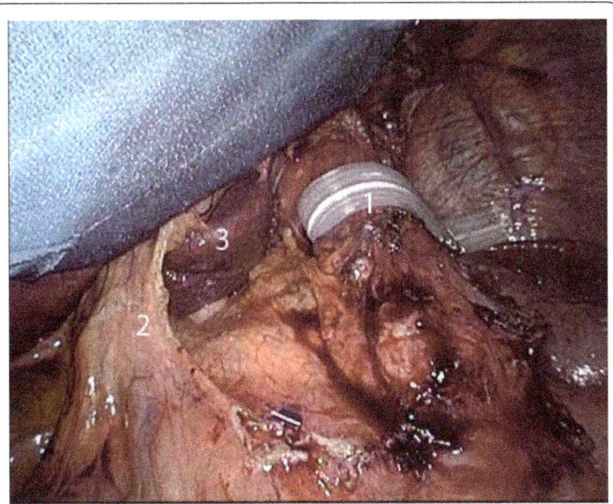

Figure 2 Situs after en-bloc resection of the gastric pouch and the gastrojejunostomy. (1 = esophagus, 2 = hepatoduodenal ligament, 3 = caudate lobe).

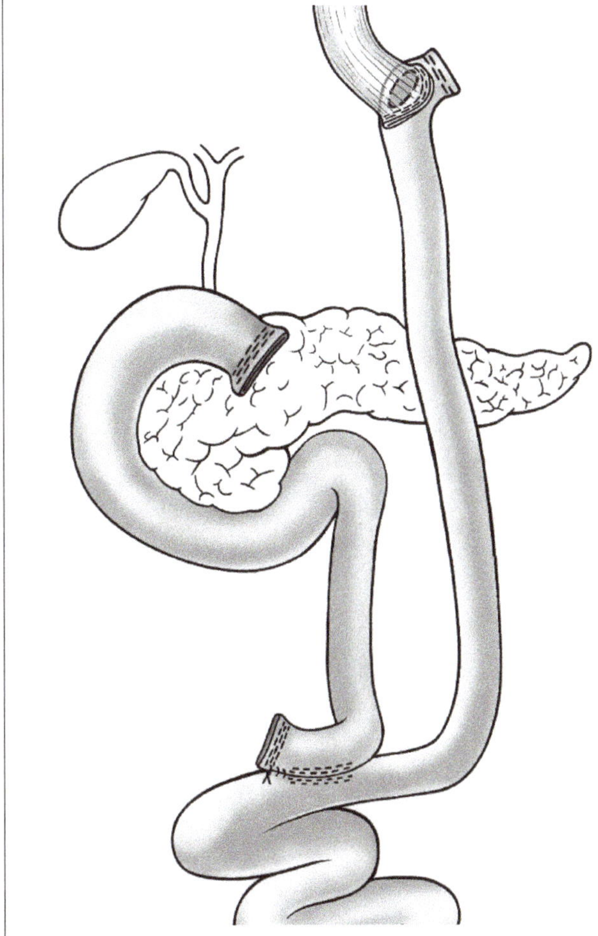

Figure 3 Roux-Y reconstruction with esophagojejunostomy.

discharged on postoperative day 10. Six months later the patient was free of symptoms, he was able to start opioid weaning and had regained 6 kg of weight. Finally, endoscopy showed a regular esophagojejunostomy.

Discussion and conclusion

Our case of a persistently recurring AU is representative for the current shortcomings in understanding the pathogenesis and thus optimal treatment of AU. We describe a successful approach for the management of intractable AU.

After LRYGB up to 7% of patients develop upper GI symptoms. Analysis and management of this condition is often challenging as 32% of symptomatic patients show a normal anatomy at endoscopy [13]. Conservative therapy has been reported to be successful in 68%-88% of the cases [8,12]. In our case, endoscopy showed no abnormalities apart from a short Roux limb at the time of referral. As a short Roux limb may facilitate biliary reflux causing postoperative pain and AU [14], we decided to lengthen the alimentary limb. Despite improvement of regurgitation symptoms, epigastric pain and AU recurred.

Approximately one third of AU recur after medical therapy. For these cases a redo of the gastrojejunostomy with a success rate of 87% has been advised [8]. Before we embarked on this strategy, we reevaluated whether putative factors leading to a recurrence were present. Endoscopy and GI contrast series excluded potential operative risk factors. Therefore a resection of the gastrojejunostomy with subsequent PPI therapy was performed. However, the ulcer recurred potentially due to the inability of the patient to quit smoking.

After revision surgery for AU, a recurrence rate of 8% has been described. In these cases, revision of the gastrojejunostomy combined with gastric remnant resection has been advocated reducing gastrin-producing- and parietal cells [8].

In contrast to the proposed simple revision of the anastomosis, we opted for a laparoscopic resection of the entire gastric pouch and the gastric remnant. By this means, the risk to leave a suboptimally vascularised or even ischemic pouch in situ was avoided since the resection was taken back to esophageal tissue. The circular esophagojejunostomy was then created in healthy, good vascularised tissue. Subsequently, the patient was free of symptoms and no recurrence was observed after a follow-up of 6 months. Hence, in our case this novel approach was effective in the management of a refractory AU and might represent a rescue option when simple revision of the gastrojejunostomy fails.

Consent

Written informed consent was obtained from the patient for publication of this case report and any accompanying images. A copy of the written consent is available for review by the Editor-in-Chief of this journal.

Acknowledgements
We thank Marco Bueter and Paul Schneider of the Department of Visceral and Transplantation Surgery, University Hospital Zurich, for the critical review of the manuscript. This study is not externally funded by government or charity foundations. No funding or assistance is received from commercial organizations.
Permissions
None of the material has been previously published.

Author details
[1]Department of Visceral and Transplantation Surgery, University Hospital Zurich, Raemistrasse 100, 8091 Zurich, Switzerland. [2]Department of Surgery, Cantonal Hospital Bruderholz, 4104 Bruderholz, Switzerland.

Authors' contributions
DCS drafted and finalized the manuscript, MS and PAC reviewed the manuscript, AN performed the surgery, monitored the drafting and critically reviewed the manuscript and has given final approve for publication. All authors read and approved the final manuscript.

Competing interests
The authors declare that they have no competing interests. No financial support has been received.

References

1. Garrido AB Jr, Rossi M, Lima SE Jr, Brenner AS, Gomes CA Jr: **Early marginal ulcer following Roux-en-Y gastric bypass under proton pump inhibitor treatment: prospective multicentric study.** *Arq Gastroenterol* 2010, **47(2)**:130-134.
2. Csendes A, Burgos AM, Altuve J, Bonacic S: **Incidence of marginal ulcer 1 month and 1 to 2 years after gastric bypass: a prospective consecutive endoscopic evaluation of 442 patients with morbid obesity.** *Obes Surg* 2009, **19(2)**:135-138.
3. Vasquez JC, Wayne Overby D, Farrell TM: **Fewer gastrojejunostomy strictures and marginal ulcers with absorbable suture.** *Surg Endosc* 2009, **23(9)**:2011-2015.
4. D'Hondt MA, Pottel H, Devriendt D, Van Rooy F, Vansteenkiste F: **Can a short course of prophylactic low-dose proton pump inhibitor therapy prevent stomal ulceration after laparoscopic Roux-en-Y gastric bypass?** *Obes Surg* 2010, **20(5)**:595-599.
5. Wheeler AA, de la Torre RA, Fearing NM: **Laparoscopic repair of perforated marginal ulcer following Roux-en-Y gastric bypass: a case series.** *J Laparoendosc Adv Surg Tech A* 2011, **21(1)**:57-60.
6. Avgerinos DV, Llaguna OH, Seigerman M, Lefkowitz AJ, Leitman IM: **Incidence and risk factors for the development of anemia following gastric bypass surgery.** *World J Gastroenterol* 2010, **16(15)**:1867-1870.
7. Sapala JA, Wood MH, Sapala MA, Flake TM Jr: **Marginal ulcer after gastric bypass: a prospective 3-year study of 173 patients.** *Obes Surg* 1998, **8(5)**:505-516.
8. Patel RA, Brolin RE, Gandhi A: **Revisional operations for marginal ulcer after Roux-en-Y gastric bypass.** *Surg Obes Relat Dis* 2009, **5(3)**:317-322.
9. Nguyen NT, Hinojosa M, Fayad C, Varela E, Wilson SE: **Use and outcomes of laparoscopic versus open gastric bypass at academic medical centers.** *J Am Coll Surg* 2007, **205(2)**:248-255.
10. Sacks BC, Mattar SG, Qureshi FG, Eid GM, Collins JL, Barinas-Mitchell EJ, Schauer PR, Ramanathan RC: **Incidence of marginal ulcers and the use of absorbable anastomotic sutures in laparoscopic Roux-en-Y gastric bypass.** *Surg Obes Relat Dis* 2006, **2(1)**:11-16.
11. Wilson JA, Romagnuolo J, Byrne TK, Morgan K, Wilson FA: **Predictors of endoscopic findings after Roux-en-Y gastric bypass.** *Am J Gastroenterol* 2006, **101(10)**:2194-2199.
12. Carrodeguas L, Szomstein S, Soto F, Whipple O, Simpfendorfer C, Gonzalvo JP, Villares A, Zundel N, Rosenthal R: **Management of gastrogastric fistulas after divided Roux-en-Y gastric bypass surgery for morbid obesity: analysis of 1,292 consecutive patients and review of literature.** *Surg Obes Relat Dis* 2005, **1(5)**:467-474.
13. Lee JK, Van Dam J, Morton JM, Curet M, Banerjee S: **Endoscopy is accurate, safe, and effective in the assessment and management of complications following gastric bypass surgery.** *Am J Gastroenterol* 2009, **104(3)**:575-582, quiz 583.
14. Swartz DE, Mobley E, Felix EL: **Bile reflux after Roux-en-Y gastric bypass: an unrecognized cause of postoperative pain.** *Surg Obes Relat Dis* 2009, **5(1)**:27-30.

2

Impact of comorbidities on postoperative complications in patients undergoing laparoscopy-assisted gastrectomy for gastric cancer

Mikito Inokuchi[1*], Keiji Kato[1], Hirofumi Sugita[1], Sho Otsuki[1] and Kazuyuki Kojima[2]

Abstract

Background: Comorbidity is a predictor of postoperative complications (PCs) in gastrectomy. However, it remains unclear which comorbidities are predictors of PCs in patients who undergo laparoscopy-assisted gastrectomy (LAG). Clinically, insufficient lymphadenectomy (LND) is sometimes performed in high-risk patients, although the impact on PCs and outcomes remains unclear.

Methods: We retrospectively studied 529 patients with gastric cancer (GC) who underwent LAG. PCs were defined as grade 2 or higher events according to the Clavien-Dindo classification. We evaluated various comorbidities as risk factors for PCs and examined the impact of insufficient LND on PCs in patients with risky comorbidities.

Result: A total of 87 (16.4%) patients had PCs. There was no PC-related death. On univariate analysis, heart disease, central nervous system (CNS) disease, liver disease, renal dysfunction, and restrictive pulmonary dysfunction were significantly associated with PCs. Both liver disease and heart disease were significant independent risk factors for PCs on multivariate analysis (odds ratio [OR] = 3.25, p = 0.022; OR = 2.36, p = 0.017, respectively). In patients with one or more risky comorbidity, insufficient LND did not significantly decrease PCs (p = 0.42) or shorten GC-specific survival (p = 0.25).

Conclusion: In patients who undergo LAG for GC, the presence of heart disease or liver disease is an independent risk factor for PC. Insufficient LND (for example, D1+ for advanced GC) might be permissible in high-risk patients, because although it did not reduce PCs, it had no negative impact on GC-specific survival.

Background

Gastric cancer (GC) is the fourth most common malignancy [1]. At present, the worldwide treatment of choice for GC is complete surgical removal of the tumor and adjacent lymph nodes. Surgical outcomes are influenced by various factors, including patients' characteristics and concurrent disease, type of operation, and quality of care. Postoperative complications (PCs) negatively affect the quality of life of patients who undergo gastrectomy and can even be life-threatening. Identification of risk factors for PCs might help to reduce such complications, and many studies have attempted to evaluate risk factors for PCs associated with various procedures. Comorbidity has been reported to be a predictor of PCs in patients who receive gastrectomy for GC [2-5]. However, what types of comorbidities are associated with the highest risk of PCs in patients who undergo gastrectomy remains to be fully defined. Risk factors probably differ between abdominal (surgical) and non-abdominal (medical) PCs. The primary objective of study was to clarify comorbidities associated with PCs in laparoscopy-assisted gastrectomy (LAG), a procedure for less invasive surgery increasingly used throughout the world. Clarifying specific comorbidities might contribute to improved treatment strategies for GC.

Scoring systems such as the Estimation of Physiologic Ability and Surgical Stress (E-PASS) score and the Physiologic and Operative Severity Score for the enUmeration of Mortality and morbidity (POSSUM) are useful for predicting the risks of mortality and morbidity after various operations [6,7], although they are not commonly used in clinical practice. In patients with comorbidities

* Correspondence: m-inokuchi.srg2@tmd.ac.jp
[1]Department of Surgical Oncology, Tokyo Medical and Dental University, Tokyo, Japan
Full list of author information is available at the end of the article

likely to adversely affect postoperative outcomes, standardized treatments, such as gastrectomy with D2 lymphadenectomy (LND) for advanced GC, tend to be avoided by surgeons. However, criteria for the selection of patients who should undergo insufficient LND and the impacts of insufficient LND on PCs and survival in high-risk patients remain to be defined. The secondary objective of this study was to evaluate the outcomes of high-risk patients who underwent insufficient LND. We verified whether insufficient LND negatively affects postoperative survival in this retrospective study.

Methods

We retrospectively identified 529 consecutive patients who underwent LAG with LND for pathological stage I to III GC in our hospital between 2003 and 2012. Patients who underwent thoracolaparotomy, emergency surgery, incomplete tumor resection, and combined operations for other malignancies were excluded. The present study was in compliance with the Declaration of Helsinki, and was approved by the ethics committee of Tokyo Medical and Dental University. In principle, early-stage GC was treated by LAG in accordance with the treatment guidelines of the Japanese Gastric Cancer Association [8]. The extent of LND was retrospectively classified as D1, D1+ (α or β), or D2 in accordance with the treatment guidelines, version 2 [8]. However, reduced LND was performed in patients with severe comorbidities. In patients who underwent LAG, carbon dioxide pneumoperitoneum was maintained at 10 mm Hg, and a 4- to 5-cm incision was made in the upper abdomen or navel to remove tissue specimens and conduct anastomosis. For lymph node dissection, we used harmonic scissors and monopolar and bipolar electric cautery devices. All patients received systemic antibiotics (a first-generation cephem) several times on the day of surgery. The nasogastric tube was left in place until postoperative day 1 according to our protocol.

All patients preoperatively underwent venous blood analysis (including hemoglobin, serum albumin, and creatinine), electrocardiography, chest radiography, and pulmonary function testing, including vital capacity (VC), forced expiratory volume in 1 second (FEV1), and forced vital capacity (FVC). The results of these examinations were retrieved from the patients' electronic medical records. The following variables were obtained from our prospective GC database: patient age and gender; body mass index (BMI); comorbidities; regular use of steroids; tumor characteristics; extent of lymph-node dissection; operation time; estimated blood loss; and PCs. All comorbidities other than pulmonary and renal dysfunction were defined as conditions that required treatment. For example, heart disease included ischemic disease treated by interventional procedures, atrial fibrillation requiring anticoagulant treatment, and congenital cardiac failure treated by medication. Liver disease included both cirrhosis and chronic hepatitis treated by medication. Pulmonary dysfunction was classified into two categories on basis of the results of preoperative spirometry. Restrictive pulmonary dysfunction was defined as a predicted VC of less than 80%, and chronic obstructive pulmonary disease (COPD) was defined as an FEV1/FVC ratio of less than 0.70. Renal dysfunction was defined as a serum creatinine concentration higher than the upper limit of normal according to our hospital's criteria (>1.1 mg/dL in males and >0.8 mg/dL in females). Anemia was defined according to the World Health Organization (WHO) criteria (<13 g/dL in males and <12 g/dL in females). Hypoalbuminemia was defined as a serum albumin concentration of less than 3.5 g/dL. In addition, some comorbidities were classified into two groups according to severity.

All patients were followed up until June 2013. The median follow-up was 52 months (5.5-126). A total of 59 (11.1%) patients died, 19 (3.6%) had recurrence of GC, and 40 (7.6%) died of other causes. Thirty-two patients (6.0%) died of benign diseases, such as cardiac, pulmonary, hepatic, and renal disease.

Patients' characteristics and surgical outcomes are shown in Table 1. In this study, PCs were defined as grade 2 or higher events according to the Clavien-Dindo classification that occurred within 30 days after gastrectomy [9]. In addition, PCs were classified into either abdominal or non-abdominal complications.

Next, we identified patients who had comorbidities that were risk factor for PCs. They were divided into two groups: patients underwent insufficient LND and those underwent sufficient LND. Insufficient LND included both insufficient D1+ dissection in pathological stage IA cancer with submucosal invasion and insufficient D2 dissection in pathological stage IB or more advanced cancer. We compared clinical outcomes between the patients who underwent insufficient LND and those underwent sufficient LND.

Statistical analysis

All variables were classified into two categories and were compared with the use of the chi-square test or Fisher's exact test, as appropriate. Multivariate analysis was carried out by binary logistic multiple regression testing using dummy variables. Seven patients (1.3%) were excluded from the multivariate analysis because of missing data. Survival was measured from the date of performing LAG to the latest follow-up date or the date of death. Kaplan-Meier curves were plotted to assess the effect of insufficient LND for patients with any risky comorbidity on survival. Different curves of survival were compared using the log-rank test. P values of <0.05 were considered to indicate statistical significance. All analyses were performed with the statistical software package SPSS 20 (SPSS Japan Inc., Tokyo, Japan).

Table 1 Patients' characteristics and surgical outcomes

	n%
Gender	
Male	380 (71.8)
Female	149 (28.2)
Age mean ± SD	64.9 ± 11.5
Body mass index (kg/m^2) mean ± SD	22.9 ± 3.1
Comorbidities	326 (61.6)
Heart disease	50 (9.5)
Ischemic disease	24 (4.5)
Arrhythmia	24 (4.5)
Congenital cardiac failure	3 (0.6)
Others	7 (1.3)
CNS disease	39 (7.4)
Cerebrovascular disease	30 (5.7)
Neurodegenerative disease	6 (1.1)
Others	3 (0.6)
Liver disease	21 (4.0)
Liver cirrhosis	8 (1.5)
Chronic hepatitis	13 (2.4)
Renal dysfunction[a)]	54 (10.2)
Pulmonary dysfunction	124 (23.4)
Restrictive pulmonary dysfunction[b)]	25 (4.7)
COPD	112 (21.2)
Diabetes mellitus	67 (12.7)
Hypertension	184 (34.8)
Other disease	45 (8.5)
Anemia[c)]	131 (24.8)
Hyoalbuminemia[d)]	8 (1.5)
Type of gastrectomy	
Total	78 (14.7)
Proximal	34 (6.4)
Distal	417 (78.8)
Extent of LND	
D1	4 (0.8)
D1+	448 (84.7)
D2	77 (14.6)
Combined resection	54 (10.2)
Gallbladder	39 (7.4)
Spleen	13 (2.5)
Intestine or colon	2 (0.4)
Operating time (min) mean ± SD	287 ± 75
Bleeding (g) median (range)	72 (0 – 2492)
Pathological tumor stage	
I	438 (82.8)
II	60 (11.3)
III	31 (5.9)

SD standard deviation, CNS central nervous system.
COPD: chronic obstructive pulmonary disease, LND: lymph node dissection
[a)]serum creatinine concentration higher than the upper limit of normal at our hospital, >1.10 in males and >0.80 in females.
[b)]predicted vital capacity <80%.
[c)]decreased hemoglobin, <13 g/dL in males and <12 g/dL in females.
[d)]decreased serum albumin <3.5 g/dL.

Results

A total of 87 (16.4%) patients had PCs. There was no PC-related death. Overall, 66 (12.5%) patients had abdominal complications, 5 (0.9%) had cardiac complications, 10 (1.9%) had pulmonary complications, and 15 (2.8%) had other complications. The details of the PCs are shown in Table 2. As for surgical factors, D2 LND, D1+ LND, and D1 LND were performed in 77 (14.6%), 448 (84.7%), and 4 (0.8%) patients, respectively. Total gastrectomy, proximal gastrectomy, and distal gastrectomy were performed in 78 (14.7%), 34 (6.4%), and 417 (78.8%) patients.

All PCs

On univariate analysis, PCs were significantly associated with many factors: male gender, higher age (≥75 years), heart disease, CNS disease, liver disease, renal dysfunction, restrictive pulmonary dysfunction, anemia, regular use of steroids, total gastrectomy, combined resection of other organ (except gallbladder), extended operating time (≥300 minutes), and higher operative bleeding volume (≥300 g) (Table 3). Only 5 patients (0.9%) received transfusion, and transfusion was not assessed in this study. Next, we evaluated independent risk factors for PCs using a multivariate model adjusted for all of the above risk factors (Table 4). Finally, both liver disease and heart disease were independent risk factors significantly related to PCs on multivariate analysis (odds ratio [OR] = 3.25, 95% confidential interval [CI]: 1.18-8.91, $p = 0.022$; OR = 2.36, 95% CI: 1.17-4.76, $p = 0.017$, respectively). The following factors showed a trend toward being risk factors on multivariate analysis: CNS disease (OR = 2.24, 95% CI: 1.00-5.01, $p = 0.050$), renal dysfunction (OR = 2.01, 95% CI: 0.98-4.13, $p = 0.058$), male gender (OR = 1.75, 95% CI: 0.93-3.29, $p = 0.082$), higher age (OR = 1.70, 95% CI: 0.95-3.03, $p = 0.075$), combined resection (OR = 2.85, 95% CI: 0.88-9.27, $p = 0.081$), and extended operating time (OR = 1.61, 95% CI: 0.95-2.73, $p = 0.079$).

Subcategorized PCs

For analysis, PCs were subcategorized into abdominal and non-abdominal (cardiac, pulmonary, etc.) PCs. Abdominal

Table 2 Postoperative complications

	n %	Grade 2/3/4/5
Total	87 (16.4)	48/34/5/0
Abdominal	66 (12.5)	31/33/2/0
Anastomotic leakage	8 (1.5)	0/7/1/0
Pancreatic fistula	5 (0.9)	1/4/0/0
Abdominal abscess	14 (2.6)	4/10/0/0
Anastomotic stenosis	14 (2.6)	3/11/0/0
Ileus	9 (1.7)	5/3/1/0
Gastric stasis	5 (0.9)	5/0/0/0
Postoperative bleeding	4 (0.8)	3/1/0/0
Ascites	4 (0.8)	3/1/0/0
Cholecystitis	2 (0.4)	1/1/0/0
Cholerrhagia	1 (0.2)	0/1/0/0
Reflux esophagitis	2 (0.4)	2/0/0/0
Enteritis	1 (0.2)	1/0/0/0
Wound infection	6 (1.1)	6/0/0/0
Non-abdominal	30 (0.9)	25/2/3/0
Ischemic attack	1 (0.2)	0/0/1/0
Arrhythmia	4 (0.8)	4/0/0/0
Pneumonia	6 (1.1)	5/1/0/0
ARDS	2 (0.4)	0/0/2/0
Atelectasis	2 (0.4)	2/0/0/0
Urinary tract infection	2 (0.4)	2/0/0/0
Infection of venous catheter	1 (0.2)	1/0/0/0
Deep vein thrombosis	1 (0.2)	0/1/0/0
Cerebral bleeding	1 (0.2)	0/0/1/0
Delirium	12 (2.3)	12/0/0/0

ARDS acute respiratory distress syndrome.

PCs occurred in 75.9% of the patients with PCs. Abdominal PCs were significantly associated with many factors on univariate analysis (Table 3). Multivariate analysis showed 3 independent predictors of abdominal PCs: liver disease (OR = 3.10, 95% CI: 1.13-8.47, $p = 0.028$), heart disease (OR = 2.40, 95% CI: 1.20-4.82, $p = 0.013$), and renal dysfunction (OR = 2.13, 95% CI: 1.06-4.29, $p = 0.035$). Extended operating time and higher operative bleeding were not significant predictors on multivariate analysis (OR = 1.57, 95% CI: 0.93-2.64, $p = 0.093$; OR = 1.22, 95% CI: 0.54-2.76, $p = 0.64$, respectively) (Table 4).

Non-abdominal PCs were also significantly associated with many factors on univariate analysis (Table 3). Heart disease was also an independent risk factor for non-abdominal PCs (OR = 2.31, 95% CI: 1.15-4.64, $p = 0.019$) on multivariate analysis. Three other factors were independent predictors of non-abdominal PCs: higher age (OR = 1.84, 95% CI: 1.04-3.26, $p = 0.036$), regular use of steroids (OR = 4.47, 95% CI: 1.04-19.3, $p = 0.045$), and extended operating time (OR = 1.71, 95% CI: 1.02-2.86, $p = 0.043$) (Table 4).

Relation between PCs and severity of comorbidities

The severity of each comorbidity was not significantly related to an increased incidence of PCs, although a high rate of PCs was found in patients with liver cirrhosis (Table 5).

Impact of insufficient LND on PCs and survival of patients with any risky comorbidity

We assessed the impact of insufficient LND (as defined in the Methods section) on PCs and survival in patients with the following risky comorbidities: heart disease, CNS disease, liver disease, renal dysfunction, and restrictive pulmonary dysfunction, all of which were significantly associated with PCs. A total of 149 patients (28% of all patients) had these risky comorbidities, and 42 (28%) of these patients underwent insufficient LND. The characteristics of the patients included in this portion of the study are shown in Table 6. The patients who underwent insufficient LND had a more advanced stage of GC ($p < 0.001$). The incidences of all PCs and of abdominal PCs were similar in the patients who underwent insufficient LND and those who underwent sufficient LND (29% vs 30%, $p = 0.87$; 19% vs 25%, $p = 0.42$, respectively). However, the incidence of non-abdominal PCs was significantly higher in the patients who underwent insufficient LND than in those who underwent sufficient LND (21% vs 8%, $p = 0.028$) (Table 6). The overall survival rate was slightly, but not significantly lower in patients who received insufficient LND (60.6% vs 79.0%, $p = 0.24$). However, GC-specific survival was similar in the two groups (90.6% vs 94.4%, $p = 0.25$), regardless of the fact that patients who underwent insufficient LND had a significantly more advanced stage of GC than those who underwent sufficient LND (Table 7).

Discussion

Our results showed that heart, CNS, liver, renal, and pulmonary comorbidities or dysfunctions were risk factors for PCs after radical gastrectomy. Heart disease and liver disease were independent risk factors for PCs in the present study, consistent with the results of a previous study of gastrectomy with D2 LND by Jeong et al. [2]. Heart disease and liver disease might be common risk factors after gastrectomy. However, Jeong et al. did not mention renal or pulmonary dysfunction, and the rates of comorbidities such as heart disease (4.6%) and neurological disease (2.2%) were lower than those in our study. Moreover, the rate of laparoscopic surgery was only 9.0% in their study. Another study found that liver cirrhosis and hypertension were independent risk factors for PCs in patients ≥70 years of age who underwent gastrectomy [5].

Table 3 Univariate analysis for risk factors of PCs in LAG

		All			Abdominal		Non-abdominal	
		n	n (%)	p	n (%)	p	n (%)	p
Gender	male	380	71 (18.7)	0.027	53 (13.9)	0.10	27 (7.1)	0.023
	female	149	16 (10.7)		13 (10.8)		3 (2.0)	
Age	≥75	117	34(29.0)	<0.001	27 (23.1)	<0.001	12 (11.4)	0.015
	<75	412	53 (12.9)		39 (9.5)		18 (4.4)	
Body mass index	≥25 (kg/m^2)	136	18 (13.2)	0.24	15 (11.0)	0.55	6 (4.4)	0.46
	<25	393	69 (17.6)		51 (13.0)		24 (6.1)	
Heart disease	yes	50	18 (36.0)	<0.001	13 (26.0)	0.002	10 (20.0)	<0.001
	no	479	69 (14.4)		53 (11.1)		20 (4.1)	
CNS disease	yes	39	13 (33.3)	0.003	10 (25.6)	0.020	7 (17.9)	0.004
	no	490	74 (15.1)		56 (11.4)		23 (4.7)	
Liver disease	yes	21	8 (38.1)	0.013	8 (38.1	<0.001	2 (9.5)	0.34
	no	508	79 (15.6)		58 (11.4)		28 (5.5)	
Diabetes mellitus	yes	67	12 (17.9)	0.73	10 (14.9)	0.52	5 (7.5)	0.57
	no	462	75 (16.2)		56 (12.1)		25 (5.4)	
Hypertension	yes	184	34 (18.5)	0.36	25 (13.6	0.57	13 (7.1)	0.31
	no	345	53 (15.4)		41 (11.9)		17 (4.9)	
Renal dysfunction	yes	54	17 (31.5)	0.002	14 (25.9)	0.002	6 (11.1)	0.11
	no	475	70 (14.7)		52 (12.3)		24 (5.1)	
Restrictive pulmonary dysfunction	yes	25	10 (40.0)	0.003	7 (28.0)	0.026	6 (24.0)	0.001
	no	498	75 (15.0)		58 (13.2)		23 (4.6)	
	not evaluated	6	2		1		1	
COPD	yes	112	17 (15.2)	0.73	11 (9.8)	0.35	8 (7.1)	0.41
	no	411	68 (16.5)		54 (13.1)		21 (5.1)	
	not evaluated	6	2		1		1	
Anemia	yes	131	29 (22.1)	0.043	22 (16.8)	0.085	12 (9.2)	0.047
	no	398	58 (14.6)		44 (11.1)		18 (4.5)	
Hypoalbuminemia	yes	8	3 (37.5)	0.13	2 (25.0)	0.26	2 (25.0)	0.071
	no	519	84 (16.2)		64 (12.3)		28 (5.4)	
	not evaluated	2	0		0		0	
Regular use of steroid	yes	9	4 (44.4)	0.045	2 (22.2)	0.31	2 (22.2)	0.087
	no	520	83 (16.0)		64 (12.3)		28 (5.4)	
Type of resection	total or proximal	112	29 (25.9)	0.002	20 (17.9)	0.052	13 (11.6)	0.002
	distal	417	58 (13.9)		46 (12.4)		17(4.1)	
Extent of lymph node dissection	D2	77	15 (19.5)	0.44	10 (13.0)	0.88	5 (6.5)	0.79
	D1+ or D1	452	72 (15.9)		56 (12.4)		25 (5.5)	
Combined resection	yes	16	6 (37.5)	0.033	4 (25.0)	0.13	2 (12.5)	0.23
	no or gallbladder	513	81 (15.8)		62 (12.1)		28 (5.5)	
Operating time	≥300 (min)	253	52 (20.6)	0.015	39 (15.4)	0.050	19 (7.5)	0.080
	<300	276	35 (12.7)		27 (9.8)		11 (4.0)	
Estimated bleeding	≥500(g)	43	12 (27.9)	0.031	10 (23.3)	0.026	4 (9.3)	0.28
	<500	485	74 (15.2)		56 (11.5)		25 (5.2)	
	unknown	1	1		0		1	

Table 4 Multivariate analysis of risk factors for PCs in LAG

	All PCs			Abdominal PCs			Non-abdominal PCs		
	OR	95% CI	p	OR	95% CI	p	OR	95% CI	p
Male gender	1.75	0.93-3.29	0.082	1.70	0.91-3.17	0.099	1.57	0.86-2.89	0.15
Higher age (≥75)	1.70	0.95-3.03	0.075	1.66	0.93-2.96	0.086	1.84	1.04-3.26	0.036
Heart disease	2.36	1.17-4.76	0.017	2.40	1.20-4.82	0.013	2.31	1.15-4.64	0.019
CNS disease	2.24	1.00-5.01	0.050	2.11	0.94-4.73	0.070	1.99	0.88-4.49	0.097
Liver disease	3.25	1.18-8.91	0.022	3.10	1.13-8.47	0.028			
Renal dysfunction	2.01	0.98-4.13	0.058	2.13	1.06-4.29	0.035			
Restrictive pulmonary dysfunction	2.08	0.81-5.34	0.13	1.95	0.76-4.99	0.16	2.12	0.83-5.42	0.12
Anemia	0.93	0.51-1.69	0.81	1.04	0.58-1.85	0.90	1.02	0.57-1.83	0.95
Hypoalbuminemia							1.53	0.21-11.2	0.67
Regular use of steroids	2.93	0.58-14.8	0.19				4.47	1.04-19.3	0.045
Total or proximal gastrectomy	1.39	0.76-2.55	0.29	1.52	0.85-2.73	0.16	1.73	0.99-3.00	0.052
Combined resection	2.85	0.88-9.27	0.081						
Extended operating time (≥300 min)	1.61	0.95-2.73	0.079	1.57	0.93-2.64	0.093	1.71	1.02-2.86	0.043
Higher operative bleeding (≥500 g)	1.10	0.48-2.52	0.83	1.22	0.54-2.76	0.64			

PCs postoperative complications, LAG laparoscopy-assisted gastrectomy.

Most patients underwent D1+ LND and distal gastrectomy in our study, because the Japanese guidelines recommend LAG for the treatment of early GC. Therefore, our results would most likely differ somewhat from those of similar studies performed in Western countries owing to differences in the most common sites of GC and the disease stage at diagnosis as compared with Japan.

In previous studies of only LAG in patients with mainly early gastric cancer, higher age (≥60 years), male gender of the patient, and type of resection or reconstruction procedure were predictors of local PCs, and inadequate experience of the operator was a predictor of systemic PCs [3,4]. Higher age was not a significant predictor of PCs in other studies of LAG [10-13], while higher age was significantly associated with non-abdominal PCs in this study. In the present study, 4 surgeons qualified in LAG performed all LAG procedures. The experience of the surgeons thus did not affect clinical outcomes. Our study had several limitations. Most important, it was a single-center study performed by experts in LAG. Our results thus might not be applicable to general hospitals. A pooled analysis or a multicenter study involving surgeons with various degrees of experience is necessary to identify common risk factors for gastrectomy.

In three studies of D2 LND including many patients who underwent OG, multiple-organ resection, advanced disease stage, extended operating time (≥180 or 200 minutes), higher age (≥50 years), male gender, higher BMI (≥25), and type of reconstruction were significant independent predictors of PCs [2,14,15]. In a randomized clinical trial of OG with D2 or more extended LND, higher age (>65 years), pancreatectomy, and extended operating time (>297 minutes) were independent risk factors for PCs [16]. In another study of open gastrectomy with various extents of lymph-node dissection, splenectomy or an extended operative time (≥360 minutes) was a risk factor for abdominal PCs [17].

Obesity is an established operative risk factor, but patients with a BMI of ≥30, defined as obese by the WHO, are uncommon in Asia. Obesity has therefore been an uncertain predictor of PCs in patients who undergo LAG [18-21]. Diabetes mellitus is a known risk factor for PCs after pancreaticoduodenectomy and

Table 5 Relationship between severity of each comorbidity and PCs

Comorbidity	Classification by severity	PCs		
		n	n (%)	p
Heart disease	surgical or interventional	19	5 (26)	0.26
	only medication	31	13 (42)	
COPD	stage 3 or 4*	8	0 (0)	0.60
	stage 1 or 2	104	17 (16)	
CNS disease	paralysis	8	2 (25)	0.69
	no paralysis	31	11 (35)	
Liver disease	cirrhosis	8	5 (63)	0.16
	hepatitis	13	3 (23)	
Renal dysfunction	dialysis	5	2 (40)	0.65
	no dialysis	49	15 (31)	
Diabetes mellitus	regular use of insulin	16	4 (25)	0.46
	oral medication	51	8 (16)	

*The stage of COPD is defined by Global Initiative for Chronic Obstructive Lung Disease.

Table 6 Comparison between insufficient LND and sufficient LND in patients with any risky comorbidity

		Insufficient LND n = 42 n (%)	Sufficient LND n = 107 n (%)	p
Age	≥75	18 (43)	45 (42)	0.93
	<75	24 (57)	62 (58)	
Gender	male	34 (81)	76 (71)	0.22
	female	8 (19)	34 (29)	
Tumor stage	I	22 (52)	96 (90)	<0.001
	II	14 (33)	7 (7)	
	III	6 (14)	4 (4)	
LND	D1	2 (5)	1 (0.9)	0.015
	D1+	40 (95)	91 (85)	
	D2	0 (0)	15 (14)	
No. of risky comorbidity	1	32 (76)	83 (78)	0.73
	2	9 (21)	19 (18)	
	≥3	1 (2)	5 (5)	
All PCs		12 (29)	32 (30)	0.87
Abdominal PCs		8 (19)	27 (25)	0.42
Non-abdominal PCs		9 (21)	9 (8)	0.028

hepatectomy [22,23], while Jeong et al. found no relation between diabetes mellitus and PCs after gastrectomy [5]. Preoperative strict diabetic control by diabetologists for about 2 weeks in patients with severe diabetes mellitus in our hospital might have resulted in the favorable postoperative course. COPD is a risk factor for postoperative pulmonary complications after non-thoracic surgery [24]. COPD was not associated with postoperative pulmonary complications in our study or in a previous study including patients who received open gastrectomy [25].

Table 7 OS and DSS in patients with any risky comorbidity

		5-year OS (%)	p	5-year DSS (%)	p
Age	<75	77.3	0.069	92.6	0.94
	≥75	44.9		94.4	
Gender	male	76.5	0.43	100.0	0.22
	female	68.5		80.8	
Tumor stage	I	81.8	<0.001[a]	100.0	<0.001[a,b]
	II	64.6	0.006[c]	80.8	0.022[c]
	III	25.0		42.2	
No. of risky comorbidity	1	73.3	0.19	92.8	0.61
	≥2	45.1		95.0	
LND	sufficient	79.0	0.24	94.4	0.25
	insufficient	60.6		90.6	

OS; overall survival, DSS; disease-specific survival.
[a]stage I vs III, [b]stage I vs II, [c]stage II vs III.

Preoperative smoking cessation for about 3 to 4 weeks in all patients and breathing exercises in patients with severe COPD might have contributed to the low incidence of pulmonary complications (10 patients, 1.8%), and 8 (1.5%) patients with 3 or more severe COPDs had no pulmonary complications in this study.

Nomograms established from preoperative data can facilitate the design of treatment strategies, but require a large volume of data from multiple centers. The Charlson comorbidity index (CCI) was developed to predict 10-year mortality for patients with a range of comorbidities [26]. Park et al. showed that the age-adjusted CCI was a useful predictor of systemic complications after LAG [27]. E-PASS and POSSUM predict the risks of mortality and morbidity after various operations, and the latter has been employed in patients undergoing gastrectomy [6,7]. However, these systems have not been routinely used in clinical practice, and many surgeons base treatment strategies on the severity of comorbidities or age of the patient. Clinically, reduced insufficient LND is often performed in patients with severe comorbidity or higher age, although criteria defining the need for more conservative procedures remain unclear. The indications for insufficient LND in risky patients were decided by consensus among a team of gastrointestinal surgeons in our hospital and were primarily based on the general condition of risky patients; we had no predefined criteria for such indications. We performed at least D1+ LND in risky patients who had a preoperative diagnosis of advanced GC. Insufficient LND did not reduce PCs in patients with risky comorbidities. In contrast, cardiac or pulmonary PCs increased in this study. However, if all patients had undergone sufficient LND, more PCs might have occurred. In addition, insufficient LND did not significantly shorten GC-specific survival in patients with any risky comorbidity. Insufficient LND, such as D1+ LND for advanced cancer, may thus be permissible in high-risk patients. A prospective randomized controlled trial would be the most reliable means of objectively evaluating the advantages and disadvantages of insufficient LND, but would be risky to perform in patients with severe comorbidities. A multicenter study or a pooled analysis is considered a better means of resolving this issue in the future. In the present study, the severity of comorbidities was not significantly related to the incidence of PCs. This finding might be attributed to the fact that few patients with severe comorbidities were allowed to receive prolonged general anesthesia. In such patients, we performed local resection with limited sampling of lymph nodes, endoscopic resection without LND, or sometimes withheld anticancer treatments.

Conclusions

Heart, CNS, liver, renal, and pulmonary comorbidities or dysfunctions were risk factors for PCs after LAG in patients with GC. Heart disease and liver disease were independent risk factors for PCs. In high-risk patients, insufficient LND did not decrease PCs, but had no negative impact on GC-specific survival. Insufficient LND, such as D1+ LND for advanced GC, might thus be permissible in this subgroup of patients.

Competing interests
The authors declare that they have no competing interests.

Authors' contributions
MI was responsible for drafting the manuscript. KK, KK, SO and HS contributed to data analysis and interpretation. All authors read and approved the final manuscript.

Acknowledgements
We thank K. Watanabe for inputting information of patients.

Author details
[1]Department of Surgical Oncology, Tokyo Medical and Dental University, Tokyo, Japan. [2]Department of Minimally Invasive Surgery, Tokyo Medical and Dental University, Tokyo, Japan.

References
1. Ferlay J, Shin HR, Bray F, Forman D, Mathers C, Parkin DM: **Estimates of worldwide burden of cancer in: GLOBOCAN 2008.** *Int J Cancer* 2010, **127:**2893–2917.
2. Jeong SH, Ahn HS, Yoo MW, Cho JJ, Lee HJ, Kim HH, Lee KU, Yang HK: **Increased morbidity rates in patients with heart disease or chronic liver disease following radical gastric surgery.** *J Surg Oncol* 2010, **101:**200–204.
3. Kim MC, Kim W, Kim HH, Ryu SW, Ryu SY, Song KY, Lee HJ, Cho GS, Han SU, Hyung WJ, Korean Laparoscopic Gastrointestinal Surgery Study (KLASS) Group: **Risk factors associated with complication following laparoscopy-assisted gastrectomy for gastric cancer: a large-scale korean multicenter study.** *Ann Surg Oncol* 2008, **15:**2692–2700.
4. Kim W, Song KY, Lee HJ, Han SU, Hyung WJ, Cho GS: **The impact of comorbidity on surgical outcomes in laparoscopy-assisted distal gastrectomy: a retrospective analysis of multicenter results.** *Ann Surg* 2008, **248:**793–799.
5. Hwang SH, Park do J, Jee YS, Kim HH, Lee HJ, Yang HK, Lee KU: **Risk factors for operative complications in elderly patients during laparoscopy-assisted gastrectomy.** *J Am Coll Surg.* 2009, **208:**186–192.
6. Haga Y, Ikejiri K, Wada Y, Takahashi T, Ikenaga M, Akiyama N, Koike S, Koseki M, Saitoh T: **A multicenter prospective study of surgical audit systems.** *Ann Surg* 2011, **253:**194–201.
7. Dutta S, Horgan PG, McMillan DC: **POSSUM and its related models as predictors of postoperative mortality and morbidity in patients undergoing surgery for gastro-oesophageal cancer: a systematic review.** *World J Surg* 2010, **34:**2076–2082.
8. Japanese Gastric Cancer Association: *Gastric cancer treatment guidelines for doctor's reference, version 2.* Tokyo (in Japanese): Kanehara Press; 2004.
9. Dindo D, Demartines N, Clavien PA: **Classification of surgical complications: a new proposal with evaluation in a cohort of 6336 patients and results of a survey.** *Ann Surg* 2004, **240:**205–213.
10. Kim HH, Hyung WJ, Cho GS, Kim MC, Han SU, Kim W, Ryu SW, Lee HJ, Song KY: **Morbidity and mortality of laparoscopic gastrectomy versus open gastrectomy for gastric cancer: an interim report–a phase III multicenter, prospective, randomized Trial (KLASS Trial).** *Ann Surg* 2010, **251:**417–420.
11. Tokunaga M, Hiki N, Fukunaga T, Miki A, Ohyama S, Seto Y, Yamaguchi T: **Does age matter in the indication for laparoscopy-assisted gastrectomy?** *J Gastrointest Surg* 2008, **12:**1502–1507.
12. Kunisaki C, Makino H, Takagawa R, Oshima T, Nagano Y, Ono HA, Akiyama H, Shimada H: **Efficacy of laparoscopy-assisted distal gastrectomy for gastric cancer in the elderly.** *Surg Endosc* 2009, **23:**377–383.
13. Yamada H, Kojima K, Inokuchi M, Kawano T, Sugihara K: **Laparoscopy-assisted gastrectomy in patients older than 80.** *J Surg Res* 2010, **161:**259–263.
14. Park DJ, Lee HJ, Kim HH, Yang HK, Lee KU, Choe KJ: **Predictors of operative morbidity and mortality in gastric cancer surgery.** *Br J Surg* 2005, **92:**1099–1102.
15. Jeong O, Park YK, Ryu SY, Kim YJ: **Effect of age on surgical outcomes of extended gastrectomy with D2 lymph node dissection in gastric carcinoma: prospective cohort study.** *Ann Surg Oncol* 2010, **17:**1589–1596. B.
16. Kodera Y, Sasako M, Yamamoto S, Sano T, Nashimoto A, Kurita A, Gastric Cancer Surgery Study Group of Japan Clinical Oncology Group: **Identification of risk factors for the development of complications following extended and superextended lymphadenectomies for gastric cancer.** *Br J Surg* 2005, **92:**1103–1109.
17. Ichikawa D, Kurioka H, Yamaguchi T, Koike H, Okamoto K, Otsuji E, Shirono K, Shioaki Y, Ikeda E, Mutoh F, Yamagishi H: **Postoperative complications following gastrectomy for gastric cancer during the last decade.** *Hepatogastroenterology* 2004, **51:**613–617.
18. Yoshikawa K, Shimada M, Kurita N, Iwata T, Nishioka M, Morimoto S, Miyatani T, Komatsu M, Mikami C, Kashihara H: **Visceral fat area is superior to body mass index as a predictive factor for risk with laparoscopy-assisted gastrectomy for gastric cancer.** *Surg Endosc* 2011, **25:**3825–3830.
19. Kawamura H, Tanioka T, Funakoshi T, Takahashi M: **Surgical effects of obesity on laparoscopy-assisted distal gastrectomy.** *Surg Laparosc Endosc Percutan Tech* 2011, **21:**155–161.
20. Yamada H, Kojima K, Inokuchi M, Kawano T, Sugihara K: **Effect of obesity on technical feasibility and postoperative outcomes of laparoscopy-assisted distal gastrectomy–comparison with open distal gastrectomy.** *J Gastrointest Surg* 2008, **12:**997–1004.
21. Kim KH, Kim MC, Jung GJ, Kim HH: **The impact of obesity on LADG for early gastric cancer.** *Gastric Cancer* 2006, **9:**303–307.
22. Cheng Q, Zhang B, Zhang Y, Jiang X, Zhang B, Yi B, Luo X, Wu M: **Predictive factors for complications after pancreaticoduodenectomy.** *J Surg Res* 2007, **139:**22–29.
23. Pessaux P, van den Broek MA, Wu T, Olde Damink SW, Piardi T, Dejong CH, Ntourakis D, van Dam RM: **Identification and validation of risk factors for postoperative infectious complications following hepatectomy.** *J Gastrointest Surg* 2013, **17:**1907–1916.
24. McAlister FA, Bertsch K, Man J, Bradley J, Jacka M: **Incidence of and risk factors for pulmonary complications after nonthoracic surgery.** *Am J Respir Crit Care Med* 2005, **171:**514–517.
25. Inokuchi M, Kojima K, Kato K, Sugita H, Sugihara K: **Risk factors for post-operative pulmonary complications after gastrectomy for gastric cancer.** *Surg Infect* 2014, **15:**314–321.
26. Charlson M, Szatrowski TP, Peterson J, Gold J: **Validation of a combined comorbidity index.** *J Clin Epidemiol* 1994, **47:**1245–1251.
27. Park HA, Park SH, Cho SI, Jang YJ, Kim JH, Park SS, Mok YJ, Kim CS: **Impact of age and comorbidity on the short-term surgical outcome after laparoscopy-assisted distal gastrectomy for adenocarcinoma.** *Am Surg* 2013, **79:**40–48.

3

Current status of robotic bariatric surgery: a systematic review

Roberto Cirocchi[1], Carlo Boselli[2], Alberto Santoro[3], Salvatore Guarino[3], Piero Covarelli[2], Claudio Renzi[2*], Chiara Listorti[2], Stefano Trastulli[1], Jacopo Desiderio[1], Andrea Coratti[4], Giuseppe Noya[2], Adriano Redler[3] and Amilcare Parisi[1]

Abstract

Background: Bariatric surgery is an effective treatment to obtain weight loss in severely obese patients. The feasibility and safety of bariatric robotic surgery is the topic of this review.

Methods: A search was performed on PubMed, Cochrane Central Register of Controlled Trials, BioMed Central, and Web of Science.

Results: Twenty-two studies were included. Anastomotic leak rate was 8.51% in biliopancreatic diversion. 30-day reoperation rate was 1.14% in Roux-en-Y gastric bypass and 1.16% in sleeve gastrectomy. Major complication rate in Roux-en-Y gastric bypass resulted higher than in sleeve gastrectomy (4,26% vs. 1,2%). The mean hospital stay was longer in Roux-en-Y gastric bypass (range 2.6-7.4 days).

Conclusions: The major limitation of our analysis is due to the small number and the low quality of the studies, the small sample size, heterogeneity of the enrolled patients and the lack of data from metabolic and bariatric outcomes. Despite the use of the robot, the majority of these cases are completed with stapled anastomosis. The assumption that robotic surgery is superior in complex cases is not supported by the available present evidence. The major strength of the robotic surgery is strongly facilitating some of the surgical steps (gastro-jejunostomy and jejunojejunostomy anastomosis in the robotic Roux-en-Y gastric bypass or the vertical gastric resection in the robotic sleeve gastrectomy).

Keywords: Morbid obesity, Bariatric surgery, Robotic, Roux-en-Y gastric bypass, Robot assisted, Gastric bypass, Sleeve gastrectomy, Gastric banding, Duodenal switch, Surgical outcomes, Complications, Anastomotic leak

Background

The increased prevalence of obesity in the general population over the past 30 years encouraged researches focused on the development of new treatment options to achieve long-lasting weight loss. Besides noninvasive conservative treatments (e.g. lifestyle modifications, medical treatment, and behavioral therapy), bariatric surgery is now playing an important role in the treatment for obesity. In 1991 the National Institutes of Health Conference Statement on Gastrointestinal Surgery for Severe Obesity developed a consensus stating that bariatric surgery was the most effective treatment for obesity since it is associated with good long-term results in terms of weight loss, glycemic control and decreased mortality [1]. It is widely recognized the growing incidence of obesity and diabetes mellitus as one of the major public burden in the western countries [2]. Current pharmacotherapy provides improvements in only less than 50% of patients with moderate to severe type 2 diabetes mellitus (T2DM). In the United States Roux-en-Y gastric bypass (RYGB) represents the most common bariatric surgical procedure [3]. Adam et al., in their Clinical Controlled Trial, enrolled 1.156 severely obese patients (BMI ≥ 35 kg/m2); they demonstrated that the RYGB surgery induced a significant weight loss, the best health-related quality of life and reduction of major obesity-related complications [4]. The only limit of bariatric surgery is represented by elevate peri-operative morbidity and mortality; in the attempt to reduce and limit this

* Correspondence: renzicla@virgilio.it
[2]Department of General and Oncologic Surgery, University of Perugia, Perugia, Italy
Full list of author information is available at the end of the article

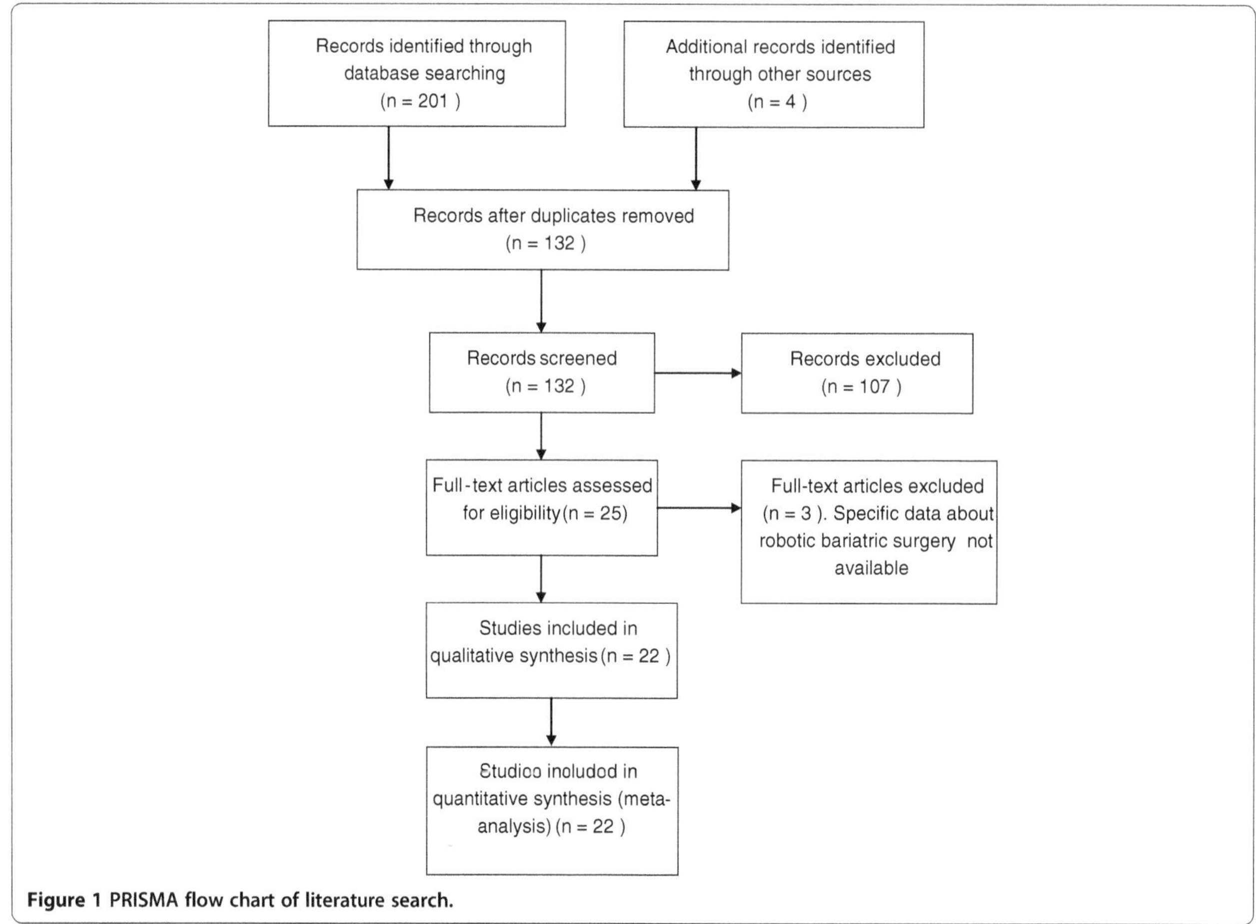

Figure 1 PRISMA flow chart of literature search.

important issue, Minimally Invasive Surgical techniques, initially laparoscopic and then robotic, are becoming more and more frequent [5]. The feasibility and safety are still debated. In 2011 a meta-analysis by Markar highlighted a decreased anastomotic stricture rate in patients undergoing Robotic RYGB (RRYGB) compared to the traditional laparoscopic approach (P = 0.04) [6]. Recently Hagen et al. demonstrated that RRYGB reduced cost of surgery by avoiding the anastomosis-related complications [7]; this was in contrast with the results presented by Scozzari et al. [8]. In their study they concluded that RRYGBP does not associate with significant shorter hospital stay and fewer complications compared to the traditional laparoscopic procedure [7,8]. Recently, a number of studies were published on this subject, for this reason, despite three systematic review were already published [9-11], a new systematic one was needed in order to evaluate the present state of the literature on robotic bariatric surgery.

Methods

A systematic literature search was performed on PubMed, Cochrane Central Register of Controlled Trials, BioMed Central and on Web of Science from January 2003 to November 2012. The Preferred Reporting Items for Systematic Reviews and Meta-analyses (PRISMA) was followed 005B [12]. Additional file 1. The following *search strategies* were used in PubMed:

- Robot-assisted [All Fields] AND ("bariatric surgery"[MeSH Terms] OR ("bariatric"[All Fields] AND "surgery"[All Fields]) OR "bariatric surgery"[All Fields])
- Robot-assisted [All Fields] AND ("gastric bypass"[MeSH Terms] OR ("gastric"[All Fields] AND "bypass"[All Fields]) OR "gastric bypass" [All Fields] OR "roux en y gastric bypass"[All Fields]) Robot-Assisted[All Fields] AND Sleeve[All Fields] AND ("gastrectomy"[MeSH Terms] OR "gastrectomy"[All Fields])
- ("robotics"[MeSH Terms] OR "robotics"[All Fields] OR "robotic"[All Fields]) AND ("bariatric surgery"[MeSH Terms] OR ("bariatric"[All Fields] AND "surgery" [All Fields]) OR "bariatric surgery"[All Fields])
- ("robotics"[MeSH Terms] OR "robotics" [All Fields] OR "robotic"[All Fields]) AND ("Band"[Journal] OR "band"[All Fields])

All titles and abstracts were assessed to select those focusing on robotic bariatric surgery. Subsequently,

Table 1 Characteristics of the included studies: setting and technique

Study*	Years of the study	City Nation	Type of trial	N. of patients	Author's definition of Robotic treatment	Type of treatment	Type of technique
Abdalla [15] 2012	2008-2011	São Paulo, Brasil	Case series	27	Robotic assisted gastric band placements Robotic assisted vertical gastrectomies Robotic asssisted gastric by-pass in Roux-en-Y	6 Gastric band placements, 5 Vertical gastrectomies and 16 Gastric by-pass in Roux-en-Y	NR[1]
Buchs [16] 2012	2006-2010	Geneva, Switzerland	Case series	167	Robotic-assisted Roux-en-Y gastric bypass	Roux-en-Y gastric bypass	Laparoscopic-Robotic
Hagen [7] 2012	1997-2010	Geneva, Switzerland	CCT	143	Robotic-assisted Roux-en-Y gastric bypass	Roux-en-Y gastric bypass	Laparoscopic-Robotic
Tieu [17] 2012	2002-2010	Houston, USA	Case series	1100	Robotic-assisted Roux-en-Y gastric bypass	Roux-en-Y gastric bypass	Laparoscopic-Robotic
Vilallonga [18] 2012	2010-2011	Barcelona, Spain	Case series	32	Robot-Assisted Sleeve Gastrectomy	Sleeve Gastrectomy	Fully Robotic
Ayloo [19] 2011	2007 - 2010	Chicago, USA	CCT	30	Robot-Assisted Sleeve Gastrectomy	Sleeve Gastrectomy	Fully Robotic
Diamantis [20] 2011	2008-2009	Athens, Greece	CCT	19	Robotic Sleeve Gastrectomy	Sleeve Gastrectomy	Fully Robotic
Edelson [21] 2011	2006-2009	Philadelphia, USA	CCT	287	Robotic gastric banding	Gastric banding	Fully Robotic
Park [22] 2011	2007-2009	Honolulu, USA	CCT	105	Robotic-assisted Roux-en-Y gastric bypass	Roux-en-Y gastric bypass	NR
Scozzari [8] 2011	2006-2009	Torino, Italy	CCT	110	Robotic-assisted Roux-en-Y gastric bypass	Roux-en-Y gastric bypass	Fully Robotic
Curet [23] 2009	2005	Stanford, USA	CCT	21	Robotic Roux-en-Y gastric bypass	Roux-en-Y gastric bypass	Fully Robotic
Deng [24] 2008	2006-2007	Pasadena, USA	Case series	100	Robotic-assisted Laparoscopic Roux-en-Y gastric bypass	Roux-en-Y gastric bypass	Fully Robotic
Hubens [25] 2008	2004-2006	Antwerpen, The Netherlands	CCT	45	Robotic Roux-en-Y gastric bypass	Roux-en-Y gastric bypass	Fully Robotic
Sudan [26] 2007	NR	Omaha, USA	Case series	47	Robotically assisted biliopancreatic diversion with duodenal switch	Biliopancreatic diversion with duodenal switch	Laparoscopic-Robotic
Parini [27] 2006	2000-2004	Aosta, Italy	Case series	17	Laparoscopic gastric bypass performed with the Da Vinci Intuitive Robotic System	Roux-en-Y gastric bypass	Laparoscopic-Robotic
Mohr [28] 2006	2004-2005	Stanford, USA	Case series	75	Totally Robotic Laparoscopic Roux-en-Y Gastric Bypass	Roux-en-Y gastric bypass	Fully Robotic
Yu [29] 2006	2003-2005	Houston, USA	Case series	100	Robotic assistance for laparoscopic Roux-en-Y gastric bypass	Roux-en-Y gastric bypass	Laparoscopic-Robotic
Ali [30] 2005	2002-2003	Sacramento, USA	Case series	50	Robot-assisted laparoscopic Roux-en-Y gastric bypass	Roux-en-Y gastric bypass	Laparoscopic-Robotic
Artuso [31] 2005	2001-2002	New York, USA	Case series	41	Laparoscopic gastric bypass performed with robotics	Roux-en-Y gastric bypass	Laparoscopic-Robotic

Table 1 Characteristics of the included studies: setting and technique *(Continued)*

Galvani [32] 2005	2000-2004	Chicago, USA	Case series	140	Robot-assisted surgery	110 Gastric bypass procedures 30 Lap band	Laparoscopic-Robotic
Sanchez [33] 2005	2004-2005	Stanford, USA	RCT	25	Totally robotic laparoscopic Roux-en-Y gastric bypass	Roux-en-Y gastric bypass	Fully Robotic
Muhlmann [34] 2003	NR	Innsbruck, Austria	CCT	10	Robotic-assisted laparoscopic silicone adjustable gastric banding Robotic implantable gastric stimulator	4 silicone adjustable gastric banding 2 implantable gastric stimulator 4 silicone adjustable gastric banding reoperation	Laparoscopic-Robotic

* Listed in chronological order.
[1]NR: not reported.

the full-text of the selected trials were independently screened by two authors (RCand ST) for eligibility. When there was overlapping between multiple articles published by the same authors and no difference in the examined time, only the most recent trial was enclosed to avoid double counting. The Pubmed function "related articles" and Google Scholar database were used to search further articles. We also searched the online database of relevant high-impact journals such as Surgery for Obesity and Related Diseases, Obesity, Obesity review, International Journal of Obesity, Obesity Surgery and Surgical Endoscopy. The references of the included studies were evaluated for other potential trials. The two screening authors evaluated the eligibility of each trial.

Inclusion criteria

In this systemic review, we considered both comparative and non-comparative studies, irrespectively of their size, publication status and language, which included patients who underwent robotic bariatric surgery . Comparative studies were included if they focused on selected outcomes of interest, irrespectively of the type of surgical approach used for comparative group (laparoscopic or open).

Exclusion criteria

Studies in which the outcomes of interest were neither reported nor directly or indirectly inferable.

Data extraction

Primary outcomes

surgical (conversion to open surgery, anastomotic leakage, re-intervention for complications, mortality), bariatric (postoperative Body Mass Index), and metabolic (type 2 DM remission) outcomes were considered.

Secondary outcomes

- Surgical ones (major and minor complication rate, pulmonary embolism rate, deep venous thrombosis, 30-days re-admission rate, anastomotic bleeding, gastrojejunostomy anastomotic stricture, post-operative small bowel obstruction, length of hospital stay, operative time).
- metabolic ones (number of patients able to discontinue medical treatment for T2DM at the follow-up and other obesity related morbidities resolution or improvement such as hypertension, sleep apnoea, gastroesophageal reflux and degenerative arthritis).

The included CCT studies were assessed for their methodological quality using the revised and modified grading system of the Scottish Intercollegiate Guidelines Network (SIGN) [13]; the case series assessment was carried out using the checklist for the quality of case series of the National Institute for Health and Clinical Excellence (NICE) [14]. Two authors (RC and CR) independently extracted data for the listed outcomes and assessed the methodological quality of each study, without masking the authors' names.

Results

The PRISMA flow chart for systematic review is presented in Figure 1. The initial search produced 132 potentially relevant articles. After the titles and abstracts were screened for relevance, 25 remaining articles were further assessed for eligibility and 3 were excluded; 22 trials whose characteristics are reported in Tables 1 and 2, were included in this systematic review: 1 Randomized Controlled Trial (RCT), 9 Clinical Controlled Trial (CCT) and 12 case series [7,8,15-34]. We excluded the abstract of the largest series trial of robotic-assisted bypass performed in three high-volume centers and presented by Wilson at the American Society for Metabolic & Bariatric

Table 2 Characteristics of the patients in the included studies

Study*	Mean preoperative age (years)	Mean weight [kg]	Mean Body Mass Index [kg/m^2]
Abdalla [15]	NR[1]	NR	NR
Buchs [16]	43	122.8	44
Hagen [7]	42.6	NR	44.5
Tieu [17]	46.9	131.9	47.9
Vilallonga [18]	44.7	NR	48.3
Ayloo [19]	38	152	57
Diamantis [20]	39.4	NR	48.2
Edelson [21]	45	NR	45.4
Park [22]	42.2	NR	46.77
Scozzari [8]	42.6	127.5	46.7
Curet [23]	46.5	NR	45.6
Deng [24]	41.7	NR	48
Hubens [25]	42	NR	44.2
Sudan [26]	38	NR	45
Parini [27]	42.9	NR	50.3
Mohr [28]	44	NR	46.1
Yu [29]	42	NR	50
Ali [30]	42	NR	47
Artuso [31]	42.5	146.2	52.8
Galvani [32]	NR	NR	NR
Sanchez [33]	43.3	NR	45.5
Muhlmann [34]	NR	NR	41.5

*Listed in chronological order.
[1]NR: not reported.

Table 3 Evaluation of methodological qualities of comparative included studies

Items/author*	[7]	[19]	[20]	[21]	[22]	[8]	[23]	[25]	[33]	[34]
Inclusion criteria	0	1	0	0	1	0	1	1	1	0
Exclusion criteria	0	0	0	0	0	0	0	0	0	0
Comparable demographics?	1	1	0	1	1	1	1	1	1	1
Could the number of participating centres be determined?	1	1	1	1	1	1	1	1	1	1
Could the number of surgeons who participated be determined?	1	1	1	1	1	0	0	1	1	1
Could the reader determine where the authors were on the learning curve for the reported procedure?	0	0	1	0	0	1	0	1	1	0
Were diagnostic criteria clearly stated for clinical outcomes if required?	1	1	1	1	1	1	1	1	1	1
Was the surgical technique adequately described?	1	1	1	0	0	1	0	1	0	1
Did they try to standardize the surgical technique?	1	0	1	0	0	1	0	1	0	1
Did they try to standardize perioperative care?	0	0	0	0	0	0	0	0	0	0
Was the age and range given for patients in the Robotic group?	1	0	1	1	1	1	0	1	1	1
Did the authors address whether there were any missing data?	1	1	1	1	1	0	1	0	1	0
Was the age and range given for patients in the comparative group?	1	0	0	1	1	1	0	1	1	1
Were patients in each group treated along similar timelines?	1	1	1	1	1	1	1	1	1	0
The patients asking to enter the study, did they actually take part to it?	0	0	0	0	0	0	0	0	1	0
Were drop-out rates stated?	0	0	0	0	0	0	0	0	1	0
Were outcomes clearly defined?	1	1	1	1	1	1	1	1	1	1
Were there blind assessors?	0	0	0	0	0	0	0	0	0	0
Were there standardized assessment tools?	1	0	0	0	0	0	0	0	1	0
Was the analysis by intention to treat?	0	0	0	0	0	0	0	0	1	0
Score	12	9	10	9	10	10	7	12	15	9

Total score, 21; <8, poor quality; 8–14, fair quality; ≥15, good quality.
* Named by reference number and listed in chronological order.

Surgery Annual Meeting in San Diego (2012) due to the limited data available in the abstract. [35]. The methodological quality according to the modified grading system of the Scottish Intercollegiate Guidelines Network resulted of fair quality for each of the 10 comparative studies included (mean score 10.3 points) (Table 3). The methodological quality assessment of the case series included proved a fair quality of the selected items evaluated with the NICE checklist (mean score 4.9 points) (Table 4). The pooled data included 2.781 (patients range per study:

Table 4 Evaluation of methodological qualities of observational included studies

Items/author*	[15]	[16]	[17]	[18]	[24]	[26]	[27]	[28]	[29]	[30]	[31]	[32]
Case series collected in more than one centre, i.e. multi-centre study	0	0	1	0	0	0	0	0	0	0	0	0
Is the hypothesis/aim/objective of the study clearly described?	1	1	1	1	1	1	1	1	1	1	1	1
Are the inclusion andexclusion criteria **(case definition) clearly reported?**	1	1	1	1	1	1	1	0	1	0	0	0
Is there a clear definition of the outcomes **reported?**	1	1	1	1	1	1	1	1	1	1	1	0
Were data collected prospectively?	0	1	1	0	0	0	0	0	1	1	0	0
Is there an explicit statement that patients were recruited consecutively?	0	0	1	1	1	0	1	1	1	0	0	0
Are the main findings of the study clearly **described?**	0	1	1	1	1	1	1	1	1	1	1	0
Are outcomes stratified? (e.g., by disease stage, abnormal test results, patient characteristics)	0	0	0	1	1	0	1	1	1	1	1	0
Total Score	3	5	7	6	6	4	6	5	7	5	4	1

Yes = 1 No(not reported, not available) = 0.
Total score, 8; ≤3, poor quality; 4–6, fair quality; ≥7, good quality.
* Named by reference number and listed in chronological order.

10–1.100 patients) who were planned to receive Robotic bariatric surgical treatment: 2.225 RRYGB, 86 Robotic Sleeve gastrectomy (RSG), 421 silicone adjustable gastric band, 47 bilio-pancreatic diversion with a duodenal switch and 2 implantable gastric stimulator. We excluded from our analysis implantable gastric stimulator (2 patients) and silicone adjustable gastric band reoperation (2 patients). The definition of the robotic approach given in the included studies was very heterogeneous: fully robotic, robotic, robotic-assisted and robot-assisted laparoscopy. The dissection and the resection were also heterogeneous and sequentially combining different approaches: laparoscopic/robotic and only robotic.

Primary outcomes

- Surgical Outcomes: The data listed in Table 5 suggest that robotic bariatric surgery is feasible, regardless of the type of treatment (99.9% in RYGB – 100% in RSG, 100% in silicone adjustable gastric band, 93.62% in biliary pancreatic diversion with duodenal switch). The analysis revealed a very low anastomotic leak rate (0.29% of gastrojejunostomy and 0.05% of jejunojejunostomy in RYGB, 0% in SG, 0.25% in silicone adjustable gastric band, 8.51% in biliary pancreatic diversion with duodenal switch). The 30-day post-operative reoperation rate was very low (1.14% in RYGB and 1.16% in SG) (Table 5). No study reported any case of 30-day postoperative mortality (Table 5).
- Bariatric outcome (postoperative Body Mass Index): only few trials reported the reduced mean BMI after 3 months from the RYGB [7,8,18,24,27,28] and SG [20] (Table 5).
- Metabolic outcomes: none of the studies reported data on the metabolic outcome.

Secondary outcomes

- Surgical Outcomes: major complication rates were 4,26% in RYGB and 1,2% in SG; minor complication rates were 1% in RYGB and 0% in SG; Pulmonary embolism rates were 0,71% in RYGB 0% in RSG; deep venous thrombosis rates were 0,37% in RYGB and 0% in SG; 30-day re-admission rates were 4,84% in RYGB and 0% in SG (Table 6). 15 cases of

Table 5 Primary outcomes

Study	Intraoperative conversions	30-day reoperations	30-day postoperative mortality	Mean body mass index 3 months after surgery
Abdalla [15]	0	1	0	NR[1]
Buchs [16]	2	2	0	NR
Hagen [7]	2	1	0	44.5
Tieu [17]	0	NR	0	39.8
Vilallonga [18]	0	0	0	NR
Ayloo [19]	0	1	0	NR
Diamantis [20]	0	0	0	reduced of 31.3%
Edelson* [21]	0	11	0	NR
Park [22]	1	1	0	NR
Scozzari [8]	0	2	0	reduced of 33.6%
Curet [23]	NR	NR	0	NR
Deng [24]	NR	0	0	17.5%
Hubens [25]	9	2	0	NR
Sudan [26]	3	NR	0	NR
Parini [27]	0	0	0	39.07
Mohr [28]	4	NR	0	reduced of 48%
Yu [29]	0	2	0	NR
Ali [30]	NR	NR	NR	NR
Artuso [31]	NR	NR	NR	NR
Galvani [32]	NR	NR	NR	NR
Sanchez [33]	1	NR	NR	NR
Muhlman [34]	NR	NR	0	NR

* Listed in chronological order.
[1]NR: not reported.

Table 6 postoperative complications and 30 day readmission in the included studies

Study*	30-day major complications	30-day minor complications	Pulmonary embolism	Deep venous thrombosis	Readmissions in the first 30 postoperative days
Abdalla [15]	1	5	0	0	NR[1]
Buchs [16]	24 (not classified)		7	2	2
Hagen [7]	23 (not classified)		NR	NR	NR
Tieu [17]	45	102	2	3	67
Vilallonga [18]	1 case	NR	NR	NR	NR
Ayloo [19]	NR		NR	NR	0
Diamantis [20]	0 (not classified)		0	0	0
Edelson [21]	NR		NR	NR	NR
Park [22]	10 (not classified)		0	0	0
Scozzari [8]	4	14	1	NR	NR
Curet [23]	3 (not classified)		NR	NR	NR
Deng [24]	4	7	NR	NR	3
Hubens [25]	NR	NR	NR	NR	NR
Sudan [26]	NR	NR	NR	NR	NR
Parini [27]	0	0	0	0	0
Mohr [28]	6	7	NR	NR	NR
Yu [29]	NR	NR	1	NR	NR
Ali [30]	NR	NR	NR	NR	NR
Artuso [31]	NR	NR	NR	NR	NR
Galvani [32]	NR	NR	NR	NR	NR
Sanchez [33]	NR	NR	NR	NR	NR
Muhlmann [34]	NR	NR	NR	NR	NR

* Listed in chronological order.
[1]NR: not reported.

anastomotic bleeding were reported over a total of 1.873 RYGB while none were reported in SG (Tables 7, 8). Gastrojejunostomy anastomotic stricture rate was 1,23% in RYGB. Post-operative small bowel obstruction rates were 1,17% in Roux-en-Y gastric bypass and 0% in sleeve gastrectomy (Tables 7, 8). The mean hospital stay ranged between 2.72 and 7.4 days in RYGB and between 2.6 and 4 days in SG (Table 9). The mean operative time ranged between 130.8 and 295 min. in RYGB and between 95 and 135 min. in SG (Table 9).

- Metabolic outcomes: none of the studies reported this outcome.

Discussion

The present study revealed slightly different outcomes and complication rates between the traditional laparoscopic approach and the robotic one. Data from a RCT collected after laparoscopic gastric bypass showed that 1-year mortality is about 0.9%, Major perioperative complications (hemorrhage, obstruction, internal herniation, or renal insufficiency) occur in 6.3% of patients and late (> 30 days postoperatively) major complications, more often stenosis or strictures, in 26.1% of them [36]. The results of this review demonstrated that the robotic approach is safe and feasible in all types of bariatric surgical procedures. The overall post-operative complication rate was very low; in particular the anastomotic leak rate (gastro-jejunostomy and jejuno-jejunostomy in RYGB) and the gastric staple line leak rate were very low and no deaths were reported. The analysis of these selected trials on the robotic bariatric surgery did not show any significant results about the bariatric and the metabolic outcomes. Our results were in line with the ones presented in 2012 by Wilson et al. at the Annual Meeting of the American Society for Metabolic & Bariatric Surgery in San Diego [35]. In this trial the authors enrolled 1,695 patients undergoing robotic-assisted RYGB surgery; the post-operative complications were 17 bowel obstructions, 5 wound infections and 18 cases of bleeding. The hospital readmissions rate was 4.8% and re-intervention rate was 2.7%. Leak and anastomotic stricture rates were very low: 0.3% and 0.2% respectively. No death was reported. "This report of the largest series of robotic-assisted bypasses from

Table 7 Surgical complications after gastric bypass

Study*	Post-operative anastomotic leak		Anastomotic stricture Gastro-jejunostomy	Anastomotic bleeding	Post-operative bowel obstruction
	g-j	j-j			
Abdalla [15]	0	0	0	0	0
Buchs [16]	0	0	3	NR[3]	1
Hagen [7]	0	0	0	3	NR
Tieu [17]	1	1	7	9	19
Park [22]	2	0	2	0	0
Scozzari [8]	2	0	3	0	1
Curet [23]	0	0	0	0	0
Deng [24]	1	0	4	3	0
Hubens [25]	0	0	2	0	1
Parini [27]	0	0	0	0	0
Mohr [28]	0	0	2	0	0
Yu [29]	0	0	2	0	0
Ali [30]	NR	NR	NR	NR	NR
Artuso [31]	1	0	0	0	0
Galvani [32]	NR	NR	NR	NR	NR
Sanchez [33]	NR	NR	NR	NR	NR

* Listed in chronological order.
[3]NR: not reported.

three high-volume centers reveals very low complication rates in the first 30 days. It reveals zero 30-day mortality, an exceptionally low leak rate, and provides strong evidence that Robot-Assisted RYGB (RARYGB) has extremely safe and reproducible outcomes" [35]. Robotic surgery allowed the reduction of the postoperative complications, especially the anastomotic dehiscence. The low anastomotic leak rate after robotic bypass can be partially explained by the improved accuracy and precision of intracorporeal suturing compared to the traditional laparoscopic approach. 5 cm proximal to the anastomosis, an antireflux longitudinal valve is fashioned with suture stitches 1 cm apart from each other. In USA the RARYGB represent the first line choice of bariatric surgery, but because of its "complexity", this operation has always been challenged by alternative surgical procedures [37].

Safety of gastric bypass was demonstrated and its effectiveness in the long term weight loss maintenance as well, nevertheless it associates with a long learning curve and it is not free from complications [38,39]. Kim et al. concluded that the use of the robot is ideal in performing RYGB [40]. This technique associates with shorter learning curve especially in performing delicate and precise manoeuvres such as fine dissections and suturing. Indeed it is widely recognized that robotic bariatric surgery, in particular RRYGB, has a steeper learning curve than laparoscopic approach and 20 cases may be enough to pass the basic learning phase [41]. Moreover this technique, unlike laparoscopic surgery, can be used in high-risk obese patients with difficult anatomy without compromising the surgical performance and outcomes [40]. The best results derived from the RSG that showed even fewer postoperative complications and no mortality, but the use of the robot in performing sleeve gastrectomy is still controversial, and not largely spread among bariatric surgeons yet. Recently few case series on this technique were published [19,20]. Robotic approach was demonstrated associating with shorter learning curve compared to the traditional laparoscopic techniques [37]. A poster presented

Table 8 Surgical complications after sleeve gastrectomy and duodenal switch

Surgical treatment	Study	Suture leak	Suture stricture	Suture bleeding	Bowel obstruction/internal hernia
Sleeve gastrectomy	Vilallonga [18]	0	0	0	0
	Ayloo [19]	0	1	0	0
	Diamantis [20]	0	0	0	0
Duodenal switch	Sudan [26]	4	0	0	0

Table 9 Secondary outcomes: mean operative time and mean hospital stay

Study*	Mean operative time (min.)	Length of hospital stay Mean ± Standard deviation (days)
Abdalla [15]	NR[1]	NR
Buchs [16]	295.2	7.2 ± 2.5
Hagen [7]	293	7.4 ± 2.6
Tieu [17]	155	NR
Vilallonga [18]	130.2	NR
Ayloo [19]	135	2.6
Diamantis [20]	95.5	4
Edelson [21]	91.5	1.3
Park [22]	169	3.41 ± 7.03
Scozzari [8]	247.5	7.8
Curet [23]	181.7	3
Deng [24]	186.3	1.5
Hubens [25]	242.2	4.7
Sudan [26]	514	NR
Parini [27]	201	9
Mohr [28]	140	2.9
Yu [29]	254	NR
Ali [30]	NR	NR
Artuso [31]	289	4.6
Galvani [32]	NR	NR
Sanchez [33]	130.8	2.72
Muhlman [34]	137	3

*Listed in chronological order.
[1]NR: not reported.

in by Miller et al. at the annual meeting of the Society of American Gastrointestinal and Endoscopic Surgeons (SAGES) compared 277 laparoscopic sleeve Gastrectomy (LSG) to 40 RSG. The mean operative time was significantly shorted (91 minutes) for LSG compared to the RSG (113 minutes) (p-0.002) No differences were revealed in overall mean hospital stay (2.4 days in the LSG group and 2.5 in the RSG group) (p = 0.86). The overall mean 90-day complication rate requiring readmission was significantly lower in patients who had undergone RSG (12.3% in the LSG group and 5% in RSG group) (p = <.001) [42].

Conclusion

Robotic assistance is used in a small percentage of bariatric procedures in the US. The major limitation of our analysis is the lack of studies and their low quality, small sample size,, heterogeneity of enrolled patients and the lack of data from metabolic and bariatric outcomes. Despite the use of the robot, the majority of these cases are completed with stapled anastomosis. The assumption that robotic surgery is superior in complex cases is not supported from actual evidence. According to our experience the major strength of the robotic surgery is strongly facilitating some of the surgical steps (gastro-jejunostomy and jejunojejunostomy anastomosis in the robotic Roux-en-Y gastric bypass or the vertical gastric resection in the robotic sleeve gastrectomy). According to our experience the major disadvantage of the robotic bariatric surgery "still remains the high operational and acquisition cost of the system" [37].

Competing interest
The Authors all report no conflicts of interest. Furthermore for the writing of this paper the Authors didn't benefit of any source of funding.

Authors' contributions
RC designed and concepted the manuscript, performed the interpretation of data, drafted and revised critically the manuscript. CB designed, concepted and revised critically the manuscript. AS analyzed the data and revised the manuscript. SG designed, drafted and revised the paper. PC took part to the interpretation of data and revised the manuscript. CR was involved in the acquisition of data, in their analysis and in drafting the manuscript. CL contributed to the acquisition of data and she took part in drafting the manuscript. ST performed the interpretation of data, drafted and revised critically the manuscript. JD took part to the acquisition of data, in their analysis and in drafting the manuscript. AC was involved in the interpretation of data and revised the manuscript. GN designed, concepted and revised critically the manuscript. AR designed, concepted and revised critically the manuscript. AP concepted and revised critically the manuscript. All authors read and approved the final manuscript and they agree to be accountable for all aspects of the work in ensuring that questions related to the accuracy or integrity of any part of the work are appropriately investigated and resolved.

Acknowledgments
The authors are the only ones responsible for the content and writing of the paper.

Author details
[1]Department of Digestive and Liver Surgery Unit, St Maria Hospital, Terni, Italy. [2]Department of General and Oncologic Surgery, University of Perugia, Perugia, Italy. [3]Department of Surgical Sciences, "Sapienza" University of Rome, Rome, Italy. [4]Department of General Surgery, Misericordia Hospital, Grosseto, Italy.

References

1. Gastrointestinal surgery for severe obesity: **National Institutes of Health consensus development conference statement.** *Am J Clin Nutr* 1992, **55**(2):615S–619S.
2. Gregg EW, Cheng YJ, Narayan KM, Thompson TJ, Williamson DF: **The relative contributions of different levels of overweight and obesity to the increased prevalence of diabetes in the United States: 1976-2004.** *Prev Med* 2007, **45**:348–52.
3. Davis MM, Slish K, Chao C, Cabana MD: **National trends in bariatric surgery. 1996-2002.** *Arch Surg* 2006, **141**(1):71–74.
4. Adams TD, Pendleton RC, Strong MB, *et al*: **Health outcomes of gastric bypass patients compared to nonsurgical, nonintervened severely obese.** *Obesity* 2010, **18**(1):121–130.
5. Schirmer B: **Laparoscopic gastric bypass.** In *Surgical pitfalls.* Edited by Evans SRT. Philadelphia: Saunders Elsevier; 2009:197–222.
6. Markar SR, Karthikesalingam AP, Venkat-Ramen V, Kinross J, Ziprin P: **Robotic vs laparoscopic Roux-en-Y gastric bypass in morbidly obese patients: systematic review and pooled analysis.** *Int J Med Robot* 2011, **7**(4):393–400.

7. Hagen ME, Pugin F, Chassot G, *et al*: **Reducing cost of surgery by avoiding complications: the model of robotic Roux-en-Y gastric bypass.** *Obes Surg* 2012, **22**(1):52–61.
8. Scozzari G, Rebecchi F, Millo P, Rocchietto S, Allieta R, Morino M: **Robot-assisted gastrojejunal anastomosis does not improve the results of the laparoscopic Roux-en-Y gastric bypass.** *Surg Endosc* 2011, **25**(2):597–603.
9. Fourman MM, Saber AA: **Robotic bariatric surgery: a systematic review.** *Surg Obes Relat Dis* 2012, **8**(4):483–488.
10. Gill RS, Al-Adra DP, Birch D, *et al*: **Robotic-assisted bariatric surgery: a systematic review.** *Int J Med Robot* 2011. doi: 10.1002/rcs.400.
11. Markar SR, Penna M, Hashemi M: **Robotic bariatric surgery: bypass, band and sleeve. Where are we now? And what is the future?** *Minerva Gastroenterol Dietol* 2012, **58**(3):181–190.
12. Moher D, Liberati A, Tetzlaff J, Altman DG: **Preferred reporting items for systematic reviews and meta-analyses: the PRISMA statement.** *PLoS Med* 2009, **6**(7):e1000097.
13. *Scottish Intercollegiate Guidelines Network (SIGN) guidelines, methodology checklist 3.* [http://www.sign.ac.uk/methodology/checklists.html]
14. *National Institute for Health and Clinical Excellence.* NICE clinical guidelines, Appendix 4 Quality of case series form. [http://www.nice.org.uk/ nicemedia/pdf/Appendix_04_qualityofcase_series_form_preop.pdf]
15. Abdalla RZ, Garcia RB, Luca CR, Costa RI, Cozer CO: **Brazilian experience in obesity surgery robot-assisted.** *Arq Bras Cir Dig* 2012, **25**(1):33–35.
16. Buchs NC, Bucher P, Pugin F, *et al*: **Value of performing routine postoperative liquid contrast swallow studies following robot-assisted Roux-en-Y gastric bypass.** *Swiss Med Wkly* 2012, **142**:w13556. doi:10.4414/smw.2012.13556.
17. Tieu K, Allison N, Snyder B, Wilson T, Toder M, Wilson E: **Robotic-assisted Roux-en-Y gastric bypass: update from 2 high-volume centers.** *Surg Obes Relat Dis* 2013, **9**(2):284–288.
18. Vilallonga R, Fort JM, Gonzales O, *et al*: **The initial learning curve for Robot-Assisted Sleeve Gastrectomy: a surgeon's experience while introducing the robotic technology in a bariatric surgery department.** *Minimally Invasive Surgery* 2012. doi:10.1155/2012/347131.
19. Ayloo S, Buchs NC, Addeo P, Bianco FM, Giulianotti PC: **Robot-assisted sleeve gastrectomy for super-morbidly obese patients.** *J Laparoendosc Adv Surg Tech A* 2011, **21**(4):295–299.
20. Diamantis T, Alexandrou A, Nikiteas N, Giannopoulos A, Papalambros E: **Initial experience with robotic sleeve gastrectomy for morbid obesity.** *Obes Surg* 2011, **21**(8):1172–1179.
21. Edelson PK, Dumon KR, Sonnad SS, Shafi BM, Williams NN: **Robotic vs. conventional laparoscopic gastric banding: a comparison of 407 cases.** *Surg Endosc* 2011, **25**(5):1402–1408.
22. Park CW, Lam EC, Walsh TM, *et al*: **Robotic-assisted Roux-en-Y gastric bypass performed in a community hospital setting: the future of bariatric surgery?** *Surg Endosc* 2011, **25**(10):3312–3321.
23. Curet MJ, Solomon H, Liu G, Morton JM: **Comparison of hospital charges between robotic, laparoscopic stapled, and laparoscopic handsewn Roux-en-Y gastric bypass.** *J Robot Surg* 2009, **3**(3):199.
24. Deng JY, Lourié DJ: **100 robotic-assisted laparoscopic gastric bypasses at a community hospital.** *Am Surg* 2008, **74**(10):1022–1025.
25. Hubens G, Balliu L, Ruppert M, Gypen B, Van Tu T, Vaneerdeweg W: **Roux-en-Y gastric bypass procedure performed with the da Vinci robot system: is it worth it?** *Surg Endosc* 2008, **22**(7):1690–1696.
26. Sudan R, Puri V, Sudan D: **Robotically assisted biliary pancreatic diversion with a duodenal switch: a new technique.** *Surg Endosc* 2007, **21**(5):729–733.
27. Parini U, Fabozzi M, Contul RB, *et al*: **Laparoscopic gastric bypass performed with the Da Vinci Intuitive Robotic System: preliminary experience.** *Surg Endosc* 2006, **20**(12):1851–1857.
28. Mohr CJ, Nadzam GS, Alami RS, *et al*: **Totally robotic laparoscopic Roux-en-Y gastric bypass: results from 75 patients.** *Obes Surg* 2006, **16**:690–696.
29. Yu SC, Clapp BL, Lee MJ, Albrecht WC, Scarborough TK, Wilson EB: **Robotic assistance provides excellent outcomes during the learning curve for laparoscopic Roux-en-Y gastric bypass: results from 100 robotic-assisted gastric bypasses.** *Am J Surg* 2006, **192**(6):746–749.
30. Ali MR, Bhaskerrao B, Wolfe BM: **Robot-assisted laparoscopic Roux-en-Y gastric bypass.** *Surg Endosc* 2005, **19**:468–472.
31. Artuso D, Wayne M, Grossi R: **Use of robotics during laparoscopic gastric bypass for morbid obesity.** *JSLS* 2005, **9**(3):266–268.
32. Galvani C, Horgan S: **Robots in general surgery: present and future.** *Cir Esp* 2005, **78**(3):138–147.
33. Sanchez BR, Mohr CJ, Morton JM, *et al*: **Comparison of totally robotic laparoscopic Roux-en-Y gastric bypass and traditional laparoscopic Roux-en-Y gastric bypass.** *Surg Obes Relat Dis* 2005, **1**:549–554.
34. Mühlmann G, Klaus A, Kirchmayr W, *et al*: **DaVinci robotic-assisted laparoscopic bariatric surgery: is it justified in a routine setting?** *Obes Surg* 2003, **13**(6):848–854.
35. Wilson EB, Toder M, Snyder BE, Wilson TD, Kim K: *Favorable early complications of robotic assisted gastric bypass from three high volume centers: 1,695 consecutive cases.* San Diego, CA: Presented at the 29 th American Society for Metabolic & Bariatric Surgery Annual Meeting; 2012.
36. Nguyen NT, Slone JA, Nguyen XM, Hartman JS, Hoyt DB: **A prospective randomized trial of laparoscopic gastric bypass versus laparoscopic adjustable gastric banding for the treatment of morbid obesity: Outcomes, quality of life, and costs.** *Ann Surg* 2009, **250**(4):631–41.
37. Garza U, Echeverria A, Galvani C: **Robotic-Assisted Bariatric Surgery.** In *Advanced Bariatric and Metabolic Surgery.* Edited by Huang CK. Shanghai: InTech; 2012:297–316.
38. Podnos YD, Jimenez JC, Wilson SE, Stevens CM, Nguyen NT: **Complications after laparoscopic gastric bypass: a review of 3464 cases.** *Arch Surg* 2003, **138**(9):957–961.
39. Trastulli S, Desiderio J, Guarino S, *et al*: **Laparoscopic sleeve gastrectomy compared with other bariatric surgical procedures: a systematic review of randomized trials.** *Surg Obes Relat Dis* 2013, **9**(5):816–29.
40. Kim KC, Buffington C: **Totally robotic gastric bypass: approach and technique.** *J Robot Surg* 2011, **5**(1):47–50.
41. Buchs NC, Pugin F, Bucher P, *et al*: **Learning curve for robot-assisted Roux-en-Y gastric bypass.** *Surg Endosc* 2012, **26**(4):1116–21.
42. Miller N, Wilson E, Snyder B, *et al*: *Comparison of Laparoscopic vs. Robotic Assisted Longitudinal Sleeve Gastrectomy.* San Diego, CA: Presented at the Society of American Gastrointestinal and Endoscopic Surgeons (SAGES) annual meeting; 2012.

4

Changes in obesity-related diseases and biochemical variables after laparoscopic sleeve gastrectomy: a two-year follow-up study

Villy Våge[1*], Vetle Aaberge Sande[2], Gunnar Mellgren[2,4], Camilla Laukeland[1], Jan Behme[1] and John Roger Andersen[1,3]

Abstract

Background: To evaluate changes in obesity-related diseases and micronutrients after laparoscopic sleeve gastrectomy (LSG).

Methods: We started the procedure in May 2007, and by December 2011, 117 patients could be evaluated for a two year follow-up. Comparisons of preoperative status with 12 and 24 months postoperative status were made for body mass index (BMI), obesity-related diseases and micronutrients.

Results: Major complications included bleeding requiring transfusion at 5.1%, leak at 1.7% and abscess without a visible leak at 0.9%. Mean BMI was reduced from 46.6 (standard deviation (SD) 6.0) kg/m^2 to 30.6 (SD 5.6) kg/m^2 at two years, and resolution occurred for 80.7% of patients with type 2 diabetes, 63.9% with hypertension, 75.8% with hyperlipidemia, 93.0% with sleep apnea, 31.4% with musculoskeletal pain, 85.4% with snoring and 73.3% with urinary incontinence. Amenorrhea resolved in all premenopausal females. The proportion of patients with symptomatic gastroesophageal reflux disease increased from 12.8% to 27.4%. The prevalence of patients with low ferritin-levels increased, while 25-hydroxyvitamin D (25(OH)D) deficiency decreased postoperatively.

Conclusions: LSG is an effective procedure for morbid obesity and obesity-related diseases, but the technique should be further explored particularly to avoid gastroesophageal reflux.

Keywords: Sleeve gastrectomy, Obesity, Comorbidities, Complications

Background

Between 1980 and 2008, the age-standardized mean global body mass index (BMI) increased by 0.4–0.5 kg/m^2 per decade in men and women [1], and worldwide obesity more than doubled. Obesity, and particularly morbid obesity (BMI ≥ 40) is known as a strong risk factor for several diseases and premature death [2].

Bariatric surgery is the only evidence-based treatment of morbid obesity with proven, sustained weight loss and improvement in comorbidities [3-5]. Laparoscopic sleeve gastrectomy (LSG) was introduced as the first stage in a two-staged bariatric surgical approach on super-obese or high-risk patients [6], but has now gained acceptance as a stand-alone bariatric procedure [7-11]. Physiologically it is an attractive procedure because it reduces the gastric volume while preserving the continuity of the gastrointestinal tract. Data on complications and weight loss after LSG have been increasingly published in the surgical literature, but data for the effects on comorbidities and micronutrients should be further explored [12,13].

Our bariatric surgical program started in 2001 with open Biliopancreatic diversion with duodenal switch (BPDDS), and LSG as a stand-alone procedure was started in May 2007. We had no experience with laparoscopic bariatric surgery prior to May 2007, and this prospective study reviews our first patients focusing on procedure complications, comorbidity resolution and changes in biochemical variables at 12 and 24 months postoperatively.

* Correspondence: villy.vage@helse-forde.no
[1]Department of Surgery, Førde Central Hospital, 6807 Førde, Norway
Full list of author information is available at the end of the article

Methods

After having obtained written informed consent from the patients, data was prospectively collected and stored in our database from the first LSG in May 2007 when LSG was introduced as a part of our standard bariatric program. The database is part of our continuous surveillance-program and approved by the Norwegian Data Inspectorate. This present study is a prospective cohort study with data extracted from the database. By December 2011 we had 117 patients eligible for a two year follow-up. Indications for LSG were either a BMI ≥ 40 kg/m^2 or a BMI ≥ 35 kg/m^2 with obesity-related diseases. Contraindications for operation were alcohol or drug abuse and active psychosis.

Preoperative evaluation and care included a one day seminar with information about morbid obesity, bariatric surgery and its risks, and estimated results as well as projected possibilities about life changes after surgery. This was followed by an individual consultation with the bariatric surgeon and other health-personnel if needed. Preoperative advice included smoking cessation, increased physical activity and weight loss.

On the evening before the operation all patients received low molecular weight heparin subcutaneously (enoxaparin), 40 mg if < 160 kg or 60 mg if ≥ 160 kg, and an H_2 blocker (cimetidine 300 mg) orally. Intravenous antibiotic prophylaxis (400 mg doxycycline, 1.5 g metronidazole) was started just prior to the operation. The operation was performed through six ports. Pneumoperitoneum was established through the upper part of the left rectal sheet using a 10 mm port containing the camera and the CO2-insufflator. A 15 mm port was introduced at the same level through the right rectal sheet. Four 5 mm ports were used: One at the right subcostal area, one just below the xiphoid process and two towards the left subcostal area. All ports were reusable (Karl Storz™) except for the 15 mm port which was non-reusable (Ethicon™).

The greater curvature was freed from the pylorus to the cardia, dividing all vessels by Ligasure (Covidien™). To ensure a good overview of the left crus and the gastro esophageal junction the periesophageal fat-pad was generally freed from both the diaphragm and the cardia. The stomach was divided along a 32 Fr bougie by the Tri-Stapler (Covidien™) from 1-2 cm proximal to the pylorus to the cardia. Over-sewing of the staple line was performed for visible bleeding. Attention was paid to avoid twisting or otherwise disrupting the gastric tube. The resected part of the stomach was removed without a bag through the incision for the 15 mm port. The abdominal fascia at this point was closed by two Polydioxanon (PDS) number 1 sutures. All skin-incisions were closed by intracutaneous reabsorbable sutures. Patients were allowed to drink freely from the first postoperative day, and discharged when tolerating a liquid diet. The enoxaparin was continued for ten days after discharge.

Postoperative advice included a low carbohydrate - high protein diet, intake of one multivitamin tablet daily, high frequency of water intake and physical activity. The first 61 patients were also routinely recommended to take Calcigran Forte (NycoMed Pharma™) containing one gram of calcium carbonate and 800IE 25-hydroxyvitamin D (25(OH)D) daily. Controls and data collection took place at the outpatient clinic 3, 12 and 24 months postoperatively. In addition, the patients were advised to see their general practitioner at 6 and 18 months. Pregnancy was strongly discouraged during the first 12 months after the operation.

Surgical complications were defined as complications occurring within 90 days after the surgical procedure. Obesity-related diseases were defined as diseases that were under medical care, and considered resolved when the patient no longer needed medical care for the actual disease (dichotomous variables). Diseases evaluated were type 2 diabetes mellitus (T2DM), hypertension, hyperlipidemia, sleep apnea, obstructive lung disease, musculoskeletal pain, anxiety, depression and gastroesophageal reflux. In addition, obesity-related problems as snoring, urinary leakage, amenorrhea and infertility were included independently of whether the patient received treatment or not. Infertility was defined as attempting to get pregnant over a period of two years without success.

Biochemical variables were selected according to our empirical experience, and were all analyzed by the Department of Clinical Biochemistry at our hospital except for the vitamin D-analyses (Hormone Laboratory, Haukeland University Hospital). The biochemical variables were converted into dichotomous variables, as either within the reference range or outside the reference range.

Statistical Package for the Social Sciences (SPSS) version 19.0 was used to perform the statistical analysis. Paired t- test was used in comparing paired means for change in BMI, and the McNemar's test was used for categorical variables. Statistical significance was set conventionally at $p < 0.05$.

Results

For the 117 patients studied (87 women and 30 men), the mean weight prior to the operation was 135.6 kg ± 23.7 kg (standard deviation (SD)), mean BMI 46.6 ± 6.0 kg/m^2, and mean age 40.3 ± 10.7 years (Table 1).

Complications

Major complications included bleeding (5.1%, n = 6), leak (1.7%, n = 2) and abscess without a visible leak (0.9%, n = 1) (Table 2). One patient had both bleeding and leak. The two patients who had a leak were treated with nil by mouth and a nasojejunal feeding tube for two and five months respectively before it healed. Both leaks were at the cardiac region. Two of the patients with bleeding had

Table 1 Overview of the patients (n = 117)

Variables	Mean ± SD
Age (years)	40.3 ± 10.7
Sex (Women/Men)	87/30
Weight (kg)	135.6 ± 23.7
BMI (kg/m^2)	46.6 ± 6.0
Operation time (min)	134.6 ± 27.5
Concurrent operations*	4

SD = Standard deviation. BMI = body mass index.
**Concurrent operations were cholecystectomi (2), appendectomy (1) and hiatal hernia repair (1).*

relaparoscopy with evacuation of blood (1.7%). There was no conversion of laparoscopic to open surgery and no mortality.

Obesity-related diseases

LSG significantly lowered the BMI to 30.3 ± 5.9 kg/m2 and 30.6 ± 5.6 kg/m2 at 12 and 24 months respectively, and resolved obesity-related diseases (Table 3). At two years, the remission-rate for Type 2 Diabetes Mellitus (T2DM) was 80.7%, hypertension 63.9%, hyperlipidemia 75.8%, sleep apnoea 93.0%, musculoskeletal pain 31.4%, snoring 85.4% and urinary leakage 73.3%. Amenorrhea was resolved for all premenopausal female patients with two years data. We lacked two year data for three of our twelve patients with preoperative amenorrhea. The prevalence of gastroesophageal reflux disease (GERD) increased from 12.8% prior to the operation to 27.4% at two years (p = 0.011).

Biochemical variables

Of the biochemical variables, ferritin was lowered while 25 (OH)-vitamin D, albumin and alanine amino transferase (ALT) improved significantly postoperatively (Table 4). We found a high prevalence of patients with Parathyroid hormone (PTH) above reference-level both preoperatively and postoperatively. Hemoglobin-, folic acid-, cobalamine-, 1, 25-dihydroxyvitamin D (1,25(OH)$_2$D), alkaline phosphatase (ALP), PTH and calcium levels did not change significantly after the procedure but 87% of the patients were taking vitamin and/or mineral supplements 24 months after the operation (Table 5). There was no difference in the vitamin or mineral status when comparing patients using supplements (n = 83) with patients not using supplements (n = 12) (chi-square test and t-test).

Table 2 90-day morbidity after surgery (n = 117)

Complications	Patients, n (%)
Bleeding (given transfusion)	6 (5.1%)
Reoperated	2 (1.7%)
Leak	2 (1.7%)
Reoperated	0 (0%)
Abscess without leak	1 (0.9%)
Reoperated	0 (0%)
Minor complications:	
Wound infection	3 (2.6%)
Incisional hernia	1 (0.9%)
Relaparoscopy for retained drain	1 (0.9%)

Discussion

In the present study we find LSG to have acceptable morbidity-rates and to be an effective procedure for weight loss and resolution of comorbidities. LSG had high resolution rates for T2DM, hypertension, hyperlipidemia, sleep apnea, musculoskeletal pain, snoring, urinary leakage and amenorrhea. The BMI and the prevalence of obesity-related diseases were stable between 12 and 24 months postoperatively. Between 85 and 90% of patients were taking some kind of vitamin and/or mineral supplement at follow-up.

In general, the reported complication rates for LSG are low despite high surgical risks in this patient group [8]. Shi et. al. systematically reviewed major perioperative complications for LSG and found a mean ± SD of 1.17 ± 1.86% for leaks and 3.57 ± 5.15% for bleeding respectively [14]. In order to reduce our leak-rate we have become particularly careful not to use heat-creating instruments close to the stomach wall at the cardia where both leaks occurred. In an attempt to reduce bleeding, we have changed our regime for prophylaxis against thrombosis in that the prophylaxis is started postoperatively and at reduced dosage. Other measures that could influence the rate of bleeding would be the use of different stapler cartridges and buttress material. There is currently no clear consensus on how the surgical technique is optimally performed [14], which makes it even more important to continuously evaluate the results at different centers.

We are only presenting resolution and not changes in the degree of severity of the obesity-related diseases or conditions, these results therefore represent an underreporting of the patients' improvement. Remission rates for T2DM, hypertension, hyperlipidemia and sleep apnea are higher among our patients than among sleeve- and gastric bypass operated patients in the study by Zhang et al., but our gastroesophageal reflux-rate is also higher [12]. This could be due to differences in the surgical technique as we used a somewhat smaller boogie (32 versus 38/40 Fr), and we start the resection closer to the pylorus. For infertility, we observed a reduction in infertility rate of 55.0% at two years, but as pregnancy was strongly discouraged for the first 12 months after the operation, the study is dependent on 36 months data for completion of the infertility data according to the definition. The regain of a normal menstrual cycle in all amenorrheic premenopausal females is remarkable.

Table 3 Proportion of patients (%) with obesity-related diseases prior to, and at 12 and 24 months after laparoscopic sleeve gastrectomy

Variable	Preoperative	12 months	24 months	P value		
				12 vs 0 months	24 vs 0 months	24 vs 12 months
No. with available data/total no.	117/117	116/117	109/117			
BMI (kg/m^2, mean ± SD)	46.6 ± 6.0	30.3 ± 5.9	30.6 ± 5.6	<0.001	<0.001	0.936
Treated for	*No. with disease/no. with available data (%)*					
T2DM	23/117 (19.7%)	5/114 (4.4%)	4/105 (3.8%)	<0.001	<0.001	1
Hypertension	50/117 (42.7%)	17/111 (15.3%)	16/104 (15.4%)	<0.001	<0.001	1
Hyperlipidemia	14/117 (12.0%)	5/114 (4.4%)	3/104 (2.9%)	0.039	0.021	1
Sleep apnea	15/117 (12.8%)	3/116 (2.9%)	1/109 (0.9%)	<0.001	<0.001	0.5
Obstructive lung disease	19/117 (16.2%)	19/114 (16.7%)	13/105 (12.4%)	1	0.063	0.063
Musculoskeletal pain	41/115 (35.7%)	29/114 (25.4%)	26/106 (24.5%)	0.067	0.026	0.804
Anxiety	18/117 (15.4%)	13/113 (11.5%)	11/103 (10.7%)	0.219	0.375	1
Depression	25/117 (21.4%)	18/113 (15.9%)	15/103 (14.6%)	0.109	0.125	1
GERD	15/117 (12.8%)	34/112 (30.4%)	29/106 (27.4%)	0.001	0.011	0.629
Suffering from (treated or not)						
Snoring	89/114 (78.1%)	28/112 (25%)	13/102 (12.8%)	<0.001	<0.001	0.002
Premenopausal/total no. of women	71/87	67/87	63/87			
Urinary leakage	33/87 (37.9%)	11/84 (13.1%)	8/79 (10.1%)	<0.001	<0.001	0.453
Amenorrhea	12/70 (17.1%)	3/65 (4.6%)	0/51 (0%)	0.021	0.016	1
Infertility	12/70 (17.1%)	*	4/52 (7.7%)		0.180	

BMI = Body mass index. SD = Standard deviation. No = Number. T2DM = Type 2 diabetes mellitus. GERD = Gastroesophageal reflux disease.
*Pregnancy was strongly discouraged during the first 12 months. At 24 months, two of the 12 women defined as infertile preoperatively had given birth to two healthy children.

Table 4 Proportion of patients (%) with important biochemical variables below or above reference value prior to, and at 12 and 24 months after laparoscopic sleeve gastrectomy

Variable	Preoperative	12 months	24 months	P value		
				12 vs. 0 months	24 vs. 0 months	24 vs. 12 months
No. with available data/total no:	95-117/117	98-107/117	65-95/117			
	No. below or above reference/no with available data (%)					
Hb<ref. (11,5-16,0 g/dl)	7/117 (6%)	5/105 (4.8%)	4/95 (4.2%)	1	1	1
Ferritin<ref. (25-300 ug/l)	13/116 (11.2%)	20/101 (19.8%)	28/85 (32.9%)	0.021	0.001	0.118
Folic acid<ref. (> 5 nmol/l)	8/106 (7.5%)	8/100 (8.0%)	2/91 (2.2%)	1	0.453	0.125
Cobalamin<ref. (145–540 pmol/l)	4/111 (3.6%)	7/107 (6.5%)	3/94 (3.2%)	0.508	1	0.727
25(OH)D<ref. (30-150 nmol/l)	29/110 (26.4%)	5/105 (4.8%)	8/79 (10.1%)	<0.001	<0.001	0.289
25(OH)D<50 nmol/l)	73/110 (66.4%)	39/105 (37.1%)	24/79 (30.4%)	<0.001	<0.001	0.839
1,25(OH)$_2$D>ref. (50-145 pmol/l)	0/104 (0.0%)	3/98 (3.1%)	1/65 (1.5%)	0.250	1	1
ALP>ref. (< 105 U/l)	6/116 (5.2%)	5/107 (4.7%)	7/94 (7.4%)	1	1	0.688
PTH>ref. (1.6-7.0 pmol/l)	35/95 (36.8%)	42/105 (40.0%)	36/85 (42.4%)	0.719	0.571	0.664
Calcium<ref. (2.15 – 2.55 mmol/l)	6/117 (5.1%)	1/108 (0.9%)	1/93 (1.1%)	0.124	0.125	1
Albumin<ref. (35-50 g/l)	16/117 (13.7%)	4/107 (3.7%)	8/94 (8.5%)	0.008	0.180	0.453
ALT>ref (35 U/l)	50/117 (42.7%)	11/107 (10.3%)	11/93 (11.8%)	<0.001	<0.001	1

No = Number. Hb = Hemoglobin. Ref = Reference value. 25(OH)D = 25 hydroxyvitamin D. 1,25(OH)$_2$D = 1,25 dihydroxyvitamin D. ALP = Alkaline Phosphatase. PTH = Parathyroid hormone. ALT = Alanine aminotransferase.

Table 5 Number of patients (%) using supplements prior to, and at 12 and 24 months after laparoscopic sleeve gastrectomy

Variable	Preoperative	12 months	24 months
no. with available data/total no:	115/117	107/117	96/117
No supplement	99 (86.1%)	16 (15.0%)	12 (12.5%)
Multivitamin	11 (9.6%)	79 (73.8%)	70 (72.9%)
Cobalamin	4 (3.5%)	26 (24.3%)	29 (30.2%)
Folic acid	5 (4.4%)	23 (21.5%)	18 (18.8%)
Calcium	2 (1.8%)	28 (26.2%)	35 (36.5%)
Iron	2 (1.8%)	3 (2.8%)	16 (16.7%)

No = Number.

Association between LSG and GERD has been systematically reviewed, finding both a significant increase and a significant decrease in GERD after LSG [15]. Our study shows a significant increase in GERD after the operation, even though five of our fifteen patients who were treated for GERD symptoms preoperatively had resolution of their GERD symptoms postoperatively. Our advice has been to have smaller meals at increased frequency and consume foods at slower rates with sufficient chewing, which might have some effect in reducing GERD-symptoms as Melissas et. al. have also experienced [16]. In accordance to the experience of Nocca et. al. [17] it is also our experience that the patients with GERD subjectively have a good effect of proton pump inhibitors. Howard et. al. [18], who had a one year GERD rate of 21.0%, declare that all of their GERD patients were "extremely happy with their surgery" and "would choose the procedure again". Despite Howard et. al.´s findings, GERD is a potential drawback for the LSG and more work is being done in order to reduce the risk for GERD after LSG [15,19,20].

A high prevalence of micronutrient deficiencies among morbidly obese prior to bariatric surgery has been observed, a proposed consequence of malnutrition and/or altered bioavailability to micronutrients due to reduced dietary intake, reduced levels of hydrochloric acid and intrinsic factor [21]. The number of patients with ferritin levels below reference range in our data increased significantly, similar to the findings of Himpens et. al. [22]. Himpens et. al. also found cobalamin deficiency one and three years after LSG, which together with iron-related deficiencies are the most common deficiencies after bariatric surgery [22,23]. The number of patients with cobalamin-deficiency was not altered in our study, but 27% and 29% of the patients were substituted with folic acid or cobalamin respectively already one year after surgery. Unfortunately, we do not know whether this substitution was based on low serum values for these vitamins or not. Our findings highlight a need for further exploring the necessity of folic acid, cobalamin, iron and possibly calcium-substitution in LSG patients before making any general recommendations.

Values for albumin and ALT showed significant improvement after the operation, and ALT levels remained significantly lowered at 24 months. Obesity is associated with non-alcoholic fatty liver disease (NAFLD) [24], and resolution of NAFLD has been proven after bariatric surgery [25]. Improvement of liver-associated biochemical variables due to resolution of NAFLD is therefore a probable explanation of our finding.

LSG has been found to be equally as safe and effective for weight loss and resolution of comorbidities as the Roux-en-Y gastric bypass (RYGBP) in the short term [12,23], and as the small bowel is not transected and no mesenteric defects are created, the risk for long term complications as jejunal ulcers and internal hernias are avoided. Also, further conversion to BPDDS or RYGBP if inadequate weight loss or weight regain should occur makes LSG a good option among the bariatric procedures. Long term effects of LSG are, however, still limited in terms of possible weight regain, side effects and persistence of comorbidity resolution [14,17,26].

Conclusion

We find LSG to have acceptable morbidity-rates and to be an effective procedure for weight loss and remission of obesity-related diseases. Further development of the technique should be attempted, particularly to reduce the risk for postoperative gastroesophageal reflux.

Competing interests

Villy Våge has had travel expenses for two international conferences covered by Covidien and Johnson & Johnson. Vetle Aaberge Sande, Gunnar Mellgren, Camilla Laukeland, Jan Behme and John Roger Andersen do not have any commercial associations that might be a conflict of interest in relation to this article.

Authors' contributions

W was responsible for the surgery, collection, and extraction of data, and participated in the statistical analysis and writing of the article. VAS participated in the extraction and analysis of data, and in writing of the article. GM participated in the design of the study, analysis of the blood-samples and writing the manuscript. CL was responsible for the dietary advices to the patients and participated in writing the manuscript. JB operated about half of the patients and participated in writing the manuscript. JRA participated in the statistical analysis and writing of the article. All authors read and approved the final manuscript.

Acknowledgement

We acknowledge Ronny Gåsdal, Helse Førde for collection of data and Jonathan Butcher, Helse Førde for reading through and commenting the English version of the manuscript.

Author details

[1]Department of Surgery, Førde Central Hospital, 6807 Førde, Norway. [2]Department of Clinical Science, University of Bergen, 5020 Bergen, Norway. [3]Department of Health, Sogn og Fjordane University College, 6803 Førde, Norway. [4]Hormone Laboratory, Haukeland University Hospital, 5021 Bergen, Norway.

References

1. Finucane MM, Stevens GA, Cowan MJ, Danaei G, Lin JK, Paciorek CJ, Singh GM, Gutierrez HR, Lu Y, Bahalim AN, *et al*: **National, regional, and global trends in body-mass index since 1980: systematic analysis of health examination surveys and epidemiological studies with 960 country-years and 9.1 million participants.** *Lancet* 2011, **377**(9765):557–567.
2. Whitlock G, Lewington S, Sherliker P, Clarke R, Emberson J, Halsey J, Qizilbash N, Collins R, Peto R: **Body-mass index and cause-specific mortality in 900 000 adults: collaborative analyses of 57 prospective studies.** *Lancet* 2009, **373**(9669):1083–1096.
3. Pories WJ, Swanson MS, MacDonald KG, Long SB, Morris PG, Brown BM, Barakat HA, de Ramon RA, Israel G, Dolezal JM, *et al*: **Who would have thought it? An operation proves to be the most effective therapy for adult-onset diabetes mellitus.** *Ann Surg* 1995, **222**(3):339–350. discussion 350-332.
4. Sjostrom L, Narbro K, Sjostrom CD, Karason K, Larsson B, Wedel H, Lystig T, Sullivan M, Bouchard C, Carlsson B, *et al*: **Effects of bariatric surgery on mortality in Swedish obese subjects.** *N Engl J Med* 2007, **357**(8):741–752.
5. WHO: *Obesity: preventing and managing the global epidemic.* Geneva: Worlds Health Organization; 2000.
6. Cottam D, Qureshi FG, Mattar SG, Sharma S, Holover S, Bonanomi G, Ramanathan R, Schauer P: **Laparoscopic sleeve gastrectomy as an initial weight-loss procedure for high-risk patients with morbid obesity.** *Surgical Endoscopy* 2006, **20**(6):859–863.
7. Baltasar A, Serra C, Perez N, Bou R, Bengochea M, Ferri L: **Laparoscopic sleeve gastrectomy: a multi-purpose bariatric operation.** *Obes Surg* 2005, **15**(8):1124–1128.
8. Brethauer SA, Hammel JP, Schauer PR: **Systematic review of sleeve gastrectomy as staging and primary bariatric procedure.** *Surgery for obesity and related diseases: official Journal of the American Society for Bariatric Surgery* 2009, **5**(4):469–475.
9. Mognol P, Chosidow D, Marmuse JP: **Laparoscopic sleeve gastrectomy as an initial bariatric operation for high-risk patients: initial results in 10 patients.** *Obesity Surgery* 2005, **15**(7):1030–1033.
10. Rice RD, Simon TE, Seery JM, Frizzi JD, Husain FA, Choi YU: **Laparoscopic sleeve gastrectomy: outcomes at a military training center.** *The American Surgeon* 2010, **76**(8):835–840.
11. Silecchia G, Boru C, Pecchia A, Rizzello M, Casella G, Leonetti F, Basso N: **Effectiveness of laparoscopic sleeve gastrectomy (first stage of biliopancreatic diversion with duodenal switch) on co-morbidities in super-obese high-risk patients.** *Obes Surg* 2006, **16**(9):1138–1144.
12. Zhang N, Maffei A, Cerabona T, Pahuja A, Omana J, Kaul A: **Reduction in obesity-related comorbidities: is gastric bypass better than sleeve gastrectomy?** *Surgical Endoscopy* 2013, **27**(4):1273–1280.
13. Committee ACI: **Updated position statement on sleeve gastrectomy as a bariatric procedure.** *Surgery for obesity and related diseases: official Journal of the American Society for Bariatric Surgery* 2012, **8**(3):e21–26.
14. Shi X, Karmali S, Sharma AM, Birch DW: **A review of laparoscopic sleeve gastrectomy for morbid obesity.** *Obesity Surgery* 2010, **20**(8):1171–1177.
15. Chiu S, Birch DW, Shi X, Sharma AM, Karmali S: **Effect of sleeve gastrectomy on gastroesophageal reflux disease: a systematic review.** *Surg Obes Relat Dis* 2011, **7**(4):510–515.
16. Melissas J, Daskalakis M, Koukouraki S, Askoxylakis I, Metaxari M, Dimitriadis E, Stathaki M, Papadakis JA: **Sleeve gastrectomy-a "food limiting" operation.** *Obesity Surgery* 2008, **18**(10):1251–1256.
17. Nocca D, Krawczykowsky D, Bomans B, Noel P, Picot MC, Blanc PM, de Seguin, de Hons C, Millat B, Gagner M, Monnier L, *et al*: **A prospective multicenter study of 163 sleeve gastrectomies: results at 1 and 2 years.** *Obesity Surgery* 2008, **18**(5):560–565.
18. Howard DD, Caban AM, Cendan JC, Ben-David K: **Gastroesophageal reflux after sleeve gastrectomy in morbidly obese patients.** *Surg Obes Relat Dis* 2011, **7**(6):709–713.
19. Soricelli E, Iossa A, Casella G, Abbatini F, Cali B, Basso N: **Sleeve gastrectomy and crural repair in obese patients with gastroesophageal reflux disease and/or hiatal hernia.** *Surg Obes Relat Dis* 2013, **9**(3):356–361.
20. Daes J, Jimenez ME, Said N, Daza JC, Dennis R: **Laparoscopic sleeve gastrectomy: symptoms of gastroesophageal reflux can be reduced by changes in surgical technique.** *Obes Surg* 2012, **22**(12):1874–1879.
21. Snyder-Marlow G, Taylor D, Lenhard MJ: **Nutrition care for patients undergoing laparoscopic sleeve gastrectomy for weight loss.** *Journal of the American Dietetic Association* 2010, **110**(4):600–607.
22. Himpens J, Dapri G, Cadiere GB: **A prospective randomized study between laparoscopic gastric banding and laparoscopic isolated sleeve gastrectomy: results after 1 and 3 years.** *Obes Surg* 2006, **16**(11):1450–1456.
23. Kehagias I, Karamanakos SN, Argentou M, Kalfarentzos F: **Randomized clinical trial of laparoscopic Roux-en-Y gastric bypass versus laparoscopic sleeve gastrectomy for the management of patients with BMI < 50 kg/m2.** *Obesity surgery* 2011, **21**(11):1650–1656.
24. Farrell GC, Larter CZ: **Nonalcoholic fatty liver disease: from steatosis to cirrhosis.** *Hepatology* 2006, **43**(2 Suppl 1):S99–S112.
25. Kral JG, Thung SN, Biron S, Hould FS, Lebel S, Marceau S, Simard S, Marceau P: **Effects of surgical treatment of the metabolic syndrome on liver fibrosis and cirrhosis.** *Surgery* 2004, **135**(1):48–58.
26. Deitel M, Gagner M, Erickson AL, Crosby RD: **Third international summit: current status of sleeve gastrectomy.** *Surgery for obesity and related diseases: official journal of the American Society for Bariatric Surgery* 2011, **7**(6):749–759.

5

Retrograde stapling of a free cervical jejunal interposition graft: a technical innovation and case report

Christina Hackl[1], Felix C Popp[1], Katharina Ehehalt[2], Lena-Marie Dendl[3], Volker Benseler[1], Philipp Renner[1], Martin Loss[1], Jurgen Dolderer[4], Lukas Prantl[4], Thomas Kühnel[5], Hans J Schlitt[1] and Marc H Dahlke[1*]

Abstract

Background: Free jejunal interposition is a useful technique for reconstruction of the cervical esophagus. However, the distal anastomosis between the graft and the remaining thoracic esophagus or a gastric conduit can be technically challenging when located very low in the thoracic aperture. We here describe a modified technique for retrograde stapling of a jejunal graft to a failed gastric conduit using a circular stapler on a delivery system.

Case presentation: A 56 year-old patient had been referred for esophageal squamous cell carcinoma at 20 cm from the incisors. On day 8 after thoracoabdominal esophagectomy with gastric pull-up, an anastomotic leakage was diagnosed. A proximal-release stent was successfully placed by gastroscopy and the patient was discharged. Two weeks later, an esophagotracheal fistula occurred proximal to the esophageal stent. Cervical esophagostomy was performed with cranial closure of the gastric conduit, which was left in situ within the right hemithorax. Three months later, reconstruction was performed using a free jejunal interposition. The anvil of a circular stapler (Orvil®, Covidien) was placed transabdominally through an endoscopic rendez-vous procedure into the gastric conduit. A free jejunal graft was retrogradely stapled to the proximal end of the conduit. Microvascular anastomoses were performed subsequently. The proximal anastomosis of the conduit was completed manually after reperfusion.

Conclusions: This modified technique allows stapling of a jejunal interposition graft located deep in the thoracic aperture and is therefore a useful method that may help to avoid reconstruction by colonic pull-up and thoracotomy.

Keywords: Gastric pull-up, Esophageal cancer, Conduit, Esophageal reconstruction

Background

Indications for cervical esophageal resection and short-distance reconstruction include limited cervical esophageal cancer, hypopharyngeal cancer invading the cervival esophagus and traumatic injury or dysfunction caused by congenital disorders, corrosive inury, or radiation damage [1,2]. Furthermore, reconstruction may be indicated as salvage surgery for failed gastric or colonic interposition grafts after prior esophagectomy when the remnant of the conduit is in good condition. While gastric pull-up and colonic interposition are standard reconstruction methods after extended esophagectomy, these techniques are invasive and less suitable for localized high cervical or hypopharyngeal reconstructions [1]. A cervical esophageal interposition graft, if technically feasible, implies lower perioperative mortality and morbidity, such as fistula or anastomotic leakage, and leads to fast postoperative recovery of functional GI continuity without reduction of quality of life by reflux, dysphagy or choking [1,2].

History of jejunal interposition grafts

In 1907, Carrel first described the technique of an autologous free jejunal graft transplanted into the neck of dogs with microvascular anastomosis to the common carotid artery and internal jugular vein [3]. In the same year, the first successful use of jejunum for esophageal reconstruction in a human patient was described by Roux, using a

* Correspondence: marc.dahlke@ukr.de
[1]Department of Surgery, University Medical Center Regensburg, Regensburg 93042, Germany
Full list of author information is available at the end of the article

pedicled jejunal graft [4]. In a review by Ochsner and Owens, losses of jejunal grafts using this technique were seen in 22%, mortality being as high as 46%, mainly as a result of inadequate blood supply to the jejunal flap [5]. Due to limited vascular length, vascularization was preserved in only 16 of 80 cases reported by Yudin in 1944 [6]. Inspired by this challenge, Longmire was the first to describe a modified technique adding microvascular anastomoses between the mesenteric vessels of the pedicled jejunal flap and the internal thoracic vessels [7]. After further refinement of microvascular surgery, Seidenberg was the first to describe the technique of a free jejunal flap [8], which at the same time was the first free flap described in humans. After further refinements, the method of free jejunal interposition shows an overall success rate of 91% today with flap survival in up to 97% of cases, an acceptable overall mortality of <5%, low prevalence of persisting leakage, fistulae or stricture (all <12%) and fast recovery of functional oral alimentation (60-90% within 16 days after surgery) [9-12].

Technical description of jejunal interposition grafts

For free cervical jejunal interposition of limited esophageal cancer, a unilateral or bilateral incision medial to the sternocleidomastoid muscle is performed and the platysma is transsected upwards. After retraction of the sternocleidomastoid muscle and division of the omohyoid muscle, lymphadenectomy around the internal jugular vein, the common carotid artery and the vagal nerve can be performed if necessary. The cervical esophagus is dissected posteriorly and mobilized from the hypopharynx down to the upper thoracic aperture. Retaining sutures can be placed and resection is completed. After confirmation of tumor-free resection margins by frozen section, a laparotomy is performed and a jejunal loop with appropriately long vessels is identified by diaphanoscopy. After graft excision, the artery is flushed with heparinized saline. An end-to-end jejunojejunostomy is then performed to restore GI continuity in the abdomen. The graft is transferred into the cervical site in isoperistaltic direction and venous and arterial anastomoses are completed using the internal jugular vein and the superior thyroid artery, the thyrocervical trunk or the common carotid trunk [2]. Due to the high metabolic rate of the jejunum and therefore limited ischemic tolerance, reperfusion must be achieved as fast as possible [1]. After reperfusion, the lower and upper esophago-jejunal anastomoses are performed end-to-end or end-to-side by hand suture or stapler [13].

Brief history of circular staplers and introduction of the OrVil® stapler (Covidien)

A first stapler-prototype, weighing 3.6 kg and needing approximately 2 hours of assembly time, was introduced in 1908 [14,15]. Production of commercially available staplers for intestinal and vascular anastomoses did not start before the 1950s [15]. The OrVil® stapling device (Covidien, USA) can be applied to create end-to-end, end-to-side or side-to-side anastomoses in both open and laparoscopic surgery. After assembly and staple formation, the stapler knife blade resects the excess tissue, creating a circular anastomosis of 21 mm or 25 mm in diameter. The anvil of the device is mounted on a 90 cm long PVC tube, thus enabling delivery through the esophagus and by endoscopic rendezvous procedures [16].

We here describe the case of a patient with a failed gastric conduit after leakage of the cervical anastomosis and development of a tracheal fistula. Three months after discontinuity resection of the anastomosis and formation of a cervical esophagostomy, reconstruction of the continuity with a free jejunal interposition graft was planned. This was difficult due to the location of the remaining gastric conduit deep in the thoracic aperture. Feasibility of a retrograde stapling procedure after endoscopic rendez-vous is described.

Case presentation

A 56 year-old caucasian female patient was referred with the diagnosis of esophageal squamous cell carcinoma (ESSC). The patient had a history of smoking (55 pack-years) and moderate alcohol consumption. Work-up including fluoroscopy, thoraco-abdominal CT scan, gastroscopy, bronchoscopy and blood works confirmed the diagnosis of a circular ESSC at 20-25 cm from the incisors (Figure 1A) with no suspect lymph nodes and no distant metastasis. After case discussion in an interdisciplinary disease management board, the patient underwent 2 cycles of neoadjuvant radiochemotherapy (cisplatin 60 mg/m2; 5-FU 1000 mg/m2; 45 Gy). A re-staging thoracoabdominal CT scan showed significant decrease in tumor size. Ivor-Lewis thoracoabdominal esophagectomy with gastric pull-up and circular end-to-side stapled cervical anastomosis (21 mm) was then performed as planned (Figure 1B). The operation included three-field lymphadenectomy, resection of the Azygos vein, cholecystectomy and insertion of a fine-needle catheter jejunostomy (FCJ) for early postoperative enteral nutrition. Histologic analysis confirmed a ypT2, ypN0, L0, V0, R0 G2 ESCC. The patient was transferred from surgical ICU to the normal surgical ward on post-operative day 5, eating strained food, supplemented by FCJ-feeding. Due to increasing CRP and leucocytosis on post-operative day 8, a thoraco-abdominal CT scan and EGD transit were performed and an anastomotic leakage with viable perfusion of the conduit was diagnosed. A proximal-release stent was successfully placed by endoscopy. After prolonged recovery from the resulting sepsis, the patient could be discharged in good clinical condition and eating regular diet on post-

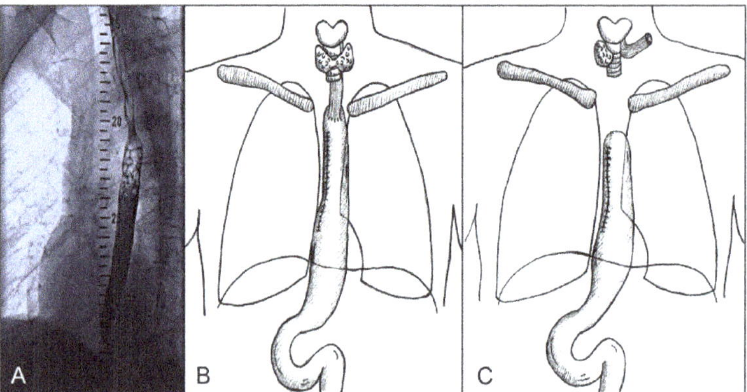

Figure 1 Diagnosis of ESSC, Esophagectomy and Esophagostomy after conduit failure. A) Workup including esophageal fluoroscopy at first presentation of the patient revealed an ESSC at 20-25 cm from the incisors. **B)** Status post Ivor-Lewis thoraco-abdominal esophagectomy with gastric pull-up and circular end-to-side stapled cervical anastomosis. **C)** Status post cervical esophagostomy and stump closure of the gastric pull-up conduit, which remained in situ within the right hemithorax.

operative day 56. Two weeks after discharge, the patient presented with symptoms of pneumonia and was readmitted. Workup including blood-works, thoraco-abdominal CT scan, bronchoscopy and gastroscopy revealed an esophagotracheal fistula cranial to the esophageal stent, not associated with the primary cervical anastomosis. After unsuccessful tracheal stenting and no possible further interventional improvement, the fistula was resected and cervical esophagostomy was performed with tracheal reconstruction by a sternoflap. The stump of the gastric pull-up conduit was closed using 3/0 monocryl handsewn interrupted suture and the intrathoracic part of the conduit remained in situ within the right hemithorax (Figure 1C). The patient could be transferred from surgical ICU to the normal ward on post-operative day 4 and was discharged on post-operative day 27. At routine follow-up three months later, the patient presented in good general condition. Restaging remained without new evidence of disease and free jejunal interposition was scheduled.

Operative Technique modifying the Free Jejunal Interposition

Angiography of SMA, IMA, ECA and subclavian arteries showed no pathological findings. Intraoperatively, the proximal stump of the gastric interposition was exposed after cervical incision. Exposition was challenging due to the very deep intrathoracic position of the conduit stump (Figure 2). Therefore, a laparotomy was performed and an endoscopy of the pull-up gastric interposition was performed after gastroscope insertion via the distal part of the gastric conduit (Figure 3A). After endoscopic diaphanoscopy, a guide-wire was placed by endoscopic rendezvous from the cervical incision into the gastric pull-up conduit (Figure 3B) and the OrViL® delivery tube was attached to the guide-wire (Figure 3C). Then, a suitable jejunal loop with vascular pedicle was identified, excised, flushed with ice-cold heparine/saline, kept on ice and transferred to the cervical operation site. The OrViL® circular stapler was inserted into the aboral part of the free jejunal graft (Figure 3D,E) and stapling of the jejunogastrostomy was performed (Figure 3E). Venous and arterial anastomoses were then performed by side-to end venous anastomosis using the internal jugular vein and end-to end arterial anastomosis using the left superior thyroid artery. Total ischemic time of the graft was less than 60 minutes with continuous cooling. After reperfusion, the jejunal graft appeared viable pink with increased peristalsis. The small incision at the distal gastric conduit used to insert the gastroscope was closed with 3/0 monocryl hand-sewn interrupted suture. Pharyngojejunal end-to-side anastomosis was then performed by hand with interrupted sutures after reperfusion (Figure 3F). Three centimeters of the cervical incision were left open to monitor the graft. The patient could be transferred from

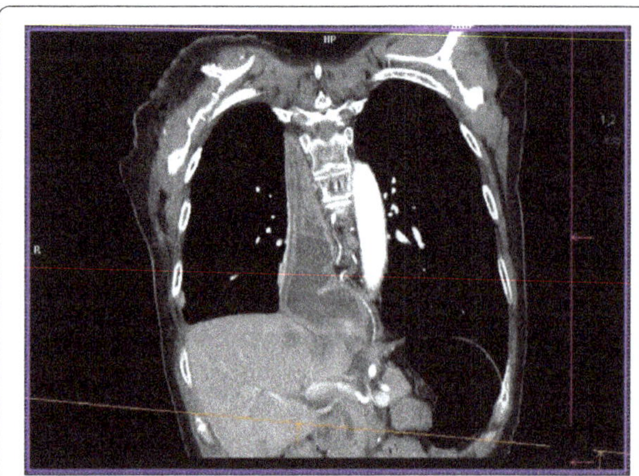

Figure 2 Position of the gastric pull-up conduit retracted into the right hemithorax before reconstruction.

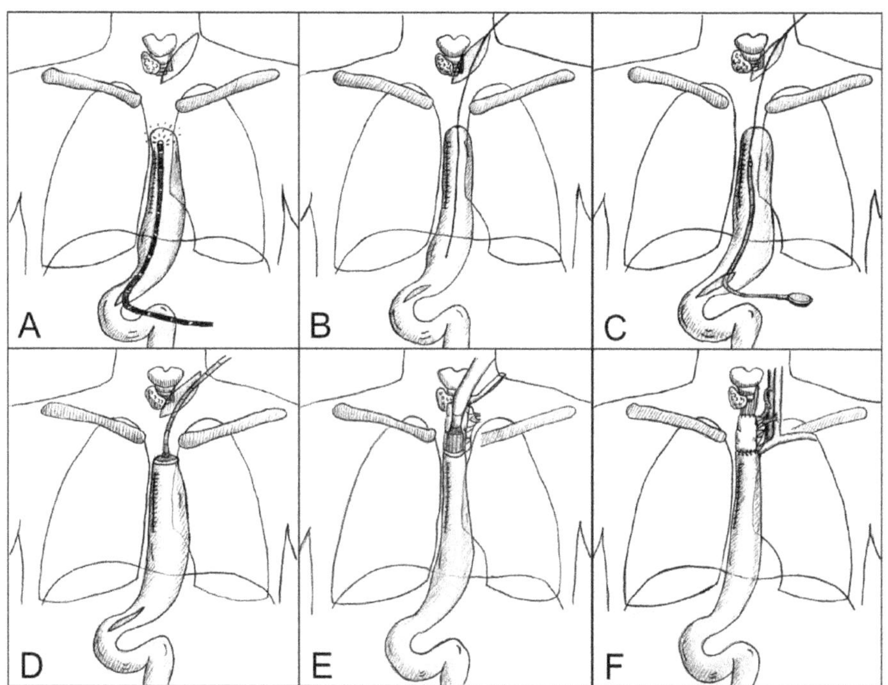

Figure 3 Reconstruction with free jejunal interposition. A) Gastroscopy and diaphanoscopy of the pull-up gastric interposition after gastroscope insertion via the distal conduit. **B)** Guide-wire positioning from the cervical incision into the gastric pull-up conduit by endoscopic rendez-vous. **C)** Attachment of the OrViL® delivery tube to the guide-wire. **D)** Insertion of the OrViL® circular stapler into the pull-up gastric interposition **E)** Stapling of the jejunogastrostomy. **F)** Revascularization and proximal anastomosis of the free jejunal interposition.

surgical ICU to the surgical ward on post-operative day 8. On day thirteen, a secondary wound closure was undertaken, which resulted in minimal leakage of the proximal anastomosis. The patient was discharged home on post-operative day 44 with regular EGD transit (Figure 4). Two weeks after discharge, the patient presented with stricture of the jejunal interposition at the distal anastomosis, which could successfully be resolved by single endoscopic balloon dilation therapy. Another three weeks later, the cervical incision had completely healed and the patient tolerated small portions of regular diet with slow weight gains. One year after final discharge, the patient presented tumor-free and eating regular diet.

Conclusions

We here describe a modified technique for retrograde stapling of a free jejunal interposition graft for a failed gastric pull-up. The gastric conduit had remained in situ within the right hemi-thorax, its proximal end deep in the thoracic aperture, opening the possibility of limited-length reconstruction by free jejunal interposition. During reconstruction, cervical exposition of the proximal

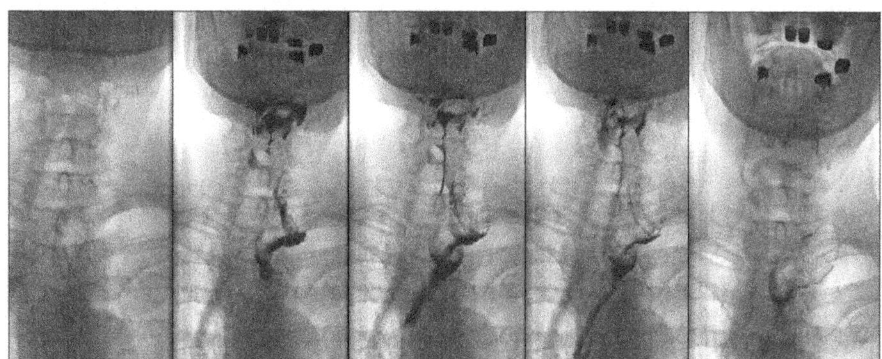

Figure 4 Regular EGD transit before discharge of the patient.

gastric stump was challenging due to its position deep in the thoracic aperture. Preparation for hand-sewn distal anastomosis would have meant a traumatizing access by sternotomy and/or thoracotomy, including a significant risk of surgical damage and yet accepting a high risk of anastomotic leakage. Instead, a laparotomy was performed with subsequent distal gastrostomy and insertion of a gastroscope followed by retrograde gastroscopy of the pull-up gastric interposition. By diaphanoscopy, the proximal stump of the gastric conduit was safely identified and a guide-wire was inserted from the cervival incision site. Then, the anvil of the OrViL circular stapler was introduced via the conduit and the jejuno-gastrostomy was stapled prior to microvascular reconstruction of the graft vessels. Concerning esophagogastric surgery with jejunal interposition, an ongoing controversy exists, whether esophago-jejunal or pharyngo-jejunal anastomoses should preferably be performed as end-to-side circular stapling or be hand-sewn end-to-end [13,17]. Up until now, no significant differences in anastomotic leakage rates are seen whereas the influence on long-term anastomotic strictures is a matter of debate [17].

In our case, revascularisation was performed after the jejuno-gastrostomy, thus enabling adaptation of an ideal vessel-length with the jejunal interpostion already in situ. Vice versa, stapling of the jejunogastrostomy, being a fast and safe procedure, did not necessitate prior microvascular anastomosis of the ischemia-intolerant jejunal flap. Leaving the gastric conduit in situ thus enabled salvage surgery by interposition of a short jejunal segment, offering the benefits of excellent peristalsis, absence of alkaline or acidic reflux and excellent size match of the two conduits [1].

Alternative methods for reconstruction of the cervical esophagus after failure of a gastric conduit are pectoralis major flaps or free tissue transfers such as the radial forearm flap or the anterolateral thigh flap or colonic interposition [1,18]. The pectoralis major flap as well as free tissue transfers offer excellent length, are resistant to reflux, allow functional swallowing and show low cardiopulmonary co-morbidity. Furthermore, no abdominal surgery is needed for flap harvest. In contrast, pectoralis major or free tissue flaps do not enable peristalsis, often show long long-term redundancy and significant risk of strictures and fistulas in the longer term [1,18]. Colonic interpositions offer the benefits of excellent length and long-term function and would be ideal for bridging long defects of the thoracic esophagus. On the other hand, colonic interposition implies the risk of extended abdominal surgery, complicated blood supply, intrinsic diseases such as cancer or bleeding, and long-term redundancy with a reduced overall quality of life [1,19].

Taken together, we here describe a modified technique of retrograde stapling of a jejunal interposition graft to a gastric conduit that had remained in situ after a leaking esophageal anastomosis. This technique may be of value for a selected group of patients with this unique surgical problem and may help to avoid then unnecessary thoracotomies or colonic pull-ups.

Competing interests

The authors declare that they have no competing interests.

Authors' contributions

CH drafted, wrote an edited the manuscript and edited the figures. FCP helped to dritically revise the manusript and performed parts of the surgeries. KE and LMD created the figures presented in this manuscript. VB and PR helped drafting and critically revising the manuscript. ML, JD, LP, TK, HJS and MHD were the surgeons performing this new technique of retrograde stapling of a jejunal interposition graft to a gastric conduit. Furthermore, MHD drafted and critically revised the manuscript and HJS critically revised the manuscript. All authors read and approved the final manuscript.

Author details

[1]Department of Surgery, University Medical Center Regensburg, Regensburg 93042, Germany. [2]Department of Anaesthesia, University Medical Center Regensburg, Regensburg, Germany. [3]Department of Radiology, University Medical Center Regensburg, Regensburg, Germany. [4]Department of Trauma, Plastic and Hand Surgery, University Medical Center Regensburg, Regensburg, Germany. [5]Department of Otorhinolaryngology, University Medical Center Regensburg, Regensburg, Germany.

References

1. Evans KFKMS, Salgado CJ, Chen H: **Esophagus and Hypopharyngeal Reconstruction.** *Semin Plast Surg* 2010, **24**(2):219–226.
2. Clavien PA, Sarr MG, Fong YE: **Atlas of Upper Gastrointestinal and Hepato-Pancreato-Biliary Surgery.** *Springer* 2007, **XXVIII**:48ff.
3. Carrel A: **The surgery of blood vessels.** *Johns Hopkins Hosp Bull* 1907, **190**:18–28.
4. Roux C: **A new operation for intractable obstruction of the esophagus (L'oesophagp-jejunogastrosiose, nouvelle operation pour retreciccement infrachissable del'oesophagus).** *Semin Med* 1907, **27**:34–40.
5. Ochsner AON: **Antethoracic oesophagoplasty for impermeable stricture of the oesophagus.** *Ann Surg* 1934, **100**:1055–1091.
6. Yudin S: **The surgical construction of 80 cases of artificial esophagus.** *Surg Gynecol Obstet* 1944, **78**:561–583.
7. Longmire W: **A modification of Roux technique for antethoracic esophageal reconstruction.** *Surgery* 1947, **22**:94–100.
8. Seidenberg B, Rosenak SS, Hurwitt ES, Som ML: **Immediate reconstruction of the cervical esophagus by a revascularized isolated jejunal segment.** *Ann Surg* 1959, **149**(2):162–171.
9. Nagasao T, Shimizu Y, Kasai S, Hatano A, Ding W, Jiang H, Kishi K, Imanishi N: **Extension of the jejunum in the reconstruction of cervical oesophagus with free jejunum transfer using the thoracoacrominal vessels as recipients.** *J Plast Reconstr Aesthet Surg* 2012, **65**(2):156–162.
10. Clark JR, Gilbert R, Irish J, Brown D, Neligan P, Gullane PJ: **Morbidity after flap reconstruction of hypopharyngeal defects.** *Laryngoscope* 2006, **116**(2):173–181.
11. Smith DF, Ott DJ, McGuirt WF, Albertson DA, Chen MY, Gelfand DW: **Free jejunal grafts of the pharynx: surgical methods, complications, and radiographic evaluation.** *Dysphagia* 1999, **14**(3):176–182.

12. Coleman JJ 3rd, Tan KC, Searles JM, Hester TR, Nahai F: **Jejunal free autograft: analysis of complications and their resolution.** *Plast Reconstr Surg* 1989, **84**(4):589–595. discussion 596-588.
13. Hsu HH, Chen JS, Huang PM, Lee JM, Lee YC: **Comparison of manual and mechanical cervical esophagogastric anastomosis after esophageal resection for squamous cell carcinoma: a prospective randomized controlled trial.** *Eur J Cardiothorac Surg* 2004, **25**(6):1097–1101.
14. Zeebregts CJ, Heijmen RH, van den Dungen JJ, Van Schilfgaarde R: **Non-suture methods of vascular anastomosis.** *Br J Surg* 2003, **90**(3):261–271.
15. Konstantinov IE: **Circular vascular stapling in coronary surgery.** *Ann Thorac Surg* 2004, **78**(1):369–373.
16. **Covidien circular staplers.** http://www.autosuture.com/autosuture/pagebuilder.aspx?topicID=153252: Date of web archive 25/1/2013.
17. Yasuda T, Shiozaki H: **Esophageal reconstruction using a pedicled jejunum with microvascular augmentation.** *Ann Thorac Cardiovasc Surg* 2011, **17**(2):103–109.
18. Maier A, Pinter H, Tomaselli F, Sankin O, Gabor S, Ratzenhofer-Komenda B, Smolle-Juttner FM: **Retrosternal pedicled jejunum interposition: an alternative for reconstruction after total esophago-gastrectomy.** *Eur J Cardiothorac Surg* 2002, **22**(5):661–665.
19. Doki Y, Okada K, Miyata H, Yamasaki M, Fujiwara Y, Takiguchi S, Yasuda T, Hirao T, Nagano H, Monden M: **Long-term and short-term evaluation of esophageal reconstruction using the colon or the jejunum in esophageal cancer patients after gastrectomy.** *Dis Esophagus* 2008, **21**(2):132–138.

6

Morpho-functional gastric pre-and post-operative changes in elderly patients undergoing laparoscopic cholecystectomy for gallstone related disease

Giovanni Aprea[1*], Alfonso Canfora[1], Antonio Ferronetti[1], Antonio Giugliano[1], Francesco Guida[1], Antonio Braun[1], Melania Battaglini Ciciriello[1], Federica Tovecci[1], Giovanni Mastrobuoni[1], Fabrizio Cardin[2], Bruno Amato[1]

Abstract

Background: Cholecystectomy, gold standard treatment for gallbladder lithiasis, is closely associated with increased bile reflux into the stomach as amply demonstrated by experimental studies. The high prevalence of gallstones in the population and the consequent widespread use of surgical removal of the gallbladder require an assessment of the relationship between cholecystectomy and gastric mucosal disorders.

Morphological evaluations performed on serial pre and post – surgical biopsies have provided new acquisitions about gastric damage induced by bile in the organ.

Methods: 62 elderly patients with gallstone related disease were recruited in a 30 months period. All patients were subjected to the most appropriate treatment (Laparoscopic cholecystectomy). The subjects had a pre-surgical evaluation with:

- dyspeptic symptoms questionnaire,
- gastric endoscopy with body, antrum, and fundus random biopsies,
- histo-pathological analysis of samples and elaboration of bile reflux index (BRI).

The same evaluation was repeated at a 6 months follow-up.

Results: In our series the duodeno-gastric reflux and the consensual biliary gastritis, assessed histologically with the BRI, was found in 58% of the patients after 6 months from cholecystectomy. The demonstrated bile reflux had no effect on H. pylori's gastric colonization nor on the induction of gastric precancerous lesions.

Conclusions: Cholecystectomy, gold standard treatment for gallstone-related diseases, is practiced in a high percentage of patients with this condition. Such procedure, considered by many harmless, was, in our study, associated with a significant risk of developing biliary gastritis after 6 months during the postoperative period.

* Correspondence: giovanni.aprea@yahoo.it

[1]Department of General, Geriatric, Oncologic Surgery and Advanced Technologies, University "Federico II" of Naples, Via Pansini, 5 - 80131 – Naples, Italy

Full list of author information is available at the end of the article

Background

A thorough review of literature has shown that cholecystectomy is accompanied, in the years following surgery, by an increase in duodenal-gastric reflux (DGR) [1-3], however, there is only partial data on the incidence of bile reflux gastritis in patients undergoing cholecystectomy [4-7].

Numerous studies have also shown an association between cholecystectomy and gastric cancer [8-12]; the increased bile reflux may be a determining factor, if this risk was confirmed.

It is common, in patients who undergo cholecystectomy, to observe a persistence of upper abdominal symptoms often labeled as post-cholecystectomy syndrome [3,13-17]; these symptoms are likely related to a post-surgical duodenal-gastric reflux.

There are still conflicting reports on the possible effects of duodenal-gastric reflux on Helicobacter pylori's gastric infection.

We therefore decided to perform a prospective study on elderly patients which refer to our general surgery department in order to evaluate whether cholecystectomy increases the risk of gastritis, induces the onset of dyspeptic symptoms, alters the incidence of *H. pylori* infection or increases the risk of gastric cancer.

Methods

The primary objective of our study was to evaluate the incidence of postoperative biliary gastritis through the prospective evaluation of patients with symptomatic gallbladder lithiasis treated with laparoscopic cholecystectomy.

Among the secondary objectives were:

- Assessment of changes in prevalence of *H. pylori* gastritis resulting from the eventual bile reflux gastritis
- Assessment of the presence of lesions, in the follow-up, considered as risk factors for gastric cancer

The study was carried out with the following modalities:

1) recruitment of elderly patients (over 70) with symptomatic gallstones and ultrasound documentation of the stones for which there was indication for cholecystectomy and who gave informed consent for the study participation.

2) exclusion of all patients exposed to other risk factors such as NSAIDs or alcohol who are able to determine gastric symptoms and / or reactive gastritis.

3) pre-surgical evaluation:

• dyspeptic symptoms questionnaire subministration (Table 1),

• gastric endoscopy in order to assess the absence of macroscopically visible lesions and to provide multiple biopsies of the gastric antrum, body and fundus,

• histo-pathological analysis of samples and elaboration of bile reflux index (BRI). This index is elaborated grading the following four histological parameters on a scale from 0 to 3: lamina propria edema (Oed), chronic inflammation (CI), intestinal metaplasia (IM), *Helicobacter pylori* colonization density (Hp). Subsequently the following formula is applied to obtain the BRI:(7xOed) + (3xIM) + (4xCI) - (6xHp).

Table 1 Dyspeptic symptoms questionnaire

Symptom	Pre-operative score(0-3)	Post-operative score(0-3)
Epigastric pain		
Nausea		
Bilious vomiting		
Upper abdominal quadrant swelling		
Post-prandial fullness		
Heartburn		
Frequent belching		

A value of BRI equal to or greater than 14 is indicative of reflux gastritis and if used as a single diagnostic investigation for pathological DGR has a sensitivity of 70% and a specificity of '85% to detect a bile level > 1.00 mmol / L in the stomach (upper limit of physiological bile reflux) [18-20]. Patients that may be positive for *H. pylori* should not perform eradication therapy at least until the first follow-up at 6 months.

4) laparoscopic cholecystectomy.

5) clinical reassessment of patients at 6 months post-operatively with the dyspeptic symptoms questionnaire and new endoscopy for BRI score evaluation.

6) Comparison of clinical and histopathological data obtained during pre-surgical phase and during follow-up at 6 months.

The study has provided so far, since January 2010, the enrollment of 62 patients. Of these, 31 completed the follow-up to 6 months, 19 were lost at follow-up, 12 patients have yet to complete the follow-up. Nineteen of 62 patients (30.64%) did not return for the post-operative follow-up ,maybe for the scant willingness to undergo an invasive follow-up endoscopy, especially if the purpose is the finding of a bile reflux gastritis, a condition that can occur without symptoms and who's long term risks are unknown. Patients who did not undergo the postoperative examination were excluded from the study.

Results and discussion

Of the 31 patients who completed follow-up (50%), 13 were men and 18 women. The age was between 70 and 85 years with an overall mean age of 74.86. The age range in the male group was between 71 and 85 years with a mean age of 75.09 years. In female subjects the minimum age was 70 years and the maximum age was 80 years, with an average of 74.70 years.

The clinical evaluation showed, in pre-operative phase, in all cases, the presence of dyspeptic symptoms. However we must remember that symptoms such as upper abdominal pain, nausea and bilious vomiting are also attributable to episodes of "biliary colic" related to the gallstone disease.

However, it results difficult to attach any dyspeptic symptom found to a possible pathological DGR present in the pre-surgical phase and to its associated morphological changes cause in 23 of 31 examined subjects a coexisting *H. pylori* infection could have been responsible for similar symptoms.

The persistence in some subjects (13 of total 31 examined), after surgical removal of the gallbladder, of the previous symptoms could, on the other hand, be related to the onset of a pathological DGR and the associated morphological changes. However, resulting the *H.pylori* infection prevalence unchanged , it remains difficult, based on clinical observations, to attribute these symptoms solely to DGR. Final results would require assessments of groups of subjects negative for *Helicobacter pylori* infection that we have chosen not to follow exclusively to evaluate the in vivo effect of bile acid levels on the *H. pylori* infection in subjects after cholecystectomy.

Preoperative histo-pathological findings showed the following:

Of the 31 patients examined 23 were positive for *Helicobacter pylori* infection in pre-operative and in all these subjects the antrum was always affected alone or in the context of a pan-gastritis. The infection was associated with morphological features of a mild or moderate chronic gastritis.

In all studied subjects , even in *H. pylori* negative areas, chronic inflammatory changes were highlighted; such thing could be explained by an abnormal duodenal-gastric reflux related to the gallbladder exclusion operated by lithiasis. In 8 cases these modifications were such that, also pre-operatively, in one or more portions of the stomach, the BRI exceeded the threshold value of 14.

Since the calculation of the BRI gives a different weight to the various evaluated morphological entities and in particular requires the subtraction of the density of *Helicobacter pylori* colonization in order to detect the presence of chronic inflammation related to duodenal-gastric reflux, it is easy to understand that, although there is an antrum-body-fundus gradient for the damage caused by DGR, because the antrum is the most common site of bacterial colonization, the average BRI value calculated in this site is going to be lower than that of the body and of the fundus (Table 2).

In the post-operative phase at 6 months there is an increase of the mean values of BRI in all patients and in all portions of the stomach, while the incidence of *Helicobacter pylori* results unchanged (Table 3 and 4).

Table 2 Pre-operative BRI values.

	BRI mean value	SD
Antrum	8.5	5.2
Body	10.69	7.06
Fondus	10.15	6.33

As a result,the number of individuals with one or more locations with a BRI value > 14 increases from 8 subjects in the preoperative phase to 18 patients in the postoperative one.

This data was statistically tested in order to demonstrate the existence of an association between the surgical removal of the gallbladder and the occurrence of bile reflux gastritis. In first instance we organized a table for observed frequencies (Table 5). Using the $\chi 2$ test we compared the observed frequencies with the expected ones if the two conditions in question were independent.

The value of the $\chi 2$ obtained from processing our data, with one degree of freedom, is 5.365 with a p value of 0.0205, and since the critical value of $\chi 2$ for one degree of freedom and with a probability of 5% is 3, 84 is possible to establish with this level of security the existence of an association between cholecystectomy and the onset of biliary gastritis.

In our sample there was no finding of intestinal metaplasia in either preoperative or postoperative phase. This result is consistent with the theory that intestinal metaplasia, although a precancerous lesion, requires a longer time (more than six months) to develop.

Conclusions

Cholecystectomy, gold standard treatment for gallstone-related diseases, is practiced in a high percentage of patients with this condition. Such procedure, considered by many harmless, was, in our study, associated with a significant risk of developing biliary gastritis after 6 months during the postoperative period. This occurrence was found in our series in 58% of patients who underwent cholecystectomy (Fig. 1). However, the presence of symptoms in post-operative timing does not reflect the histological findings in these same patients: while, in fact, a positive histological BRI was found in 58% of patients after cholecystectomy, clinical symptoms were found in 41.9% of them .In addition these symptoms could also be related to the persistence of *H. pylori* infection.

Table 3 Post-operative BRI values.

	BRI mean value	SD
Antrum	15.82	7.83
Body	17.24	7.72
Fondus	16.93	7.48

Table 4 H. pylori positivity in pre e post-operative phase

	H. pylori -	H.pylori +
Pre-operative	8	23
Post-operative	8	23

Table 5 Observed frequencies

	BRI < 14	BRI > 14
Pre-operative	23	8
Post-operative	13	18

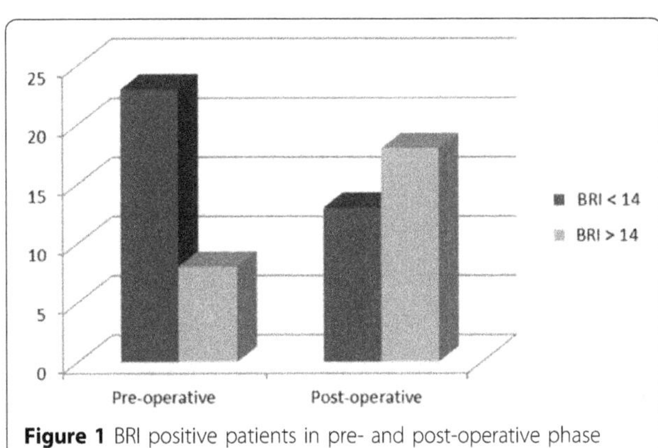

Figure 1 BRI positive patients in pre- and post-operative phase

Infection by *H. pylori* detected preoperatively in 23 of 31 patients resulted unchanged at the 6 months post-operative follow-up. In our series the duodeno-gastric reflux, assessed histologically with the BRI in 58% of the patients after cholecystectomy, seems to have no effect or, at least, no ability to eradicate *H. pylori* from the gastric mucosa.

Although in our series we have not found the presence of intestinal metaplasia of the gastric mucosa in any of the postoperative samples, studies such as the Swedish study [12] are only partially refuted, and associate cholecystectomy with an increased incidence of gastric cancer, potentially attributable to chronic inflammatory insults such as bile reflux gastritis; this condition is all but uncommon in our series of patients who undergo cholecystectomy.

Although these findings remain to be confirmed on a wider coverage, pending further clarification, a clinical and endoscopic follow-up in relation to the suspected potential transformation is recommended in patients who undergo cholecystectomy and in which a chronic bile reflux gastritis is diagnosed. We planned, therefore, to continue our experimental investigation for the next three years, aiming to gather a wider sample of individuals in order to draw further conclusions.

List of abbreviations

BRI: Bile Reflux Index; DGR: duodenal-gastric reflux.

Acknowledgements

This article has been published as part of *BMC Surgery* Volume 12 Supplement 1, 2012: Selected articles from the XXV National Congress of the Italian Society of Geriatric Surgery. The full contents of the supplement are available online at http://www.biomedcentral.com/bmcsurg/supplements/12/S1.

Author details

[1]Department of General, Geriatric, Oncologic Surgery and Advanced Technologies, University "Federico II" of Naples, Via Pansini, 5 - 80131 – Naples, Italy. [2]Department of Surgical and Gastroenterological Sciences, Padova University Hospital, Italy Via Giustiniani n.2, 35126 Padova, Italy.

Authors' contributions

FG, AG, AC, AF, AB, MBC, FT, GM:acquisition of data, drafting the manuscript, given final approval of the version to be published, GA,BA: conception and design, interpretation of data, given final approval of the version to be published, FC: acquisition of data, drafting the manuscript, given final approval of the version to be published.

Competing interests

The authors declare that they have no competing interests.

References

1. Svennson JO, Gelin J, Svanvik : **Gallstones, cholecystectomy and duodenogastric reflux of bile acid.** *Scand J Gastroenterol* 1986, **21**:181-7.
2. Chen MF, Wang Cs: **A prospective study of the effect of cholecystectomy on duodenogastric reflux in humans using 24h gastric hydrogen monitoring.** *Surg Gynecol Obstet* 1992, **175**:52-56, Stefănescu G, Bălan G, Stanciu C The relationship between bile reflux and symptoms in patients with gallstones before and after cholecystectomy. Rev Med ChirSoc Med Nat Iasi 2009,113(3):698-703.
3. Wilson P, Jamieson JR, Hinder RA, Anselmino M, Perdikis G, Ueda RK, DeMeester TR: **Pathologic duodenogastric reflux associated with persistence of symptoms after cholecystectomy.** *Surgery* 1995, **117**:421-428.
4. Lo Russo D, Pezzola F, Cavallini A, Messa C, Giorgio P, Caruso ML, Piccioli E, Guerra V, Misciagna G: **A prospective study on duodenogastric reflux and on histological changes in gastric mucosa after cholecystectomy.** *Gastroenterol Clin Biol* 1992, **16**:328-333.
5. Lo Russo D, Pezzola F, Linsalata M, Caruso ML, Giorgio P, Guerra V, Misciagna G, Piccioli E, Di Leo A: **Duodenogastric reflux, histology and cell proliferation of the gastric mucosa bifore and six months after cholecystectomy.** *Acta Gastro-enterologica Belgica* 1995, **LVIII.**
6. Santarelli L, Gabrielli M, Candelli M, Cremonimi F, Nista EC, Cammarota G, *et al*: **Post-cholecystectomy alkaline reactive gastritis: a randomized trial comparing sucralfate versus rabeprazole or no treatment.** *Eur J Gastroenterol Hepatol* 2003, **15**:975-979.
7. Kuran S, Parlak E, Aydog G, Kacar S, Sasmaz N, Ozden A, Sahin B: **Bile reflux index after therapeutic biliary procedures.** *BMC Gastroenterol* 2008, **11**:8-4.
8. Miwa K, Hattori T, Miyazaki I: **Duodenogastric reflux and foregut carcinogenesis.** *Cancer* 1995, **75**:1426-1432.
9. Freedman J, Lagergren J, Bergström R, Näslund E, Nyrén O: **Cholecystectomy, peptic ulcer disease and the risk of adenocarcinoma of the oesophagus and gastric cardia.** *Br J Surg* 2000, **87(8)**:1087-93.
10. Gustavsson S, Adami HO, Meirik O, Nyrén O, Krusemo UB: **Cholecystectomy as a risk factor for gastric cancer. A cohort study.** *Dig Dis Sci* 1984, **29(2)**:116-20.
11. Guida F, Antonino A, Conte P, Formisano G, Esposito D, Bencivenga M, Aprea G, Amato B, Avallone U, Persico G: **Gastric cancer in elderly: clinico-pathological features and surgical treatment.** *BMC Geriatrics* 2009, **9(suppl)**:A66.
12. Fall K, *et al*: **Risk for gastric cancer after cholecystectomy.** *Am J Gastroenterol* 2007, **102**:1180-4.
13. Wilson P, Jamieson JR, Hinder RA, Anselmino M, Perdikis G, Ueda RK, DeMeester TR: **Pathologic duodenogastric reflux associated with persistence of symptoms after cholecystectomy.** *Surgery* 1995, **117(4)**:421-8.
14. Tamhankar AP, Mazari F, Olubaniyi J, Everitt N, Ravi K: **Postoperative Symptoms, after-care, and return to routine activity after laparoscopic cholecystectomy.** *JSLS* 2010, **14(4)**:484-9.

15. Jaunoo SS, Mohandas S, Almond LM: **Postcholecystectomy syndrome (PCS).** *Int J Surg* 2010, **8(1)**:15-7.
16. Farsakh A, Stietieh M, Farsakh FA: **The postcholecystectomy syndrome. A role for duodenogastric reflux.** *J ClinGastroenterol* 1996, **22**:197-201.
17. Aprea G, Coppola Bottazzi E, Guida F, Masone S, Persico G: **Laparoendoscopic single site (LESS) versus classic video-laparoscopic cholecystectomy: a randomized prospective study.** *J Surg Res* 2011, **166(2)**:e109-12.
18. Dixon MF, Mapstone NP, Neville PM, Moayyedi P, Axon AT: **Bile reflux gastritis and intestinal metaplasia at the cardia.** *Gut* 2002, **51(3)**:351-5.
19. Zullo A, Rinaldi V, Hassan C, Lauria V, Attili AF: **Gastric pathology in cholecystectomy patients: role of Helicobacter pylori and bile reflux.** *J Clin Gastroenterol* 1998, **27(4)**:335-8.
20. Mathai E, Arora A, Cafferkey M, Keane CT, O'Morrain C: **The effect of bile acid on growth and adherence of Helicobacter Pylori.** *Aliment Pharmacol Ther* 1991, **5**:653-658.

7

Cervical lymph node metastasis classified as regional nodal staging in thoracic esophageal squamous cell carcinoma after radical esophagectomy and three-field lymph node dissection

Junqiang Chen[1*†], Sangang Wu[2†], Xiongwei Zheng[3], Jianji Pan[1], Kunshou Zhu[4], Yuanmei Chen[4], Jiancheng Li[1], Lianming Liao[5], Yu Lin[1] and Zhongxing Liao[6]

Abstract

Background: Lymph node metastasis (LNM) is most common in esophageal squamous cell carcinoma (SCC). The bi-directional spread is a key feature of LNM in patients with thoracic esophageal SCC (TE-SCC). The purpose of this study was to analyze the prognostic factors of survival in patients with TE-SCC with cervical lymph node metastasis (CLM) and validate the staging system of the current American Joint Committee on Cancer (AJCC) in a cohort of Chinese patients.

Methods: Of 1715 patients with TE-SCC who underwent radical esophagectomy plus three-field lymph node dissection at a single hospital between January 1993 and March 2007, 547 patients who had pathologically confirmed CLM (296 had surgery only and 251 had surgery + postoperative radiotherapy) were included in this study. The locations of the lymph nodes (LNs) were classified based on the guidelines of the Japanese Society for Esophageal Diseases.

Results: The rate of CLM was 31.9% for all patients and was 44.2%, 31.5%, and 14.4% for patients with upper, middle, and lower TE-SCC, respectively ($P < 0.0001$). The rates of metastasis to 101 (paraesophageal lymph nodes), 104 (supraclavicular lymph nodes), 102 (deep cervical lymph nodes) and 103 (retropharyngeal lymph nodes) areas were 89.0%, 25.6%, 3.7% and 0.5%, respectively. The 5-year overall survival (OS) rate with CLM was 27.7% (median survival, 27.5 months). The 5-year OS rates were 21.3% versus 34.2% (median survival, 21.9 months versus 35.4 months) for after surgery only versus surgery + postoperative radiotherapy, respectively ($P < 0.0001$ for both). Multivariate analysis showed that the independent prognostic factors for survival were sex, pT stage, pN stage, number of fields with positive LNs, and treatment modality. In surgery only group, the 5-year OS rates were 24.1%, 16.2% and 11.7%, respectively, when there was metastasis to 101 LN alone, 104 LN alone or both 101 LN and 104 LN. The 5-year OS rates were 17.7%, 22.5% and 31.7%, for patients with upper, middle and lower TE-SCC , respectively ($P = 0.112$). The 5-year OS rates were 43.0%, 25.5%, 10.2% in patients with 1 field (cervical LNs), 2 fields (cervical + mediastinal, and/or cervical + abdominal LNs), and 3 fields (cervical + mediastinal + abdominal LNs) positive LNs, respectively ($P < 0.0001$). The number of fields of positive LNs did not impact the OS according to different pN stage (all $P > 0.05$).

(Continued on next page)

* Correspondence: junqiangc@163.com
†Equal contributors
[1]Department of Radiation Oncology, The Teaching Hospital of Fujian Medical University, Fujian Provincial Cancer Hospital, 91 Maluding, Fuma Road, Fuzhou, Fujian 350014, China
Full list of author information is available at the end of the article

(Continued from previous page)

Conclusion: Patients with TE-SCC with CLM have better prognosis, which supports the current AJCC staging system for esophageal SCC.

Keywords: Esophageal cancer, Radiotherapy, Cervical lymph node metastasis, Prognosis, Tumor staging

Background

Lymph node metastasis (LNM) is most common in esophageal squamous cell carcinoma. The bi-directional or skip node spread is a key feature of LNM in patients with thoracic esophageal squamous cell carcinoma (TE-SCC), with a metastasis rate of 23.4-49.5% in the cervical node [1-4].

In the past two decades, advances in esophageal cancer surgery have been remarkable. Radical esophagectomy with extensive lymphadenectomy in the mediastinum, abdomen, and neck (so-called three-field lymphadenectomy, 3FL) has been the mainstay treatment for TE-SCC. The surgical approach can sufficiently expose the surgical field and completely dissect related lymph nodes with metastasis [1-5].

According to the Guidelines for Clinical and Pathologic Studies on Carcinoma of the Esophagus issued by the Japanese Society for Esophageal Diseases, the cervical lymph nodes (LNs) were classified into 101 (paraesophageal nodes), 102 (deep cervical nodes), 103 (retropharyngeal LNs), and 104 (supraclavicular LNs) areas. Each area is divided into left and right parts [6]. In the seventh edition of the American Joint Committee on Cancer tumor node metastasis (AJCC TNM) staging system for esophageal squamous cell carcinoma issued in 2009, LNs from the neck to the abdomen are defined as regional LNs. In the sixth edition AJCC TNM staging system, the subdivision of "M" classification into M1A and M1B according to the presence of nonregional LN involvement is not longer used [5]. In addition, whether metastasis to the cervical LNs, especially supraclavicular LNs (104), should be classified as local or distant metastasis has not be proposed. In the present retrospective study, the prognostic factors were analyzed in 547 patients with TE-SCC with cervical LNM after receiving extended esophagectomy with 3FL.

Methods

Patient population

From January 1993 to March 2007, 1715 consecutive patients with biopsy-proven TE-SCC were treated with 3FL at the Fujian Province Cancer Hospital, Fujian Medical University, Fuzhou, Fujian, China. Medical records of these patients were retrieved. Patients meeting the following criteria were selected for this study: (1) pathologically confirmed as squamous cell carcinoma of the esophagus and underwent extended esophagectomy plus 3FL, (2) the number of dissected LNs was ≥15, (3) presurgical enhanced computed tomography scan did not reveal LN with a diameter >1 cm in the cervical area (including supraclavicular area), (4) did not undergo chemotherapy and radiotherapy before esophagectomy and did not undergo chemotherapy after esophagectomy, and (5) did not have distant metastasis. According to the seventh edition of the AJCC TNM staging system released in 2009, N is subclassified based on the number of positive regional LNs (N1, 1-2 positive LNs; N2, 3-6 positive LNs; and N3, ≥7 positive LNs) [5]. This study was performed in accordance with the Declaration of Helsinki and was approved by the ethics committee of Fujian Provincial Cancer Hospital. All patients provided written informed consent form for storage of their information in the hospital database and for using this information in this study. Of the 1715 patients, 547 patients were with cervical LNM, 296 patients underwent esophagectomy only, and 251 patients underwent radiotherapy after esophagectomy. The field of LNM was in accordance with the cervical, mediastinal, and abdominal LNs.

Surgical procedures

The resection of the thoracic esophagus was performed through a cervical incision, a right thoracotomy, and a laparotomy. Details of the procedure were described elsewhere [1]. According to the guidelines for clinical and pathologic studies on carcinoma of the esophagus issued by the Japanese Society for Esophageal Diseases, the cervical LNs were classified into 101 (paraesophageal nodes), 102 (deep cervical nodes), 103 (retropharyngeal lymph nodes) and 104 (supraclavicular nodes) areas. Each area is divided into left and right parts [6].

Radiotherapy

Patients underwent radiotherapy 3-4 weeks after esophagectomy. T-shaped fields were used. The T-shaped field included bilateral supraclavicular fossi, mediastinum, left gastric nodes, and the tumor bed. The medium total radiation dose consisted of 50 Gy for the tumor bed administered in 2 Gy of daily dose fractions, 5 fractions a week, over a period of 5 weeks [7].

Follow-up

Patients were instructed to undergo follow-up evaluations every 3 months for the first year, every 6 months for the next 2 years, and annually thereafter. As of May

1, 2009, 90.1% of the patients returned for follow-up according to the schedule. Survival status of patients who did not come at the scheduled follow-up times was updated through telephone calls or letters every 6 months. Survival status of patients who could not be reached in this manner was obtained through the Fujian Public Safety Bureau's registration center system. In total, 1336, 799, and 447 patients were followed up for 1, 3, and 5 years, respectively.

Statistical analysis

Statistical analysis of group differences was performed using the Chi-square test for categorical variable data. Survival plots of patients were constructed using the Kaplan-Meier method and were compared using the log-rank test. A Cox regression proportional hazard multivariate analysis was performed to identify statistically significant factors associated with overall survival (OS). $P < 0.05$ was considered to be statistically significant. All statistical analyses were performed using the software package SPSS 15.0.

Results

Rate and pattern of LNM

In total, 547 of the 1715 patients met the inclusion criteria. The mean number of dissected LNs was 25.8 (range, 15-73). The frequency of any LNM was 31.9%. Specifically, the rates of cervical LNM for upper, middle, and lower TE-SCC were 44.2%, 31.5%, and 14.4%, respectively ($P < 0.0001$) (Table 1). The rates of LNM to 101, 104, 102, and 103 regions were 28.4%, 8.2%, 1.2%, and 0.2%, respectively. The rates of LNM from upper, middle, and lower TE-SCC to 101 and 104 were significantly different ($P < 0.05$) (Table 1). For patients with cervical metastasis, the rates of LNM to 101, 104, 102, and 103 regions were 89.0%, 25.6%, 3.7%, and 0.5%, respectively.

Relationship between cervical lymph node metastasis and survival

The 3-year and 5-year survival rates for patients (n = 547) with LNM were 41.5% and 27.7%, respectively. The median survival was 27.5 months. The 5-year survival rates and the median survival times were 21.3% versus 34.2%, and 21.9 months versus 35.4 months after surgery only (n = 296) versus surgery plus postoperative radiotherapy (n = 251), respectively [$P < 0.0001$ for both, hazard ratio (HR) (95% CI) 0.641 (0.521-0.788)] (Figure 1).

In surgery only group, the 5-year OS rates for patients' metastasis to 101 LN alone, 104 LN alone or both 101 LN and 104 LN were 24.1%, 16.2%, and 11.7%, respectively. The median survival times were 23.3 months, 20.0 months, and 17.7 months, respectively [$P = 0.117$, HR (95% CI) 1.129 (0.996-1.280)] (Figure 2). The 5-year OS for patients with upper, middle, and lower TE-SCC were 17.7%, 22.5%, and 31.7%, respectively. The corresponding median survival times were 17.3 months, 22.6 months, and 37.2 months, respectively [$P = 0.112$, HR (95% CI) 0.734 (0.549-0.980)] (Figure 3).

Analysis of prognostic factors of survival

Univariate analysis showed that sex, tumor length by x-ray, pT stage, pN stage, the number of fields with positive LNs, and treatment modality were predictors for survival. Age, tumor location, and histopathological type were not statistically significant predictors of survival ($P > 0.05$) (Table 2).

Multiple Cox regression indicated that sex, pT stage, pN stage, the number of fields with positive LNs, and treatment modality were independent predictors for survival (Table 3).

Survival of different fields of positive lymph nodes according to the pN stage

The 5-year OS rates were 43.0%, 25.5%, 10.2% in patients with 1 field (cervical LNs), 2 fields (cervical + mediastinal, and/or cervical + abdominal LNs), and 3 fields

Table 1 Characteristics of LNM in 1715 patients with TE-SCC

Variable	All patients	Location of esophageal tumor			χ^2 Value	*P*-value
		Upper	Middle	Lower		
Number of patients (%)	1715 (100)	274 (16.0)	1281 (74.7)	160 (9.3)		
Mean number of dissections						
Nodes per patient (range)	25.8 (15-73)	26.8 (15-68)	25.7 (15-71)	24.7 (15-73)		
Number of positive CLM (%)	547 (31.9)	121 (44.2)	403 (31.5)	23 (14.4)	41.698	<0.0001
Paraesophageal (101), n (%)	487 (28.4)	108 (39.4)	358 (27.9)	21 (13.1)	34.843	<0.0001
Deep cervical (102), n (%)	20 (1.2)	7 (2.6)	12 (0.9)	1 (0.6)	5.575	0.062
Retropharyngeal (103), n (%)	3 (0.2)	2 (0.7)	1 (0.1)	0 (0.0)	5.802	0.055
Supraclavicular (104), n (%)	140 (8.2)	31 (11.3)	104 (8.1)	5 (3.1)	9.049	0.011

Abbreviations: CLM cervical lymph node metastasis, *LNM* lymph node metastasis, *TE-SCC* thoracic esophageal squamous cell carcinoma.

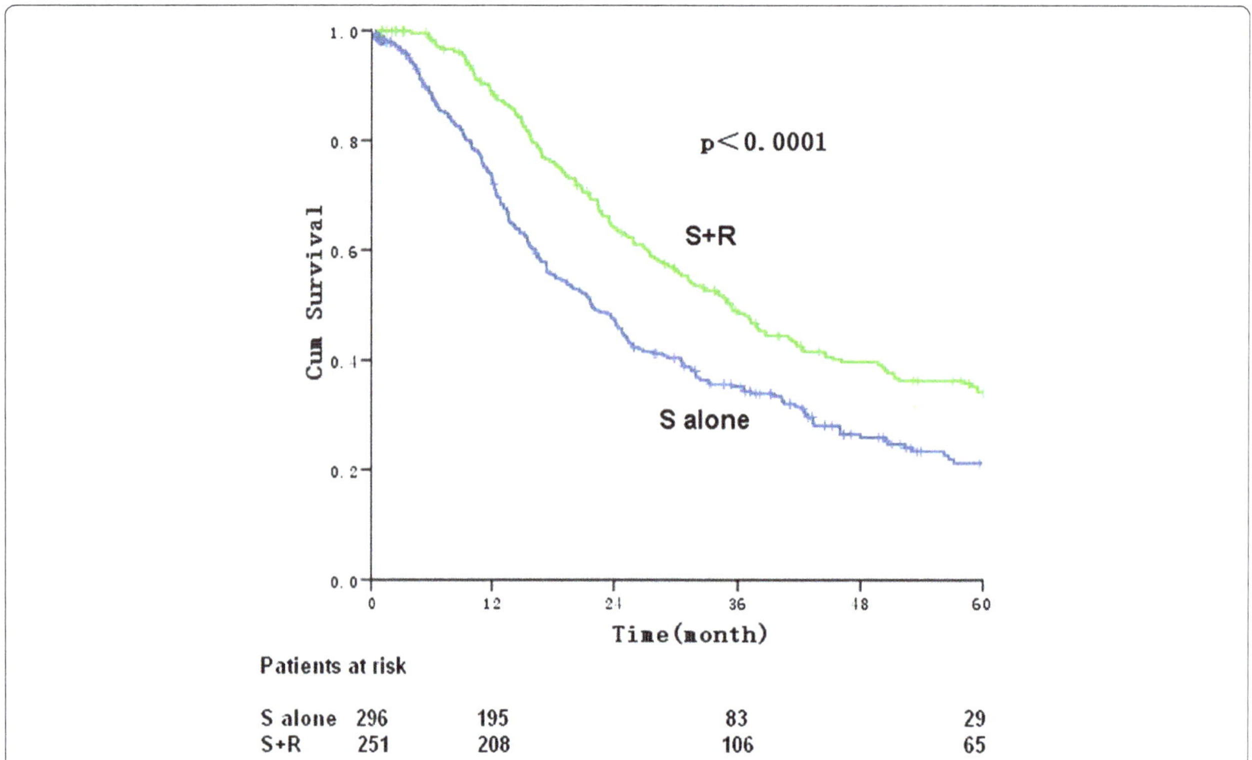

Figure 1 Overall survival of patients who underwent surgery only (S, blue line) and who underwent surgery followed by radiation (S + R, green line) for thoracic esophageal squamous cell carcinoma.

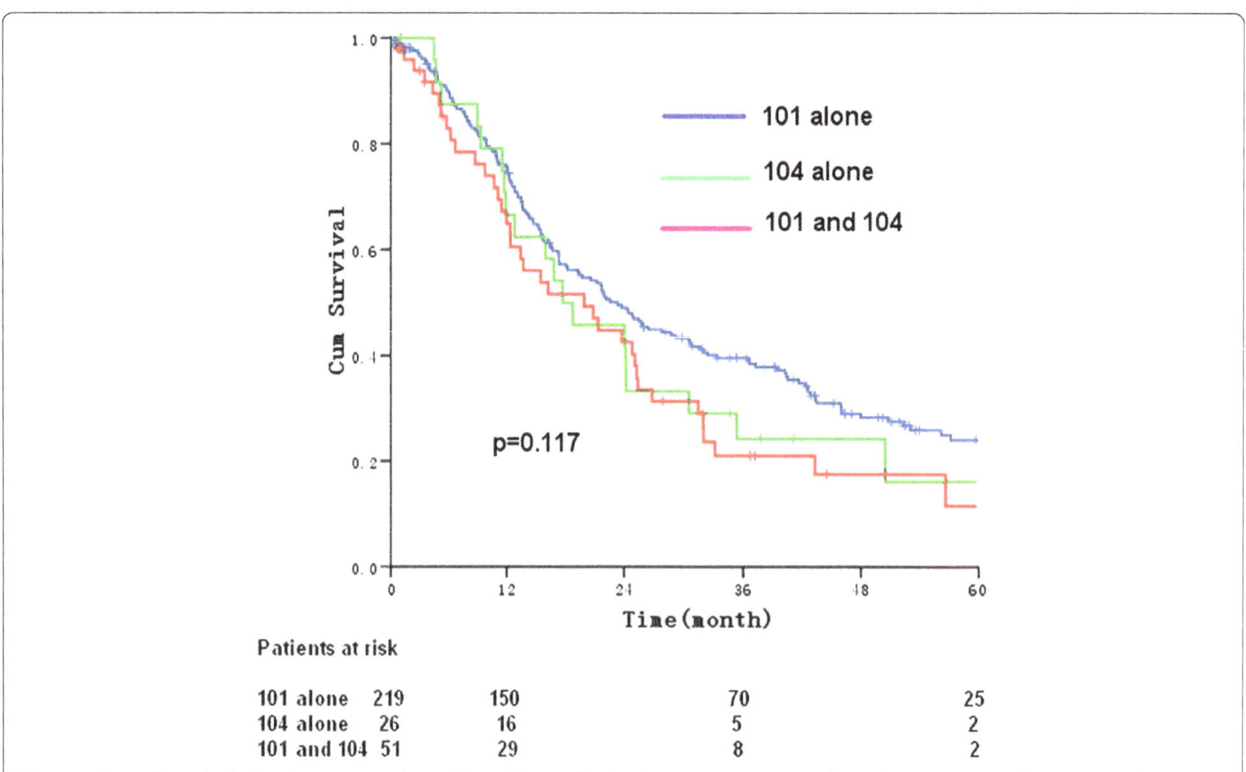

Figure 2 Overall survival of patients presenting with positive nodes in the 104 region (green line), the 101 region (blue line), and in both (red line) regions.

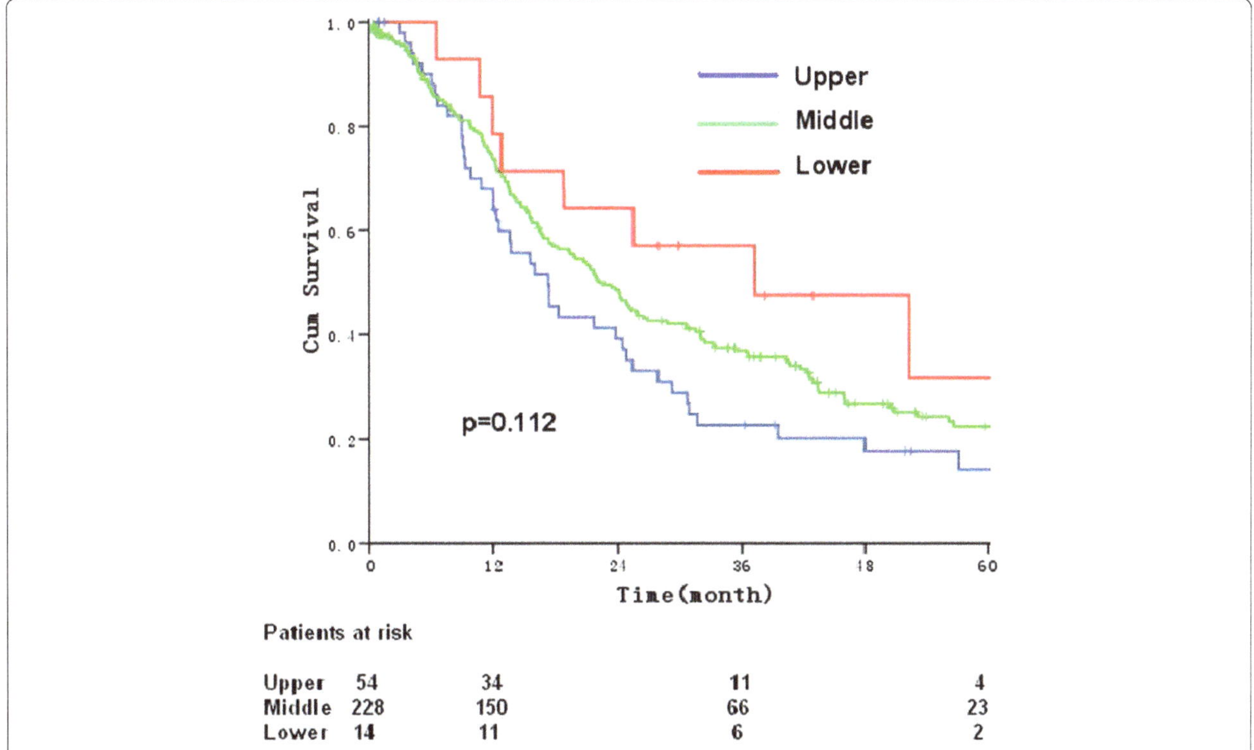

Figure 3 Overall survival of patients presenting with positive nodes in the lower region (i.e., middle and lower mediastinal and upper abdominal beds) (red line), the upper region (i.e., cervical and upper mediastinal beds) (blue line), and in the middle region (green line).

(cervical + mediastinal + abdominal LNs) positive LNs, respectively [$P < 0.0001$, HR (95% CI) 1.643 (1.437-1.878)] (Figure 4A). Subgroup analysis showed that the number of fields of positive LNs did not impact the OS according to different pN stage (all $P > 0.05$) (Table 4 and Figure 4B-D). The OS between cervical + mediastinal positive LNs and cervical + abdominal positive LNs were not significantly different (Table 4 and Figure 5).

Pattern of disease progression

Postoperative radiotherapy reduced the recurrence rate of cervical and mediastinal LN compared with surgery alone ($P < 0.05$). The pattern of disease progression in patients with and without postoperative radiotherapy is shown in Table 5.

Toxicity of postoperative radiotherapy

Early toxicities related to postoperative radiotherapy were gastrointestinal reactions (swallowing pain and loss of appetite) accounting for 28.3% (71 patients), bronchitis (cough) accounting for 21.1% (53 patients), and leukopenia accounting for 34.3% (86 patients, including 80 patients with grade 1-2 and 6 patients with grade 3).

Late toxicities were nonmalignant pleural effusion pericardial accounting for 2.4% (6 patients), radiation-induced pulmonary fibrosis accounting for 2.0% (5 patients), thoracic ulcer bleeding accounting for 1.2% (3 patients), anastomotic stricture accounting for 1.6% (4 patients), and anastomotic fistula accounting for 0.4% (1 patient).

Discussion

In the present study, pertinent results include that cervical LNM was the highest in patients with upper TE-SCC, followed by patients with middle and lower TE-SCC. Metastasis to paraesophageal nodes was most common. Metastasis to deep cervical nodes was less common. Metastasis to either retropharyngeal LNs or supraclavicular LNs was rare. The 5-year survival rates of patients undergoing surgery only were similar irrespective of whether there was metastasis to 101 LN alone, 104 LN alone, or both 101 LN and 104 LN. Multivariate factor analysis showed that the independent prognostic factors for survival were sex, pT stage, pN stage, the number of fields with positive LNs, and treatment modality. Cervical lymph node metastasis (CLM) was independent of tumor location.

There is controversy with regard to the prognostic significance and staging classification of cervical LNM in patients with TE-SCC. Most studies suggest that patients with cervical LNM have a better prognosis than those with hematogenous metastasis and thus cervical LNM should be included in "N" instead of "M" staging. Lerut

Table 2 Univariate analysis of prognostic factors of survival in patients with TE-SCC with CLM

Variable	All (%)	5-year Survival rate (%)	Median survival (Months)	χ^2 value	*P*-value
Patients	547 (100)	27.7			
Sex				8.323	0.004
Male	406 (74.2)	24.6	24.8		
Female	141 (25.8)	37.0	39.5		
Age (years)				0.225	0.635
<60	335 (61.2)	27.8	25.9		
≥60	212 (38.8)	27.1	31.5		
Thoracic tumor location				0.456	0.796
Upper	121 (22.1)	31.7	29.2		
Middle	403 (73.7)	26.6	26.8		
Lower	23 (4.2)	23.3	25.5		
Differentiation				1.623	0.444
Low	118 (21.6)	23.4	24.1		
Intermediate	349 (63.8)	29.1	27.8		
High	80 (14.6)	28.6	28.3		
Tumor length (cm)				7.638	0.006
≤5	283 (51.7)	31.7	32.0		
>5	264 (48.3)	23.4	23.6		
pT stage				20.517	<0.0001
pT1	16 (2.9)	86.7	53.6		
pT2	84 (15.4)	41.6	43.4		
pT3	386 (70.6)	23.1	26.4		
pT4	61 (11.2)	23.2	22.5		
Number of nodal metastases				63.872	<0.0001
1-2	226 (41.3)	43.3	49.7		
3-6	221 (40.4)	20.3	23.5		
≥7	100 (18.3)	9.9	16.7		
Number of fields with positive lymph nodes[a]				55.313	<0.0001
1 field	191 (34.9)	43.0	43.3		
2 fields	214 (39.1)	25.5	29.2		
3 fields	142 (26.0)	10.2	19.3		
Treatment program				18.145	<0.0001
Surgery only	296 (54.1)	21.3	21.9		
Surgery + radiation	251 (45.9)	34.2	35.4		

Abbreviations: CLM cervical lymph node metastasis, *TE-SCC* thoracic esophageal squamous cell carcinoma.
[a]1 field (cervical lymph nodes), 2 fields (cervical + mediastinal, and/or cervical + abdominal lymph nodes), 3 fields (cervical + mediastinal + abdominal lymph nodes) with positive lymph nodes.

et al. reported that the 5-year OS for patients with positive LNs was 27.2% after 3FL in patients with middle TE-SCC [8]. Fang *et al.* reported that 5-year OS for patients with positive cervical nodes was 20.0% after 3FL with TE-SCC [9]. Tachimori *et al.* reported that 3-year OS for patients with positive cervical nodes was 43.8% after 3FL with TE-SCC [10]. Hsu *et al.* enrolled 488 patients who underwent primary curative resection without neoadjuvant therapy for esophageal cancer between 1995 and 2006. They found the 3-year OS rate was 35.4%. The 3-year OS rate was equivalent among patients in N1 (23.3%), M1a (22.0%), and nonregional LNM-related M1b (18.5%). No survival difference was noted (18.5%). However, differences in survival rate were evident between patients with and without distant metastasis ($P < 0.001$) [11]. Kato *et al.* reported that in

Table 3 Multivariate analysis of prognostic factors of survival in patients with TE-SCC with CLM

Variable	Regression coefficient B	SE	Wald value	HR (95% CI)	*P*-value
Sex (male vs. female)	-0.294	0.127	5.342	0.745 (0.581-0.956)	0.021
Tumor length (≤5 cm vs. >5 cm)	0.202	0.106	3.651	1.224 (0.995-1.505)	0.056
pT category (T1, 2, 3, 4)	0.283	0.096	8.687	1.327 (1.100-1.602)	0.003
Number of nodal metastases (1-2, 3-6, ≥7)	0.332	0.102	10.533	1.393 (1.140-1.702)	0.001
Fields of LNM (1 field, 2 fields, 3 fields)	0.203	0.100	4.109	1.225 (1.007-1.490)	0.043
Treatment program (surgery only vs. surgery + radiation)	-0.414	0.107	15.025	0.661 (0.536-0.815)	<0.0001

patients who underwent 3FL, the survival of patients with cervical LNM was significantly better than that of patients with hematogenous metastasis ($P = 0.002$). In patients without hematogenous metastases, the survival curve for the patients with histologic cervical LNM did not significantly differ from that of patients with mediastinal or abdominal LNM [12]. Rice *et al.* also found that the survivals were similar between patients in M0 classification and M1 classification ($P < 0.0001$). However, the survivals were significantly different between patients in M1a subclassification and M1b subclassification ($P = 0.9$) [13].

The results from the current study are similar to those reported by other researchers and support the current AJCC staging system which considers cervical LN to be regional LN [8-12]. The patients with cervical LN metastasis are classified as one group according to the AJCC staging system, and there is no explicit deliberation on whether the LNs adjacent to the cervical esophagus and supraclavicular LNs should be included. However, the cervical LN metastasis is classified elaborately into four groups including cervical esophageal LNs, cervical posterior deep LNs, retropharyngeal LNs, and supraclavicular LNs by the Japanese Society for Esophageal Diseases, though there was no published report on the prognosis related to this classification on cervical LNM. In the present study, the patients who underwent surgery only were classified into three groups, group of cervical esophageal LN metastasis, group of supraclavicular LN metastasis, and group of both cervical esophageal and supraclavicular LN metastasis. The stratified analysis on these three groups indicated that there was no significant difference in terms of 5-year survival rate, with the rate of 24.1%, 16.2%, and 11.7%, respectively ($P = 0.117$). These findings were in accordance with the concept defined by the AJCC staging system (seventh edition) that all cervical LN metastasis shall be regarded as one common regional LN metastasis.

In the present study, the 5-year survival rates in the postoperational radiotherapy group and surgery only group were 34.2% and 21.3%, respectively ($P < 0.0001$). The improvement in survival rate by postoperational radiotherapy might be due to blood vessels, lymphatic vessels, and surrounding organs, exposure of the lower cervical area is challenging during esophagectomy and complete removal of LNs is sometimes impossible, which will cause recurrence after surgery. Postoperative radiotherapy will reduce metastasis and increase survival [14].

It was widely believed that the number of fields of cervical LN metastasis was a vital factor for prognosis of thoracic esophageal carcinoma [13,15], which was consistent with the results of the present study that the number of fields of cervical LN metastasis was an independent factor of prognosis. The further stratified analysis indicated that the number of fields of cervical LN metastasis and survival rate were not significantly different among the patients with different numbers of positive LNs ($P > 0.05$), and the possible underlying reason might be that the number of positive LNs is

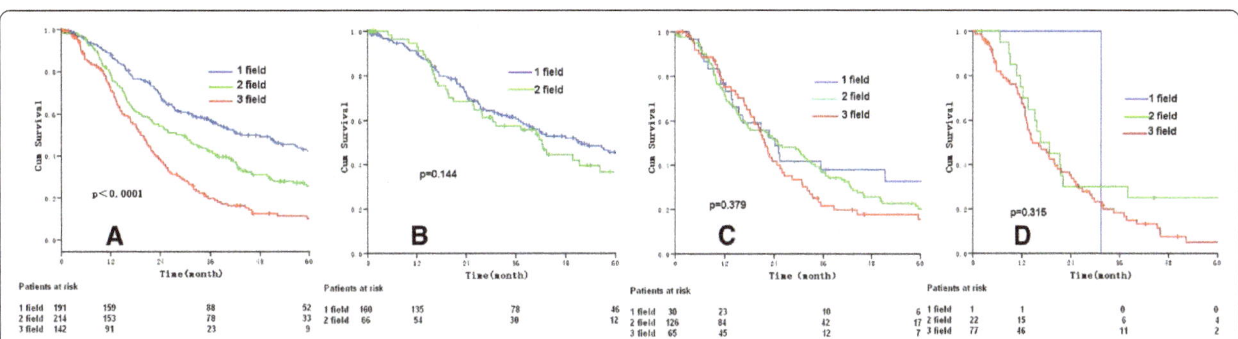

Figure 4 The survival of different fields of positive lymph nodes according to the different pN stages as entire group (A), pN1 stage (B), pN2 stage (C), and pN3 stage (D).

Table 4 Survival of different fields of positive lymph nodes according to the pN stage

Variable	All (%)	5-year Survival rate (%)	Median survival Time (months)	χ^2 value	*P*-value
pN1				2.136	0.144
1 field	160 (29.3)	45.6	51.8		
2 fields	66 (12.1)	36.8	42.3		
pN2				1.940	0.379
1 field	30 (5.5)	32.6	24.2		
2 fields	126 (23.0)	20.3	24.9		
3 fields	65 (11.9)	15.5	21.9		
pN3				2.311	0.315
1 field	1 (0.2)	0.0	31.5		
2 fields	22 (4.0)	25.0	16.7		
3 fields	77 (14.1)	5.1	14.7		
Fields of LNM				0.154	0.695
C + M	163 (76.2)	23.7	25.9		
C + A	51 (23.8)	30.1	34.0		

Abbreviations: A, abdominal; C, cervical; LNM, lymph node metastasis; M, mediastinal.
[a]1 field (cervical lymph nodes), 2 fields (cervical + mediastinal, and/or cervical + abdominal lymph nodes), 3 fields (cervical + mediastinal + abdominal lymph nodes) with positive lymph nodes.
Abbreviations: CI = confidence interval; CLM = cervical lymph node metastasis; HR = hazard ratio; LNM, lymph node metastasis; SE = standard error; TE-SCC = thoracic esophageal squamous cell carcinoma.

correlated to the number of fields of metastasis, implying that the number of positive LNs is the most critical factor for prognosis instead of number of fields of metastasis.

Conclusion

This study demonstrates that patients with TE-SCC with cervical LNM have a better prognosis. Five-year survival in patients with TE-SCC with metastasis to paraesophageal

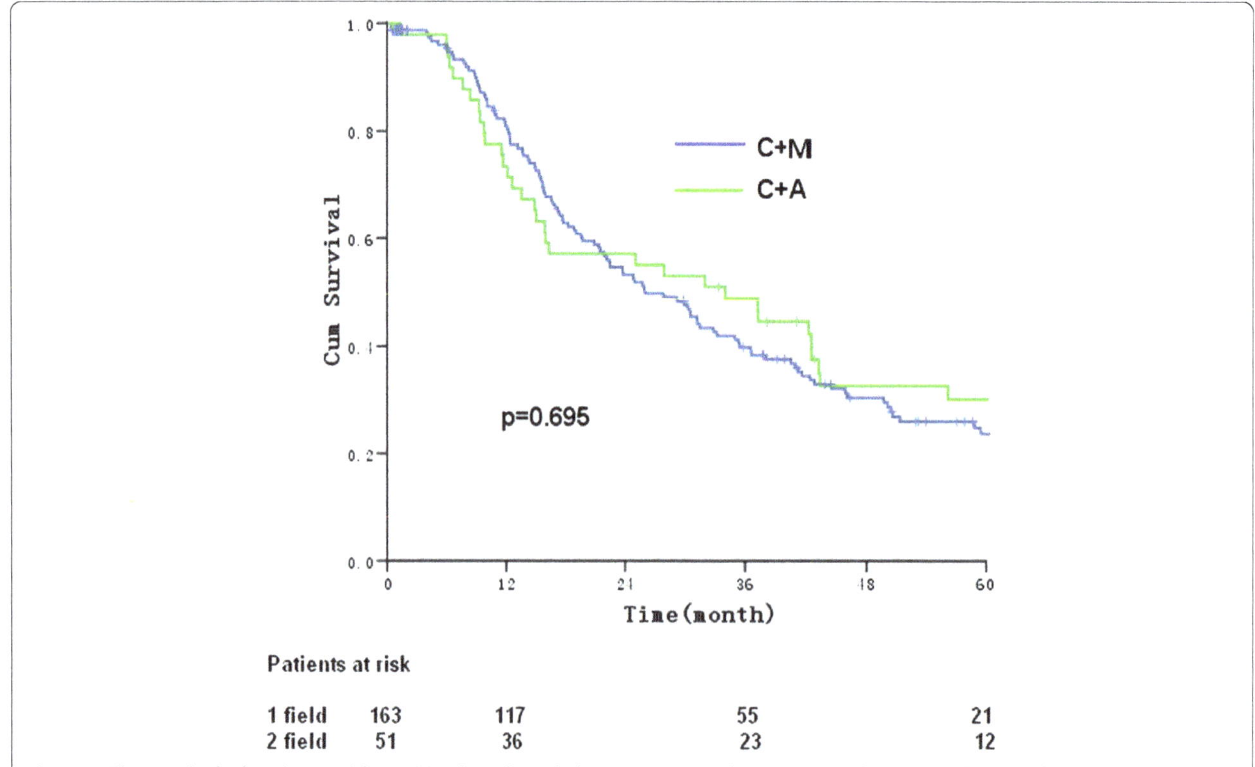

Figure 5 The survival of patients with positive lymph node between cervical + mediastinal group and cervical + abdominal group.

Table 5 Pattern of disease progression

Variable	Surgery (n = 296) (%)	Surgery + postoperative radiotherapy (n = 251) (%)	χ^2 value	*P*-value
Site of lymph node metastasis				
Cervical lymph nodes	42 (14.2)	13 (5.2)	12.192	<0.0001
Mediastinal lymph nodes	23 (7.8)	9 (3.6)	4.318	0.038
Abdominal lymph nodes	10 (3.4)	13 (5.2)	1.094	0.296
Tumor bed	6 (2.0)	2 (0.8)	1.426	0.2326
Distant metastasis	70 (23.6)	57 (22.7)	0.067	0.795
Locoregional and distant recurrence	126 (42.6)	93 (37.1)	1.721	0.190

nodes was similar to those with metastasis to supraclavicular LNs and supports the staging system of the current AJCC for esophageal squamous cell carcinoma that classifies cervical LN as regional LN. These patients will benefit from postoperative radiotherapy. Further perspective studies are needed to validate the conclusion.

Abbreviations
3-FL: Three-field lymphadenectomy; AJCC: American Joint Committee on Cancer; CLM: Cervical lymph node metastasis; LN: Lymph node; LNM: Lymph node metastasis; TE-SCC: Thoracic esophageal squamous cell carcinoma; TNM: Tumor-nodes-metastasis.

Competing interests
The authors declare that they have no competing interests.

Authors' contributions
JQC and SGW designed the study. JQC, XWZ, and JJP provided the databases. KSZ, YL, YMC,JCL, LML, and ZXL assembled and analyzed the data. JQC and SGW wrote the manuscript. All authors read and approved the final manuscript.

Acknowledgement
The authors thank the patients and their families and all the investigators, including the physicians, nurses, and laboratory technicians in this study.

Author details
[1]Department of Radiation Oncology, The Teaching Hospital of Fujian Medical University, Fujian Provincial Cancer Hospital, 91 Maluding, Fuma Road, Fuzhou, Fujian 350014, China. [2]Xiamen Cancer Center, Department of Radiation Oncology, the First Affiliated Hospital of Xiamen University, Xiamen 361003, China. [3]Departments of Pathology, The Teaching Hospital of Fujian Medical University, Fujian Provincial Cancer Hospital, Fuzhou 350014, China. [4]Departments of Surgery, The Teaching Hospital of Fujian Medical University, Fujian Provincial Cancer Hospital, Fuzhou 350014, China. [5]Center of Oncology Research, Academy of Integrative Medicine, Fujian University of Traditional Chinese Medicine, Fuzhou 350014, China. [6]Department of Radiation Oncology, The University of Texas M. D. Anderson Cancer Center, Unit 97, 1515 Holcombe Boulevard, Houston, TX, USA.

References
1. Chen J, Liu S, Pan J, Zheng X, Zhu K, Zhu J, Xiao J, Ying M: **The pattern and prevalence of lymphatic spread in thoracic oesophageal squamous cell carcinoma.** *Eur J Cardiothorac Surg* 2009, **36**(3):480–486.
2. Akiyama H, Tsurumaru M, Udagawa H, Kajiyama Y: **Radical lymph node dissection for cancer of the thoracic esophagus.** *Ann Surg* 1994, **220**(3):364–372. discussion 372-3.
3. Ando N, Ozawa S, Kitagawa Y, Shinozawa Y, Kitajima M: **Improvement in the results of surgical treatment of advanced squamous esophageal carcinoma during 15consecutive years.** *Ann Surg* 2000, **232**(2):225–232.
4. Kato H, Igaki H, Tachimori Y, Watanabe H, Tsubosa Y, Nakanishi Y: **Assessment of cervical lymph node metastasis in the staging of thoracic esophageal carcinoma.** *J Surg Oncol* 2000, **74**(4):282–285.
5. Edge SB, Byrd DR, Compton CC: *AJCC cancer staging manual.* 7th edition. New York: Springer; 2009.
6. Japanese Society for Esophageal Diseases: *Clinicopathological aspects. In: Guidelines for clinical and pathologic studies on carcinoma of the esophagus.* 9th edition. Tokyo: Kanehara & Co., Ltd; 1999:1–34.
7. Chen J, Zhu J, Pan J, Zhu K, Zheng X, Chen M, Wang J, Liao Z: **Postoperative radiotherapy improved survival of poor prognostic squamous cell carcinoma esophagus.** *Ann Thorac Surg* 2010, **90**(2):435–442.
8. Lerut T, Nafteux P, Moons J, Coosemans W, Decker G, De Leyn P, Van Raemdonck D, Ectors N: **Three-field lymphadenectomy for carcinoma of the esophagus and gastroesophageal junction in 174 R0 resections: impact on staging, disease-free survival, and outcome: a plea for adaptation of TNM classification in upper-half esophageal carcinoma.** *Ann Surg* 2004, **240**(6):962–972. discussion 972-974.
9. Fang WT, Feng J, Mao T, Fu SJ, Chen WH: **Clinical implications of the new TNM staging system for thoracic esophageal squamous cell carcinoma.** *Zhonghua Zhong Liu Za Zhi* 2011, **33**(9):687–691 [Article in Chinese].
10. Tachimori Y, Kato H, Watanabe H, Yamaguchi H: **Neck ultrasonography for thoracic esophageal carcinoma.** *Ann Thorac Surg* 1994, **57**(5):1180–1183.
11. Hsu WH, Hsu PK, Hsieh CC, Huang CS, Wu YC: **The metastatic lymph node number and ratio are independent prognostic factors in esophageal cancer.** *J Gastrointest Surg* 2009, **13**(11):19131920.
12. Kato H, Igaki H, Tachimori Y, Watanabe H, Tsubosa Y, Nakanishi Y: **Assessment of cervical lymph node metastasis in the staging of thoracic esophageal carcinoma.** *J Surg Oncol* 2000, **74**(4):282–285.
13. Rice TW, Blackstone EH, Rybicki LA, Adelstein DJ, Murthy SC, DeCamp MM, Goldblum JR: **Refining esophageal cancer staging.** *J Thorac Cardiovasc Surg* 2003, **125**(5):1103–1113.
14. Chen J, Pan J, Zheng X, Zhu K, Li J, Chen M, Wang J, Liao Z: **Number and location of positive nodes, postoperative radiotherapy, and survival after esophagectomy with three-field lymph node dissection for thoracic esophageal squamous cell carcinoma.** *Int J Radiat Oncol Biol Phys* 2012, **82**(1):475–482.
15. Shimada H, Okazumi S, Matsubara H, Nabeya Y, Shiratori T, Shimizu T, Shuto K, Hayashi H, Ochiai T: **Impact of the number and extent of positive lymph nodes in 200 patients with thoracic esophageal squamous cell carcinoma after three-field lymph node dissection.** *World J Surg* 2006, **30**(8):1441–1449.

8

Long term follow up and retrospective study on 533 gastric cancer cases

Wei-Juan Zeng[1], Wen-Qin Hu[2], Lin-Wei Wang[1], Shu-Guang Yan[2], Jian-Ding Li[3*], Hao-Liang Zhao[4], Chun-Wei Peng[1], Gui-Fang Yang[1] and Yan Li[1*]

Abstract

Background: Gastric cancer (GC) is the third leading cause of cancer death in China and the outcome of GC patients is poor. The aim of the research is to study the prognostic factors of gastric cancer patients who had curative intent or palliative resection, completed clinical database and follow-up.

Methods: This retrospective study analyzed 533 GC patients from three tertiary referral teaching hospitals from January 2004 to December 2010 who had curative intent or palliative resection, complete clinical database and follow-up information. The GC-specific overall survival (OS) status was determined by the Kaplan-Meier method, and univariate analysis was conducted to identify possible factors for survival. Multivariate analysis using the Cox proportional hazard model and a forward regression procedure was conducted to define independent prognostic factors.

Results: By the last follow-up, the median follow-up time of 533 GC patients was 38.6 mo (range 6.9-100.9 mo), and the median GC-specific OS was 25.3 mo (95% CI: 23.1-27.4 mo). The estimated 1-, 2-, 3- and 5-year GC-specific OS rates were 78.4%, 61.4%, 53.3% and 48.4%, respectively. Univariate analysis identified the following prognostic factors: hospital, age, gender, cancer site, surgery type, resection type, other organ resection, HIPEC, LN status, tumor invasion, distant metastases, TNM stage, postoperative SAE, systemic chemotherapy and IP chemotherapy. In multivariate analysis, seven factors were identified as independent prognostic factors for long term survival, including resection type, HIPEC, LN status, tumor invasion, distant metastases, postoperative SAE and systemic chemotherapy.

Conclusions: Resection type, HIPEC, postoperative SAE and systemic chemotherapy are four independent prognostic factors that could be intervened for GC patients for improving survival.

Keywords: Gastric cancer, GC-specific overall survival, Prognosis, Multivariate analysis, Clinical pathological factors

Background

Gastric cancer (GC) remains the second leading cause of cancer death worldwide [1], accounting for 8% of the total cases and 10% of total deaths in 2008 [2]. In China, GC is the third leading cause of cancer death [3] and the outcome of GC patients is poor, especially for patients at advanced stage, and the 5-year survival rate is less than 20%-25% [4].

* Correspondence: cjr.jianding@vip.163.com; liyansd2@163.com
[3]Department of Medical Imaging, The First Affiliated Hospital of Shanxi Medical University, No 85, South Jiefang Road, Taiyuan City 030001, Shangxi Province, China
[1]Departments of Oncology & Pathology, Zhongnan Hospital of Wuhan University, Hubei Key Laboratory of Tumor Biological Behaviors & Hubei Cancer Clinical Study Center, Wuhan 430071, China
Full list of author information is available at the end of the article

Early diagnosis and early treatment remain the best strategy for GC. In China, however, a majority of GC patients are not early cancer by the time when they seek medical attention [5,6]. Therefore, surgery-based multidisciplinary treatment approach is warranted in order to improve both overall survival (OS) and the quality of life.

Despite this common-sense knowledge, there is no commonly accepted multidisciplinary treatment strategy in China, primarily due to the lack of large database information reflecting the clinical reality of the current treatment situation.

In our previous studies on GC patients, we evaluated the common tumor markers for the diagnosis of gastric cancer. In these relatively large cohort studies, stage III and beyond patients accounted for over 65% of the entire patient population [6,7], a result similar to other reports from China [5,8]. For these patients, GC is no longer a local disease, but at least a regional or a systemic disease.

Currently, surgery remains the most effective therapy for GC, offering an excellent chance (90%) of a cure for early GC patients [9]. Surgical procedures have a big impact on OS and recurrence [10]. R0 resection with D2 lymphadenectomy is regarded as the standard surgical technique [11,12], as D2 lymphadenectomy had lower recurrence and GC-related death rates [13]. However, for stage III and beyond patients, the currently adopted surgical procedure only removes local tumor mass but often neglects the micro-metastases. Therefore, additional adjuvant therapies are required to ensure better treatment efficacy.

Over the past years, our database has grown bigger and more detailed information on major clinico-pathological characteristics has been accumulated. Therefore, we conducted this comprehensive analysis of the data collected from three major teaching hospitals in Central China, so as to gain deeper insights to the major features of GC in central China and to identify independent factors for prognosis that could be intervened.

Methods

Ethics statement

All patients provided written informed consent for their information to be stored in the hospital database; and we obtained separate consent for research. Study approval was obtained from independent ethics committees from Zhongnan Hospital of Wuhan University. The study was undertaken in accordance with the ethical standards of the World Medical Association Declaration of Helsinki.

Patients

This study included a total of 533 GC patients from three tertiary referral hospitals, from January 2004 to December 2010. These patients underwent resection with curative intent (D2 lymphadenectomy) or palliative resection. All the detailed clinic-pathological information was available, including demographic variables, underlying co-morbidities, surgical modality, lab and image study information, pathological reports, pre- and post-operative therapies, and follow-up information. Pathological information was mainly focused on tumor type, pathological grading, TNM stages, blood vessel or neural invasions. The pathologic staging was based on the 7th edition of AJCC staging criteria [14]. Postoperative treatments were focused on chemotherapy regimens and cycles, and radiotherapy if applicable. GC patients with T2 or higher, any N tumors should receive systemic chemotherapy except patients who declined the offer [15]. Hyperthermic intraperitoneal chemotherapy (HIPEC) and intraperitoneal chemotherapy (IP chemotherapy) were adjuvant chemotherapy, and only those who had peritoneal carcinomatosis (PC) should receive [16]. In our study, the systemic chemotherapy administered were mainly FOLFOX4 and FOLFOX6, HIPEC were mainly using lobaplatin and paclitaxel, and IP chemotherapy were docetaxel and carboplatin.

These patients were followed-up every 3 months during the first 2 years after operation, every 6 months on the third postoperative year and every year thereafter. All the follow-up information was incorporated into a standardized database.

Database construction

The above-mentioned information was incorporated into a central database, set up at the Zhongnan Hospital of Wuhan University, which undergoes regular updating every 3 months.

Statistical analysis

All eligibility cases from the central database were analyzed by SPSS 17.0 statistical package software (SPSS Inc., Chicago, IL, USA). The variables were hospital (Zhongnan Hospital, Heji Hospital or Hubei Tumor Hospital), gender (male or female), age (≤65 yr or > 65 yr), cancer site (upper third [excluding squamous cell carcinoma at gastroesophageal junction], middle third, lower third or whole stomach), pathological type (well or intermediately differentiated adenocarcinoma, poorly differentiated or undifferentiated carcinoma, signet ring cell carcinoma or mucious adenocarcinoma or others), surgery type (proximal gastrectomy, distal gastrectomy or total gastrectomy), resection type (for stomach itself) (palliative resection or curative resection), other organ resection (mainly included liver, spleen, intestines, ovarian, ovarian ducts) (0, 1, 2 or ≥ 3), HIPEC (yes or no), lymph node status (LN status) (N0, N1, N2 or N3), tumor invasion (T1, T2, T3, T4a or T4b), distant metastasis (M0 or M1), pathological stage (I, II, IIIA, IIIB, IIIC or IV) [14], postoperative serious adverse event (postoperative SAE) (defined as life threatening events after operation, including gastrointestinal obstruction, anastomotic leakage, and bleeding leading to grade 3 and above anemia, abdominal abscess) (yes or no), systemic chemotherapy (0, 1 to 6 cycles or > 6 cycles), IP chemotherapy (yes or no), GC-specific overall survival (GC-specific OS, defined as the time interval from first treatment to GC-specific death, with the last follow-up time on May 31, 2012).

The numerical data was analyzed directly. The category data was converted when necessary. The Kaplan-Meier survival curve was used to study the survival status, using log rank test to decipher the statistical significance, which was judged as $P < 0.05$ throughout this study.

To work out independent factors for survival, a Cox proportional hazard model was used to first obtain the possible factors and then used forward regression procedure to finally identify the independent factors.

Results

Characteristics of the patients

A total of 533 patients with GC were recruited from 3 tertiary referral teaching hospitals, including 194 patients from Zhongnan Hospital of Wuhan University, 182 patients from Heji Hospital and 157 patients from Hubei Tumor Hospital. By the time of last follow-up, 278 deaths (52.2%) occurred, including 126 deaths (64.9%) out of 194 enrolled patients from Zhongnan Hospital of Wuhan University, 84 deaths (46.2%) out of 182 enrolled patients from Heji Hospital, and 68 deaths (43.3%) out of 157 enrolled patients from Hubei Tumor Hospital. The median age of cases was 58 years (range 20–85 years), and male-to-female ratio was 2.7 to 1. Detailed information on major demographic and clinico-pathological characteristics was listed in Table 1.

GC-specific OS

By the time of last follow-up, the median follow-up time was 38.6 mo (range 6.9-100.9 mo), and 278 patients died out of the entire 533 assessable patients (52.2%). The median GC-specific OS was 25.3 mo (95% CI: 23.1-27.4 mo). The survival curve by stages was shown in Figure 1. The estimated 1-, 2-, 3- and 5-year GC-specific OS rates were 78.4%, 61.4%, 53.3% and 48.4%, respectively. The median survival by stages I, II, IIIA, IIIB, IIIC and IV were 85.2 mo (95% CI: 76.1-94.3 mo), 53.9 mo (95% CI: 46.6-61.3 mo), 40.0 mo (95% CI: 21.7-58.3 mo), 28.0 mo (95% CI: 14.9-41.1 mo), 14.8 mo (95% CI: 10.6-19.1 mo) and 11.1 mo (95% CI: 9.7-12.4 mo), respectively. As shown in Figure 1, significant differences in GC-specific OS were found among different clinical stages. Patients at clinical stage IIIB and beyond had much poorer GC-specific OS status than other patients.

Mortality analysis

By the time of last follow-up, 278 patients (52.2%) died among the entire 533 assessable patients. In terms of absolute number of patient death on the yearly basis, there were 114 (41.0%), 92 (33.1%), 43 (15.5%), 18 (6.5%), 8 (2.9%) deaths, respectively, in the 1st, 2ed, 3rd, 4th, and 5th postoperative year. Only 3 (1.1%) deaths occurred after 5 years. Information on GC-specific death in relationship with clinical stages was depicted in Figure 2. Putting together, there were 249 (89.6%) deaths within three years after operation.

Univariate survival analysis

In this study, all variables were analyzed by Kaplan-Meier curve and log-rank test. Among these variables, pathological type had no statistically significant impact on GC-specific OS ($P = 0.212$), but statistically significant factors were hospital ($P = 0.008$), age ($P < 0.001$), gender ($P = 0.019$), cancer site ($P = 0.004$), surgery type ($P < 0.001$), resection type ($P < 0.001$), other organ resection ($P < 0.001$), HIPEC ($P < 0.001$), LN status ($P < 0.001$), tumor invasion ($P < 0.001$), distant metastases ($P < 0.001$), TNM stage ($P < 0.001$), postoperative SAE ($P < 0.001$), systemic chemotherapy ($P = 0.001$), and IP chemotherapy ($P = 0.003$) (Table 1).

Multivariate survival analysis

After univariate survival analysis, the above significant factors were further subjected to multivariate analysis using Cox proportional hazard model and forward regression procedure. The following variables were identified as independent factors for prognosis: tumor invasion ($P < 0.001$), LN status ($P < 0.001$), distant metastases ($P < 0.001$), resection type ($P = 0.015$), HIPEC ($P = 0.049$), postoperative SAE ($P < 0.001$) and systemic chemotherapy ($P < 0.001$) (Table 2).

Discussion

Several important points should be considered from this study. First, a majority of GC patients are at advanced clinical stage. In our series of 533 patients, 354 cases (66.4%) were clinically stage III and beyond. For these patients, GC is no longer a local disease, but at least a regional or a systemic disease. Although surgery could remove the bulky tumor mass itself, it may leave some unseen cancer cells in the operating field. Therefore, more intensive adjuvant chemotherapy should be followed in order to eradicate these left-over cancer cells. Two large scale randomized clinical trials have already demonstrated the superiority of this approach over conventional surgery alone [17,18]. Another reasonable approach is to start perioperative chemotherapy, to down-stage the tumor, followed by curative resection. It has been proven that such a treat modality indeed could improve the clinical outcomes of GC patients [19].

Secondly, our analysis found that over 40% of GC death occurred in the first year after operation, and another 30% plus of GC death occurred during the second year after operation [20-22]. Therefore, it is clinically important to design rational strategies to address these problems. One key consideration is that high risk factors should be investigated and identified, so as to reduce them and reduce the death risk. Another strategy is to design a close follow-up plan and strictly implement it, so as to identify those patients with early signs of recurrence and apply appropriate therapies. Among the currently used methods, serum tumor markers study and medical imaging studies are most widely used approaches. Regular monitoring blood tumor markers carcinoembryonic antigen (CEA) and carboxyl antigen 19–9 (CA19-9) could help provide warning information on cancer recurrence [23].

Table 1 Characteristics of the 533 GC patients enrolled into this study

Variables	Total n (%)	Events n (%)	Median GC-specific OS (95% CI) (mo)	*P* value
Age (yr)				
≤ 65	380 (71.3)	178 (46.8)	51.7 (39.7-63.7)	**< 0.001**
> 65	153 (28.7)	100 (65.4)	28.0 (21.6-34.4)	
Gender				
Male	389 (73.0)	192 (49.4)	39.7 (29.9-49.5)	**0.019**
Female	144 (27.0)	86 (59.7)	28.0 (17.9-38.1)	
Cancer site				
Upper third	156 (29.3)	80 (51.3)	32.6 (25.9-39.3)	
Middle third	119 (22.3)	61 (51.3)	38.9 (9.4-68.4)	**0.004**
Lower third	222 (41.7)	112 (50.5)	42.1 (34.2-49.9)	
Whole stomach	36 (6.8)	25 (69.4)	13.2 (10.1-16.3)	
Pathological type				
Adeno WD/ID	131 (24.6)	59 (45.0)	42.1 (29.9-54.2)	
Adeno PD/UN	299 (56.1)	160 (53.5)	34.9 (27.5-42.4)	0.212
Signet ring/mucious Ca	85 (15.9)	49 (57.6)	28.0 (10.9-45.1)	
Others	18 (3.4)	10 (55.6)	33.7 (20.0-47.5)	
Surgery type				
Proximal gastrectomy	169 (31.7)	82 (48.5)	35.9 (20.5-51.3)	
Distal gastrectomy	268 (50.3)	128 (47.8)	46.6 (38.1-55.1)	**< 0.001**
Total gastrectomy	96 (18.0)	68 (70.8)	17.4 (11.3-23.4)	
Resection type				
Palliative resection	11 (2.1)	11 (100.0)	9.8 (8.0-11.6)	**< 0.001**
Curative resection	522 (97.9)	267 (51.1)	38.9 (31.8-46.0)	
Other organ resection (n)				
0	507 (95.1)	256(50.5)	39.3 (32.5-46.0)	
1	14 (2.6)	11 (78.6)	24.1 (9.6-38.7)	**< 0.001**
2	8 (1.5)	7 (87.5)	12.4 (2.7-22.2)	
≥ 3	4 (0.8)	4 (100.0)	13.6 (2.7-24.4)	
HIPEC				
No	505 (94.7)	251 (49.7)	39.7 (32.4-47.0)	**< 0.001**
Yes	28 (5.3)	27 (96.4)	13.4 (9.6-17.2)	
LN status				
N0	172 (32.3)	51 (29.7)	67.3 (59.8-74.8)	
N1	112 (21.0)	57 (50.9)	35.9 (26.8-45.0)	**< 0.001**
N2	143 (26.8)	86 (60.1)	27.0 (19.9-34.1)	
N3	106 (20.0)	84 (30.5)	14.4 (12.0-16.8)	
Tumor invasion				
T1	25 (4.7)	3 (12.0)	75.4 (66.4-84.4)	
T2	85 (15.9)	19 (22.4)	72.7 (62.2-83.2)	
T3	2 (0.4)	1 (50.0)	29.1 (10.7-47.4)	**< 0.001**
T4a	332 (62.3)	187 (56.3)	33.0 (26.6-39.4)	
T4b	89 (16.7)	68 (76.4)	14.8 (10.8-18.9)	

Table 1 Characteristics of the 533 GC patients enrolled into this study *(Continued)*

Distant metastases				
No	478 (89.7)	224 (46.9)	42.5 (34.6-50.4)	< 0.001
Yes	55 (10.3)	54 (98.2)	10.6 (9.0-12.1)	
TNM staging				
Stage I	79 (14.8)	8 (10.1)	85.2 (76.1-94.3)	< 0.001
Stage II	100 (18.8)	35 (35.0)	53.9 (46.6-61.3)	
Stage IIIA	80 (15.0)	38 (47.5)	40.0 (21.7-58.3)	
Stage IIIB	116 (21.8)	67 (57.8)	28.0 (14.9-41.1)	
Stage IIIC	117 (22.0)	90 (76.9)	14.8 (10.6-19.1)	
Stage IV	41 (7.7)	40 (97.6)	11.1 (9.7-12.4)	
Postoperative SAE				
No	458 (85.9)	205 (44.8)	49.8 (32.5-67.0)	< 0.001
Yes	75 (14.1)	73 (97.3)	14.8 (10.0-19.6)	
Systemic chemotherapy (cycles)				
0	217 (40.7)	128 (59.0)	26.3 (19.2-33.4)	0.001
1 to 6	302 (56.7)	142 (47.0)	51.7 (36.6-66.9)	
> 6	14 (2.6)	8 (57.1)	37.8 (16.9-58.7)	
IP chemotherapy				
No	521 (97.7)	267 (51.2)	37.0 (29.8-44.2)	0.003
Yes	12 (2.3)	11 (91.7)	11.1 (7.0-15.1)	

GC: gastric cancer; GC-specific OS: gastric cancer-specific overall survival; Adeno WD/ID: well differentiated or intermediately differentiated adenocarcinoma; Adeno PD/UN: poorly differentiated or undifferentiated carinoma; Signet ring/mucious Ca: Signet ring cell carcinoma or mucious adenocarcinoma; HIPEC: hyperthermic intraperitoneal chemotherapy; LN status: lymph node status; SAE: serious adverse event; IP chemotherapy: intraperitoneal chemotherapy.

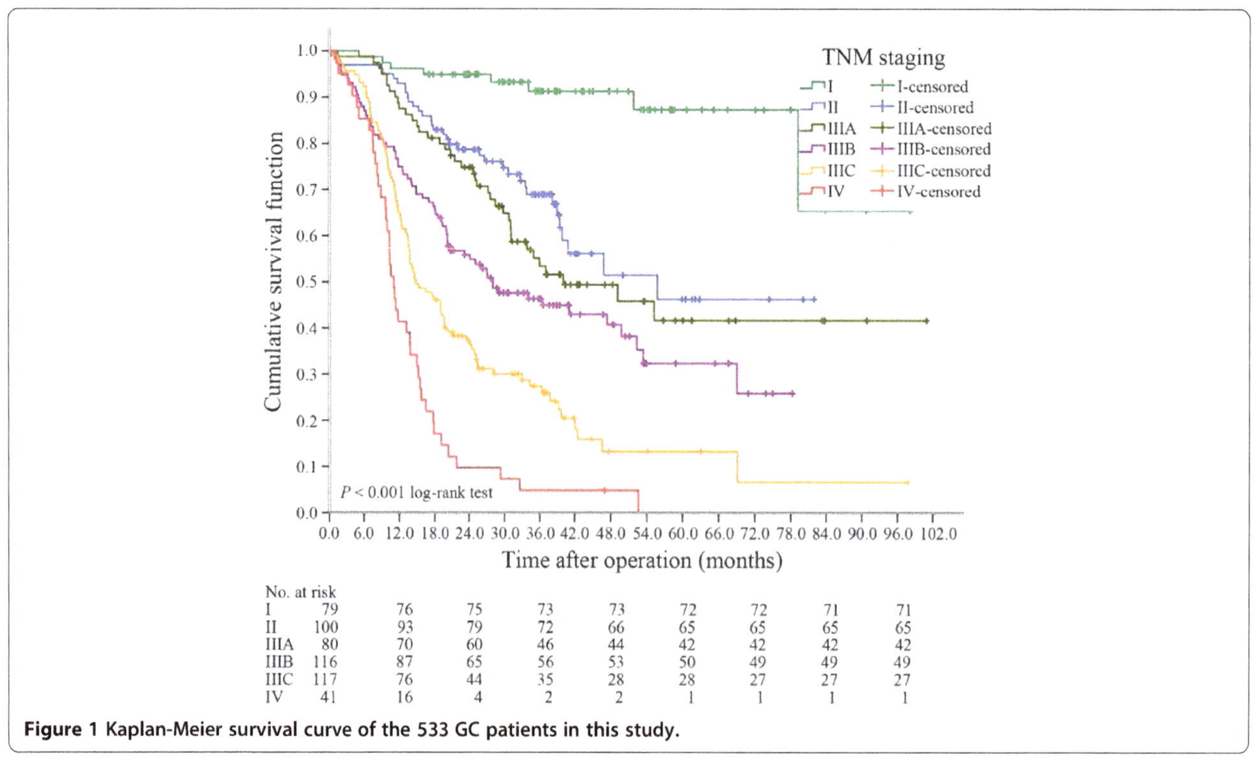

Figure 1 Kaplan-Meier survival curve of the 533 GC patients in this study.

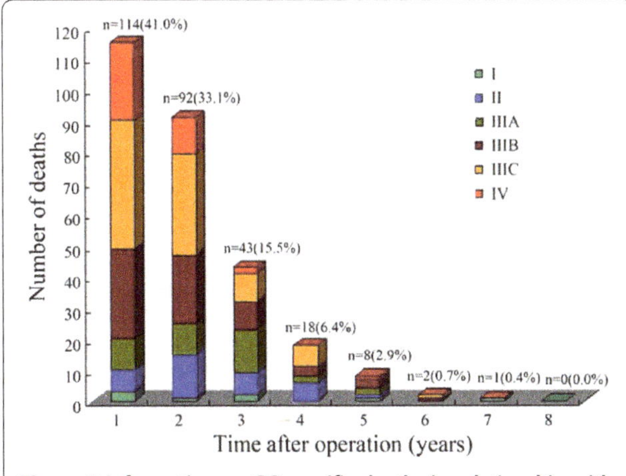

Figure 2 Information on GC-specific deaths in relationship with clinical stages.

Various clinicopathological factors have been reported to impact on GC-specific OS, such as age, gender, cancer site, surgery type, resection type, other organ resection, HIPEC, LN status, tumor invasion, distant metastases, TNM stage, postoperative SAE, systemic chemotherapy and IP chemotherapy [5,7,8,20,24-28]. These results are in accordance with our study. In our study, pathological type had no impact on GC-specific OS, which is not in conformity with several previous studies that concluded that pathological type was an important factor for prognosis and survival of GC [5,24], but is in agreement with some other studies that reported that pathological type had no influence on GC-specific OS [7,27]. This could be due to the different typing method used. It has been documented that Lauren histological classification is a simple and practical typing method to have significant correlation with survival of GC. Clinical-pathological information of this study was obtained from hospital department of pathology, and they did not adopt Lauren classification. In future studies, we should adopt this classification.

Table 2 Independent prognostic factors of 533 GC patients identified by multivariate analysis

Covariate	χ^2	*P*	HR	95% CI	
				Lower	Upper
Tumor invasion	13.008	< 0.001	1.022	1.010	1.034
LN status	36.845	< 0.001	1.462	1.293	1.653
Distant metastases	29.004	< 0.001	2.832	1.939	4.137
Resection type	5.900	0.015	0.430	0.218	0.850
HIPEC	3.863	0.049	1.707	1.001	2.910
Postoperative SAE	27.752	< 0.001	2.507	1.781	3.528
Systemic chemotherapy	24.064	< 0.001	0.521	0.402	0.676

GC: gastric cancer; HR: hazard ratio; CI: confidence interval; LN status: lymph node status; HIPEC: hyperthermic intraperitoneal chemotherapy; SAE: serious adverse event.

For cancer patients, the clinical outcomes depend on several important factors, which could be divided into those that cannot be intervened such as TNM stage, and those can be intervened such as treatment models. After the Cox proportional hazard model analysis, we worked out seven independent factors that had significant impact on survival, six of these seven factors have already been well recognized as the most important determinants of patients' survival [5,7,8,29]. What deserves special attention is the finding that HIPEC is also an independent factor for improved survival. Several phases I to III studies have already demonstrated the treatment advantage of HIPEC. Glehen et al. consecutively treated 49 advanced GC patients with HIPEC, which resulted in 10.3 months of GC-specific OS, against 6.1 months of GC-specific OS treated with only standard curative resection [30]. In another study by Yonemura et al., 107 GC patients also treated with HIPEC, and the GC-specific OS was 11.5 months [31]. More importantly, a recent phase III prospective randomized clinical trial also confirmed the survival advantage of 11.0 months in the HIPEC group against 6.5 months in the CRS group [32]. In addition, a systematic review and meta-analysis of 13 acceptable qualities randomized controlled trials also have established that HIPEC has significant survival advantage over the currently standard treatment for advanced GC [33]. Taken together, all these facts confirm the value of HIPEC for the treatment of stage III and beyond GC patients. In this study, the median survival of patients with HIPEC was 13.4 mo (95% CI: 9.6-17.2), which was shorter than others without HIPEC (39.7 mo [95% CI: 32.4-47.0]). It was due to patients with HIPEC were gastric cancer with metastasis and prognosis was not optimistic. However, the median survival of patients with HIPEC was longer than patients with metastasis (13.4 mo *vs* 10.6 mo, $P < 0.05$). It supports HIPEC has significant survival advantage even though there could be selection bias in this regard, due to the limited number of patients treated by HIPEC.

Postoperative SAE included gastrointestinal obstruction, anastomotic leakage, and bleeding leading to grade 3 and above anemia, abdominal abscess. All these have been confirmed to have a significant negative impact on GC-specific OS. In the study of Sierzega et al. [34], the median OS of patients with anastomotic leakage was significantly lower than patients with non-anastomotic leakage (4.1 mo vs. 23 mo, $P < 0.001$), and the progression-free survival of patients with anastomotic leakage was also significantly shorter than patients with non-anastomotic leakage (11 mo vs. 19 mo, $P = 0.021$). In another study by Yoo et al. [35], the mean OS of patients with anastomotic leakage was significantly lower than patients with non-anastomotic leakage (30.5 mo vs. 96.2 mo, $P < 0.001$). Anastomotic leakage could promote gastric cancer progression by prolonging inflammation [34-36]. According to Tokunaga et al. [37], GC patients with intra-abdominal infection had a poorer 5-year OS rate and 5-relapse-free survival rate than patients without intra-abdominal infectins (66.4% vs. 86.8%, $P < 0.001$ and 64.9% vs. 84.5%, $P < 0.001$). In another study by Li et al. [38], postoperative complications including gastrointestinal obstruction, anastomotic leakage, and bleeding leading and abdominal abscess all were independent and negative prognostic factors for GC. Therefore, all efforts should be made to reduce the risk for postoperative SAE, including careful patient selection for surgery and optimized perioperative patient care.

Conclusion

In summary, this study identified four independent prognostic factors that could be intervened for GC patients, including curative resection, HIPEC, postoperative SAE and systemic chemotherapy, and three independent prognostic factors that cannot be intervened: tumor invasion, LN status and distant metastasis. Therefore, increasing attention should be directed at better understanding tumor biology involved in cancer invasion and metastasis, and refining multi-disciplinary comprehensive treatment strategies to enhance efficacy and reduce SAE.

Competing interests

The authors declare that they have no competing interests.

Authors' contributions

YL, GFY and JDL conceived of the study, and participated in its design and coordination. WQH, LWW, SGY, HLZ, CWP and WJZ participated in the database collection and follow-up. WJZ performed the statistical analyses and drafted the manuscript. All authors read and approved the final manuscript.

Acknowledgements

This work is supported by Award for Excellent PhD. Candidates Funded by Ministry of Education of China (No. 5052011303014), Science Fund of the National Natural Science Foundation of China (No. 81171396), Science Fund for Creative Research Groups of the National Natural Science Foundation of China (No. 20621502, 20921062), and the Fundamental Research Funds for the Central Universities of Ministry of Education of China (No. 4103005).

Author details

[1]Departments of Oncology & Pathology, Zhongnan Hospital of Wuhan University, Hubei Key Laboratory of Tumor Biological Behaviors & Hubei Cancer Clinical Study Center, Wuhan 430071, China. [2]Department of Surgery, Heji Hospital Affiliated to Changzhi Medical College, Changzhi 046000, China. [3]Department of Medical Imaging, The First Affiliated Hospital of Shanxi Medical University, No 85, South Jiefang Road, Taiyuan City 030001, Shangxi Province, China. [4]Department of General Surgery, Shanxi University Hospital, No 99, Longcheng Street, Taiyuan City 046000, Shangxi Province, China.

References

1. Ferlay J, Shin HR, Bray F, Forman D, Mathers C, Parkin DM: **Estimates of worldwide burden of cancer in, GLOBOCAN 2008.** *Int J Cancer* 2008, **2010**(127):2893–2917.
2. Jemal A, Bray F, Center MM, Ferlay J, Ward E, Forman D: **Global cancer statistics.** *CA Cancer J Clin* 2011, **61**:69–90.
3. Yang L: **Incidence and mortality of gastric cancer in China.** *World J Gastroenterol* 2006, **12**:17–20.
4. Hartgrink HH, Jansen EP, van Grieken NC, van de Velde CJ: **Gastric cancer.** *Lancet* 2009, **374**:477–490.
5. Wang W, Sun XW, Li CF, Lv L, Li YF, Chen YB, Xu DZ, Kesari R, Huang CY, Li W, Zhan YQ, Zhou ZW: **Comparison of the 6th and 7th editions of the UICC TNM staging system for gastric cancer: results of a Chinese single-institution study of 1,503 patients.** *Ann Surg Oncol* 2011, **18**:1060–1067.
6. Chen C, Chen LQ, Chen LD, Yang GL, Li Y: **Evaluation of tumor markers biochip C12 system in the diagnosis of gastric cancer and the strategies for improvement: analysis of 100 cases.** *Hepatogastroenterology* 2008, **55**:991–997.
7. Wu HL, Tian Q, Peng CW, Liu SP, Li Y: **Multivariate survival and outcome analysis of 154 patients with gastric cancer at a single Chinese institution.** *Asian Pac J Cancer Prev* 2011, **12**:3341–3345.
8. Zhang XF, Huang CM, Lu HS, Wu XY, Wang C, Guang GX, Zhang JZ, Zheng CH: **Surgical treatment and prognosis of gastric cancer in 2,613 patients.** *World J Gastroenterol* 2004, **10**:3405–3408.
9. Li BS, Zhao YL, Guo G, Li W, Zhu ED, Luo X, Mao XH, Zou QM, Yu PW, Zuo QF, Li N, Tang B, Liu KY, Xiao B: **Plasma microRNAs, miR-223, miR-21 and miR-218, as novel potential biomarkers for gastric cancer detection.** *PLoS One* 2012, **7**:e41629.
10. Yokota T, Ishiyama S, Saito T, Teshima S, Shimotsuma M, Yamauchi H: **Treatment strategy of limited surgery in the treatment guidelines for gastric cancer in Japan.** *Lancet Oncol* 2003, **4**:423–428.
11. Diaz DLA, Yarnoz C, Aguilar R, Artieda C, Ortiz H: **Rationale for gastrectomy with D2 lymphadenectomy in the treatment of gastric cancer.** *Gastric Cancer* 2008, **11**:96–102.
12. D'Annibale A, Pende V, Pernazza G, Monsellato I, Mazzocchi P, Lucandri G, Morpurgo E, Contardo T, Sovernigo G: **Full robotic gastrectomy with extended (D2) lymphadenectomy for gastric cancer: surgical technique and preliminary results.** *J Surg Res* 2011, **166**:e113–e120.
13. Songun I, Putter H, Kranenbarg EM, Sasako M, van de Velde CJ: **Surgical treatment of gastric cancer: 15-year follow-up results of the randomised nationwide Dutch D1D2 trial.** *Lancet Oncol* 2010, **11**:439–449.
14. Washington K: **7th edition of the AJCC cancer staging manual: stomach.** *Ann Surg Oncol* 2010, **17**:3077–3079.
15. Ajani JA, Bentrem DJ, Besh S, D'Amico TA, Das P, Denlinger C, Fakih MG, Fuchs CS, Gerdes H, Glasgow RE, Hayman JA, Hofstetter WL, Ilson DH, Keswani RN, Kleinberg LR, Korn WM, Lockhart AC, Meredith K, Mulcahy MF, Orringer MB, Posey JA, Sasson AR, Scott WJ, Strong VE, Varghese TJ, Warren G, Washington MK, Willett C, Wright CD, McMillian NR, *et al.* **Gastric cancer, version 2.2013: featured updates to the NCCN Guidelines.** *J Natl Compr Canc Netw* 2013, **11**:531–546.
16. Yonemura Y, Endou Y, Sasaki T, Hirano M, Mizumoto A, Matsuda T, Takao N, Ichinose M, Miura M, Li Y: **Surgical treatment for peritoneal carcinomatosis from gastric cancer.** *Eur J Surg Oncol* 2010, **36**:1131–1138.
17. Sakuramoto S, Sasako M, Yamaguchi T, Kinoshita T, Fujii M, Nashimoto A, Furukawa H, Nakajima T, Ohashi Y, Imamura H, Higashino M, Yamamura Y, Kurita A, Arai K: **Adjuvant chemotherapy for gastric cancer with S-1, an oral fluoropyrimidine.** *N Engl J Med* 2007, **357**:1810–1820.
18. Macdonald JS, Smalley SR, Benedetti J, Hundahl SA, Estes NC, Stemmermann GN, Haller DG, Ajani JA, Gunderson LL, Jessup JM, Martenson JA: **Chemoradiotherapy after surgery compared with surgery alone for adenocarcinoma of the stomach or gastroesophageal junction.** *N Engl J Med* 2001, **345**:725–730.
19. Cunningham D, Allum WH, Stenning SP, Thompson JN, Van de Velde CJ, Nicolson M, Scarffe JH, Lofts FJ, Falk SJ, Iveson TJ, Smith DB, Langley RE, Verma M, Weeden S, Chua YJ, MAGIC TP: **Perioperative chemotherapy versus surgery alone for resectable gastroesophageal cancer.** *N Engl J Med* 2006, **355**:11–20.
20. Shiraishi N, Inomata M, Osawa N, Yasuda K, Adachi Y, Kitano S: **Early and late recurrence after gastrectomy for gastric carcinoma: Univariate and multivariate analyses.** *Cancer* 2000, **89**:255–261.
21. Kodera Y, Ito S, Yamamura Y, Mochizuki Y, Fujiwara M, Hibi K, Ito K, Akiyama S, Nakao A: **Follow-up surveillance for recurrence after curative gastric cancer surgery lacks survival benefit.** *Ann Surg Oncol* 2003, **10**:898–902.
22. Yoo CH, Noh SH, Shin DW, Choi SH, Min JS: **Recurrence following curative resection for gastric carcinoma.** *Br J Surg* 2000, **87**:236–242.
23. Yang XQ, Yan L, Chen C, Hou JX, Li Y: **Application of C12 multi-tumor marker protein chip in the diagnosis of gastrointestinal cancer: results of 329 surgical patients and suggestions for improvement.** *Hepatogastroenterology* 2009, **56**:1388–1394.

24. Yang D, Hendifar A, Lenz C, Togawa K, Lenz F, Lurje G, Pohl A, Winder T, Ning Y, Groshen S, Lenz HJ: **Survival of metastatic gastric cancer: Significance of age, sex and race/ethnicity.** *J Gastrointest Oncol* 2011, **2**:77–84.
25. Nanthakumaran S, Fernandes E, Thompson AM, Rapson T, Gilbert FJ, Park KG: **Morbidity and mortality rates following gastric cancer surgery and contiguous organ removal, a population based study.** *Eur J Surg Oncol* 2005, **31**:1141–1144.
26. Li C, Yan M, Chen J, Xiang M, Zhu ZG, Yin HR, Lin YZ: **Surgical resection with hyperthermic intraperitoneal chemotherapy for gastric cancer patients with peritoneal dissemination.** *J Surg Oncol* 2010, **102**:361–365.
27. Landry CS, Brock G, Scoggins CR, McMasters KM, Martin RN: **A proposed staging system for gastric carcinoid tumors based on an analysis of 1,543 patients.** *Ann Surg Oncol* 2009, **16**:51–60.
28. Cheong JH, Shen JY, Song CS, Hyung WJ, Shen JG, Choi SH, Noh SH: **Early postoperative intraperitoneal chemotherapy following cytoreductive surgery in patients with very advanced gastric cancer.** *Ann Surg Oncol* 2007, **14**:61–68.
29. Heise K, Bertran E, Andia ME, Ferreccio C: **Incidence and survival of stomach cancer in a high-risk population of Chile.** *World J Gastroenterol* 2009, **15**:1854–1862.
30. Glehen O, Schreiber V, Cotte E, Sayag-Beaujard AC, Osinsky D, Freyer G, Francois Y, Vignal J, Gilly FN: **Cytoreductive surgery and intraperitoneal chemohyperthermia for peritoneal carcinomatosis arising from gastric cancer.** *Arch Surg* 2004, **139**:20–26.
31. Yonemura Y, Kawamura T, Bandou E, Takahashi S, Sawa T, Matsuki N: **Treatment of peritoneal dissemination from gastric cancer by peritonectomy and chemohyperthermic peritoneal perfusion.** *Br J Surg* 2005, **92**:370–375.
32. Yang XJ, Huang CQ, Suo T, Mei LJ, Yang GL, Cheng FL, Zhou YF, Xiong B, Yonemura Y, Li Y: **Cytoreductive surgery and hyperthermic intraperitoneal chemotherapy improves survival of patients with peritoneal carcinomatosis from gastric cancer: final results of a phase III randomized clinical trial.** *Ann Surg Oncol* 2011, **18**:1575–1581.
33. Yan TD, Black D, Sugarbaker PH, Zhu J, Yonemura Y, Petrou G, Morris DL: **A systematic review and meta-analysis of the randomized controlled trials on adjuvant intraperitoneal chemotherapy for resectable gastric cancer.** *Ann Surg Oncol* 2007, **14**:2702–2713.
34. Sierzega M, Kolodziejczyk P, Kulig J: **Impact of anastomotic leakage on long-term survival after total gastrectomy for carcinoma of the stomach.** *Br J Surg* 2010, **97**:1035–1042.
35. Yoo HM, Lee HH, Shim JH, Jeon HM, Park CH, Song KY: **Negative impact of leakage on survival of patients undergoing curative resection for advanced gastric cancer.** *J Surg Oncol* 2011, **104**:734–740.
36. Kubota T, Hiki N, Sano T, Nomura S, Nunobe S, Kumagai K, Aikou S, Watanabe R, Kosuga T, Yamaguchi T: **Prognostic significance of complications after curative surgery for gastric cancer.** *Ann Surg Oncol* 2014, **21**:891–898.
37. Tokunaga M, Tanizawa Y, Bando E, Kawamura T, Terashima M: **Poor survival rate in patients with postoperative intra-abdominal infectious complications following curative gastrectomy for gastric cancer.** *Ann Surg Oncol* 2013, **20**:1575–1583.
38. Li QG, Li P, Tang D, Chen J, Wang DR: **Impact of postoperative complications on long-term survival after radical resection for gastric cancer.** *World J Gastroenterol* 2013, **19**:4060–4065.

9

Bridging the gap between gastric pouch and jejunum: a bariatric nightmare

Noëlle Geubbels*, Ingrid Kappers and Arnold W. J. M. van de Laar

Abstract

Background: Even in a large volume bariatric centre, bariatric surgeons are sometimes confronted with intraoperative anatomical challenges which force even the most experienced surgeon into a pioneering position. In this video we present how a large gap of approximately 8 cm is bridged by applying several techniques that are not part of our standardized surgical procedure.

Case presentation: After creation of a 20 mL gastric pouch we discovered that the alimentary limb could not be advanced further cranially due to a very short a thick jejunal mesentery in a 49 year old male patient during laparoscopic Roux-en-Y gastric bypass (LRYGB) surgery. By dissecting the gastro-oesophageal junction form the crus, stretching the gastric pouch, transecting the jejunal mesentery, using a retrocolic/retrogastric route, and creating a fully hand-sewn gastrojejunostomy we were able to safely complete the LRYGB. Drains were left near the gastrojejunostomy and the patient was kept nil by mouth for 5 days. On the 5th postoperative day radiographic swallow series were obtained which revealed no sign of leakage. The patient was discharged in good clinical condition on the 6th postoperative day. To date, no complications have occurred. Weight loss results are −31.5 % of the preoperative total body weight.

Conclusions: When confronted with a large distance between the gastric pouch and the alimentary limb, several techniques presented in this video may be of aid to the bariatric surgeon. We stress that only experienced bariatric surgeon should embark on these techniques. Inspecting the alimentary limb before the creation of the gastric pouch may prevent the need for such complex techniques.

Keywords: Laparoscopic Roux-en-Y gastric bypass surgery, Short mesentery, Retrocolic/retrogastric route, Intraoperative event

Background

The Slotervaart Hospital is a teaching hospital in Amsterdam, The Netherlands. We commenced our bariatric program in 2007, gradually expanding in surgical volume about 900 patients annually in 2014. Over the course of these years, many modifications were made to the bariatric program in order to facilitate this expanding number of patients. We have changed our surgical technique, implemented an enhanced recovery, or 'fast track' program and trained 2 new residents in to bariatric surgeons, all leading to improvements in patient safety and flatter surgical learning curves [1, 2]. Still, experience and standardization does not rule out that one is sometimes confronted with an exceptional surgical situation. The aim of this video is to demonstrate how a large distance between the alimentary limb and the gastric pouch can be overcome with the aid of several surgical techniques.

* Correspondence: ngeubbels@gmail.com
Department of Surgery, Slotervaart hospital, Amsterdam, The Netherlands

Case presentation

Brief description of our standardized surgical technique

A 20 mL gastric pouch is created with the use of two to three 60 mm linear staplers (Endo GIA, Covidien and Dublin, Ireland). At approximately 40 cm proximal to the ligament of Treitz the jejunum is grasped and mobilized to the gastric pouch. The posterior side of the gastrojejunostomy is stapled with a 30 mm linear stapler and the anterior side is hand sewn with an absorbable unidirectional barded 3—0 V-Loc™ suture (Covidien, Dublin, Ireland). At about 150 cm a fully stapled jejunojejunostomy is created with two linear 60 mm staplers. Then the jejunum is transected between the two anastomoses using a 60 mm linear stapler without division of the mesentery. The gastrojejunal anastomosis is tested for leakage with methylene blue through the orogastric tube. There is no routine placement of drains. The orogastric tube is removed at the end of surgery. The patients are allowed a clear fluid diet when fully recovered from anaesthesia. No routine radiographic swallow series are obtained. All patients receive subcutaneous low molecular weight heparin during the first two weeks after surgery as thromboprophylaxis. The patient's diet is gradually expanded to a full liquid during their admission and continued for two weeks. All patients receive supplementary vitamins and a proton pump inhibitor.

The patient

In December 2012, a 49 year old male was scheduled for laparoscopic Roux-en-Y gastric bypass surgery (LRYGB). At the time of surgery his weight was 138.2 kg with a Body Mass Index (BMI) of 45.1 kg/m^2. His past medical history revealed Obstructive Sleep Apnea (OSA), for which he uses Continuous Positive Airway Pressure (CPAP) therapy, Chronic Obstructive Pulmonary Disease (COPD) stage GOLD 2, Post-Traumatic Stress Disorder (PTSD) after a car accident and non-ST elevated myocardial infarction (NSTEMI) for which he underwent a successful percutaneous coronary intervention (PCI) of the ramus circumflexus of his left coronary artery. During his medical screening the patient was diagnosed with Type 2 Diabetes Mellitus (T2DM) 'de novo', which was treated with oral medication. The patient's cardiac, respiratory, and endocrinological function were well assessed prior to surgery and optimally regulated.

During the surgery of this patient we where forced to make several deviations from our standardized protocol. The subheadings correspond to the headings of the accompanying video (Additional file 1).

Identification of the ligament of Treitz and discovery of the short mesentery

After positioning the patient, the introduction of the ports, the creation of a 20 ml gastric pouch and the division of the (very bulky) omentum, the ligament of Treitz is identified. When measuring the jejunum from the ligament of Treitz is becomes apparent that the mesentery is very short. It is not possible to mobilize the jejunum over the transverse colon (antecolic route) and the remnant stomach (antegastric route). The distance between the jejunum is about 8 cm. We measured this distance with the aid of marking on our graspers.

Transection of the jejunum and division of the mesentery

In order to create the alimentary limb, the jejunum is transected at the point where the distance to the proximal gastric pouch is the shortest. To further mobilize the alimentary limb, the mesentery is divided with the ultracision harmonic scalpel.

Placement of a marker stitch in the alimentary limb

A marker stitch (vicryl 2.0, Ethicon Inc. Johnson, & Johnson, New Brunswick, New Jersey, USA) is placed to mark the alimentary limb. Later, this stitch will be used to pull the limb through the retrocolic route.

Dissection of the gastro-oesophageal junction from the crus

To lengthen the proximal gastric pouch, first the gastro-oesophageal junction is dissected from the crus by transecting the phrenoesophageal ligament on both sides. This technique lengthens the proximal pouch about 2 cm. Because of the traction caused by the gastrojejunostomy, we decided no fixation was needed.

Stretching the pouch

Consecutively the pouch is stretched. This is achieved by grasping the pouch on both sides and to pull the pouch caudally for about 1 min. This manipulation of the pouch will gain another 0.5 cm.

Creation of the retrocolic route through the mesocolon

The retrocolic route is created starting on the caudal side of the mesocolon using the ultracision harmonic scalpel.

Pulling the alimentary limb through the retrocolic/ retrogastric route

When completed, the marker stitch is placed in the retrocolic 'tunnel'. The mesocolon is folded down. Cranially of the mesocolon, the marker stitch is found. The jejunum is retracted by pulling the marker stitch whilst retracting the gastric remnant caudally.

Creation of the hand—sewn gastrojejunostomy - The posterior sutures

It becomes apparent that a stapled anastomosis between the gastric pouch and the jejunum is not preferable due to the foreseen tension on this stapler line. Therefore, we decided to make a full hand—sewn anastomosis with V-Loc™ sutures.

Creation of the gastro—and the jejunotomy

A defect is created in the gastric pouch and the jejunum using the ultracision harmonic scalpel.

Introduction of the 34 Ch orogastric tube

A 34 Ch orogastric tube is passed through the gastric pouch and into the alimentary limb of the jejunum.

Creation of the anterior hand sewn anastomosis
A running V-Loc™ suture is used to close the anterior part over the tube in order to ensure the patency of the anastomosis.

Leak test: leak at the right lateral side of the anastomosis
The first leak test with methylene blue through the oro-gastric tube shows a leak on the right lateral side of the anastomosis.

Oversewing the right lateral side of the anastomosis
The defect is over sewn with the remaining V-Loc™ sutures.

Final leak test: no leakage
The final leak test revealed no leakage.

The creation of the jejuno—jejunostomy went according to our standardized protocol. The mesenteric, mesocolic, and Petersen's defect were closed using the hernia stapler. A 27 Fr drain was left lateral to the gastrojejunostomy. The patient was kept nil by mouth for 5 days and fed parenteral.

Results

During the whole admission, the patient was in a good clinical condition: he was hemodynamically stable and showed no signs of anastomotic leakage. On the 5th postoperative day radiographic swallow series where obtained, which showed no signs of leakage. The drain was unproductive during the whole admission. After the swallow studies the drain was removed. On the 6th postoperative day, the patient was discharged with a full liquid diet. To date, no signs of any complication have emerged (we were especially watchful for signs of stricture, stenosis, and internal herniation). Weight loss results are good: 31.5 % of total preoperative body weight after 12 months. Patients' blood glucose values returned to normal with discontinuation of all anti-diabetic medications.

Discussion

This video provides a step—to—step guidance on how to solve the rare, but technically demanding intraoperative complication of a large gap between the gastric pouch and the alimentary limb of the jejunum. By dissecting the gastro-oesophageal junction form the crus, stretching the pouch, dividing the mesentery of the jejunum, using the retrocolic/retrogastric route, and the creation of a total hand—sewn gastrojejunostomy were we were able to bridge the gap.

In stark contrast to the reports elaborating the benefits of LRYGB surgery, very little is known about the intraoperative complications. In large trials and reviews conversion rates up to 4.2 % percent are reported [3, 4], but number are seldom accompanied with a reason why the decision to conversion was made. This is strange considering the occurrence of 'intraoperative events' turns out to be an individual predictor for postoperative complications in a large study by Stenberg *et al.* [5]. This study also revealed that more than one third of the conversions were due to 'difficult anatomic conditions' [5]. The lack of reports on how to cope with intraoperative events force even the most experienced bariatric surgeons in to a pioneering position.

All techniques we describe are not part of our standardized surgical technique and may have disadvantages for the patient. Dissecting the gastro-oesophageal junction from the crus can cause a hiatal hernia, but since the traction in caudal direction from the gastrojejunostomy will prevent the pouch from moving cranially, we thing this is a minor concern. Any form of manipulation of the tissue of the pouch might cause bleeding, ischemia, or tearing. Therefore, stretching of the pouch is a subject of debate. We stress that only experienced surgeons can decide whether or not to apply this technique, based on 'tissue feel', and their ability to cope with the possible complications. Division of the mesentery, especially in a situation of increased tension, may result in bleeding, and consequent ischemia of the adjoining jejunum [6]. Furthermore, some authors stress that transecting the mesentery creates a large orifice and may become a potential hernia space [7], although this was not proven in a recent anatomical study [8]. In a survey executed amongst 215 American Society for Bariatric Surgery (ASBS) affiliated surgeons 64 % of the surveyed bariatric surgeons used the antecolic/antegastric route for the alimentary limb [9]. Eleven percent preferred the retrocolic/retrogastric route [9]. An advantage of the retrocolic/retrogastric route is that it is the shortest route for the alimentary limb to cranially reach the gastric pouch. A disadvantage is the need to create an extra opening in the mesocolon of the transverse colon to facilitate this route, hereby creating an extra orifice and potential hernia space [10]. Several studies report a decrease in internal hernia (IH) incidence when using the antecolic/antegastric route in comparison to the retrocolic route [11–14], although some authors report the lowest IH incidence using a retrocolic/retrogastric technique [15]. In this case we performed a hand—sewn gastrojejunostomy whilst our standardized technique is the linear stapling technique. We chose this technique over all others due to the decrease in surgical time compared to circular and hand—sewn anastomosis [16] and the high incidence of wound infections with circular stapling technique [17]. In this case, the traction on the anastomosis did not allow us to use linear stapling. In the ASBS survey 41 % of the surgeons indicated that they used the linear stapling technique to create the gastric pouch. In addition, 43 % used a circular stapler device and 21 % reported to make a hand sewn gastrojejunostomy [9]. Some studies found a higher rate of strictures with a hand sewn suturing technique in comparison to linear or circular stapling techniques [16], others found no difference [18].

Because of the increased tension on the gastrojejunostomy the risk of leak was high. As a safety measure, we left drains near the gastrojejunostomy, kept the patient nil by mouth and we obtained radiographic swallow series on the 5th postoperative day. It is doubtful if these precautions would have prevented a leak. The aim of these precautions was rather to decrease the severity in case of a leak and to detect a possible leak in an early phase.

From above it is clear that all applied techniques are inferior to our standardized technique and that they should only be used when confronted with an intraoperative event. Maybe even better is the prevention of such situations. This can be done by switching the order of the surgical steps. In our standardized technique the gastric pouch is created at the beginning of the procedure. Schauer *et al.* suggested the formation of the gastric pouch after the inspection and creation of the alimentary limb [17]. If we had adapted this technique, we could have created a longer pouch or –maybe even better—we could have converted to a sleeve gastectomy.

Conclusion

This video report shows how a large distance between a newly created gastric pouch and the alimentary limb can be bridged, By dissecting the gastro-oesophageal junction from the crus, stretching the pouch, transecting the mesentery of the jejunum, using a retrocolic/ retrogastric route and creating a hand—sewn anastomosis we were able to bridge a 8 cm gap. All these manoeuvres are not part of our standard surgical technique as they are all associated with adverse patient outcome. We stress that only experienced bariatric surgeons should embark on these techniques. Inspection of the alimentary limb before pouch created might prevent the need for these complex techniques.

Competing interests

The authors declare that they have no competing interests.

Authors' contributions

NG made a substantial contribution in the analysis and interpretation of the presented surgical techniques, editing the video images, drafting, and revising the manuscript and gave approval for the final version to be published. IK was part of the surgical team that performed the operation and made a substantial contribution to the drafting and revising process of the article and gave approval for the final version to be published. AL made a substantial contribution in the interpretation of the described surgical techniques, drafting, and revising the video as well as the manuscript and gave approval for the final version to be published. All authors read and approved the final manuscript.

Acknowledgements

The authors would like to thank Yair I.Z. Acherman, M.D. for providing critical feedback on the video contents.

References

1. Geubbels N, Bruin SC, Acherman YIZ, van de Laar AWJM, Hoen MB, de Brauw LM. Fast track care for gastric bypass patients decreases length of stay without increasing complications in an unselected patient cohort. Obes Surg. 2014;24:390–6.
2. Geubbels N, de Brauw LM, Acherman YIZ, van de Laar AWJM, Wouters MWJM, Bruin SC. The preceding surgeon factor in bariatric surgery: a positive influence on the learning curve of subsequent surgeons. Obes Surg. 2014 [epub ahead of print].
3. Nguyen NT, Silver M, Robinson M, Needleman B, Hartley G, Cooney R, et al. Result of a national audit of bariatric surgery performed at academic centers: a 2004 University HealthSystem Consortium Benchmarking Project. Arch Surg. 2006;141(May 2006):445–9. discussion 449–450.
4. Angrisani L, Lorenzo M, Borrelli V. Laparoscopic adjustable gastric banding versus Roux-en-Y gastric bypass: 5-year results of a prospective randomized trial. Surg Obes Relat Dis. 2007;3:127–32.
5. Stenberg E, Szabo E, Agren G, Näslund E, Boman L, Bylund A, et al. Early complications after laparoscopic gastric bypass surgery: results from the scandinavian obesity surgery registry. Ann Surg. 2013;00:1–8.
6. Rodríguez A, Mosti M, Sierra M, Pérez-Johnson R, Flores S, Dominguez G, et al. Small bowel obstruction after antecolic and antegastric laparoscopic Roux-en-Y gastric bypass: could the incidence be reduced? Obes Surg. 2010;20:1380–4.
7. Pomp A. Letters to the editor. Surg Obes Relat Dis. 2006;2:591–81.
8. Ortega J, Cassinello N, Sánchez-Antúnez D, Sebastián C, Martínez-Soriano F. Anatomical basis for the low incidence of internal hernia after a laparoscopic Roux-en—Y gastric bypass without mesenteric closure. Obes Surg. 2013;23:1273–80.
9. Madan AK, Harper JL, Tichansky DS. Techniques of laparoscopic gastric bypass: on-line survey of American Society for Bariatric Surgery practicing surgeons. Surg Obes Relat Dis. 2008;4:166–72. discussion 172–3.
10. Clements RH, Harper HC, Laws HL. Facilitating retrocolic—retrogastric gastrojejunostomy in laparoscopic roux-en-y gastric bypass for morbid obesity. J Am Coll Surg. 2001;193:331–2.
11. Steele KE, Prokopowicz GP, Magnuson T, Lidor A, Schweitzer M. Laparoscopic antecolic Roux-en-Y gastric bypass with closure of internal defects leads to fewer internal hernias than the retrocolic approach. Surg Endosc. 2008;22:2056–61.
12. Escalona A, Devaud N, Pérez G, Crovari F, Boza C, Viviani P, et al. Antecolic versus retrocolic alimentary limb in laparoscopic Roux-en-Y gastric bypass: a comparative study. Surg Obes Relat Dis. 2007;3:423–7.
13. Comeau E, Gagner M, Inabnet WB, Herron DM, Quinn TM, Pomp A. Symptomatic internal hernias after laparoscopic bariatric surgery. Surg Endosc. 2005;19:34–9.
14. Taylor JD, Leitman IM, Rosser JB, Davis B, Goodman E. Does the position of the alimentary limb in Roux-en-Y gastric bypass surgery make a difference? J Gastrointest Surg. 2006;10:1397–9.
15. Carmody B, DeMaria EJ, Jamal M, Johnson J, Carbonell A, Kellum J, et al. Internal hernia after laparoscopic Roux-en-Y gastric bypass. Surg Obes Relat Dis. 2005;1:543–8.
16. Abdel-Galil E, Sabry AA. Laparoscopic Roux-en-Y gastric bypass–evaluation of three different techniques. Obes Surg. 2002;12:639–42.
17. Schauer PR, Ikramuddin S, Hamad G, Eid GM, Mattar S, Cottam D, et al. Laparoscopic gastric bypass surgery: current technique. J Laparoendosc Adv Surg Tech A. 2003;13:229–39.
18. Bendewald FP, Choi JN, Blythe LS, Selzer DJ, Ditslear JH, Mattar SG. Comparison of hand—sewn, linear-stapled, and circular—stapled gastrojejunostomy in laparoscopic Roux-en-Y gastric bypass. Obes Surg. 2011;21:1671–5.

10

Management of acute upside-down stomach

Tobias S Schiergens[1*], Michael N Thomas[1], Thomas P Hüttl[2] and Wolfgang E Thasler[1]

Abstract

Background: Upside-down stomach (UDS) is characterized by herniation of the entire stomach or most gastric portions into the posterior mediastinum. Symptoms may vary heavily as they are related to reflux and mechanically impaired gastric emptying. UDS is associated with a risk of incarceration and volvulus development which both might be complicated by acute gastric outlet obstruction, advanced ischemia, gastric bleeding and perforation.

Case presentation: A 32-year-old male presented with acute intolerant epigastralgia and anterior chest pain associated with acute onset of nausea and vomiting. He reported on a previous surgical intervention due to a hiatal hernia. Chest radiography and computer tomography showed an incarcerated UDS. After immediate esophago-gastroscopy, urgent laparoscopic reduction, repair with a 360° floppy Nissen fundoplication and insertion of a gradually absorbable GORE® BIO-A®-mesh was performed.

Conclusion: Given the high risk of life-threatening complications of an incarcerated UDS as ischemia, gastric perforation or severe bleeding, emergent surgery is indicated. In stable patients with acute presentation of large paraesophageal hernia or UDS exhibiting acute mechanical gastric outlet obstruction, after esophago-gastroscopy laparoscopic reduction and hernia repair followed by an anti-reflux procedure is suggested. However, in cases of unstable patients open repair is the surgical method of choice. Here, we present an exceptionally challenging case of a young patient with a giant recurrent hiatal hernia becoming clinically manifest in an incarcerated UDS.

Keywords: Upside-down stomach, Hiatal hernia, Paraesophageal hernia, Gastric incarceration, Gastric outlet obstruction, Gastric volvulus

Background

Upside-down stomach (UDS) is the rarest type of hiatal hernia (< 5%). It is characterized by herniation of the entire stomach or most gastric portions into the posterior mediastinum [1,2]. Both gastroesophageal junction and parts of the stomach migrate intrathoracically, thus UDS represents a large mixed type - sliding and paraesophageal (type 3) hernia [1-3]. By many authors, UDS is also referred to as type 4 hiatal hernia [4]. Other intra-abdominal organs can be involved in the herniation [5,6]. The pathophysiology of hiatal hernias remains poorly understood. Three pathogenic components are widely found in the literature which can individually exist in different proportions (1) increased intra-abdominal pressure (transdiaphragmatic pressure gradient); (2) esophageal shortening (fibrosis, vagal nerve stimulation); (3) widening of the diaphragmatic hiatus due to congenital or acquired structural changes of periesophageal ligaments and muscular crura of the hiatus [7]. The latter include abnormalities of elastin, collagens, and matrix metalloproteinases [7-10].

As hiatal and true paraesophageal hernia, UDS can manifest itself clinically in a wide variety of symptoms including substernal pain, heartburn, postprandial distress and fullness, dysphagia, postprandial nausea and vomiting [2,3]. They occur due to reflux related to the sliding component and mechanically impaired gastric emptying, thereby, the latter symptoms usually preponderate [4,11]. Chronic mucosal bleeding may cause anemia and is ascribed to venous obstruction of the migrated stomach [2]. While UDS itself is a very rare condition it is associated with a risk of incarceration as well as volvulus development. These complications can cause acute gastric outlet obstruction and thereby present clinically as acute abdomen. Further complications are acute and severe gastric bleeding, ischemia and perforation. All of these complications represent true emergencies as life-threatening conditions. Prevalence of acute symptoms or incarceration in paraesophageal hernia was reported to be 30,4% [12].

* Correspondence: Tobias.Schiergens@med.uni-muenchen.de
[1]Department of Surgery, University of Munich, Campus Grosshadern, Munich, Germany
Full list of author information is available at the end of the article

Once diagnosed, UDS should be surgically addressed by reduction of the migrated stomach, excision of hernia sac, and hiatal defect closure combined with an anti-reflux procedure as 360° or partial fundoplication. Laparoscopic repair provides benefits as reduced postoperative morbidity and hospital stay. Even if asymptomatic a surgical intervention is indicated as a conservative approach bears the risk of a high mortality rate due to complications which is significantly reduced by elective surgery [1,2,4,5,11]. In the light of only few series and cases reported, there is no clear evidence from review of the current literature for the management of acute paraesophageal hernia or UDS as very rare conditions [13]. In addition, there is an ongoing controversial discussion about whether prothetic reinforcement of the hiatus by mesh insertion is reasonable and effective. In the face of high recurrence rates several surgeons recommend the use of prosthetic meshes. However, many severe complications can be associated with mesh implantation as perforation necessitating partial esophagogastrectomy or acute erosive bleeding of the abdominal aorta [14]. In summary, there is still a considerable controversy regarding the routine mesh insertion and the quality of evidence is very low.

Management of acute incarceration - case presentation

A 32-year-old male presented to the emergency department (ED) after acute thoraco-epigastric pain had set in after dinner several hours before. On arrival in the ED, his intolerant epigastralgia and anterior chest pain had been associated with acute onset of nausea and vomiting. The patient reported on having had recurrent substernal pain and dysphagia as well as mild symptoms of reflux which had persisted for more than a year. He reported on a previous surgical intervention due to a hiatal hernia, whereupon a anterior hemifundoplication had been performed two years ago. Furthermore the patient had a history of Ebstein's anomaly which had been addressed by a reconstruction of the tricuspid valve a year ago.

A naso-gastric tube was tried to be placed but pushing it forward proved to be challenging and required repeated attempts, which all turned out to be unsuccessful. On admission the patient's lactate level was mildly elevated (2.4 mmol/L) and besides a slightly increased WBC (12 / nL) unremarkable. Notably, no elevation of cardiac enzymes was detected. Electrocardiogram on admission showed sinus tachycardia, an incomplete right bundle branch block and a distinct S1Q3-pattern. Echocardiography revealed a normal left-ventricular ejection fraction, however the right ventricle was dilated. Upright chest radiography showed no subdiaphragmatic free air but visceral gas was seen in projection on the posterior mediastinum. Adjacent contrast-enhanced computer tomography disclosed a giant hiatal hernia (Figure 1). Most portions of the stomach and some of the greater omentum had migrated into the posterior mediastinum, whereas parts of the greater curvature appeared to be incarcerated in the diaphragmatic hiatus. Immediate esophago-gastroscopy showed a kinking-stenosis of the cardia and a stenosis caused by the strangling diaphragm which could hardly be passed. A naso-gastric tube was then positioned endoscopically and food residue and gas were sucked off for therapeutic decompression of the incarcerated stomach. Altogether mucosa appeared unremarkable and there were no signs of ischemia or restrained perfusion (Figure 2). After endoscopy the patient's complains were attenuated but not resolved.

Emergent surgery for reduction of the incarcerated stomach and repair of the hiatal defect was performed through five trocars evenly dispersed to the upper abdomen (Figure 3). First, retracting the left liver lobe laparoscopic reduction of the stomach and attached portions of the greater omentum was conducted (Figure 3A–C) opening the view to a giant hiatal defect (Figure 3D). After preparation of the diaphragmatic crura and the distal esophagus preserving the rami of N. vagus a hiatoplasty was performed by anterior and posterior approximation of the diaphragmatic crura (Figure 3E–G). Given the fact of a recurrent hernia and a very wide defect of approimately 8 cm, a gradually absorbable GORE® BIO-A®-mesh (W.L. Gore & Associates Inc., Flagstaff, AZ) of biocompatible synthetic polymers was inserted enlacing the gastro-esophageal transition (Figure 3H–I). In a final step, a 360° floppy Nissen fundoplication was accomplished (Figure 3J–L). Postoperatively the patient recovered very well and was discharged five days later without any complication. He is to be followed up by the surgical outpatient department and is presently free of any complaints.

Discussion

Surgery for incarcerated paraesophageal hernia or UDS has to be performed emergently as incarceration can become irreversible and severe bleeding can occur due to distension and vascular dilation. Moreover, ischemia and gastric perforation are on the verge. However, there are no clear evidence or existing guidelines on the management of acute paraesophageal hernia or UDS. Referring to this, Bawahab and colleagues have proposed algorithms based on the results of a series of 20 patients with acute presentation of paraesophageal hernia [13]. From this data and our experience, we suggest prompt open surgery in cases of unstable patients [4,13]. However, from our point of view, in case of gastric perforation or if there is any gastroscopic evidence of advanced gastric ischemia in stable patients, an initial laparoscopic approach is justifiable in case of adequate expertise, otherwise emergent open repair is suggested. In stable patients with acute presentation and mechanical gastric outlet obstruction due to incarceration

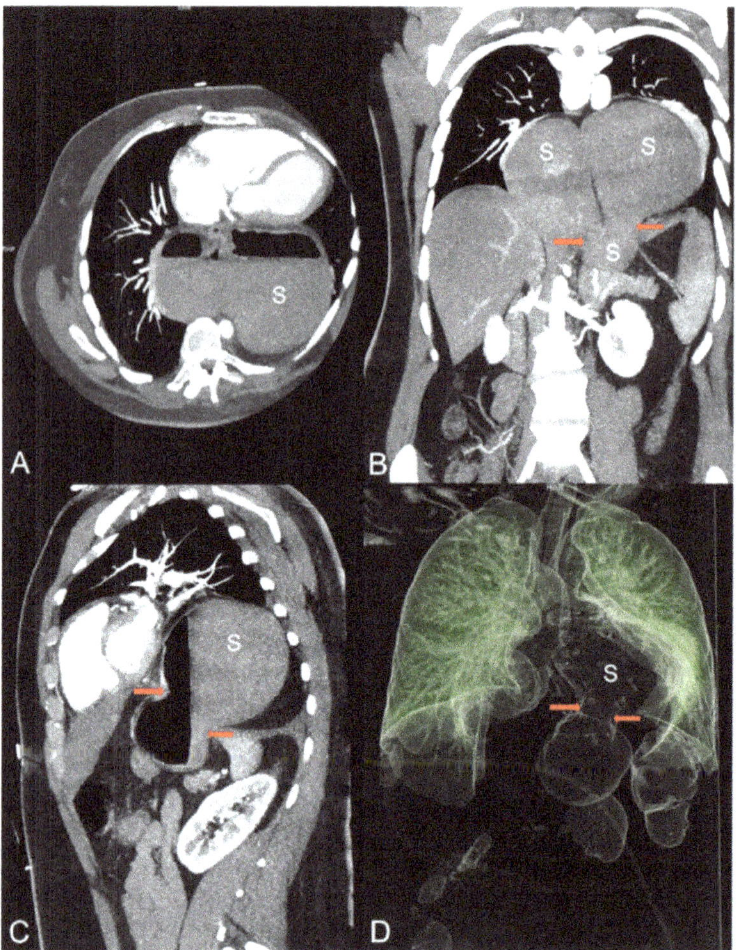

Figure 1 Contrast-enhanced computer tomography. (A–C) Giant mixed-type hernia (upside-down stomach (S)) with an incarcerated portion of the stomach (red arrows). **(D)** Visceral gas distribution seen from the *3D*-reconstruction showing the proximal gastric portion (S) in the posterior mediastinum (incarceration: red arrows).

as in the presented case, emergent laparoscopic reduction and repair is reasonable and prudent after urgent contrast-enhanced computer tomography and decompressing gastroscopy. For patients with acute presentation but without mechanical gastric obstruction and without gastric ischemia, we suggest a semi-elective repair. In summary, laparoscopic reduction and repair of acute paraesophageal hernia and UDS was shown to be safe in patients without gastric perforation or ischemia as well as feasible with low morbidity and mortality affording the benefits of minimally-invasive

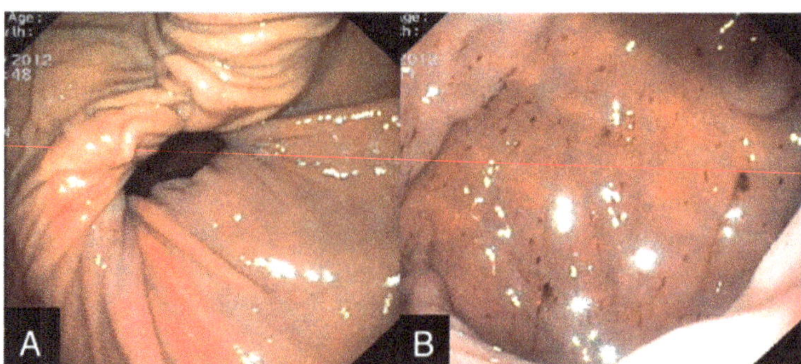

Figure 2 Esophago-gastroscopy. (A) Distended stomach migrated intrathoracically exhibiting the stenosis caused by the strangling diaphragm which could hardly be passed endoscopically. **(B)** Gastric mucosa appearing unremarkable aside from minor petechial bleedings.

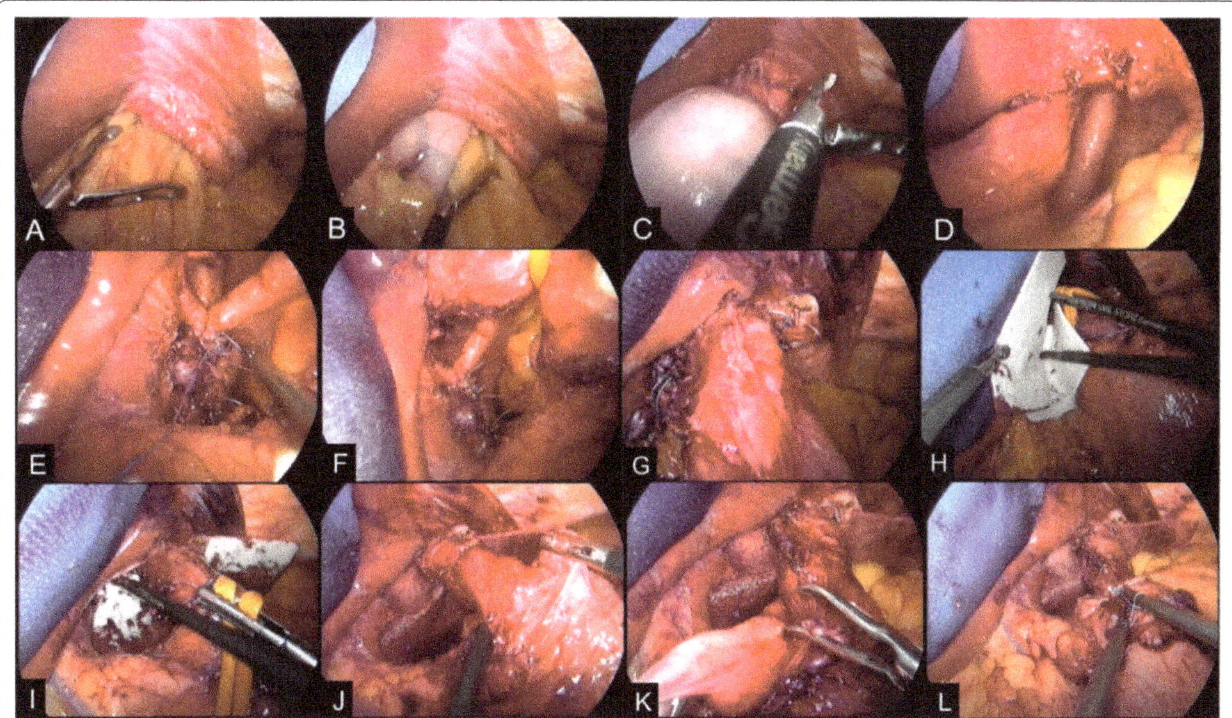

Figure 3 Laparoscopic reduction (A–D) and repair (E–G) of the incarcerated upside-down-stomach with insertion of a gradually absorbable mesh (H–I) and accomplishment of a 360° floppy Nissen fundoplication (J–L).

surgery [4,13]. Moreover, studies have been published reporting on percutaneous endoscopic gastrostomy (PEG) as useful and feasible approach [15-18]. Tabo *et al.* described a method facilitating the endoscopic reposition of the stomach by inserting a gastric balloon and to fixate the stomach subsequently applying the PEG-method (intraabdominal fixation of the stomach by gastrostomy) [18]. It may be an effective approach in elderly patients as the periprocedural risk is very low. In our young patient, however, we decided in favor of a laparoscopic approach repairing the hernia gate as sustainable therapy. In a series of 40 patients we could show that laparoscopic treatment of UDS is safe and highly effective using a laparoscopic hiatoplasty and anterior hemifundoplication [4].

As to the diagnosis in the ED, a high index of suspicion is essential when patients present acutely with epigastralgia and symptoms of upper gastrointestinal obstruction indicating mechanical gastric outlet obstruction. In our series, 5 of 50 patients with UDS (10%) presented with acute symptoms, two of them with gastric incarceration, one with upper gastrointestinal bleeding and one patient with omentum incarceration [4]. In another series of 147 patients, Allen and colleagues revealed that in 95% of all patients with UDS symptoms occurred which were primarily obstructive [11]. Complications of hiatal hernia are rarely considered in patients presenting with acute chest or epigastric pain as well as acute gastric outlet obstruction. Obstructive symptoms can range from mild nausea, bloating, postprandial fullness, dysphagia, retching or vomiting but rarely lead to the diagnosis in the ED. Hence, there is a high risk to mis- and underdiagnose an incarcerated UDS. Treatment as acute coronary syndrome (ACS) can have fatal consequences as gastric perforation [19,20]. Although information and sensitivity are low, plain chest radiography should be the first diagnostic tool whereby other differential diagnoses can be considered or ruled out. As a more reliable tool to work out the details of this important differential diagnosis contrast-enhanced thoracoabdominal computer tomography is suitable especially for the detection of complications as well as the decision for indicating surgery [19]. Impossibility of naso-gastric tube application as in our patient can be an evidence for gastric incarceration or volvulus as it is described by the *Borchardt's Triad* consisting of the inability to pass a naso-gastric tube, usually unproductive retching as well as epigastric pain and distension [21]. The presented case shows the diagnostic challenge of acute presentation of paraesophageal hernia or UDS as they rarely feature one's lists of differential diagnoses of acute epigastralgia or chest pain. Having confirmed the correct diagnosis, immediate decompressing esophago-gastroscopy and emergent surgery with reduction, hernia repair and antireflux procedure are able to prevent life-threatening complications.

Conclusions

We present an exceptionally challenging case of a young patient with a history of Ebstein's anomaly and a giant recurrent hiatal hernia becoming clinically manifest in an incarcerated UDS. In spite of anterior hemifundoplication two years ago the patient presented with this clinically and patho-anatomically impressive recrudescence. A genetically related common cause for cardiac and hiatal tissue defect can be hypothesized but was not assessed for lack of therapeutic consequences in this patient. However, given the fact of a recurring and very large hernia in spite of previous surgical repair as well as the postulated underlying tissue deficiency, we decided in favor of insertion of an absorbable mesh for hiatal reinforcement and tension-free repair. However, in the view of the above described complications associated with mesh implantation, we are exceedingly reserved regarding routine use of meshes and recommend thorough indication.

Competing interests

The authors declare that they have no competing interests.

Authors' contributions

TSS and WET collected the patient's history data. TSS drafted the manuscript with committed and dedicated review and discussion of MNT, TPH and WET. All authors contributed substantially to the patient's care and therapy. All authors read and approved the final manuscript.

Author details

[1]Department of Surgery, University of Munich, Campus Grosshadern, Munich, Germany. [2]Department of Surgery, Chirurgische Klinik München-Bogenhausen, Munich, Germany.

References

1. Hill LD, Tobias JA: **Paraesophageal hernia.** *Arch Surg* 1968, **96**:735–744.
2. Krahenbuhl L, Schafer M, Farhadi J, Renzulli P, Seiler CA, Buchler MW: **Laparoscopic treatment of large paraesophageal hernia with totally intrathoracic stomach.** *J Am Coll Surg* 1998, **187**:231–237.
3. Wo JM, Branum GD, Hunter JG, Trus TN, Mauren SJ, Waring JP: **Clinical features of type III (mixed) paraesophageal hernia.** *Am J Gastroenterol* 1996, **91**:914–916.
4. Obeidat FW, Lang RA, Knauf A, Thomas MN, Huttl TK, Zugel NP, *et al*: **Laparoscopic anterior hemifundoplication and hiatoplasty for the treatment of upside-down stomach: mid- and long-term results after 40 patients.** *Surg Endosc* 2011, **25**:2230–2235.
5. Skinner DB, Belsey RH: **Surgical management of esophageal reflux and hiatus hernia. Long-term results with 1,030 patients.** *J Thorac Cardiovasc Surg* 1967, **53**:33–54.
6. Landreneau RJ, Del PM, Santos R: **Management of paraesophageal hernias.** *Surg Clin North Am* 2005, **85**:411–432.
7. Weber C, Davis CS, Shankaran V, Fisichella PM: **Hiatal hernias: a review of the pathophysiologic theories and implication for research.** *Surg Endosc* 2011, **25**:3149–3153.
8. Curci JA, Melman LM, Thompson RW, Soper NJ, Matthews BD: **Elastic fiber depletion in the supporting ligaments of the gastroesophageal junction: a structural basis for the development of hiatal hernia.** *J Am Coll Surg* 2008, **207**:191–196.
9. Asling B, Jirholt J, Hammond P, Knutsson M, Walentinsson A, Davidson G, *et al*: **Collagen type III alpha I is a gastro-oesophageal reflux disease susceptibility gene and a male risk factor for hiatus hernia.** *Gut* 2009, **58**:1063–1069.
10. Melman L, Chisholm PR, Curci JA, Arif B, Pierce R, Jenkins ED, *et al*: **Differential regulation of MMP-2 in the gastrohepatic ligament of the gastroesophageal junction.** *Surg Endosc* 2010, **24**:1562–1565.
11. Allen MS, Trastek VF, Deschamps C, Pairolero PC: **Intrathoracic stomach. Presentation and results of operation.** *J Thorac Cardiovasc Surg* 1993, **105**:253–258.
12. Hill LD: **Incarcerated paraesophageal hernia. A surgical emergency.** *Am J Surg* 1973, **126**:286–291.
13. Bawahab M, Mitchell P, Church N, Debru E: **Management of acute paraesophageal hernia.** *Surg Endosc* 2009, **23**:255–259.
14. Zugel N, Lang RA, Kox M, Huttl TP: **Severe complication of laparoscopic mesh hiatoplasty for paraesophageal hernia.** *Surg Endosc* 2009, **23**:2563–2567.
15. Criblez DH: **Percutaneous endoscopic gastrostomy to treat upside-down stomach before stent insertion in a patient with distal esophageal carcinoma.** *Am J Gastroenterol* 1998, **93**:1938–1941.
16. Januschowski R: **Endoscopic repositioning of the upside-down stomach and its fixation by percutaneous endoscopic gastrostomy.** *Dtsch Med Wochenschr* 1996, **121**:1261–1264.
17. Lukovich P, Dudas I, Tari K, Jonas A, Herczeg G: **PEG fixation of an upside-down stomach using a flexible endoscope: case report and review of the literature.** *Surg Laparosc Endosc Percutan Tech* 2013, **23**:e65–e69.
18. Tabo T, Hayashi H, Umeyama S, Yoshida M, Onodera H: **Balloon repositioning of intrathoracic upside-down stomach and fixation by percutaneous endoscopic gastrostomy.** *J Am Coll Surg* 2003, **197**:868–871.
19. Chang CC, Tseng CL, Chang YC: **A surgical emergency due to an incarcerated paraesophageal hernia.** *Am J Emerg Med* 2009, **27**:135. el-3.
20. Trainor D, Duffy M, Kennedy A, Glover P, Mullan B: **Gastric perforation secondary to incarcerated hiatus hernia: an important differential in the diagnosis of central crushing chest pain.** *Emerg Med J* 2007, **24**:603–604.
21. Johnson JA III, Thompson AR: **Gastric volvulus and the upside-down stomach.** *J Miss State Med Assoc* 1994, **35**:1–4.

11

Prognostic analysis of combined curative resection of the stomach and liver lesions in 30 gastric cancer patients with synchronous liver metastases

Yan-Na Wang[1], Kun-Tang Shen[1*], Jia-Qian Ling[1], Xiao-Dong Gao[1], Ying-Yong Hou[2], Xue-Fei Wang[1], Jing Qin[1], Yi-Hong Sun[1] and Xin-Yu Qin[1]

Abstract

Background: Gastric cancer with synchronous liver metastasis remains a clinical treatment challenge. There has been a longstanding debate on the question whether surgical resection could be beneficial to long-term survival. This study is to investigate the effectiveness and prognostic factors of combined curative resection of the stomach and liver lesions in gastric cancer patients with synchronous liver metastases.

Methods: A total of 30 patients who underwent simultaneous curative gastric and liver resection from March 2003 to April 2008 were analyzed retrospectively. Univariate and multivariate analyses were performed to select independent factors for survival.

Results: The overall 1-, 2-, 3- and 5-year survival rates of 30 patients were 43.3%, 30.0%, 16.7% and 16.7%, respectively, with a median survival of 11.0 months and 5 patients still living by the time of last follow-up. Single liver metastasis ($p = 0.028$) and an absence of peritoneal dissemination ($p = 0.007$) were significantly independent prognostic factors for these gastric cancer patients with synchronous liver metastases. Major adverse events were protracted stomach paralysis in 2 patients and pulmonary infection in another 2 patients, all of whom recovered after conservative treatment.

Conclusions: This descriptive study without control group found that patients with solitary liver metastasis and absence of peritoneal dissemination could have better survival benefit from simultaneous curative resection of the gastric cancer and liver metastases.

Keywords: Gastric cancer, Liver metastases, Clinicopathological factors, Prognosis

Background

Liver is one of the most frequent sites of cancer metastasis from gastrointestinal origin, and the major cause of disease death from stomach cancer [1]. The 5-year survival rate could be up to 29% for metachronous liver metastasis and only 6% for synchronous liver metastasis, from gastric cancer [2]. Therefore, it has long been thought by many that surgical treatment could not bring any substantial survival benefit for gastric cancer patients with synchronous liver metastasis. However, there has also been longstanding debate on the question whether surgical resection could be beneficial to long-term survival. Some believe that if R0 resection could be performed for both gastric cancer and synchronous liver metastasis, such simultaneous resection could significantly improve survival [3,4]. On the other hand, gastric cancer patients with liver metastasis usually have multiple intrahepatic lesions, peritoneal metastasis, regional lymph nodes metastasis and adjacent organs involvements [5-7], making it questionable whether simultaneous resection could bring any survival benefit. From March 2003 to April 2008, we performed simultaneous

* Correspondence: shen.kuntang@zs-hospital.sh.cn
[1]Department of General Surgery, Zhongshan Hospital of Fudan University, No 180 Fenglin Road, Shanghai 200032, China
Full list of author information is available at the end of the article

resection of both the gastric cancer and liver metastasis on 30 patients. This study is to summarize our experience and to analyze the efficacy and prognosis on these patients.

Methods

The study complied with the declaration of Helsinki and was approved by Biomedical Research Ethics Committee of Zhongshan Hospital of Fudan University (NO.2009-160). All subjects gave written informed consent.

Patients and treatment

From March 2003 to April 2008, a total of 2942 patients with gastric cancer were treated at our institution. From the archived medical records, a complete database was established on 30 gastric cancer patients with synchronous liver metastasis, who had simultaneous complete resection of both gastric cancer and liver metastasis. The database covered all clinico-pathological characteristics. Lymph node grouping was based on Japanese classification on cancer typing [8] and TNM classification was base on AJCC 7th edition [9].

Of these 30 patients were 27 males and 3 females, with age ranging from 33 to 72 years old (median 60 yr). The primary stomach cancer was located at the antrum in 11 cases, at the gastric body in 9 cases and at the cardia-fundus region in 10 cases. On local invasion status, 4 cases had tumor invasion beneath the serosa, and the remaining 26 cases all had tumor invasion beyond the serosa. On lymph nodes status, 7 cases did not have lymph nodes metastasis while the remaining 23 cases were lymph nodes positive. In terms of liver metastasis, 22 patients had one intrahepatic metastasis lesion and 8 patients had 2–3 liver metastases. There were 27 patients with metastasis limited to one lobe of the liver (H1), and 3 cases with metastasis on both lobes of the liver (H2). Simultaneous peritoneal metastasis was found in 5 patients. Of surgical approaches, 11 patients had curative distal gastrectomy, 10 patients had curative proximal gastrectomy and 9 cases had total gastrectomy. For liver resection, 7 patients had lobectomy and 23 patients had partial hepatectomy. These patients did not receive any preoperative chemotherapy, but all patients had postoperative adjuvant chemotherapy by experienced oncologists.

Follow-up

All patients were regularly followed-up by telephone, with the last follow-up on April 14, 2012. The survival was calculated from the date of surgery to the date of death or last follow-up. There were 25 cases died, all due to cancer recurrence.

Statistical analysis

All the data were analyzed with SPSS 16.0 software. The survival was analyzed by Kaplan-Meier and log rank test. Cox regression model analysis was performed for univariate and multivariate analysis, so as to discover

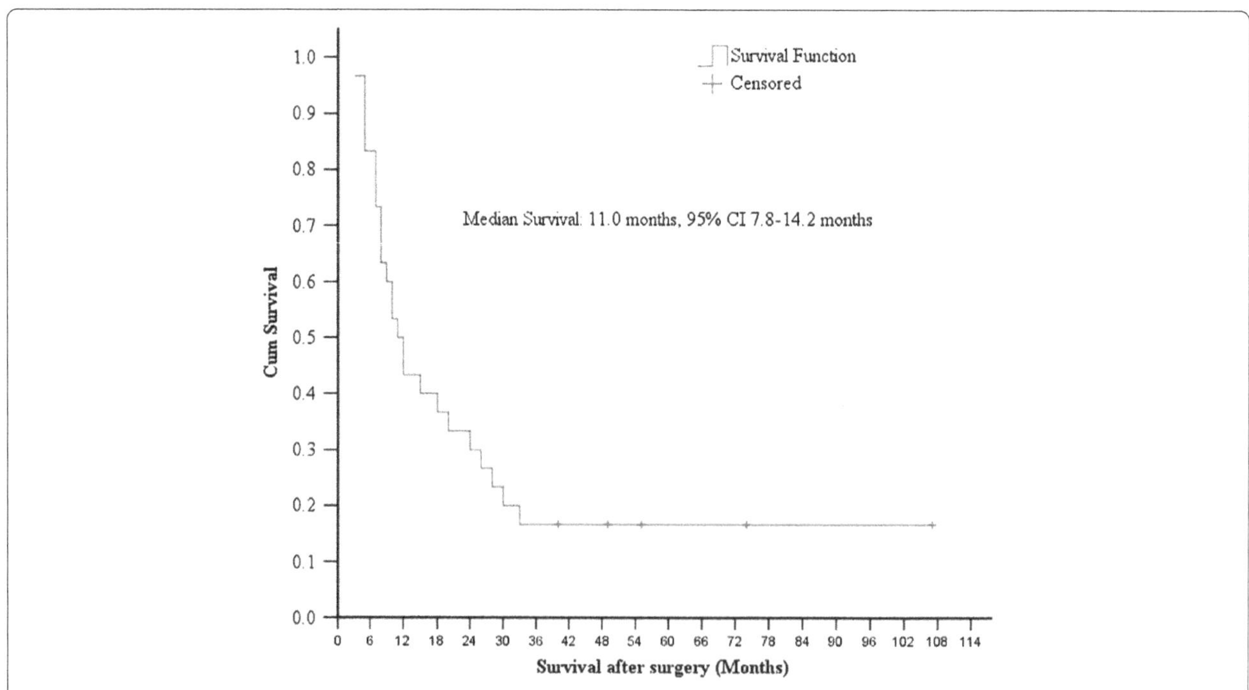

Figure 1 Median survival in 30 patients. Kaplan-Meier survival curve of the 30 patients in this study showed a median survival of 11.0 months after the simultaneous curative resection of the stomach and liver metastases.

Table 1 Clinico-pathological features on 30 patients in this study

Age (yr)	
Median (Range)	60 (33—72)
Gender: n (%)	
Male	27 (90.0%)
Female	3 (10.0%)
Gastric cancer site: n (%)	
Gastric antrum	11 (36.7%)
Gastric body	9 (30.0%)
Gastric cardia-fundus	10 (33.3%)
Elevated tumor markers: n (%)	
CEA	7 (23.3%)
AFP	6 (20.0%)
CA19-9	8 (26.7%)
Gastric cancer diameter: cm	
Median (Range)	3.7 (1.0—11.0)
Pathological type: n (%)	
Papillary adenocarcinoma	13 (43.3%)
Tubular adenocarcinoma	10 (33.3%)
Poorly differentiated adenocarcinoma	4 (13.3%)
Mucinous adenocarcinoma	3 (10.0%)
Number of intrahepatic metastases: n (%)	
Single metastastic lesion	22 (73.3%)
Multiple metastatic lesions	8 (26.7%)
Diameter of intrahepatic metastasis lesions: cm	
Median (Range)	3.1 (0.5—16.0)
Surgical approaches: n (%)	
Distal gastrectomy	11 (36.7%)
Total gastrectomy	9 (30.0%)
Proximal gastrectomy	10 (33.3%)
T classification: n(%)	
T1	1 (3.3%)
T2	3 (10.0%)
T4a	26 (86.7%)
N classification: n (%)	
N0	7 (23.3%)
N1	3 (10.0%)
N2	5 (16.7%)
N3	15 (50.0%)
Peritoneal metastasis	
P0	25 (83.3%)
P1	5 (16.7%)
Tumor embolus	
Yes	13 (43.3%)
No	17 (56.7%)
Tumor differentiation: n (%)	
Well differentiated	2 (6.67%)
Intermediately differentiated	5 (16.7%)
Poorly differentiated	23 (76.7%)
Survival status: n (%)	
Survived	5 (16.7%)
Died	25 (83.3%)

independent prognostic factors. Two-sided $p < 0.05$ was considered as statistically significant.

Results

Perioperative features

There were 14 (46.7%) cases with blood transfusion (300–1000 mL, median 520 mL), 24 (80.0%) cases with albumin transfusion (20–100 g, median 43 g), and 12 (40.0%) cases with parenteral nutrition support. Two (6.7%) patients had gastric paralysis after operation and subsequently recovered after nasogastric tube depression for 19 and 22 days, respectively. Two (6.7%) patients had pulmonary infection, one with A. baumanii and treated with antibiotics for 49 days, and the other one infected with Klebsiella pneumoniae and treated for 10 days with anti-infection agents, and both were recovered well. There were no perioperative deaths.

Follow-up Results

All 30 patients had complete follow-up data. By the time of last follow-up, 25 (83.3%) patients died and 5 (16.7%) patients were living, with median survival of 11.0 months (95% CI 7.8 to 14.2 months). The 1-, 2-, 3- and 5-year survival rates were 43.3%, 30.0%, 16.7% and 16.7%, respectively (Figure 1). One patient with gastric ulcerative hepatoid adenocarcinoma (pT2N2M1) lived for 107 months without evidence of recurrence.

Analysis on survival related independent factors

Table 1 summarized the correlation of major clinicopathological factors with survival status. Age, gender, tumor marker levels (CEA, AFP and CA19-9), primary tumor size, liver metastasis lesion size, tumor emboli, ascites, T staging and N staging all had no significant correlation with survival, but the number of liver metastatic lesions (log rant test, $p = 0.028$, Table 2, Figure 2) and peritoneal metastasis (log rant test, $p = 0.007$, Table 2, Figure 3) were significantly correlated with survival. Multivariate Cox regression survival analysis also confirmed that number of liver metastasis and peritoneal metastasis were independent prognostic factors (Table 3).

Table 2 Survival analysis

Items	N (survival rate)	Log rank *p*	HR	95% CI	*P*
Age: (yr)					
≤ 60 yr	15 (13.3%)	0.617	0.822	0.374-1.808	0.627
> 60 yr	15 (20.0%)				
Gender: n(%)					
Male	27 (18.5%)	0.725	0.809	0.238-2.748	0.734
Female	3 (0)				
CEA					
Normal	23 (13.0%)	0.499	0.716	0.265-1.936	0.497
Increased	7 (28.6%)				
AFP					
Normal	24 (16.7%)	0.728	1.185	0.443-3.172	0.736
Increased	6 (16.7%)				
CA19-9					
Normal	22 (13.6%)	0.527	0.748	0.297-1.886	0.538
Increased	8 (25.0%)				
Ascites					
Yes	7 (17.4%)	0.793	1.127	0.449-2.833	0.799
No	23 (14.3%)				
Primary tumor size					
< 5cm	18 (22.2%)	0.984	1.008	0.454-2.236	0.985
≥ 5cm	12 (8.3%)				
Number of liver metastasis					
Single	22 (22.2%)	***0.028**	2.456	1.048-5.756	***0.039**
Multiple	8 (8.3%)				
Liver metastasis size					
< 5cm	14 (21.4%)	0.766	1.124	0.509-2.482	0.772
≥ 5cm	16 (12.5%)				
Peritoneal metastasis					
P1	5 (20.0%)	***0.007**	3.836	1.292-11.383	***0.015**
P0	25 (0)				
Liver surgery					
Lobectomy	23 (17.4%)	0.944	1.032	0.411-2.593	0.946
Partial hepatotrectomy	7 (14.3%)				
T stage: n(%)					
T1, T2	4 (50.0%)	0.508	0.757	0.324-1.767	0.519
T3, T4	26 (11.5%)				
N metastasis: n(%)					
Negative	7 (14.3%)	0.574	1.293	0.515-3.249	0.584
Positive	23 (17.4%)				
Tumor embolus					
Yes	13 (15.4%)	0.650	1.196	0.541-2.647	0.658
No	17 (17.6%)				
Tumor differentiation					
Well-intermediately differentiation	7 (28.6%)	0.379	1.535	0.573-4.112	0.394
Poorly differentiated	23 (13.0%)				

Discussion and conclusions

Liver is one of the most frequent sites of cancer metastasis from gastrointestinal origin, and the major cause of disease death from stomach cancer. The incidence of synchronous liver metastasis from gastric cancer is about 2.0%-9.6%, which is lower than that from colorectal cancer. Approximately 0.4%-1.0% of these patients could be treated by liver resection [7,10-12], with median survival of 5–31 months, 1-year survival rate of 15%-77%, and 5-year survival rate of 0%-38%, after hepatectomy [6,7,13-17].

In the current study, 30 gastric cancer patients with synchronous liver metastasis were simultaneously treated by both gastrectomy and hepatectomy, resulting a median overall survival of 11.0 months, and 1-, 2-, 3- and 5-year survival rates of 43.3%, 30.0%, 16.7% and 16.7%, respectively. Of particular note, 1 patient has a disease-free survival of 107 months. Our multivariate analysis found that preoperative tumor marker levels, primary tumor size, tumor invasion depth, lymph nodes metastasis, histological types, tumor emboli, ascites, liver metastasis sizes all had no significant impact on survival, but the number of liver metastasis and peritoneal metastasis did have significant impact on survival.

It has been reported that gastric cancer prognosis could be heavily influenced by many tumor pathological features such as tumor invasion depth, lymph nodes metastasis, pathological types and tumor emboli [2,7,16,18].This study, however, did not find any significant survival impact of these features, most probably due to the fact that most previous studies included patients with both synchronous and metachronous metastases, but our study only focused on gastric cancer patients with synchronous liver metastasis. Many other studies since 2001 [2,3,6,13,16,19] also suggested that pathological staging of the primary tumor did not have significant impact on postoperative survival. Based on these results, we believe that the routine clinicopathological features of the primary gastric cancer are not major factors to impact on postoperative survival in such patients with simultaneous resection of the gastric cancer the liver metastasis.

In our study, we found that the number of liver metastases and peritoneal metastasis are independent prognostic factors for such patients with simultaneous resection. Okano et al. [11] also found that patients with

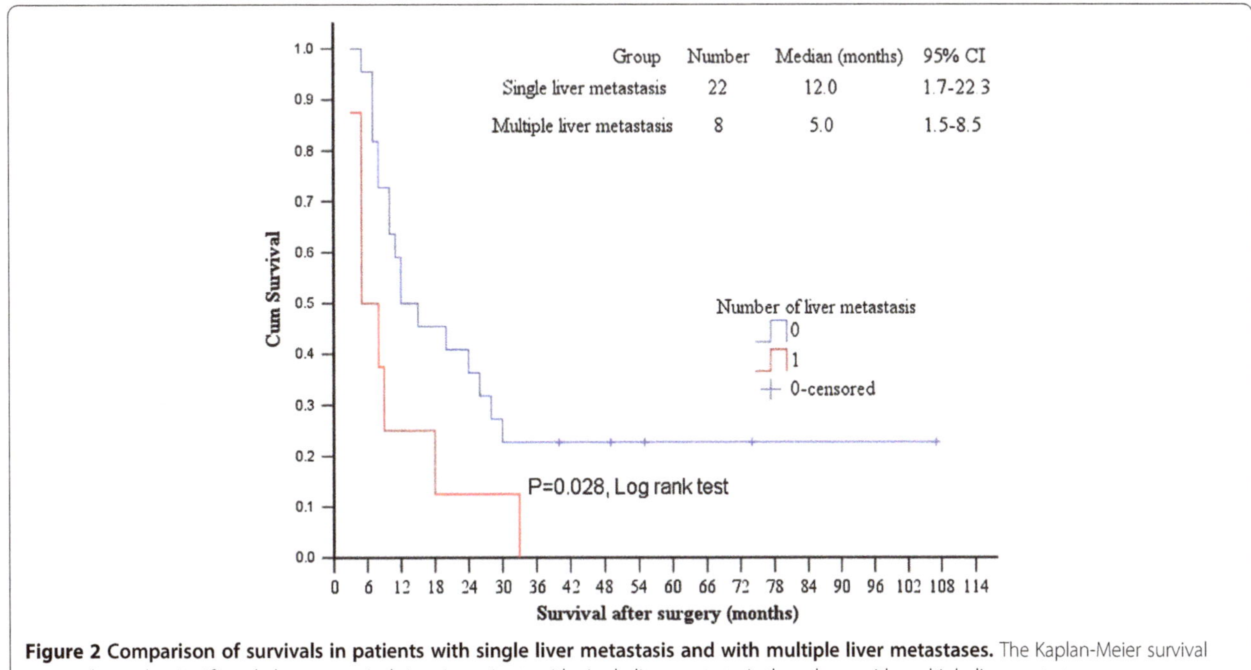

Figure 2 Comparison of survivals in patients with single liver metastasis and with multiple liver metastases. The Kaplan-Meier survival curves showed a significantly longer survival time in patients with single liver metastasis than those with multiple liver metastases.

single liver metastasis had significantly higher 3-year survival rate than those with multiple liver metastases. In addition, several other reports [6,16,20] also confirmed that the number of liver metastases is a major prognostic factor. Ueda et al. [21] also found in 72 gastric cancer patients with liver metastasis who had simultaneous resection, that patients with H1 and no peritoneal metastasis had better survival, and such result was repeated in a another similar study [19]. Because the number of liver cancer metastases had strong correlation with distribution of liver metastases (one lobe or two lobes), the prognostic significance of liver cancer metastasis distribution should be further investigated in large scale clinical studies.

This study did not find any independent survival impact of conventional pathological factors such as T stage and N stage. Two major reasons may account for such difference. The first concerns the disease status in our series. This study included 30 patients of gastric cancer with synchronous liver metastasis. In addition, there were also 5 patients with peritoneal metastasis. Therefore, all these patients were clinical stage IV. So it is not surprising that the multivariate analysis found that the number of liver metastases and peritoneal metastases were the only two independent factors influencing survival. The second concerns the number of patients at different T and N stages in this study. There were only 4 T1 and T2 cases, and 26 T4a cases. Similarly, there were only 10 N0 and N1 cases out of the total 30 cases. The smaller the number, the less statistical power they had. The much smaller number of early T and early N cases may also account for reason why they seemed not to have influence on overall survival after multivariate analysis.

Among the 30 cases in this cohort, 6 patients had increased AFP levels. These patients may had gastric hepatoid carcinoma, which is a special subtype of gastric cancer having very aggressive evolution. As the number was not large enough, it is not possible to reach definite conclusions on such patients. Accumulation of more patients is warranted to make a more comprehensive study of this patient subpopulation.

To our knowledge, our study is the largest series from China to report on the simultaneous resection of gastric cancer and liver metastasis. Our conclusion is that patients with single liver metastasis and no peritoneal metastasis could have better prognosis after simultaneous resection of both lesions. Although this was a retrospective observational study without control group, the results could be helpful to form rational treatment approaches for such patients in China.

Liver metastasis is not the absolute contraindication for gastric cancer surgery, but the following conditions should be considered in selecting patients. First, the primary tumor could be resectable, and there should be no superclavicular lymph nodes metastases or abnominal aorta lymph nodes metastasis, no extrahepatic metastasis

Table 3 Multivariate Cox regression analysis

	HR	95% CI	P value
Peritoneal metastasis (P0 *vs* P1)	3.481	1.159-10.458	*0.026
Number of liver metastasis (1 *vs* 2–3)	2.262	1.056-5.349	*0.043

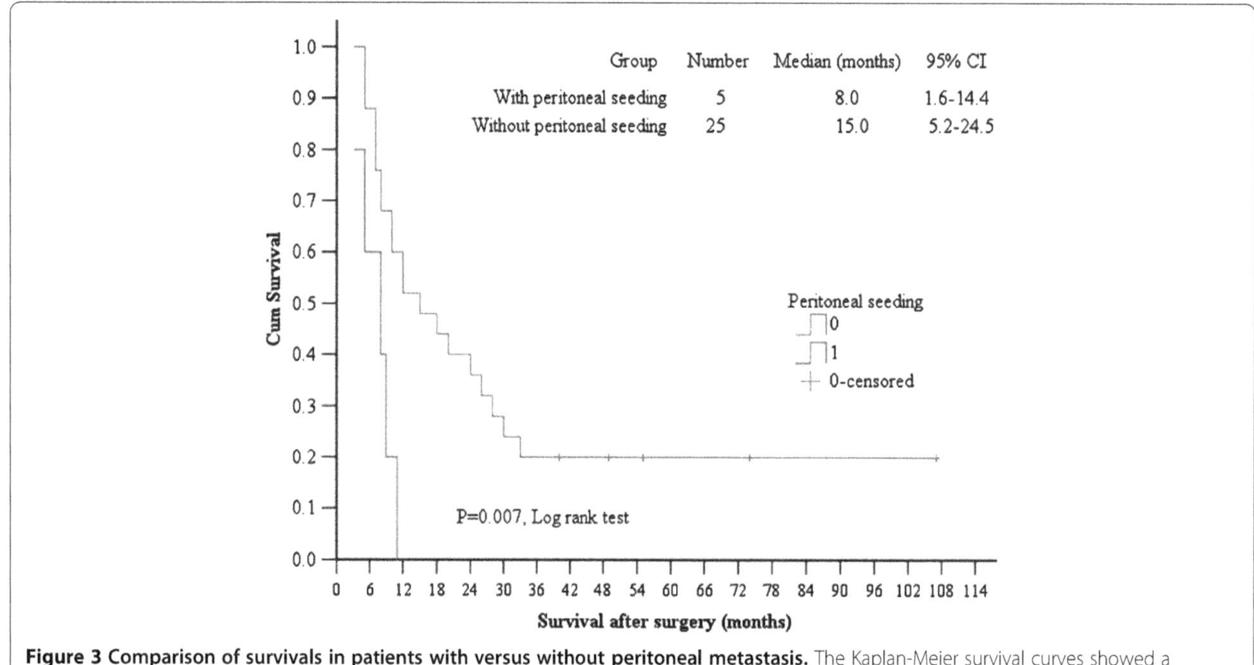

Figure 3 Comparison of survivals in patients with versus without peritoneal metastasis. The Kaplan-Meier survival curves showed a significantly shorter survival time in patients with versus without peritoneal metastasis.

or peritoneal metastasis. Secondly, there exists single liver metastatic lesion, or lesions confined to one lobe of the liver. Thirdly, the patient should have good organ function reserve, with basically normal cardiac, pulmonary, hepatic and renal functions. Absolute contraindications are extrahepatic metastases and unresectable liver metastases. Whether preoperative chemotherapy could be helpful to reduce liver metastasis or to enhance the possibility of a clean margin resection, we did not conduct any study on this point. Future work should consider this option.

Based on our results and literature study, we concluded the for gastric cancer patients with liver metastasis: (1) careful preoperative evaluation should be performed to consider if curative resection is possible, and laparoscopy could be considered if necessary; (2) for patients with synchronous single liver metastasis, curative resection should be the treatment of choice; (3) patients with peritoneal metastasis had poor survival; (4) preoperative tumor marker levels should not be the criteria to judge whether surgery should be performed; and (5) the pathological staging of the primary tumor does on have significant impact on postoperative survival.

Competing interests

The authors declare that they have no competing interests.

Authors' contributions

KTS, XYQ, YHS and JQ designed research; YNW, JQL, XDG and XFW conducted research; YYH provided pathological databases; YNW and XFW analyzed data or performed statistical analysis; YNW and KTS wrote paper; KTS had primary responsibility for final content; All authors read and approved the final manuscript.

Acknowledgements

This project was supported by the National Natural Science Foundation for Young Scholars of China (Grant No. 81101809).

Author details

[1]Department of General Surgery, Zhongshan Hospital of Fudan University, No 180 Fenglin Road, Shanghai 200032, China. [2]Department of Pathology, Zhongshan Hospital of Fudan University, No 180 Fenglin Road, Shanghai 200032, China.

References

1. Moon YH, Jeung HC, Rha SY, Yoo NC, Roh JK, Noh SH, Kim BS, Chung HC: **Changing patterns of prognosticators during 15-year follow-up of advanced gastric cancer after radial gastrectomy and adjuvant chemotherapy: a 15-year follow-up study at a single Korean institute.** *Ann Surg Oncol* 2007, **14**(10):2730–2737.
2. Ambiru S, Miyazaki M, Ito H, *et al*: **Benefits and limits of hepatic resection for gastric metastases.** *Am J Surg* 2001, **181**(3):279–83.
3. Garancini M, Uggeri F, Degrate L, *et al*: **Surgical treatment of liver metastases of gastric cancer: is local treatment in a systemic disease worthwhile?** *HPB (Oxford)* 2012, **14**(3):209–15.
4. Miki Y, Fujitani K, Hirao M, *et al*: **Significance of surgical treatment of liver metastases from gastric cancer.** *Anticancer Res* 2012, **32**(2):665–70.
5. Bines SD, England G, Deziel DJ, *et al*: **Synchronous, metachronous, and multiple hepatic resections of liver tumors originating from primary gastric tumors.** *Surgery* 1993, **114**(4):799–805.
6. Miyazaki M, Itoh H, Nakagawa K, *et al*: **Hepatic resection of liver metastases from gastric carcinoma.** *Am J Gastroenterol* 1997, **92**(3):490–3.
7. Ochiai T, Sasako M, Mizuno S, *et al*: **Hepatic resection for metastatic tumours from gastric cancer: analysis of prognostic factors.** *Br J Surg* 1994, **81**(8):1175–8.
8. Japanese Gastric Cancer A: **Japanese Classification of Gastric Carcinoma - 2nd English Edition.** *Gastric Cancer* 1998, **1**(1):10–24.
9. Edge SB, Compton CC: **The American Joint Committee on Cancer: the 7th edition of the AJCC cancer staging manual and the future of TNM.** *Ann Surg Oncol* 2010, **17**(6):1471–4.

10. Rafique M, Adachi W, Kajikawa S, *et al*: **Management of gastric cancer patients with synchronous hepatic metastasis: a retrospective study.** *Hepatogastroenterology* 1995, **42**(5):666–71.
11. Okano K, Maeba T, Ishimura K, *et al*: **Hepatic resection for metastatic tumors from gastric cancer.** *Ann Surg* 2002, **235**(1):86–91.
12. Sakamoto Y, Ohyama S, Yamamoto J, *et al*: **Surgical resection of liver metastases of gastric cancer: an analysis of a 17-year experience with 22 patients.** *Surgery* 2003, **133**(5):507–11.
13. Sakamoto Y, Sano T, Shimada K, *et al*: **Favorable indications for hepatectomy in patients with liver metastasis from gastric cancer.** *J Surg Oncol* 2007, **95**(7):534–9.
14. Imamura H, Matsuyama Y, Shimada R, *et al*: **A study of factors influencing prognosis after resection of hepatic metastases from colorectal and gastric carcinoma.** *Am J Gastroenterol* 2001, **96**(11):3178–84.
15. Elias D, Cavalcanti De Albuquerque A, Eggenspieler P, *et al*: **Resection of liver metastases from a noncolorectal primary: indications and results based on 147 monocentric patients.** *J Am Coll Surg* 1998, **187**(5):487–93.
16. Shirabe K, Shimada M, Matsumata T, *et al*: **Analysis of the prognostic factors for liver metastasis of gastric cancer after hepatic resection: a multi-institutional study of the indications for resection.** *Hepatogastroenterology* 2003, **50**(53):1560–3.
17. Tiberio GAM, Coniglio A, Marchet A, Marrelli D, Giacopuzzi S, Baiocchi L, Roviello F, de Manzoni G, Nitti D, Giulini SM: **Metachronous hepatic metastases from gastric carcinoma: A multicentric survey.** *EJSO.* 2009, **35**(5):486–491.
18. Dicken BJ, Bigam DL, Cass C, *et al*: **Gastric adenocarcinoma: review and considerations for future directions.** *Ann Surg* 2005, **241**(1):27–39.
19. Liu J, Li JH, Zhai RJ, *et al*: **Predictive factors improving survival after gastric and hepatic surgical treatment in gastric cancer patients with synchronous liver metastases.** *Chin Med J.* 2012, **125**(2):165–71.
20. Cheon SH, Rha SY, Jeung HC, *et al*: **Survival benefit of combined curative resection of the stomach (D2 resection) and liver in gastric cancer patients with liver metastases.** *Ann Oncol* 2008, **19**(6):1146–53.
21. Ueda K, Iwahashi M, Nakamori M, *et al*: **Analysis of the prognostic factors and evaluation of surgical treatment for synchronous liver metastases from gastric cancer.** *Langenbecks Arch Surg* 2009, **394**(4):647–53.

12

Jejunal obstruction due to a variant of transmesocolic hernia: a rare presentation of an acute abdomen

Duminda Subasinghe[1], Chathuranga Tisara Keppetiyagama[2] and Dharmabandhu N Samarasekera[3*]

Abstract

Background: Internal hernias include paraduodenal, pericecal, through foramen of Winslow, intersigmoid and retroanastomotic hernias. These hernias could be either congenital or acquired after abdominal surgery. They account for approximately 0.5-5 % of all cases of intestinal obstruction.

Case presentation: A 48-year-old female was admitted to casualty with a history of abdominal distension and vomiting of 3 days duration. An abdominal X-ray supine film showed multiple small bowel loops with air fluid levels. On surgery she was found to have a transmesocolic hernia. The defect in the transverse mesocolon was repaired.

Conclusion: The clinical signs and symptoms of lesser sac hernia are non-specific. These rare lesser sac hernias can be lethal. Therefore, immediate diagnosis and surgery is essential. Although a rare entity, they account for significant mortality form intestinal obstruction. We report an extremely rare case of an internal abdominal hernia through the transverse mesocolon, in a young woman.

Keywords: Internal hernia, Transmesocolic, Intestinal obstruction

Background

Internal hernia is protrusion of a viscus or part of a viscus through anatomical or pathological opening within the limits of peritoneal cavity. They could be either congenital or acquired. There are several main types of internal hernias based on the location as described by Meyers [1]. Specifically these include paraduodenal, pericecal, foramen of Winslow, transmesocolic, inter sigmoid and retroanastomotic hernias. Although the overall incidence of internal hernias are low (0.2–0.9 %) and they accounts only for 0.5 %–5 % of cases of intestinal obstruction, the overall mortality exceeds 50 % if strangulation is present [2, 3]. Transmesocolic hernia is an extremely rare type of internal hernia. Transmesocolic hernia accounts for approximately 5–10 % of all internal hernias [4]. The defects of the mesentery are mostly due to congenital, surgical, traumatic, inflammatory or idiopathic in origin. Although a rare entity, they account for significant mortality form intestinal obstruction. Usually these are detected during surgery for acute abdomen or during an autopsy [5].

Case presentation

We report a case of transmesocolic herniation of jejunal loops into supracolic compartment with intestinal obstruction which was diagnosed intraoperatively.

A 48-year-old female was admitted to casualty with a history of abdominal distension and vomiting of 3 days duration. She had no past history of any gastrointestinal surgery but had undergone lower segment caesarean section 21 years earlier. The caesarean section was uneventful without any iatrogenic injury. On admission, she had bilious vomiting. Physical examination revealed tachycardia, generalized abdominal distension, rebound tenderness and rigidity over left upper quadrant. There was no evidence of organomegaly or free fluid and her external hernia orifices were normal. Her bowel sounds

* Correspondence: samarasekera58@yahoo.co.uk
[3]University Surgical Unit, The National Hospital of Sri Lanka, 28/1, Ishwari road, Colombo 06 Colombo, Sri Lanka
Full list of author information is available at the end of the article

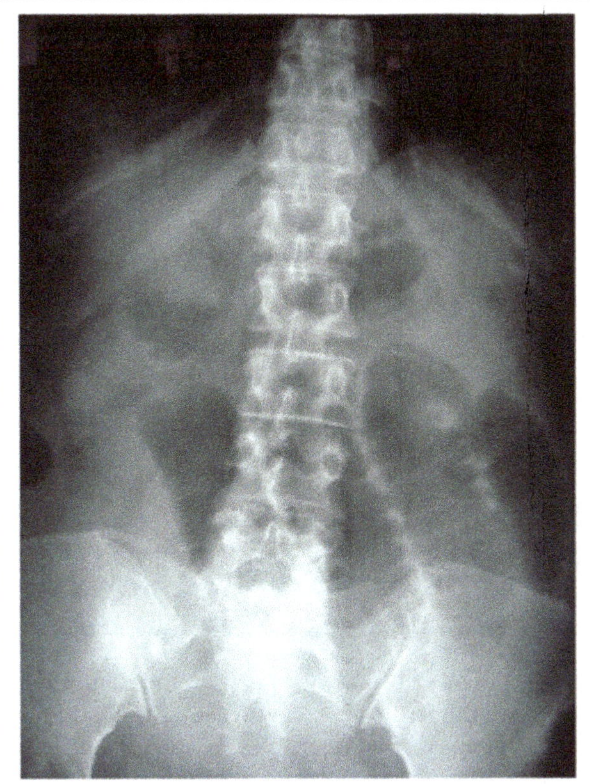

Fig. 1 Dilated jejunal loops on X ray abdomen supine film

were sluggish. Digital rectal examination revealed an empty rectum. Laboratory investigation on admission revealed a normal full blood count with a white blood cell count of 5000/mm3 and normal renal and liver functions. Her serum potassium on admission was 3.5 mmol/l and she was started in intravenous potassium supplements. An abdominal X-ray supine film showed multiple small bowel loops with air fluid levels without free air under the dome of the diaphragm (Fig. 1). Surgical exploration revealed significant amount of free fluid in the peritoneal cavity and ischemic small intestine. On further exploration, we found the DJ flexure in the supracolic compartment and almost all the jejunum and proximal ileum herniating through a small defect about 5 × 6 cm in the transverse mesocolon. Jejunal loops were contained inside a thick walled hernial sac (Fig. 2) which was extending in to the supracolic compartment. The hernia sac with contents was extending into the lesser sac. The contents were reduced and the sac was opened and repaired (Fig. 3). Paraduodenal fossae were found to be normal during the surgery (Fig. 4). The defect in the transverse mesocolon was repaired. Small bowel showed features of viability and therefore, was not resected. The patient was discharged on post operative day 14. Her post operative period was uneventful. She also underwent a contrast study of the small bowel at post op day 10 which showed normal small intestine (Fig. 5).

Discussion and conclusion

The clinical signs and symptoms of lesser sac hernia are non-specific and include abdominal pain, nausea, vomiting and distension. These rare lesser sac hernias can be lethal. Therefore, immediate diagnosis and surgery is essential. In the literature, only few cases of internal hernias have been documented [6]. The anomaly of transmesocolic herniation, which was first reported by Rokitansky in 1836 is an extremely rare type of internal hernia [2]. According to the literature, herniation into the lesser

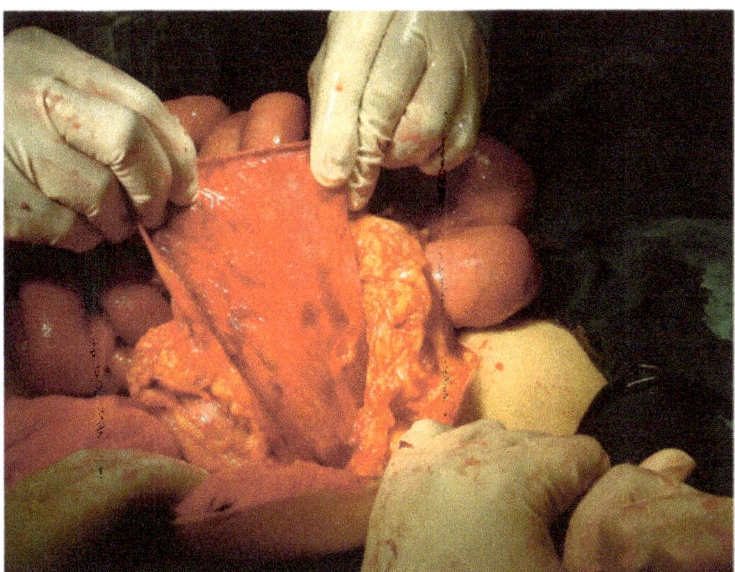

Fig. 2 Sac of the transmesocolic hernia

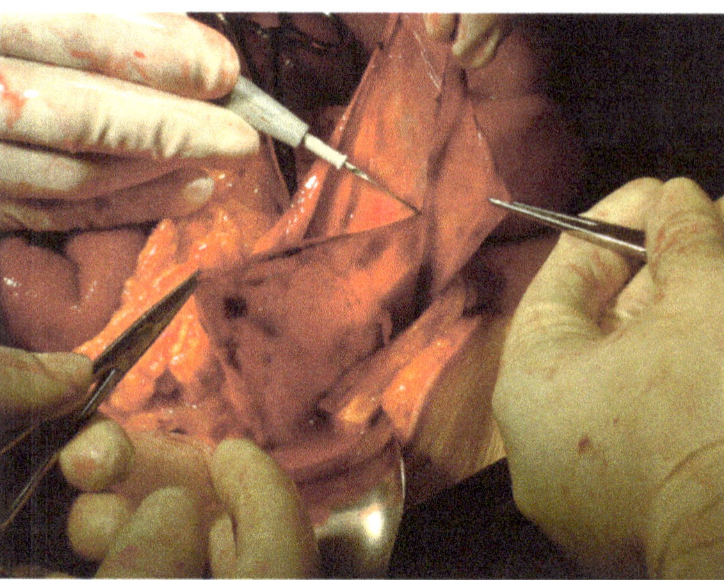

Fig. 3 opening and repair of the hernia sac in the supracolic compartment

sac can be classified into three basic types according to the site of the aperture [7, 8]. Type 1 is a hernia through the foramen of Winslow, type 2 is a hernia through a defect in the lesser or greater omentum and type 3 is a hernia through a defect in the transverse mesocolon. Our patient had type 3 transmesocolic hernia. Type 3 is usually secondary to abdominal trauma or prior abdominal surgery with the creation of a Roux-en-Y loop [9, 10]. Approximately 5–10 % of all internal hernias occur through defects in the mesentery of the small bowel and almost 35 % of transmesocolic hernias are observed among paediatric age group, mainly those aged between 3 and 10 years [3]. In adults, however most mesenteric defects are the result of previous gastrointestinal operations, abdominal trauma or intra peritoneal inflammation [11–13]. Our case was a rare presentation in an adult without a history of trauma or previous bowel surgery. Gomes et al. [3] and described a patient with congenital transmesenteric type internal hernia presented with intractable colick epigastric pain. Frediani et al. [6] has described a transmesocolic hernia presented with small intestinal obstruction. Agresta et al. [4] has described two patients presented with acute small intestinal obstruction due to internal hernia during

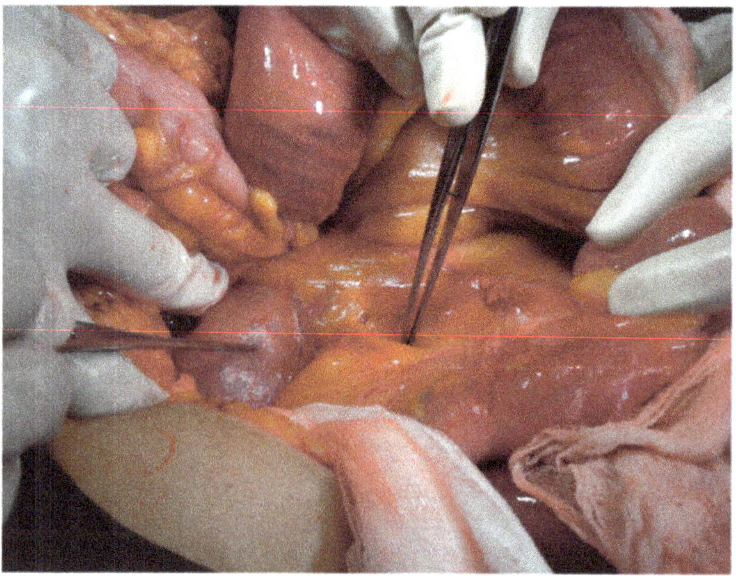

Fig. 4 Paraduodenal fossa

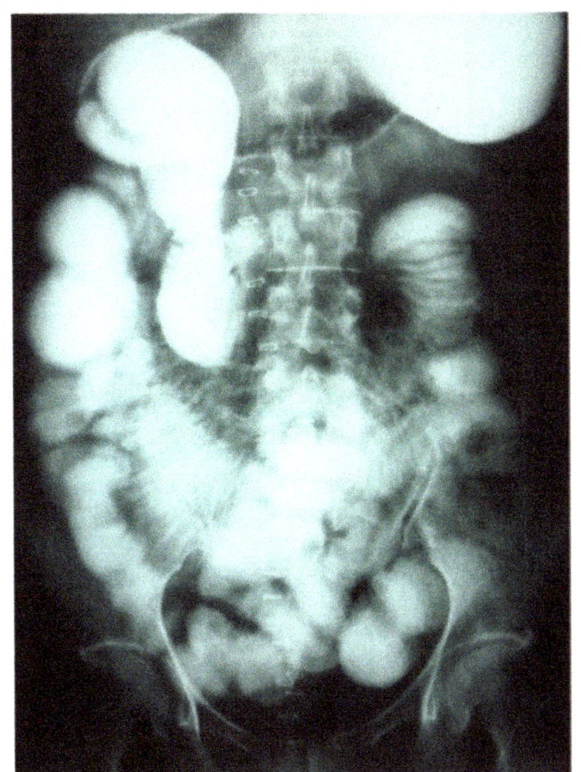

Fig. 5 Post operative barium meal and follow through showing normal small intestines

immediate post operative period following laparoscopic hernia repair.

Although tansmesocolic hernia is a difficult preoperative diagnosis, CT abdomen might help the diagnosis by peripherally located small bowel, and lack of omental fat between the loops and the anterior abdominal wall [14, 15]. Congenital tansmesocolic hernias are extremely rare and todate only few cases of transmesocolic hernias were reported in the literature [3, 6, 16].

In conclusion, diagnosis of intestinal obstruction caused by a congenital mesocolic hernia remains difficult preoperatively despite the techniques currently available, so it is important to consider the possibility of a transmesocolic hernia in a patient with ileus even with no past history of gastrointestinal surgery.

Competing interests
The authors declare that they have no competing interests.

Authors' contributions
All authors contributed to management of the patient and contributed equally towards drafting of the manuscript. DNS and DS provided overall supervision and edited the final version of the manuscript. All authors have read and approved the final manuscript.

Acknowledgement
The authors acknowledge all the ward staff who took care of our patient.

Author details
[1]General Surgery, University Surgical Unit, The National Hospital of Sri Lanka, Colombo, Sri Lanka. [2]Gastrointestinal Surgery, University Surgical Unit, The National Hospital of Sri Lanka, Colombo, Sri Lanka. [3]University Surgical Unit, The National Hospital of Sri Lanka, 28/1, Ishwari road, Colombo 06 Colombo, Sri Lanka.

References

1. Meyers MA. Dynamic radiology of the abdomen:normal and pathologic anatomy. 4th ed. New York, NY: Springer; 1994.
2. Newsom BD, Kukora JS. Congenital and acquired internal hernias: unusual causes of small bowel obstruction. Am J Surg. 1986;152:279–85.
3. Gomes R, Rodrigues J. Spontaneous adult transmesenteric hernia with bowel gangrene. Hernia. 2011;15:343–5.
4. Agresta F, Mazzarolo G, Bedin N. Incarcerated internal hernia of the small intestine through a re-approximated peritoneum after a trans-abdominal pre-peritoneal procedure – apropos of two cases: review of the literature. Hernia. 2011;15:347–50.
5. Parsons PB. Paraduodenal hernias. Am J Roentgenol Radium Ther Nucl Med. 1953;69:563–89.
6. Frediani S, Almberger M, Iaconelli R, Avventurieri G, Manganaro F. An unusual case of congenital mesocolic hernia. Hernia. 2010;14:105–7.
7. Li JC, Chu DW, Lee DW, Chan AC. Small-bowel intestinal obstruction caused by an unusual internal hernia. Asian J Surg. 2005;28:62–4.
8. Okayasu K, Tamamoto F, Nakanishi A, Takanashi T, Maehara T. A case of incarcerated lesser sac hernia protruding simultaneously through both the gastrocolic and gastrohepatic omenta. Radiat Med. 2002;20:105–7.
9. Blachar A, Federle MP, Dodson SF. Internal hernia: clinical and imaging findings in 17 patients with emphasis on CT criteria. Radiology. 2001;218:68–74.
10. Blachar A, Federle MP, Brancatelli G, Peterson MS, Oliver 3rd JH, Li W. Radiologist performance in the diagnosis of internal hernia by using specific CT findings with emphasis on transmesenteric hernia. Radiology. 2001;221:422–8.
11. Uchiyama S, Imamura N, Hidaka H, Maehara N, Nagaike K, Ikenaga N, et al. An unusual variant of a left paraduodenal hernia diagnosed and treated by laparoscopic surgery: report of a case. Surg Today. 2009;39:533–5.
12. Shaffner Lde S, Pennell TC. Congenital internal hernia. Surg Clin North Am. 1971;51:1355–9.
13. Mock CJ, Mock Jr HE. Strangulated internal hernia associated with trauma. AMA Arch Surg. 1958;77:881–6.
14. Tauro LF, Vijaya G, D'Souza CR, Ramesh HC, Shetty SR, Hegde BR. Mesocolic hernia: an unusual internal hernia. Saudi J Gastroenterol. 2007;13:141–3.
15. Blachar A, Federle MP. Internal hernia: an increasingly common cause of small bowel obstruction. Semin Ultrasound CT MR. 2002;23:174–83.
16. Wu SY, Ho MH, Hsu SD. Meckel's diverticulum incarcerated in a transmesocolic internal hernia. World J Gastroenterol. 2014;20(37):13615–9.

Heterotopic pancreas in excluded stomach diagnosed after gastric bypass surgery

Marta Guimarães[1†], Pedro Rodrigues[1†], Gil Gonçalves[1], Mário Nora[1] and Mariana P Monteiro[2,3*]

Abstract

Background: Heterotopic pancreas is defined as finding of pancreatic tissue without anatomic and vascular continuity with the normal pancreas. Heterotopic pancreas is a rare condition difficult to diagnose and with controversial clinical management.

Case presentation: We describe a 43 year old female patient previously submitted to laparoscopic gastric bypass for primary treatment of morbid obesity; 5 years later, the patient was discovered to have a mass in the antrum of the excluded stomach that was found to be heterotopic pancreatic tissue. Before gastric bypass surgery, the presence of the pancreatic mass in the gastric wall was unnoticed in the imagiologic records.

Conclusion: This is the first reported case of pancreatic heterotopy diagnosed in the excluded stomach after gastric bypass. A putative role of incretin hormones in mediating pancreatic cell hyperplasia of heterotopic pancreatic remnants should be considered an additional hypothesis that requires further research.

Keywords: Heterotopic pancreas, Gastric bypass, Excluded stomach, Incretins

Background

Heterotopic pancreas was first described in 1727 by Schultz and is defined as the presence of pancreatic tissue whithout anatomic and vascular continuity with the normal pancreas [1]. It is found in 0.55-15% of autopsy specimens [2] being more common at the age of 30–50 years with a male predominance [3]. The heterotopic tissue can be found anywhere from the distal end of the esophagus to the colon, but mostly occurs in upper gastrointestinal tract: stomach(25%), duodenum(30%) and jejunum(15%), but also in liver, gallbladder, distal small intestine, colon, appendix, omentum, fallopian tube, common bile duct, cystic duct, ampulla of Vater, spleen, lymph nodes and Meckel's diverticula. Extra-abdominal sites included mediastinal cysts, bronchi, lung, umbilicus and brain [4-8]. The most common heterotopic site is the stomach (25-40%), especially antrum and prepyloric region on the greater curvature or posterior wall [9].

* Correspondence: mpmonteiro@icbas.up.pt
†Equal contributors
2Endocrinology Unit of Hospital São Sebastião, Hospital de São Sebastião, Santa Maria da Feira, Portugal
3Department of Anatomy, Multidisciplinary Unit for Biomedical Research (UMIB), ICBAS, University of Porto, Porto, Portugal
Full list of author information is available at the end of the article

Heterotopic pancreas is thought to take place when the foregut rotates between weeks 5 and 8 of gestation, while pancreatic fragments detach from the pancreas and are deposited ectopically [10]. Heterotopic pancreatic tissue in the gastro-intestinal tract generally occurs as discrete firm, irregular, yellow nodules located in the submucosa. Histologically heterotopic pancreatic tissue is not a true neoplasm but rather a hamartoma of fat glandular tissue with pancreatic acinar formation and duct development [8]. In the majority of cases the patients are asymptomatic and the condition is incidentally discovered [11]. Almost all changes which can occur in the pancreas itself may develop in heterotopic pancreas [12], although malignant transformation is extremely rare [10].

There are several cases of heterotopic pancreases described in the literature, but to date none of them was diagnosed in the excluded stomach after gastric bypass.

Case presentation

A 43 years old female patient was previously submitted to laparoscopic gastric bypass for morbid obesity without co-morbidities. Seven months after the bariatric surgery the patient showed intense episodic epigastric abdominal pain that was aggravated by food ingestion and led to multiple visits to the emergency room.

One month after the onset of pain complaints, the patient was offered hospital admission for further evaluation. Physical examination was unremarkable and routine blood assessment of liver and pancreatic functions were normal. The upper endoscopy and esophageal-gastro-jejunal transit were normal; the abdominal CT and MRI were considered normal despite the presence of a mass in the excluded stomach, as it was ascribed to the anatomical rearrangement after the bypass surgery (Figure 1A). During hospital stay the patient did present any evidence of abdominal pain, complaints or need for analgesia; after formal psychiatric evaluation, a major depression was diagnosed and the patient was started on anti-depressants.

Five years after gastric bypass, due to ongoing epigastric pain complaints, abdominal CT and MRI were repeated, with subsequent diagnosis of a 4.5 cm of greater diameter subserosal neoplasm in the antrum (Figure 1B).

The patient underwent laparoscopic gastrectomy of the excluded stomach for suspected gastrointestinal stromal tumor (GIST) (Figure 2A). Gross examination of the specimen revealed a subserosal polypoid mass in the gastric antrum, which corresponded to a 4.5 cm cystic cavity of greater diameter with creamy yellowish thick content, growing in dependency of the gastric muscular layer (Figure 2B). The histology of the mass showed a flap of gastric wall with antral mucosa and a heterotopic pancreatic cist, while in the adipose tissue of the root of the greater omentum six other yellow and lobulated nodules were identified and dissected. All fragments corresponded histologicaly to pancreatic tissue with normal exocrine and endocrine distribution, as displayed by the immunohistochemistry staining for chromogranin A, insulin and glucagon expressing cells, as well as a low proliferation index as revealed by the Ki-67 staining, which are characteristic of the normal pancreatic tissue (Figure 3, A-F). After gastrectomy, the patient became asymptomatic and so has remained ever since.

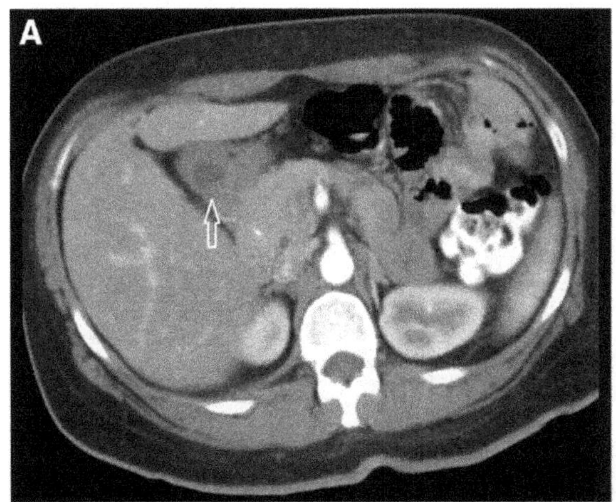

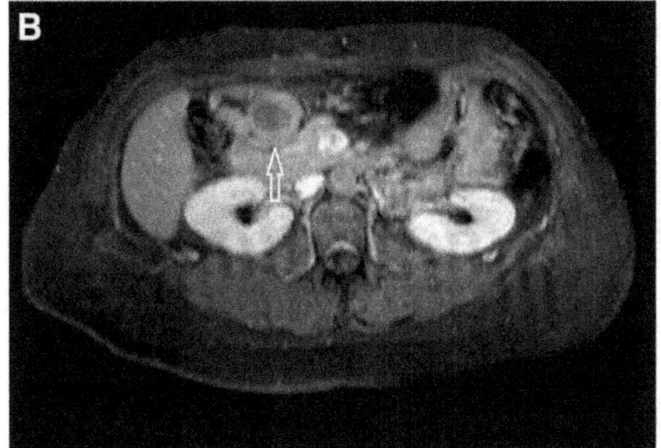

Figure 1 Abdominal MRI shortly after (A) and 5 years after gastric bypass (B) displaying the subserosal mass in the gastric antrum (arrows), the former previously unnoticed.

Discussion

Most patients with heterotopic pancreas are asymptomatic; when present, the reported symptoms include abdominal pain, epigastric discomfort, bleeding, nausea and vomiting; sometimes symptoms are related to complications, such as mechanical occlusion - intussusceptions and obstruction of the small bowel, obstructive jaundice and pyloric stenosis [8,13]. Other complications include: pancreatitis, pseudocyst formation, carcinomas, islet-cell tumors and inflammatory pseudotumors [6]. Most cases of gastric heterotopic pancreas are incidental findings during surgery, gastrointestinal exam or autopsy.

The differential diagnosis includes GIST, gastrointestinal autonomic nerve tumor (GANT), carcinoid, lymphoma or gastric carcinoma which can be misinterpreted on imaging studies or endoscopic examinations [14,15].

Since heterotopic pancreas is an uncommon condition, unlike GIST, it is rarely considered a diagnostic hypothesis. Five CT features were pointed as significant predictors in the differential diagnosis of heterotopic pancreas from GIST and leiomyomas, namely: 1) prominent enhancement of the overlying mucosa, 2) location, 3) long diameter/short diameter ratio of the lesion, 4) growth pattern and 5) lesion border [16]. At endoscopy the heterotopic pancreas generally appears as a well-defined dome-shaped filling defect with central umbilication. Definitive diagnosis requires histological confirmation.

Management of this condition is controversial. Most cases undergo surgery due to diagnostic uncertainty. Reasons for surgical treatment depend on the presence of symptoms, as well as need of definitive diagnosis, excluding malignancy or avoiding complications [17].

This patient had both normal abdominal ultrasound and gastroduodenoscopy before gastric bypass, and the presence of a mass in the excluded stomach had been unnoticed in the abdominal CT and MRI performed four years before gastrectomy. In the herein case presented, GIST of the excluded stomach was the first diagnostic

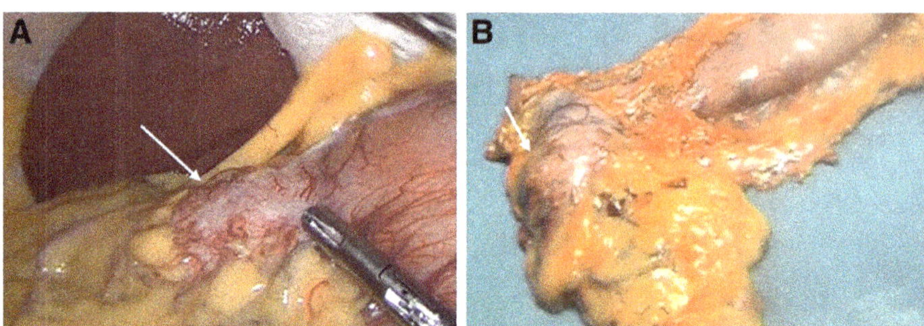

Figure 2 Macroscopic appearance of the subserosal mass at laparoscopy (A) and in the excluded stomach removed after partial gastrectomy (white arrows) (B).

hypothesis, due to the previous history of gastric bypass, endoscopic ultra-sound (EUS) could not be useful.

There was no evidence of acute pancreatitis in any recurrency of episodic abdominal pain that lead patient to visit the emergency room, as suggested from serum amylase and lipase levels, however, since the heterotopic pancreas included a cystic cavity with a thick liquid content, the formation of a cyst in result of retention of exocrine secretions in the absence of communication between the glandular epithelium and the gastric lumen cannot be excluded.

Gastric bypass is known to induce changes in the secretion of insulinotropic enteric hormones, which may be involved in metabolic changes, remission of diabetes mellitus [18,19] and have a role in inducing pancreatic exocrine and endocrine cell proliferation [20]. Thus, it is conceivable that microscopic heterotopic nodules of pancreatic tissue can grow in result of gastric bypass surgery, similarly to what has been hypothesized to occur with regards to orthotic pancreatic tissue. Notwithstanding, the action of incretin hormones in stimulation the growth of pancreatic tissue still needs further research.

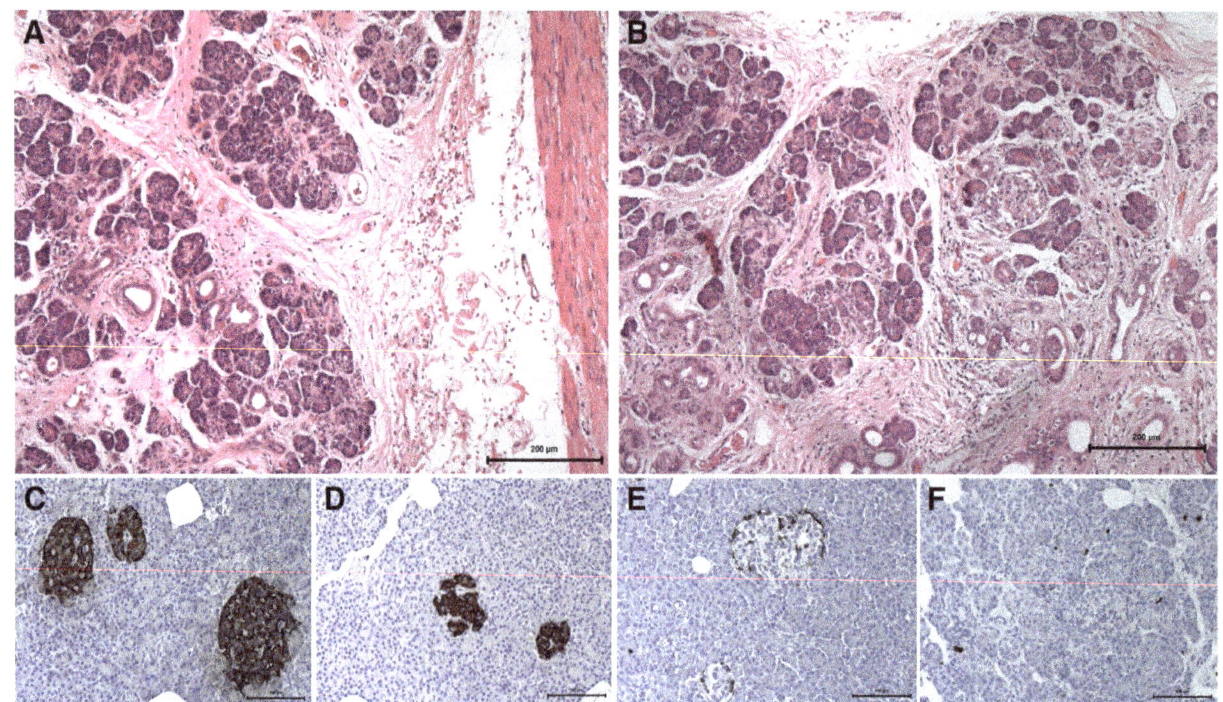

Figure 3 Histology of the muscular gastric wall and the normal heterotopic pancreatic tissue in the subserosa (A) and tissue nodule in the omentum (B), with respective imunostaining for the neuro-endocrine markers chromogranin A (C), insulin (D) and glucagon (E), showing normal exocrine pancreas and Langerhans islets, with normal distribution of neuroendocrine cells, as well as insulin and glucagon expressing cells; the proliferation index was also normally low as displayed by the Ki-67 staining (F) (immune staining in brown).

Conclusion

Heterotopic pancreas is a rare condition, difficult to diagnose and with controversial management. We present the first case of pancreatic heterotopy diagnosed after gastric bypass surgery. The role of incretin hormones in stimulating the growth of pancreatic cells and its consequences justifies further investigation.

Abbreviations

CT: Computed tomography; EUS: Endoscopic ultra-sound; GANT: Gastrointestinal autonomic nerve tumor; GIST: Gastrointestinal stromal tumor; MRI: Magnetic resonance Imaging.

Competing interests

The authors declare that they have no competing interests.

Authors' contributions

MG, PR, MN, GG have been made substantial contributions to diagnosis and treatment of the patient; MPM contributed with patient data analysis and interpretation; MG and MPM wrote the manuscript. All authors read and approved the final manuscript.

Acknowledgements

The authors acknowledge the contributions of Madalena Costa, Sofia Pereira and Tiago Morais ICBAS-UP, for technical support with histology and immunohistochemistry of the pancreatic tissue as well as picture art work. UMIB is funded by grants from FCT POCTI/FEDERFcomp-01-0124-FEDER-015893.

Author details

[1]Department of General Surgery, Hospital de São Sebastião, Santa Maria da Feira, Portugal. [2]Endocrinology Unit of Hospital São Sebastião, Hospital de São Sebastião, Santa Maria da Feira, Portugal. [3]Department of Anatomy, Multidisciplinary Unit for Biomedical Research (UMIB), ICBAS, University of Porto, Porto, Portugal.

References

1. Guillou L, Nordback P, Gerber C, Schneider RP: **Ductal adenocarcinoma arising in a heterotopic pancreas situated in a hiatal hernia.** *Arch Pathol Lab Med* 1994, **118**(5):568–571.
2. Hill I, Lebenthal E: **Congenital abnormalities of the exocrine pancreas.** In *The Pancreas: Biology, Pathobiology and Disease.* New York: Raven; 1993:1029–1040.
3. Mulholland KC, Wallace WD, Epanomeritakis E, Hall SR: **Pseudocyst formation in gastric ectopic pancreas.** *JOP* 2004, **5**(6):498–501.
4. Caberwal D, Kogan SJ, Levitt SB: **Ectopic pancreas presenting as an umbilical mass.** *J Pediatr Surg* 1977, **12**(4):593–599.
5. Heller RS, Tsugu H, Nabeshima K, Madsen OD: **Intracranial ectopic pancreatic tissue.** *Islets* 2010, **2**(2):65–71.
6. Jaschke W, Aleksic M, Aleksic D: **Heterotopic pancreatic tissue in a bronchogenic cyst-diagnosis and therapy.** *Thorac Cardiovasc Surg* 1982, **30**(1):58–60.
7. Szabados S, Lenard L, Tornoczky T, Varady E, Verzar Z: **Ectopic pancreas tissue appearing in a mediastinal cyst.** *J Cardiothorac Surg* 2012, **7**:22.
8. Wang C, Kuo Y, Yeung K, Wu C, Liu G: **CT appearance of ectopic pancreas: a case report.** *Abdom Imaging* 1998, **23**(3):332–333.
9. Papaziogas B, Koutelidakis I, Tsiaousis P, Panagiotopoulou K, Paraskevas G, Argiriadou H, Atmatzidis S, Atmatzidis K: **Carcinoma developing in ectopic pancreatic tissue in the stomach: a case report.** *Cases J* 2008, **1**(1):249.
10. Seifert G: **Congenital anomalies.** In *Pancreatic pathology.* Edited by Klöppel G, Heitz PU. London: Churchill Livingstone; 1984:69–94.
11. Armstrong CP, King PM, Dixon JM, Macleod IB: **The clinical significance of heterotopic pancreas in the gastrointestinal tract.** *Br J Surg* 1981, **68**(6):384–387.
12. Huang YC, Chen HM, Jan YY, Huang TL, Chen MF: **Ectopic pancreas with gastric outlet obstruction: report of two cases and literature review.** *Chang Gung Med J* 2002, **25**(7):485–490.
13. Megibow AJ, Balthazar EJ, Cho KC, Medwid SW, Birnbaum BA, Noz ME: **Bowel obstruction: evaluation with CT.** *Radiology* 1991, **180**(2):313–318.
14. O'Reilly DJ, Craig RM, Lorenzo G, Yokoo H: **Heterotopic pancreas mimicking carcinoma of the head of the pancreas: a rare cause of obstructive jaundice.** *J Clin Gastroenterol* 1983, **5**(2):165–168.
15. Christodoulidis G, Zacharoulis D, Barbanis S, Katsogridakis E, Hatzitheofilou K: **Heterotopic pancreas in the stomach: a case report and literature review.** *World J Gastroenterol* 2007, **13**(45):6098–6100.
16. Kim JY, Lee JM, Kim KW, Park HS, Choi JY, Kim SH, Kim MA, Lee JY, Han JK, Choi BI: **Ectopic pancreas: CT findings with emphasis on differentiation from small gastrointestinal stromal tumor and leiomyoma.** *Radiology* 2009, **252**(1):92–100.
17. Ura H, Denno R, Hirata K, Saeki A, Natori H: **Carcinoma arising from ectopic pancreas in the stomach: endosonographic detection of malignant change.** *J Clin Ultrasound* 1998, **26**(5):265–268.
18. Kashyap SR, Daud S, Kelly KR, Gastaldelli A, Win H, Brethauer S, Kirwan JP, Schauer PR: **Acute effects of gastric bypass versus gastric restrictive surgery on beta-cell function and insulinotropic hormones in severely obese patients with type 2 diabetes.** *Int J Obes (Lond)* 2010, **34**(3):462–471.
19. Nora M, Guimaraes M, Almeida R, Martins P, Goncalves G, Freire MJ, Ferreira T, Freitas C, Monteiro MP: **Metabolic laparoscopic gastric bypass for obese patients with type 2 diabetes.** *Obes Surg* 2011, **21**(11):1643–1649.
20. Butler AE, Campbell-Thompson M, Gurlo T, Dawson DW, Atkinson M, Butler PC: **Marked expansion of exocrine and endocrine pancreas with incretin therapy in humans with increased exocrine pancreas dysplasia and the potential for glucagon-producing neuroendocrine tumors.** *Diabetes* 2013, **62**(7):2595–2604.

Local recurrence of gastric cancer after total gastrectomy: an unusual presentation

Bruno Martella[1*], Fabrizio Cardin[1], Renata Lorenzetti[1], Claudio Terranova[2], Bruno Amato[3], Carmelo Militello[1]

From XXV National Congress of the Italian Society of Geriatric Surgery
Padova, Italy. 10-11 May 2012

Abstract

A 71 years old Italian man had type 3 gastric cancer of the greater curvature. Total gastrectomy with splenectomy and D2 lymph node dissection were performed. After discharge chemotherapy ELF regimen was administred for 6 months. After 16 months from the operation a local recurrence was discovered by CT scan. Surgical en-bloc resection was performed removing pancreatic tail, splenic colic flexure and a portion of left diaphragm. Histological examination confirmed local recurrence of gastric adenocarcinoma infiltrating pancreas, colon and diaphragm with lymph node metastasis.

Introduction

In Western countries gastric cancer still represents a disabling disease: unfortunately late diagnosis is common and loco-regional recurrence rate after surgery alone is high especially in patients with advanced stage disease at the time of diagnosis (gastric wall penetration and lymph node metastasis). Local recurrence may occur also in those patient which had R0 resection: management of these cases is extremely difficult for the involvement of regional structures resulting in poor surgical chances. Therefore multidisciplinary therapeutic approach is necessary to achieve better results. The aim of this report is to refer about an unusual presentation of local relapse in an old patient submitted to a total gastrectomy in which surgical approach permitted a good control of the disease.

Case report

Male, 71 years old; on July 27, 2004, he was submitted to total gastrectomy with splenectomy and lymph-node dissection (D2) for an ulcerated adenocarcinoma of the greater curvature of the upper third of the stomach. Roux-en-Y stapled esofago-jejunoanastomosis was performed and oral food intake resumed in 7th post-operative day after X-ray control with hydro-soluble contrast. Hospital stay was prolonged by left basal pneumonia associated to pleural effusion; discharge occurred after one month. Histological examination demonstrated an adenocarcinoma (Laurèn intestinal type, Ming infiltrating type) extended to all layers of gastric wall and metastasis to greater curvature lymph-nodes (station 4 of JGCA) [1]; the others stations of JGCA (from 1 to 12, excluded 4) were non metastatic (43 lymph-nodes were examined); it was stage IIIA according to TNM classification (T3 N1 M0) [2]. After discharge chemotherapy was given (Etoposide/Leucovorin/5-fluorouracil, ELF-regimen) from September 2004 to March 2005. Follow-up was uneventful till December 2005. In this period patient suffered of left hypochondriac pain, mild dyspnoea and anorexia. Esophagojejunoscopy was unremarkable. X-Ray confirmed left basal pleural effusion; blood examination resulted only in CEA increase (19.3 ug/L). CT scan demonstrated a bulk in splenic area of about 8 cm in diameter and infiltrating pancreatic tail with adhesions to left diaphragm, left colic flexure and left kidney fascia (Fig. 1). On 7 February 2006, he was submitted to explorative laparotomy that confirmed CT scan report. The bulk was resected en-bloc with pancreatic tail, left colic flexure, a portion of left diaphragm and kidney fascia; bowel continuity was restored by side-to-side stapled anastomosis; diaphragm was directly sutured (Fig. 2). Accurate inspection of abdominal cavity excluded others localizations of the disease. Post-operative period was uneventful as regards surgical problems. Angina attack compared in 9th post-operative day;

* Correspondence: bruno.martella@sanita.padova.it
[1]Department of Molecular Medicine, University of Padua, Italy
Full list of author information is available at the end of the article

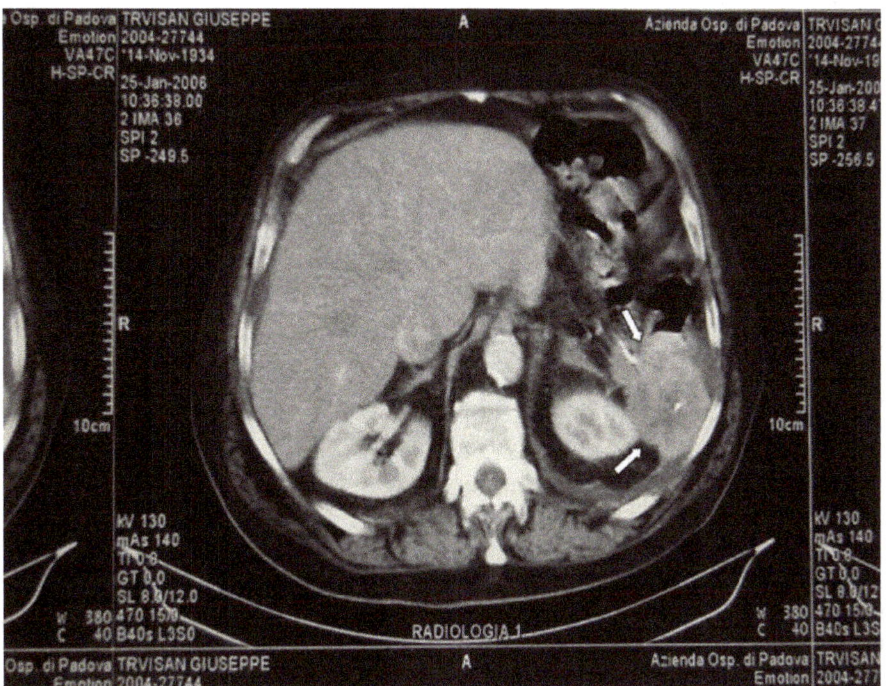

Figure 1 CT scan demonstrating a bulk in splenic area of about 8 cm in diameter and infiltrating pancreatic tail with adhesions to left diaphragm, left colic flexure and left kidney fascia.

after resolution of this complication patient was discharged. Histological examination resulted in poor differentiated gastric carcinoma infiltrating colic wall and pancreas with metastasis in one of nine peri-colic lymphnodes examinated.

Discussion

Loco-regional recurrence and distant metastases are common events after surgery for gastric adenocarcinoma.

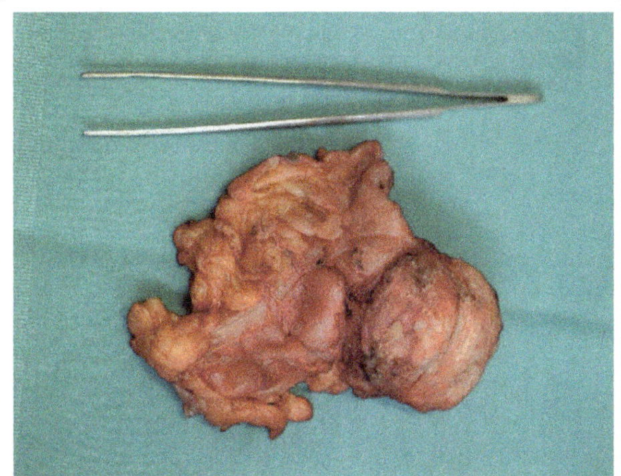

Figure 2 Surgical specimen comprehensive of the bulk resected en-bloc with pancreatic tail, left colic flexure, a portion of left diaphragm and kidney fascia.

Abdominal extraluminal recurrence of gastric cancer is a disarmimg condition because of poor therapeutic chances. Generally it is a matter of peritoneal carcinosis or multiple liver metastasis; in these cases surgery has little opportunities to be useful. Literature reports rare cases of single localization in abdominal cavity that may be resected. Menzel [3] reported a case of infrarenal aortic aneurysm whose detection permitted to discover gastric carcinoma. A similar condition is reported by Shimoyama [4] who diagnosed gastric cancer after nephroureterectomy for hydronephrosis due to ureteral metastasis. Imachi [5] referred about metastatic adenocarcinoma to the uterine cervix. Rare extrabdominal localizations are reported: intramuscular gluteal tumour [6], scalp and forehead [7], testis [8], axillary lymph node [9]. Yoo and Colleagues [8] reported a multivariate analysis of risk factors involved in the recurrence of gastric cancer; in order they are lymph node metastasis, serosal invasion, infiltrative or diffuse type, larger tumour size (4 cm or greater), undifferentiated tumour and proximally located tumour. Serosal invasion and lymph node metastasis were common risk factors for all recurrence patterns. Buzzoni [10] underlined the role of radical surgery respect more conservative surgery to reduce the rate of loco-regional recurrence: particularly the pT stage was related to loco-regional recurrence whereas pN stage had importance on distant metastases. Motoori [11] developed a diagnostic system based on systematic analysis of gene expression profiling to predict the recurrence at clinically meaningful level: the prediction accuracy was high especially in patients with small tumours in I and II stage. Marrelli [12] obtained a scoring system with a regression model based on follow-up data to define subgroups of patients at risk for recurrence after radical surgery for gastric cancer. On the other hand, Bennet [13] affirmed that follow-up did not identify no symptomatic recurrence earlier than symptomatic one.

Our case is unusual in its presentation: an isolated bulk involving neighbouring organs suitable for surgical resection. The result after the en-bloc resection is very amazing. Considering the primary surgical specimen we may suppose the modalities of the local relapse: the spleen and local lymph-nodes were radically removed, but in spite of that, local contamination during the first operation remains the most reasonable interpretation. All risk factors suggested by Yoo and Colleagues [8] were present in the initial specimen: serosal invasion and nodal metastases, large tumour size (7 x 5 cm on the specimen) infiltrative and undifferentiated type and proximally located tumour. We can speculate that chemotherapy has favoured the delay of the clinical presentation of the recurrence. Recently developed new agents such as irinotecan, taxanes and capecitabine, provide more promising results also in metastatic gastric cancer such as new molecular targeting agents [14]. Encouraging perspectives may result from IORT by virtue of its technical properties which permits to exceed conventional doses [15]. We believe that an appropriate association between varies therapeutic option [16,17] (surgery, chemo and radiotherapy – EBRT and/or IORT-) may bring about a change for a better management of recurrent gastric cancer.

Acknowledgements

This article has been published as part of *BMC Surgery* Volume 12 Supplement 1, 2012: Selected articles from the XXV National Congress of the Italian Society of Geriatric Surgery. The full contents of the supplement are available online at http://www.biomedcentral.com/bmcsurg/supplements/12/S1.

Author details

[1]Department of Molecular Medicine, University of Padua, Italy. [2]Department of Surgical and Gastroenterological Sciences, University of Padua, Italy. [3]University of Naples Federico II - Department of General Surgery, Italy.

Authors' contributions

BM, CM and RL have studied the patient and performed the surgical operation. FC performed the endoscopic preoperative study of the patient and contributed to the literature review. CT contributed to the discussion of medico-legal issues and to the writing of the paper. BA and CM gave their contribution to the analysis of the data and contributed to the writing of the paper. All the authors read and approved the final manuscript.

Competing interests

The authors declare that they have no competing interests.

References

1. Japanese Gastric Cancer Association. **Japanese Classification of Gastric Carcinoma - 2nd English Edition.** *Gastric Cancer* 1998, **1**:10-24.
2. Sobin LH, Wittekind CH: **International Union Against Cancer (UICC). TNM classification of malignant tumours.** New York: John Wiley & Sons;, 5 1997.
3. Menzel T, Peters K, Hammerschimdt S, Ritter O: **Metastatic signet ring cell gastric carcinoma presenting as an infrarenal aortic aneurysm.** *Gastric Cancer* 2005, **8(1)**:47-49.
4. Shimoyama Y, Ohashi M, Hashiguchi N, Ishihara M, Sakata M, Tamura A, *et al*: **Gastric cancer recognized by metastasis to the ureter.** *Gastric Cancer* 2000, **3(2)**:102-105.
5. Imachi M, Tsukamoto N, Amagase H, Shigematsu T, Amada S, Nakano H: **Metastatic adenocarcinoma to the uterine cervix from gastric cancer.** *Cancer* 1993, **71**:3472-3477.
6. Kondo S, Onodera H, Kan S, Uchida S, Toguchida J, Imamura M: **Intramuscular metastasis from gastric cancer.** *Gastric Cancer* 2002, **5(2)**:107-111.
7. Lifshitz OH, Berlin JM, Taylor JS, Bergfeld WF: **Metastatic gastric adenocarcinoma presenting as an enlarging plaque on the scalp.** *Cutis* 2005, **76(3)**:194-196.
8. Yoo CH, Noh SH, Shin DW, Choi SH, Min JS: **Recurrence following curative resection for gastric carcinoma.** *Br J Surg* 2000, **87**:236-242.
9. Kobayashi O, Sugiyama Y, Konishi K, Kanari M, Cho H, Tsuburaya A, *et al*: **Solitary metastasis to teh left axillary lymph node after curative gastrectomy in gastric cancer.** *Gastric Cancer* 2002, **5**:173-6.
10. Buzzoni R, Bajetta E, Di Bartolomeo M, Miceli R, Beretta E, Ferrario E, *et al*: **Pathological features as predictors of recurrence after radical resection of gastric cancer.** *Br J Surg* 2006, **93(2)**:205-209.
11. Mootori M, Takemasa I, Yano M, Saito S, Miyata H, Takiguchi S, *et al*: **Prediction of recurrence in advanced gastric cancer patients after curative resection by gene expression profiling.** *Int J Cancer* 2005, **114(6)**:963-968.
12. Marrelli D, De Stefano A, De Manzoni G, Morgagni P, Di Leo A, Roviello F: **Prediction of recurrence after radical surgery for gastric cancer: a scoring system obtained from a prospective multicenter study.** *Ann Surg* 2005, **241(2)**:247-255.
13. Bennett JJ, Gonen M, D'Angelica M, Jaques DP, Brennan MF, Coit DG: **Is detection of asymptomatic recurrence after curative resection associated with improved survival in patients with gastric cancer?** *J Am Coll Surg* 2005, **201(4)**:503-510.
14. Ohtsu A: **Current status and future prospects of chemotherapy for metastatic gastric cancer: a review.** *Gastric Cancer* 2005, **8(2)**:95-102.
15. Tomio L, Pani G, Agugiaro S, Valentini A, Fellin G, Mussari S: **Intraoperative radiotherapy in gastric adenocarcinoma: a long tem analysis on 26 patients.** *Tumori (supplementi)* 2005, **4(6)**:s43-47.
16. Rispoli C, Rocco N, Iannone L, Compagna R, De Magistris L, Braun A, Amato B: **Developing guidelines in geriatric surgery: Role of the grade system.** *BMC Geriatrics* 2009, **9(SUPPL. 1)**, Article n.A99.
17. Guida F, Antonino A, Conte P, Formisano G, Esposito D, Bencivenga M, Aprea G, Amato B, Avallone U, Persico G: **Gastric cancer in elderly: Clinico-pathological features and surgical treatment.** *BMC Geriatrics* 2009, **9(SUPPL. 1)**, Article n.A66.

15

Gastrointestinal stromal tumor: 15-years' experience in a single center

Ming Wang[1], Jia Xu[1], Yun Zhang[1], Lin Tu[1], Wei-Qing Qiu[1], Chao-Jie Wang[1], Yan-Ying Shen[2], Qiang Liu[2] and Hui Cao[1*]

Abstract

Background: Gastrointestinal stromal tumor (GIST) is known for its wide variability in biological behaviors and it is difficult to predict its malignant potential. The aim of this study is to explore the characteristics and prognostic factors of GIST.

Methods: Clinical and pathological data of 497 GIST patients in our center between 1997 and 2012 were reviewed.

Results: Patients were categorized into very low-, low-, intermediate- and high-risk groups according to modified National Institutes of Health (NIH) consensus classification system. Among the 401 patients untreated with imatinib mesylate (IM), 5-year overall survival (OS) in very low-, low-, intermediate- and high-risk groups was 100%, 100%, 89.6% and 65.9%; and 5-year relapse-free survival (RFS) was 100%, 98.1%, 90.9% and 44.5%, respectively. Univariate analysis revealed that sex, tumor size, mitotic rate, risk grade, CD34 expression, and adjacent involvement were predictors of OS or RFS. COX hazard proportional model (Forward LR) showed that large tumor size, high mitotic rate, and high risk grade were independent risk factors to OS, whereas high mitotic rate, high risk grade and adjacent organ involvement were independent risk factors to RFS. The intermediate-high risk patients who received IM adjuvant therapy (n = 87) had better 5-year OS and RFS than those who did not (n = 188) (94.9% vs. 72.1; 82.3% vs. 56.3%, respectively). Similarly, advanced GIST patients underwent IM therapy (n = 45) had better 3-year OS and 1-year progression-free survival (PFS) than those who didn't (n = 42) (75.6% vs. 6.8%; 87.6% vs. 12.4%, respectively).

Conclusions: Very low- and low-risk GISTs can be treated with surgery alone. Large tumor size, high mitotic rate, high risk grade, and adjacent organ involvement contribute to the poor outcome. IM therapy significantly improves the survival of intermediate-high risk or advanced GIST patients.

Keywords: Gastrointestinal stromal tumor, Survival, Imatinib

Background

Gastrointestinal stromal tumor (GIST) is the most common mesenchymal neoplasm in the gastrointestinal (GI) tract [1]. Mazur and Clark [2] first introduced the concept of "stromal tumor" in 1983. Advance in pathology, immunohistochemistry and molecular biology in recent years has greatly improved the diagnosis of GIST. It is now considered that GISTs arise from interstitial Cajal cells (ICCs), expressing CD117 (product of c-kit proto-oncogene), and harboring c-kit or platelet-derived growth factor receptor alpha (PDGFRA) gain-of-function mutation [3-5].

* Correspondence: caohuishcn@hotmail.com
[1]Department of General Surgery, Ren Ji Hospital, School of Medicine, Shanghai Jiao Tong University, Floor 11, Building 7, NO. 1630, Dongfang Road, Shanghai 200127, China
Full list of author information is available at the end of the article

GIST is known for its wide variability in biological behaviors and it is difficult to predict its malignant potential [6,7]. Tumor size, mitotic rate and tumor site are considered as the most important prognostic parameters for patients after surgery [8]. However, neither small size nor low mitotic rate could exclude malignant potential [9]. On the other hand, some enormous tumor with high mitotic rate could also achieve long-term survival, even without adjuvant therapy [10]. The post-operation outcome of GIST is highly variable, with 5-year survival rate ranging from 48% to 80% [11,12]. The variability is mainly due to the introduction of a tyrosine kinases inhibitor (TKI), imatinib mesylate, which was used in metastatic/recurrent GISTs since 2000 and had been proved as an adjuvant therapy several years ago [13,14].

The purpose of this study is to share our latest 15 years of experience and to explore the prognostic factors of GISTs.

Methods

The clinicopathological and follow-up data of 497 operable GIST patients admitted to Department of General Surgery, Ren Ji Hospital, School of Medicine, Shanghai Jiao Tong University between 1997 and 2012 were reviewed. Each diagnosis of "GIST" was confirmed by postoperative histopathology and immunohistochemistry assay (IHCA). The results of histopathological features and IHCA findings of every case were reviewed by 2 experienced pathologists. Those diagnosed as "gastrointestinal stromal mesenchymal tumor" prior to 2000 were re-examined by IHCA to confirm the diagnosis of GIST. The tumors were categorized into very low, low, intermediate and high risk groups according to the modified NIH risk classification criteria [7] (Table 1). Only the cases with complete medical records and pathological data were involved in present study. The following parameters were reviewed and analyzed: age, sex, clinical presentation, surgical detail, tumor site, tumor size, mitotic rate, IHCA (CD117, CD34, vimentin, smooth muscle actin (SMA), S-100, Discovered On GIST 1 (DOG1)), TKI therapy and outcome. Survival outcome in terms of overall survival (OS), relapse-free survival (RFS), and progression-free survival (PFS) were assessed. OS was defined as the period from surgery to the last follow-up or death. RFS was defined as the period from surgery to the time of clinical or radiological evidence of disease relapse. PFS in patients who had metastatic or recurrent disease was defined as the period from the time when relapse was diagnosed to clinical or radiological evidence of progression or death.

Table 1 Risk classification of GISTs

Risk classification	Tumor size (cm)	Mitotic rate per 50 HPF	Tumor site
Very low risk	<2	<=5	Any
Low risk	2.1-5.0	<=5	Any
	2.1-5.0	>5	Gastric
Intermediate risk	<5	6-10	Any
	5.1-10	<=5	Gastric
High risk	Any	Any	Tumor rupture
	>10	Any	Any
	Any	>10	Any
	>5	>5	Any
	2.1-5.0	>5	Non gastric
	5.1-10.0	<=5	Non gastric

HPF = high power field.

All patients provided written informed consent for their information to be stored in the hospital database, and we obtained separate consent for use of research. Study approval was obtained from independent ethics committees from Ren Ji Hospital, School of Medicine, Shanghai Jiao Tong University. The study was undertaken in accordance with the ethical standards of the World Medical Association Declaration of Helsinki.

χ^2 test and Fisher's exact test were performed to analyze qualitative parameters and Kaplan-Meier method with log rank test was used for postoperative survival analysis. Independent factors were identified in multivariate analysis by COX proportional hazard analysis with forward selection at $P < 0.05$. Odds ratios (ORs) and 95% confidence intervals (CIs) were determined using unconditional multiple logistic regression models. Two-sided P values of 0.05 or less were considered to indicate statistical significance.

Results

The incidence of GIST ranges from 11 to 15 per million per year [15-18]. Growing evidence indicates the incidence is considerably underestimated [19,20]. The number of GIST patients admitted to our center is on the rise. In the past two year, it has approached 100 cases a year (Figure 1).

Clinical and pathological characteristics

Total 497 GIST patients were involved in present study, with a median age of 60 years (range 23–90) and 55.9% was male. Stomach and small bowel were the most common sites of primary disease (59.0% and 22.5%, respectively). The most common clinical presentation was abdominal discomfort, followed by GI bleeding. Distribution of risk groups: 8.0%, very low; 36.4%, low; 15.7%, intermediate; and 39.8%, high risk. IM adjuvant therapy was given to 96 of the patients to prevent disease relapse. Recurrence or metastases were observed in 89 patients during the follow-up period. Among which, IM was used to control disease in 46 patients.

Of all the cases, 87.3% was CD117 (+); 80.3%, CD34 (+); 23.6%, SMA (+); and 21.5%, S-100 (+). DOG1 was a newly developed IHCA marker, which was positive in 139 out of 149 cases (93.3%). The diagnosis of GIST in patients presented as both CD117 and DOG1 negative was confirmed by detection of mutation in c-kit/PDGFRA gene. Their clinical and pathological characteristics are listed in Table 2.

Lymph node metastasis was detected in 5 out of 497 cases (1.01%); clinical and pathological characteristics of these 5 cases were described in Table 3.

Survival analysis on patients without IM adjuvant therapy

Given the fact that imatinib is an effective drug on GIST, the first survival analysis was based on the population of

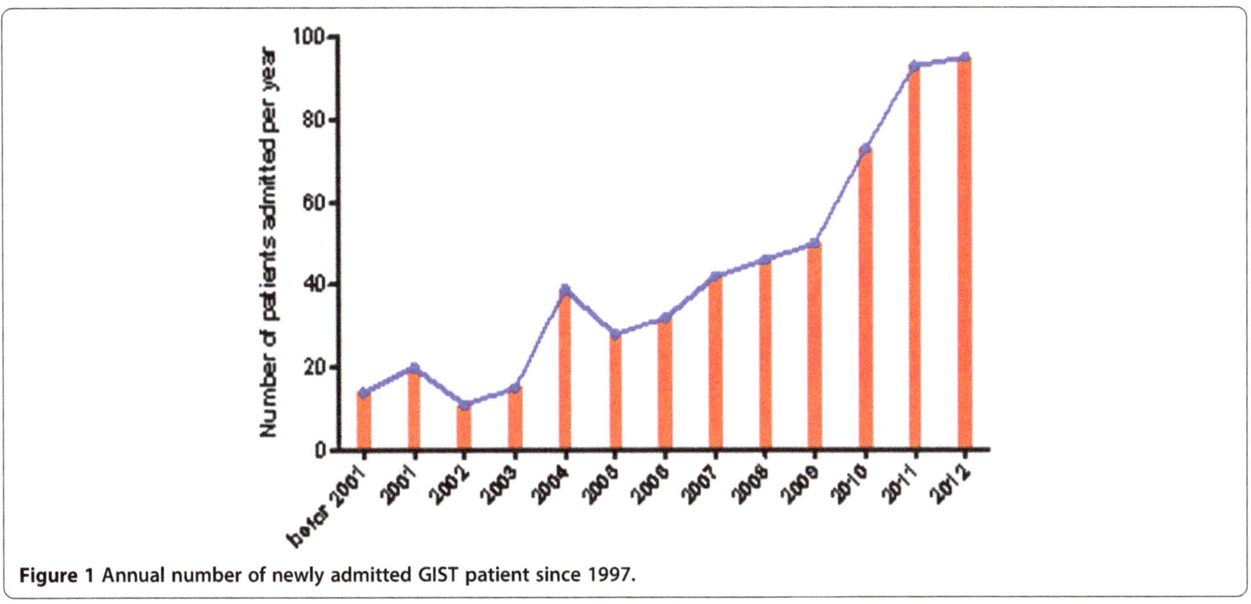

Figure 1 Annual number of newly admitted GIST patient since 1997.

patients who were not given IM adjuvant therapy. Therefore, 401 patients with operable GIST were enrolled in the cohort, with a median duration of 50 months (range, 7–187 months). Recurrence or metastasis occurred in 79 patients (19.7%). The abdominopelvic cavity was the most common site of metastases (51 cases), followed by liver (22 cases), lung (3 cases), vertebral column (1 case), umbilicus (1 case), and fossa axillaris (1 case). Forty-five patients died of GIST progression, and 4 died of other diseases. The 1-, 3-, 5-year OS of 401 GISTs was 97.7%, 92.6% and 84.8%, respectively; The 1-, 3-, 5-year RFS was 93.2%, 82.1% and 77.4%, respectively.

The 1-, 3-, 5-year OS according to risk grade was: 100%, 100%, 100% (very low risk); 100%, 100%, 100% (low risk); 100%, 97.8%, 89.6% (intermediated risk); 93.5%, 80.8%, 65.9% (high risk), respectively (Figure 2).

The 1-, 3-, 5-year RFS according to risk group was: 100%, 100%, 100% (very low risk); 100%, 100%, 98.1% (low risk); 100%, 93.8%, 90.9% (intermediated risk); 80.6%, 53.1%, 44.5% (high risk), respectively (Figure 3).

Univariate analysis revealed that male gender, non-gastric origin, larger tumor size, higher mitotic rate, higher risk grade, CD34 negative expression, and adjacent organ involvement contributed to poorer outcome (lower OS and RFS), whereas age and expression of CD117, SMA, and S-100 were not associated with prognosis (see Table 4 and Additional files 1 and 2).

Multivariate analysis by Cox proportional hazards regression (Forward LR) model indicated that tumor size, mitotic rate, and risk grade were independent risk factors to OS for GISTs, and that mitotic rate, risk grade, and adjacent involvement were independent risk factors to RFS (Tables 5 and 6).

Survival analysis of patients received IM therapy

From 2007 to 2012, 87 patients with intermediate-high risk GIST received IM adjuvant therapy after radical resection (Adjuvant group). Compared with those patients who were with same risk GIST (intermediate-high risk) while were not given IM adjuvant therapy (Non-adjuvant group, n = 188), adjuvant group had better 5-year RFS (82.3% vs. 56.3%, $P < 0.001$) and 5-year OS (94.9% vs. 72.1%, $P = 0.001$) (Figure 4). In addition, there was no statistical difference in other clinicopathological features (sex, age, tumor site, tumor size, mitotic rate, risk grade, etc.) between the two groups (see Additional file 3), indicating that these features had no impact on the effect of IM.

In the cohort, 87 patients developed recurrence of metastasis after surgery for the primary disease. Among them, c-kit/PDGFRA mutation status was screened in 39 patients. Their mutational characteristics were demonstrated in our previous report [21]. Mutations in c-kit exon 11, c-kit exon 9, and PDGFRA exon 18 were identified in 29, 4, and 1 patients, respectively. And the rest 5 GISTs showed c-kit and PDGFRA wild type. Among all the 87 advanced GIST patients, 45 (including 33 c-kit mutant GISTs, 5 wild-type GISTs, and 7 GISTs with unknown mutation type) were treated with IM, and the other 42 didn't undergo any TKI therapy (10 due to personal reasons and the rest were cases prior to 2005). There was significant difference in outcome between the two groups: patients underwent postoperative IM treatment had better 1-, 3-year OS than those untreated with IM (97.6% and 75.6% vs. 58.7% and 6.8%, respectively, $P < 0.001$). IM therapy also improved 1-year progression-free survival (PFS) of these patients (87.6% vs. 12.4%, $P < 0.001$) (Figure 5).

Table 2 Clinical and pathological characteristics of 497 GIST patients

Age (years)	
Median	60
Range	23-90
Sex, n (%)	
Male	278 (55.9)
Female	219 (44.1)
Primary site of tumor, n (%)	
Stomach	293 (59.0)
Duodenum	31 (6.2)
Small bowel	112 (22.5)
Large bowel	4 (0.8)
Rectum	21 (4.2)
Esophagus	3 (0.6)
Other (omentum, mesenterium and retroperitoneum)	33 (6.6)
Clinical manifestation, n (%)	
Abdominal discomfort	184 (37.0)
GI bleeding	142 (28.6)
Diagnosed at physical examination	81 (16.3)
Abdominal mass	14 (2.8)
Other (fever, fatigue, appetite and explored at surgery for other diseases)	76 (15.3)
IM therapy	
As adjuvant therapy for primary disease	96
As therapy for advanced disease (recurrent, metastatic, unresectable, or incomplete resected)	46
Immunohistochemistry, n (%)	
CD117	434 (87.3)
CD34	399 (80.3)
SMA	119 (23.9)
S-100	107 (21.5)
DOG1	139 (93.3)*

*DOG1 was examined in 165 cases.

Discussion

Although the incidence of GISTs is rising in the oriental population, available document on this area is still limited, especially studies with large sample size in a single center. This study reviewed the clinical and pathological features of 497 GIST cases in Shanghai Ren Ji Hospital to explore the prognostic factors of the disease.

GISTs represent 80% of mesenchymal tumor of the digestive tract and constitute 5% of all sarcoma [22]. It had been reported that the annual occurrences of GIST were 11–15 per million people [15-18]. However, growing evidences have proved that the incidence of GISTs is seriously underestimated. Learn from the studies of Abraham et al. [23] and Agaimy et al. [24], we can draw a conclusion that sub-centimeter GISTs (smaller than 1 cm) are common lesions in stomach. Our epidemiologic data show the number of newly diagnosed GISTs is on the fast rise (Figure 1), probably due to the increasing awareness of the disease in clinicians.

Our data indicate that GIST occurrences culminate among people in their 50s and 60s. The youngest GIST patient is a 23-year-old female, who suffered from giant retroperitoneal GIST and died of recurrent disease 32 months after surgery. The oldest patient is a 90-year-old male with intermediate-risk gastric GIST and he was relapse-free at last follow-up, six months after surgery. Although in most published documents there is no clear sex predilection [3,25,26], some studies revealed that there was a slight male predominance [27-29]. Our data agree with the latter.

GISTs have no specific symptom, increasing the difficulty in early diagnosis and treatment. In our data, consistent with the literature, the most frequent complaint is abdominal discomfort, which may or may not be accompanied by GI bleeding [30,31].

GIST may arise anywhere in the GI tract and also in extragastrointestinal locations (extragastrointestinal stromal tumor, EGIST), including omentum, mesenterium, and retroperitoneum [32]. According to our data, the most common GI location of primary disease was stomach (59.0%), followed by small bowel (22.5%), duodenum

Table 3 Clinical and pathological characteristics of 5 GIST patients with lymph node metastasis

Case	Sex	Age	Primary site	Tumor size	Mitotic rate per 50HPF	MLN/TLN	Mutation	IM therapy	Outcome
1	M	60	S	8	23	2/4	c-kit exon9	Yes	Died of disease progression at 33 months after surgery
2	M	58	G	5	12	1/2	not available	No	DFS at 101 months after surgery
3	F	59	G	5.5	<5	4/4	c-kit exon11	Yes	DFS at 45 months after surgery
4	F	70	G	9	8	1/9	c-kit exon11	Yes	DFS at 25 months after surgery
5	M	31	D	18	<5	2/2	c-kit exon11	Yes	Survival with residual disease at 3 months after surgery

S = small intestine; G = stomach; D = duodenum MLN = metastatic lymph nodes; TLN = total examined lymph nodes; DFS = Disease-free survival.

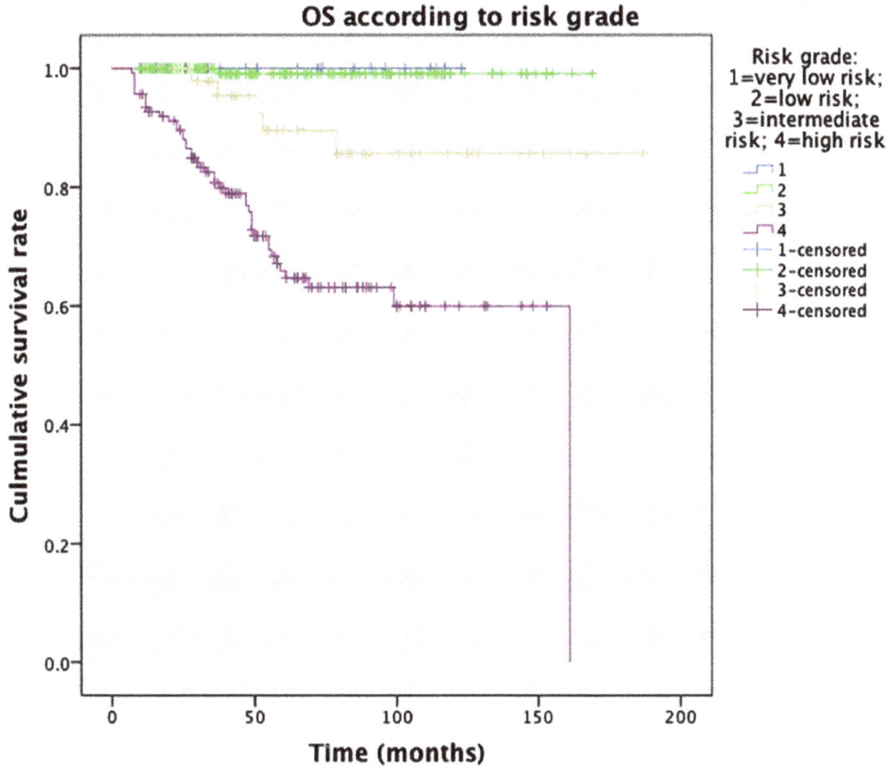

Figure 2 Overall survival in 401 GIST patients according to risk class.

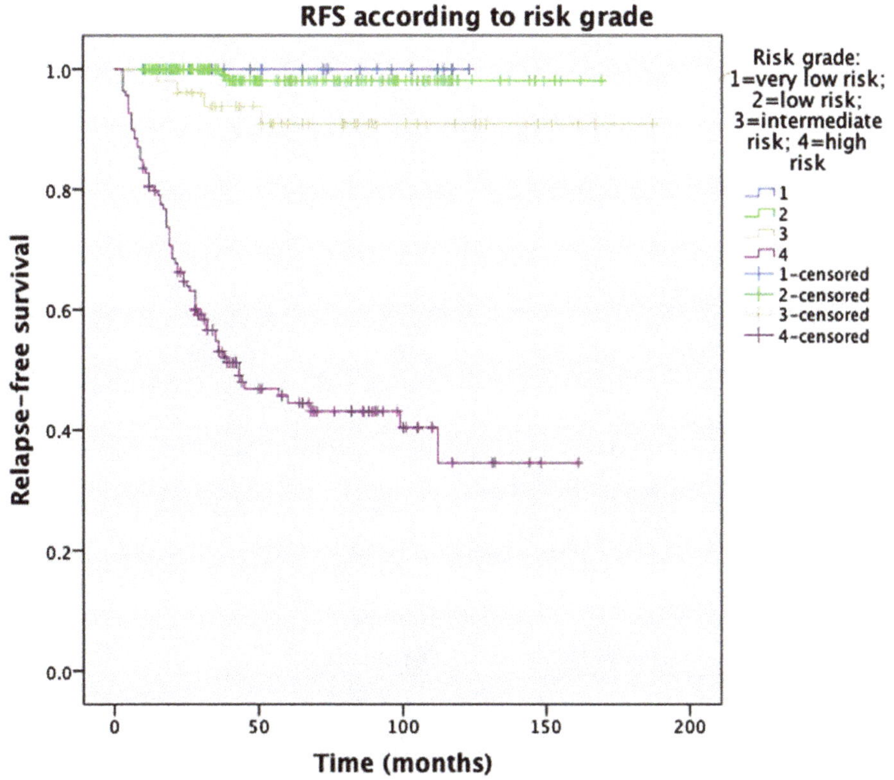

Figure 3 Relapse-free survival in 401 GIST patients according to risk class.

Table 4 Univariate analysis of OS and RFS in 401 GIST patients

Clinicopathological feature	Group	N	OS			RFS		
			5-year OS (%)	χ^2	P-value	5-year RFS (%)	χ^2	P-value
Gender	Male	221	80.2	6.590	0.010	71.6	8.914	0.003
	Female	180	90.6			84.4		
Age	<60	197	85.7	1.573	0.210	77.4	0.011	0.917
	≥60	204	84.0			77.4		
Tumor site	Gastric	241	86.5	1.969	0.161	86.1	18.876	<0.001
	Non-gastric	160	82.5			65.3		
Tumor size	≤2 cm	51	100	110.281	<0.001	100	146.144	<0.001
	2.1-5 cm	178	98.0			94.6		
	5.1-10 cm	109	80.9			66.8		
	>10 cm	63	49.2			33.5		
Mitotic rate	<5/50 HPF	296	95.9	83.348	<0.001	91.2	152.472	<0.001
	5-10/50 HPF	44	68.0			55.3		
	>10/50 HPF	61	54.2			33.7		
Risk class	Very low	39	100	66.044	<0.001	100	154.234	<0.001
	Low	172	99.1			98.1		
	Intermediate	51	89.6			90.9		
	High	139	65.9			44.5		
CD117 expression	Positive	350	83.4	3.315	0.069	76.6	1.401	0.237
	Negetive	51	95.1			82.6		
CD34 expression	Positive	322	87.2	7.564	0.006	80.6	10.777	0.001
	Negative	79	75.4			64.3		
SMA expression	Positive	101	90.6	1.559	0.212	83.2	2.246	0.134
	Negative	300	83.2			75.6		
S-100 expression	Positive	84	88.2	1.377	0.241	74.0	0.529	0.467
	Negative	317	83.7			78.5		
Adjacent involvement	Without	336	92.1	66.176	<0.001	87.2	147.885	<0.001
	With	65	53.0			30.8		

(6.2%), rectum (4.2%), large bowel (0.8%), esophagus (0.6%). EGISTs were found in 6.6% of cases.

Typical GISTs are characterized by positive immunohistochemical (IHC) staining of KIT (CD117), a transmembrane receptor tyrosine kinase. More recently the antigen DOG1 has been incorporated in the IHC panel when CD117 was negative [33]. Our data confirmed the high specificity and sensitivity of this marker: DOG1 expression was seen in 139 of 149 GISTs, including 15 CD117 negative ones.

Except for some sporadic studies [34], lymph node metastasis is reported to be extremely rare in GIST, with incidence ranging from 0 ~ 5% [11,35-37]. Although lymph node metastasis (LNM) is usually considered as a morphological feature associated with malignancy and poor prognosis [38,39], our data do not support this opinion. Three out of the 5 patients with LNM in this study achieved longer than 2 years' DFS; one of them, though untreated with IM, was still disease-free at the latest follow-up, over 8 years after surgery. This aroused the

Table 5 Multivariate COX regression analysis of OS in 401 GIST patients

Covariate	χ^2	P-value	Hazard ratio	95% CI
Tumor size (> = 10 cm vs. <10 cm)	13.224	<0.001	3.293	1.732-6.261
Mitotic rate (> = 5/50 HPF vs. <5/50 HPF)	10.619	0.001	3.841	1.710-8.628
Risk grade (high risk vs. non-high risk)	4.956	0.026	3.440	1.159-10.207

Table 6 Multivariate COX regression analysis of RFS in 401 GIST patients

Covariate	χ^2	P-value	Hazard ratio	95% CI
Adjacent involvement (with vs. without)	11.841	0.001	2.295	1.430-3.683
Mitotic rate (> = 5/50 HPF vs. <5/50 HPF)	8.895	0.003	2.406	1.351-4.284
Risk grade (high risk vs. non-high risk)	26.129	<0.001	11.794	4.579-30.379

controversy over the exact impact of LNM on GIST outcome. Further studies with larger sample size are required to solve this puzzle. Nonetheless, lymph node dissection should be considered in case of suspected or confirmed LNM.

The distribution of very low-, low-, intermediate-, high-risk groups was 8.0%, 36.4%, 15.7%, and 39.8%, respectively. Compared to most published literature [28,40,41], the proportion of very low and low risk GIST was much higher. One reason might be the improved screening system and early surgery. In addition, clinical study on minimal invasive procedure (laparoscopic/laparoscopy-endoscopy cooperative surgeries) for GIST is being conducted in our center, and offers the opportunity of early operation and further elevated the proportion. Thanks to the popularity of endoscopy, more and more GISTs can be determined at small size. In most cases, having the advantages of small incision and fast recovery, minimal invasive surgery is preferred to traditional open operation.

In our study, the outcome (both OS and RFS) of IM-naive GIST patients was better than that in most published literature [12,42,43] for the same reasons mentioned above (higher proportion of low risk GIST). Nonetheless, the high-risk group still had unsatisfactory results (5-year OS 65.9%, 5-year RFS 44.5%, respectively). However, very low- and low-risk GISTs in present study had rather better prognosis: no relapse was found in very low risk group; only one case, a rectal tumor 3.5cm in diameter with mitotic rate of <5/50HPF, occurred recurrence in low-risk group.

Prediction of biological behavior of a GIST is essential for selection of candidates for adjuvant therapy as well as determination of the frequency and intensity of post-operative surveillance. However, accurate prediction is often a difficult job. It has been widely accepted that tumor size, mitotic rate, and anatomic site are the most important factors influencing the prognosis of GISTs [8]. These factors form the basis for consensus risk classification. Our study reveals that risk grade and mitotic rate were independent prognostic factors of both OS and RFS, while tumor size and adjacent organ involvement was independent predictor of OS and RFS, respectively. Mitotic rate was described as a vital indicator for GIST staging and consequential choice of surgical and target therapeutic approach [44,45], its value in prognosis prediction was confirmed again in our study. It's worth mentioning that there is a difficulty in reproducibility among examiners when determining the mitotic rate [44]. Therefore, all specimens should be examined by specialized experts to decrease the deviation.

In present study, males had lower survival rate than females (5-yaer OS, 80.2% vs. 90.6%, P = 0.010; 5-year RFS, 71.6% vs. 84.4%, P = 0.003). This finding was in

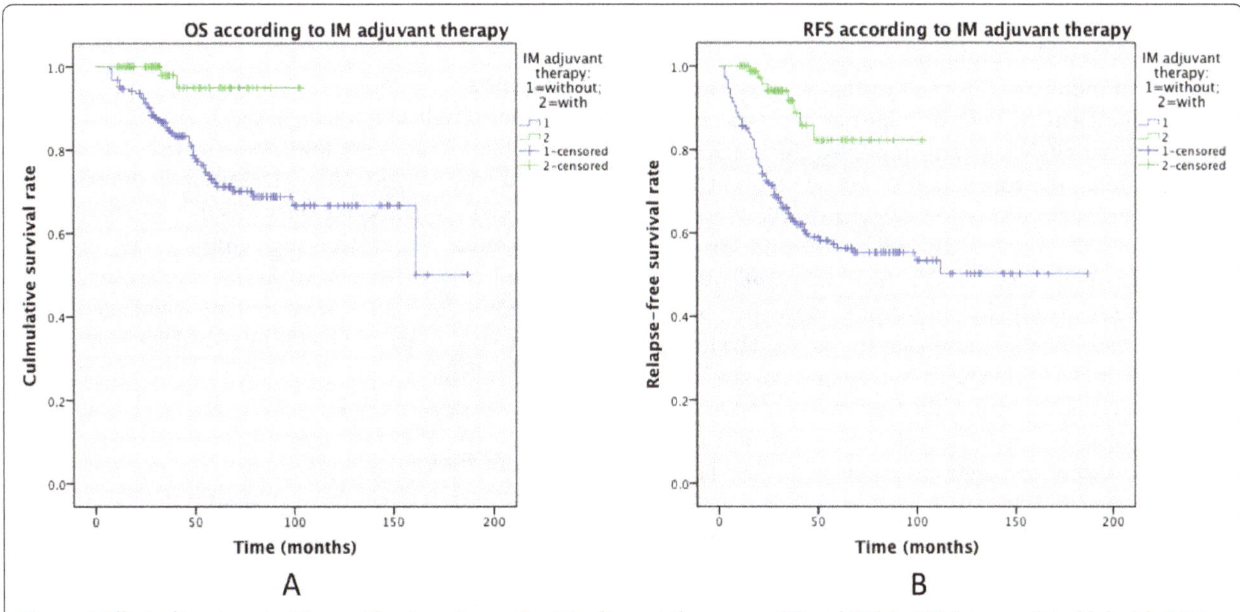

Figure 4 Effect of treatment with or without postoperative IM adjuvant therapy on OS and RFS in 275 intermediate-high risk GIST patients (A: overall survival; B: relapse-free survival).

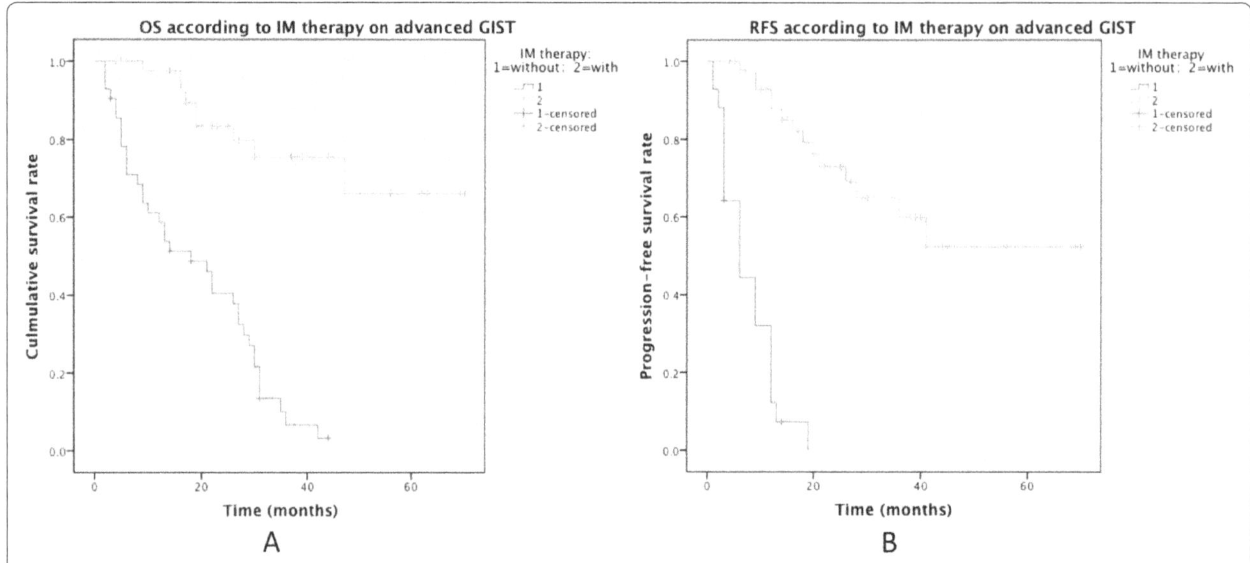

Figure 5 Effect of treatment with or without post-operation IM therapy on OS and PFS in 87 advanced GIST cases (A: overall survival; B: progression-free survival).

consistent with other retrospective studies [46-48]. However, no relationship between sex and survival was found in the multivariate analysis.

Most documents, including our previous study on a small cohort, didn't demonstrate correlation between CD34 expression and GIST patients' prognosis [49-51]. However, univariate analysis of present study revealed that CD34 positive GIST patients had better outcome than CD34 negative patients (5-yaer OS, 87.2% vs. 75.4%, P = 0.006; 5-year RFS, 80.6% vs. 64.3%, P = 0.001). Yet subsequent multivariate analysis didn't show relationship between CD34 and patients' survival. Therefore, further studies are required to determine the exact impact of sex and CD34 on GIST prognosis.

Long-term monitoring has shown that surgery alone is usually insufficient to control high-risk diseases. Introduction of imatinib has greatly improved the outcome of GIST. In China, the application of IM as adjuvant therapy was widely accepted not earlier than 2005. Presently, IM is standard therapy for advanced and primary intermediate-high risk GISTs (for adjuvant option) [14]. In present study, IM adjuvant therapy had better 5-year OS and RFS than non-adjuvant group. The limitation of this study is obvious: the selection of candidates and the interval of adjuvant therapy were not standardized. The follow-up period of adjuvant group was much shorter than that of non-adjuvant group, which highlighted the importance of persistent follow-up on those patients. The exact effect of IM on GIST can only be assessed by prospective randomized controlled trials with long-term follow-up, just like Z9001 [52] and SSGXVIII trials [53]. However, our findings still encourage the use of IM adjuvant therapy.

Undoubtedly, residual, recurrent or metastatic GISTs should be treated with imatinib according to the guidelines by European Society for Medical Oncology (ESMO) [54] or National Comprehensive Cancer Network (NCCN) [55]. In this cohort, however, some patients with advanced disease did not undergo IM therapy. Most of the cases were before 2005, when IM was not available in China. In present study, late-stage GIST (residual disease) patients underwent IM therapy had better 3-year OS and 1-year PFS than those who didn't (75.6% vs. 6.8%; 87.6% vs. 12.4%, respectively), confirming the effect of IM on advanced disease.

Conclusions

In summary, radical surgery is the treatment of choice for operable GISTs. Very low- and low-risk diseases can be treated with surgery alone. Lymph node metastasis is rare in GIST patients and may not be associated with poor prognosis. Large size, high mitotic rate, high risk group, and adjacent organ involvement all contribute to bad outcome of GISTs. IM therapy significantly improves survival of patients with intermediate-high risk or advanced GISTs.

Additional files

Additional file 1: Univariate analysis of OS. Univariate analysis of overall survival in 401 GIST patients (a: gender; b: tumor size; c: mitotic rate; d: CD34 expression; e: adjacent involvement).

Additional file 2: Univariate analysis of RFS. Univariate analysis of relapse-free survival in 401 GIST patients (a: sex; tumor site; c: tumor size; d: mitotic rate; e: CD34 expression; f: adjacent involvement).

Additional file 3: Intermediate-high risk GIST. Clinicopathological characteristics of 275 intermediate-high risk GIST patients according to whether received post-operation IM adjuvant therapy.

Abbreviations

GIST: Gastrointestinal stromal tumor; NIH: National Institutes of Health; IM: Imatinib mesylate; OS: Overall survival; RFS: Relapse-free survival; GI: Gastrointestinal; ICC: Interstitial Cajal cell; PDGFRA: Platelet-derived growth factor receptor alpha; TKI: Tyrosine kinase inhibitor; HPF: High power field; IHCA: Immunohistochemistry assay; SMA: Smooth muscle actin; DOG1: (Discovered On GIST 1); PFS: Progression-free survival; OR: Odds ratio; CI: Confidence interval; EGIST: Extragastrointestinal stromal tumor; IHC: Immunohistochemical; LNM: Lymph node metastasis; ESMO: European society for medical oncology; NCCN: National comprehensive cancer network.

Competing interests

The authors declare that they have no competing interests.

Authors' contributions

The work presented here was carried out in collaboration between all authors. HC conceived of the study, and participated in its design and coordination and helped to draft the manuscript. YYS and QL carried out the IHCA and were in charge of the pathological diagnosis of GIST. LT, WQQ, and CJW were in charge of data collection and follow-up, MW, JX, and YZ analyzed the data. MW interpreted the results and drafted the manuscript. All authors read and approved the final manuscript.

Acknowledgment

This study was supported by the grant of 1) National Science Foundation of China (no. 81272743) and 2) Projects of Shanghai Committee of Science and Technology (no. 11411950800, no. 13411950902, and no. 13XD1402500).

Author details

[1]Department of General Surgery, Ren Ji Hospital, School of Medicine, Shanghai Jiao Tong University, Floor 11, Building 7, NO. 1630, Dongfang Road, Shanghai 200127, China. [2]Department of Pathology, Ren Ji Hospital, School of Medicine, Shanghai Jiao Tong University, Shanghai, China.

References

1. Miettinen M, Lasota J: **Histopathology of gastrointestinal stromal tumor.** *J Surg Oncol* 2011, **104**:865–873.
2. Mazur MT, Clark HB: **Gastric stromal tumors. Reappraisal of histogenesis.** *Am J Surg Pathol* 1983, **7**:507–519.
3. Miettinen M, Lasota J: **Gastrointestinal stromal tumors: review on morphology, molecular pathology, prognosis, and differential diagnosis.** *Arch Pathol Lab Med* 2006, **130**:1466–1478.
4. Fletcher CD, Berman JJ, Corless C, Gorstein F, Lasota J, Longley BJ, Miettinen M, O'Leary TJ, Remotti H, Rubin BP, Shmookler B, Sobin LH, Weiss SW: **Diagnosis of gastrointestinal stromal tumors: A consensus approach.** *Hum Pathol* 2002, **33**:459–465.
5. Dei Tos AP: **The reappraisal of gastrointestinal stromal tumors: from Stout to the KIT revolution.** *Virchows Arc* 2003, **442**:421–428.
6. Grotz TE, Donohue JH: **Surveillance strategies for gastrointestinal stromal tumors.** *J Surg Oncol* 2011, **104**:921–927.
7. Joensuu H: **Risk stratification of patients diagnosed with gastrointestinal stromal tumor.** *Hum Pathol* 2008, **39**:1411–1419.
8. Dematteo RP, Gold JS, Saran L, Gönen M, Liau KH, Maki RG, Singer S, Besmer P, Brennan MF, Antonescu CR: **Tumor mitotic rate, size, and location independently predict recurrence after resection of primary gastrointestinal stromal tumor (GIST).** *Cancer* 2008, **112**:608–615.
9. Franquemont DW: **Differentiation and risk assessment of gastrointestinal stromal tumors.** *Am J Clin Pathol* 1995, **103**:41–47.
10. Rossi S, Miceli R, Messerini L, Bearzi I, Mazzoleni G, Capella C, Arrigoni G, Sonzogni A, Sidoni A, Toffolatti L, Laurino L, Mariani L, Vinaccia V, Gnocchi C, Gronchi A, Casali PG, Dei Tos AP: **Natural history of imatinib-naive GISTs: a retrospective analysis of 929 cases with long-term follow-up and development of a survival nomogram based on mitotic index and size as continuous variables.** *Am J Surg Pathol* 2011, **35**:1646–1656.
11. DeMatteo RP, Lewis JJ, Leung D, Mudan SS, Woodruff JM, Brennan MF: **Two hundred gastrointestinal stromal tumors: recurrence patterns and prognostic factors for survival.** *Ann Surg* 2000, **231**:51–58.
12. Rosa F, Alfieri S, Tortorelli AP, Di Miceli D, Papa V, Ricci R, Doglietto GB: **Gastrointestinal stromal tumors: prognostic factors and therapeutic implications.** *Tumori* 2012, **98**:351–356.
13. Dematteo RP, Heinrich MC, El-Rifai WM, Demetri G: **Clinical management of gastrointestinal stromal tumors: before and after STI-571.** *Hum Pathol* 2002, **33**:466–477.
14. Casali PG, Fumagalli E, Gronchi A: **Adjuvant therapy of gastrointestinal stromal tumors (GIST).** *Curr Treat Options Oncol* 2012, **13**:277–284.
15. Goettsch WG, Bos SD, Breekveldt-Postma N, Casparie M, Herings RM, Hogendoorn PC: **Incidence of gastrointestinal stromal tumours is underestimated: results of a nation-wide study.** *Eur J Cancer* 2005, **4**:2868–2872.
16. Tryggvason G, Gislason HG, Magnusson MK, Jónasson JG: **Gastrointestinal stromal tumors in Iceland, 1990–2003: the icelandic GIST study, a population-based incidence and pathologic risk stratification study.** *Int J Cancer* 2005, **117**:289–293.
17. Sandvik OM, Soreide K, Kvaloy JT, Gudlaugsson E, Søreide JA: **Epidemiology of gastrointestinal stromal tumours: single-institution experience and clinical presentation over three decades.** *Cancer Epidemiol* 2011, **35**:515–520.
18. Pisters PW, Blanke CD, von Mehren M, Picus J, Sirulnik A, Stealey E, Trent JC, reGISTry Steering Committee: **A USA registry of gastrointestinal stromal tumor patients: changes in practice over time and differences between community and academic practices.** *Ann Oncol* 2011, **22**:2523–2529.
19. Kawanowa K, Sakuma Y, Sakurai S, Hishima T, Iwasaki Y, Saito K, Hosoya Y, Nakajima T, Funata N: **High incidence of microscopic gastrointestinal stromal tumors in the stomach.** *Hum Pathol* 2006, **37**:1527–1535.
20. Rossi S, Gasparotto D, Toffolatti L, Pastrello C, Gallina G, Marzotto A, Sartor C, Barbareschi M, Cantaloni C, Messerini L, Bearzi I, Arrigoni G, Mazzoleni G, Fletcher JA, Casali PG, Talamini R, Maestro R, Dei Tos AP: **Molecular and clinicopathologic characterization of gastrointestinal stromal tumors (GISTs) of small size.** *Am J Surg Pathol* 2010, **34**:1480–1491.
21. Wang M, Xu J, Zhao W, Tu L, Qiu W, Wang C, Shen Y, Liu Q, Cao H: **Prognostic value of mutational characteristics in gastrointestinal stromal tumors: a single-center experience in 275 cases.** *Med Oncol* 2014, **31**:819.
22. Joensuu H, Fletcher C, Dimitrijevic S, Silberman S, Roberts P, Demetri G: **Management of malignant gastrointestinal stromal tumours.** *Lancet Oncol* 2002, **3**:655–664.
23. Abraham SC, Krasinskas AM, Hofstetter WL, Swisher SG, Wu TT: **"Seedling" mesenchymal tumors (gastrointestinal stromal tumors and leiomyomas) are common incidental tumors of the esophagogastric junction.** *Am J Surg Pathol* 2007, **31**:1629–1635.
24. Agaimy A, Wünsch PH, Hofstaedter F, Blaszyk H, Rümmele P, Gaumann A, Dietmaier W, Hartmann A: **Minute gastric sclerosing stromal tumors (GIST tumorlets) are common in adults and frequently show c-KIT mutations.** *Am J Surg Pathol* 2007, **31**:113–120.
25. Alvarado-Cabrero I, Vázquez G, Sierra Santiesteban FI, Hernández-Hernández DM, Pompa AZ: **Clinicopathologic study of 275 cases of gastrointestinal stromal tumors: the experience at 3 large medical centers in Mexico.** *Ann Diagn Pathol* 2007, **11**:39–45.
26. Mucciarini C, Rossi G, Bertolini F, Valli R, Cirilli C, Rashid I, Marcheselli L, Luppi G, Federico M: **Incidence and clinicopathologic features of gastrointestinal stromal tumors. A population-based study.** *BMC Cancer* 2007, **7**:230.
27. Bülbül Doğusoy G, Turkish GIST Working Group: **Gastrointestinal stromal tumors: A multicenter study of 1160 Turkish cases.** *Turk J Gastroenterol* 2012, **23**:203–211.
28. Brady-West D, Blake G: **Clinicopathological features and outcome of gastrointestinal stromal tumors in an Afro-Caribbean population.** *J Natl Med Assoc* 2012, **104**:72–77.
29. Bhalgami R, Manish K, Patil P, Mehta S, Mohandas KM: **Clinicopathological study of 113 gastrointestinal stromal tumors.** *Indian J Gastroenterol* 2013, **32**:22–27.
30. Caterino S, Lorenzon L, Petrucciani N, Iannicelli E, Pilozzi E, Romiti A, Cavallini M, Ziparo V: **Gastrointestinal stromal tumors: correlation between symptoms at presentation, tumor location and prognostic factors in 47 consecutive patients.** *World J Surg Oncol* 2011, **9**:13.

31. Kapoor R, Khosla D, Kumar P, Kumar N, Bera A: **Five-year follow up of patients with gastrointestinal stromal tumor: Recurrence-free survival by risk group.** *Asia Pac J Clin Oncol* 2013, **9:**40–46.
32. Steigen SE, Eide TJ: **Gastrointestinal stromal tumors (GISTs): a review.** *APMIS* 2009, **117:**73–86.
33. Wong NA: **Gastrointestinal stromal tumours–an update for histopathologists.** *Histopathology* 2011, **59:**807–821.
34. Gong N, Wong CS, Chu YC: **Is lymph node metastasis a common feature of gastrointestinal stromal tumor? PET/CT correlation.** *Clin Nucl Med* 2011, **36:**678–682.
35. Tashiro T, Hasegawa T, Omatsu M, Sekine S, Shimoda T, Katai H: **Gastrointestinal stromal tumour of the stomach showing lymph node metastases.** *Histopathology* 2005, **47:**438–439.
36. Sato T, Kanda T, Nishikura K, Hirota S, Hashimoto K, Nahagawa S, Ohashi M, Hatakeyama K: **Two cases of gastrointestinal stromal tumor of the stomach with lymph node metastasis.** *Hepatogastroenterology* 2007, **54:**1057–1060.
37. Agaimy A, Wünsch PH: **Lymph node metastasis in gastrointestinal stromal tumours (GIST) occurs preferentially in young patients < or = 40 years: an overview based on our case material and the literature.** *Langenbecks Arch Surg* 2009, **394:**375–381.
38. Hou YY, Lu SH, Zhou Y, Xu JF, Ji Y, Hou J, Qi WD, Shi Y, Tan YS, Zhu XZ: **Predictive values of clinical and pathological parameters for malignancy of gastrointestinal stromal tumors.** *Histol Histopathol* 2009, **24:**737–747.
39. Tokunaga M, Ohyama S, Hiki N, Fukunaga T, Yamamoto N, Yamaguchi T: **Incidence and prognostic value of lymph node metastasis on c-Kit-positive gastrointestinal stromal tumors of the stomach.** *Hepatogastroenterology* 2011, **58:**1224–1228.
40. Brabec P, Sufliarsky J, Linke Z, Plank L, Mrhalova M, Pavlik T, Klimes D, Gregor J: **A whole population study of gastrointestinal stromal tumors in the Czech Republic and Slovakia.** *Neoplasma* 2009, **56:**459–464.
41. Tanimine N, Tanabe K, Suzuki T, Tokumoto N, Ohdan H: **Prognostic criteria in patients with gastrointestinal stromal tumors: a single center experience retrospective analysis.** *World J Surg Oncol* 2012, **10:**43.
42. Seker M, Sevinc A, Yildiz R, Cihan S, Kaplan MA, Gokdurnali A, Dane F, Yaman E, Karaca H, Colak D, Uyeturk U, Bilici A, Ozdemir NY, Kalender ME, Uncu D, Salepci T, Isikdogan A, Benekli M, Ozkan M, Gumus M, Coskun U, Camci C, Oksuzoglu B, Buyukberber S, Anatolian Society of Medical Oncology (ASMO): **Prognostic factors in gastrointestinal stromal tumors: multicenter experience of 333 cases from Turkey.** *Hepatogastroenterology* 2012, **60:**768–775.
43. Chan KH, Chan CW, Chow WH, Kwan WK, Kong CK, Mak KF, Leung MY, Lau LK: **Gastrointestinal stromal tumors in a cohort of Chinese patients in Hong Kong.** *World J Gastroenterol* 2006, **12:**2223–2228.
44. Agaimy A: **Gastrointestinal stromal tumors (GIST) from risk stratification systems to the new TNM proposal: more questions than answers? A review emphasizing the need for a standardized GIST reporting.** *Int J Clin Exp Pathol* 2010, **3:**461–471.
45. Coccolini F, Catena F, Ansaloni L, Pinna AD: **Gastrointestinal stromal tumor and mitosis, pay attention.** *World J Gastroenterol* 2012, **18:**587–588.
46. Joensuu H, Vehtari A, Riihimäki J, Nishida T, Steigen SE, Brabec P, Plank L, Nilsson B, Cirilli C, Braconi C, Bordoni A, Magnusson MK, Linke Z, Sufliarsky J, Federico M, Jonasson JG, Dei Tos AP, Rutkowski P: **Risk of recurrence of gastrointestinal stromal tumour after surgery: an analysis of pooled population-based cohorts.** *Lancet Oncol* 2012, **13:**265–274.
47. Mrowiec S, Jabłońska B, Liszka L, Pająk J, Leidgens M, Szydło R, Sandecka A, Lampe P: **Prognostic factors for survival post surgery for patients with gastrointestinal stromal tumors.** *Eur Surg Res* 2012, **48:**3–9.
48. Cho MY, Sohn JH, Kim JM, Kim KM, Park YS, Kim WH, Jung JS, Jung ES, Jin SY, Kang DY, Park JB, Park HS, Choi YD, Sung SH, Kim YB, Kim H, Bae YK, Kang M, Chang HJ, Chae YS, Lee HE, Park do Y, Lee YS, Kang YK, Kim HK, Chang HK, Hong SW, Choi YH, Shin O, Gu M, *et al*: **Current trends in the epidemiological and pathological characteristics of gastrointestinal stromal tumors in Korea, 2003–2004.** *J Korean Med Sci* 2010, **25:**853–862.
49. Cao H, Zhang Y, Wang M, Shen DP, Sheng ZY, Ni XZ, Wu ZY, Liu Q, Shen YY, Song YY: **Prognostic analysis of patients with gastrointestinal stromal tumors: a single unit experience with surgical treatment of primary disease.** *Chin Med J (Engl)* 2010, **123:**131–136.
50. Song Z, Wang JL, Pan YL, Tao DY, Gan MF, Huang KE: **Survival and prognostic factors analysis in surgically resected gastrointestinal stromal tumor patients.** *Hepatogastroenterology* 2009, **56:**149–153.
51. Fujimoto Y, Nakanishi Y, Yoshimura K, Shimoda T: **Clinicopathologic study of primary malignant gastrointestinal stromal tumor of the stomach, with special reference to prognostic factors: analysis of results in 140 surgically resected patients.** *Gastric Cancer* 2003, **6:**39–48.
52. Dematteo RP, Ballman KV, Antonescu CR, Maki RG, Pisters PW, Demetri GD, Blackstein ME, Blanke CD, von Mehren M, Brennan MF, Patel S, McCarter MD, Polikoff JA, Tan BR, Owzar K, American College of Surgeons Oncology Group (ACOSOG) Intergroup Adjuvant GIST Study Team: **Adjuvant imatinib mesylate after resection of localised, primary gastrointestinal stromal tumour: a randomised, double-blind, placebo-controlled trial.** *Lancet* 2009, **373:**1097–1104.
53. Joensuu H, Eriksson M, Sundby Hall K, Hartmann JT, Pink D, Schütte J, Ramadori G, Hohenberger P, Duyster J, Al-Batran SE, Schlemmer M, Bauer S, Wardelmann E, Sarlomo-Rikala M, Nilsson B, Sihto H, Monge OR, Bono P, Kallio R, Vehtari A, Leinonen M, Alvegard T, Reichardt P: **One vs three years of adjuvant imatinib for operable gastrointestinal stromal tumor: a randomized trial.** *JAMA* 2012, **307:**1265–1272.
54. ESMO / European Sarcoma Network Working Group: **Gastrointestinal stromal tumors: ESMO Clinical Practice Guidelines for diagnosis, treatment and follow-up.** *Ann Oncol* 2012, **23**(Suppl 7):49–55.
55. von Mehren M, Benjamin RS, Bui MM, Casper ES, Conrad EU 3rd, DeLaney TF, Ganjoo KN, George S, Gonzalez R, Heslin MJ, Kane JM 3rd, Mayerson J, McGarry SV, Meyer C, O'Donnell RJ, Paz B, Pfeifer JD, Pollock RE, Randall RL, Riedel RF, Schuetze S, Schupak KD, Schwartz HS, Shankar S, Van Tine BA, Wayne J, Sundar H, McMillian NR: **Soft tissue sarcoma, version 2.2012: featured updates to the NCCN guidelines.** *J Natl Compr Canc Netw* 2012, **10:**951–960.

Surgery for a gastric Dieulafoy's lesion reveals an occult bleeding jejunal diverticulum: A case report

G Orlando[3], IM Luppino[1], R Gervasi[3], MA Lerose[3], B Amato[2], R Spagnuolo[1], R Marasco[1], P Doldo[1], A Puzziello[3*]

Abstract

Background: Jejunal diverticulosis is an uncommon disease and usually asymptomatic. It can be complicated not only by diverticulitis, but by hemorrhage, perforation, intussusception, volvulus, malabsorption and even small bowel obstruction due to enteroliths formed and expelled from these diverticula.

Methods: We describe a case of an occult bleeding jejunal diverticulum, casually discovered in a patient that was taken to surgery for a Dieulafoy's lesion after unsuccessful endoscopic treatment. We performed a gastric resection together with an ileocecal resection.
Macroscopic and microscopic examinations confirmed the gastric Dieulafoy's lesion and demonstrated the presence of another source of occult bleeding in asymptomatic jejunal diverticulum.

Discussion: The current case emphasizes that some gastrointestinal bleeding lesions, although rare, can be multiple and result in potentially life-threatening bleeding. The clinician must be mindful to the possibility of multisite lesions and to the correlation between results of the investigations and clinical condition of the bleeding patient.

Background

Jejunal diverticulosis (JD) is an uncommon disease and usually asymptomatic [1] with an incidence of 0.06–1.3% although the prevalence seems to increase with age. The highest incidence of JD occurs during the sixth and seventh decades of life, and the disease is thought to be more common in males. It is frequently seen in the duodenum while jejunal and ileal locations are very rare. More commonly JD is diagnosed as an incidental finding of computed tomography imaging, small bowel barium radiographic series, or during surgery [2,3].

This report presents a case of small bowel bleeding jejunal diverticulum with enteroliths formed inside casually discovered intraoperatively as another cause of bleeding in a patient with a Dieulafoy's lesion.

* Correspondence: puzziello@unicz.it
[3]Endocrine Surgery Unit, Department of Surgical and Medical Sciences, University Magna Graecia, Catanzaro, Italy
Full list of author information is available at the end of the article

Case report

A 75-years-old-man was admitted for an undiagnosed gastric bleeding lesion treated with endoscopic clips. He suffered of anemia and asthenia without nausea, abdominal pain or weight loss. Laboratory studies revealed mild anemia with hemoglobin level of 10 g/dL. An upper gastrointestinal endoscopy was performed showing a 2 cm bleeding ulceration at the corpo-antral junction in the greater curve. Endoscopic ultrasound (EUS) confirmed the presence of a single long vessel of 1 mm diameter perforating the muscular layer of the gastric wall and coming to lie in the submucosa. The arterial nature of the vessel was confirmed by pulse Doppler [4,5]. It was diagnosed a Dieulafoy's lesion (DL) according to the following diagnostic criteria: 1. active arterial spurting or micropulsatile bleeding from a minute mucosal defect less than 3 mm or normal mucosa; 2. visualization of a protruding vessel with or without bleeding within a small mucosal defect or normal mucosa; 3. appearance of a fresh, adherent clot to a minute mucosal defect or normal mucosa [6]. The first choice was endoscopic treatment. Injection of epinephrine (1:10) and the use of endoscopic clips led to complete cessation of bleeding [7]. No complications developed after the procedure and there was no recurrence of bleeding at the 90-day follow-up. After six months the patient was readmitted because of a worsening of general condition with acute upper GI bleeding. An endoscopic treatment was performed placing three clips. At the follow-up the failure of procedure needed a gastric wedge resection.

The patient suffered of a severe stage of COPD and laparoscopic procedure was contraindicated so the laparotomy was performed. Intraoperative abdominal exploration incidentally revealed a jejunal diverticulum close to caecum [Fig.1]. An ileocecal resection was performed with a double-layer side-to-side single stitches anastomosis (Vicryl*Plus 3/0SHplus). Afterwards, a gastric wedge resection was performed by a linear stapler (Covidien DST Series™ GIA™ 60-3.5) [Fig.2].

The discharge was in the 5th day post op.

Macroscopic examination showed a segment of intestine approximately 30 cm in length with JD on the antimesenteric side. Three enteroliths were founded formed inside with a smooth dark outer surface, the largest one of 3 cm in major diameter without protruding into the intestinal lumen. Histological sections of bowel showed wall thinning of the jejunal mucosal with bleeding areas and intense neutrophilic exudate that covered all the coats of the intestinal wall. The gastric gross examination confirmed a Dieulafoy's lesion.

One year after surgery the patient has a hemoglobin level of 14,5 g/dL.

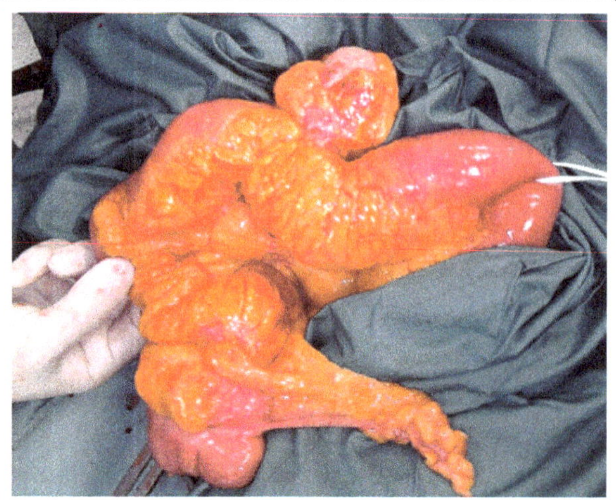

Figure 1 Intraoperative jejunal diverticulum.

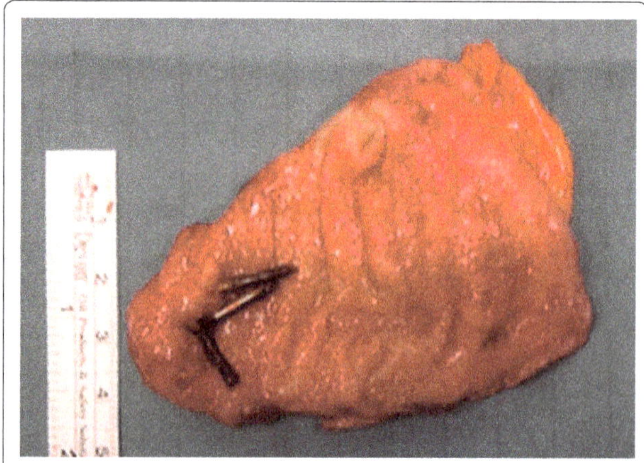

Figure 2 Opened wedge resection showing endoscopic clips.

Discussion

This case report shows in the same patient two rare causes of GI bleeding and permits a discussion about their suitable treatment.

Dieulafoy's lesion

A Dieulafoy's lesion is an aberrantly dilated and tortuous submucosal arteriole, often identified after it erodes through the mucosa of the gastrointestinal tract and begins to bleed. There is no consensus on the treatment of DL. The evolution of endoscopic methods of haemostasis has markedly reduced the need for surgery achieving more than 90% of resolution [8,9]. These procedures can be classified into three groups: electrocoagulation, regional injection and mechanical treatments [10,11]. The initial haemostasis rate of injection therapy may be close to 95%. On the other hand, the re-bleeding after injection monotherapy is reported to be up to 55%.

More studies have shown that mechanical endoscopic methods, such as the clip placement (EHP) and the band ligation (EBL), are more effective treatments than other endoscopic methods. They could be considered the first option in the management of DL. Ahn reports in a retrospective single center study both EHP and EBL are suitable for the treatment of bleeding DL. EBL can be used as an initial haemostatic method for bleeding DL because of a favorable clinical outcome comparable to that with EHP and a shorter procedure time [12].

The risk of re-bleeding has a range of 9-40% and is higher in endoscopic monotherapy compared with combined methods. Endoscopic methods are the preferred treatment if re-bleeding occurs. Angiography, more suitable for lower GI tract lesions, can be used to stop the bleeding by selective embolisation of the feeding vessel, but up to date there are conflicting data [10]. Wide-wedge resection is today the last surgical resort overtaken by advances in endoscopic procedures. Actually, surgery has a role in the 5% of uncontrolled or unidentified bleeding and in the failure of endoscopic interventions [6,13,14].

Jejunal diverticular disease

Jejunal diverticular disease is a rarely found pathology (±5% of post-mortem examinations). Despite being a rare pathology, there is a greater prevalence of JD disease in the older age population but it is often asymptomatic. Diverticular disease of the small intestine is noted in 60%-70% duodenal, 20%-25% jejunal, and 5%-10% ileal [2]. JD is diagnosed as an incidental finding of computed tomography imaging, small bowel barium radiographic series or during surgery [3,1]. Some patients have a history of chronic symptoms such as vague abdominal discomfort, fullness, pain or recurrent central and upper abdominal cramps because of pseudo-obstruction. Anemia due to iron deficiency and megaloblastic anemia have often been reported and commonly attributed to malabsorption, steatorrhea, and B12 vitamin deficiency [3]. Patients with JD can present with emergent complications such as massive gastrointestinal bleeding, intestinal obstruction or perforation [15]. Recently, the total laparoscopic approach has been used as a valid surgical strategy, even in cases of complicated diverticulitis [16].

In this case the incidental intraoperative discovery of JD imposed the choice of an ileocecal resection as prevention of complications in a patient with an high surgical risk.

Conclusion

In conclusion, these conditions, although rare, can be multiple and result in potentially life-threatening bleeding. The clinician must be mindful to the possibility of multisite lesions and to the correlation between results of the investigations and clinical condition of the bleeding patient. In this case the incidental discovery of an occult bleeding lesion and a targeted surgical approach made us to ensure a suitable therapy of GI bleeding. The follow up will be done by capsule endoscopy, a safe and effective method of intestinal post operative control [17].

Acknowledgements

This article has been published as part of *BMC Surgery* Volume 12 Supplement 1, 2012: Selected articles from the XXV National Congress of the Italian Society of Geriatric Surgery. The full contents of the supplement are available online at http://www.biomedcentral.com/bmcsurg/supplements/12/S1.

Author details

[1]Gastroenterology and Endoscopy Unit, T. Campanella Oncological Foundation, Catanzaro, Italy. [2]General Surgery Unit, Dept of General Surgery, Geriatric and Endoscopy, University Federico II, Naples, Italy. [3]Endocrine Surgery Unit, Department of Surgical and Medical Sciences, University Magna Graecia, Catanzaro, Italy.

Authors' contributions

GO: conception and design, interpetration of data, given final approval of the version to be published; IML: acquisition of data, drafting the manuscript, given final approval of the version to be published; RG: acquisition of data, drafting the manuscript, given final approval of the version to be published; MAL: acquisition of data, drafting the manuscript, given final approval of the version to be published; BA: acquisition of data, drafting the manuscript, given final approval of the version to be published; RS: acquisition of data, interpretation of data, given final approval of the version to be published; RM: acquisition of data, interpretation of data, given final approval of the version to be published; PD: acquisition of data, interpretation of data, given final approval of the version to be published; AP: conception and design, critical revision, given final approval of the version to be published.

Competing interests

The authors declare that they have no competing interests.

References

1. Chugay P, Choi J, Dong XD: **Jejunal diverticular disease complicated by enteroliths: Report of two different presentations.** *World J Gastrointest Surg* 2010, **2**:26-29.
2. Yaqub S, Evensen BV, Kjellevold K: **Massive rectal bleeding from acquired jejunal diverticula.** *World J Emerg Surg* 2011, **6**:17.
3. Butler JS, Collins CG, McEntee GP: **Perforated jejunal diverticula: a case report.** *J Med Case Reports* 2010, **4**:172.
4. Fockens P, Meenan J, Van Dullemen HM, Bolwerk CJ, Tytgat GN: **Dieulafoy's disease: endosonographic detection and endosonography-guided treatment.** *Gastrointest Endosc* 1996, **44**:437-42.
5. Jaspersen D: **Dieulafoy's disease controlled by Doppler ultrasound endoscopic treatment.** *Gut* 1993, **34**:857-858.
6. Lee YT, Walmsley RS, Leong RW, Sung JJ: **Dieulafoy's lesion.** *Gastrointest Endosc* 2003, **58**:236-243.
7. Nikolaidis N, Zezos P, Giouleme O, Budas K, Marakis G, Paroutoglou G, Eugenidis N: **Endoscopic band ligation of Dieulafoy-like lesions in the upper gastrointestinal tract.** *Endoscopy* 2001, **33**:754-760.
8. Chung IK, Kim EJ, Lee MS, Kim HS, Park SH, Lee MH: **Bleeding Dieulafoy's lesions and the choice of endoscopic method: comparing the hemostatic efficacy of mechanical and injection methods.** *Gastrointest Endosc* 2000, **52**:721-724.
9. Marangoni G, Cresswell AB, Faraj W, Shaikh H, Bowles MJ: **An uncommon cause of life-threatening gastrointestinal bleeding: 2 synchronous Dieulafoy lesions.** *J Paediatr Surg* 2009, **44**:441-443.
10. Alshumrani G, Almuaikeel M: **Angiographic findings and endovascular embolization in Dieulafoy disease: a case report and literature review.** *Diagn Interv Radiol* 2006, **12**:151-154.
11. Parra-Blanco A, Takahashi H, Mendez Jerez PV, Kojima T, Aksoz K, Kirihara K, Pamerin J, Takekuma Y, Fujita R: **Endoscopic management of Dieulafoy lesions of the stomach: a case study of 26 patients.** *Endoscopy* 1997, **29**:834-839.
12. Ahn DW, Lee SH, Park YS, Shin CM, Hwang JH, Kim JW, Jeong SH, Kim N, Lee DH: **Hemostatic efficacy and clinical outcome of endoscopic treatment of Dieulafoy's lesions: comparison of endoscopic hemoclip placement and endoscopic band ligation.** *Gastrointest Endosc* 2012, **75(1)**:32-8.
13. Cheng CL, Liu NJ, Lee CS, Chen PC, Ho YP, Tang JH, Yang C, Sung KF, Lin CH, Chiu CT: **Endoscopic Management of Dieulafoy Lesions in Acute Nonvariceal Upper Gastrointestinal Bleeding.** *Dig Dis Sci* 2004, **49(7-8)**:1139-44.
14. Baxter M, Aly EH: **Dieulafoy's lesion: current trends in diagnosis and management.** *Ann R Coll Surg Engl* 2010, **92(7)**:548-54.
15. Crace PP, Grisham A, Kerlakian G: **Jejunal diverticular disease with unborn enterolith presenting as a small bowel obstruction: a case report.** *Am Surg* 2007, **73**:703-705.
16. Garg N, Khullar R, Sharma A, Soni V, Baijal M, Chowbey P: **Total laparoscopic management of large complicated jejunal diverticulum.** *J Minim Access Surg* 2009, **5**:115-117.
17. De Palma GD, Rega M, Puzziello A, Aprea G, Ciacci C, Castiglione F, Ciamarra P, Persico M, Patrone F, Mastantuono L, Persico G: **Capsule endoscopy is safe and effective after small-bowel resection.** *Gastrointest Endosc* 2004, **60**:135-8.

17

Long-term effects of laparoscopic sleeve gastrectomy versus roux-en-Y gastric bypass for the treatment of Chinese type 2 diabetes mellitus patients with body mass index 28-35 kg/m^2

Jingge Yang, Cunchuan Wang*, Guo Cao, Wah Yang, Shuqing Yu, Hening Zhai and Yunlong Pan

Abstract

Background: To compare long term effects of two bariatric procedures for Chinese type 2 diabetes mellitus (T2DM) patients with a body mass index (BMI) of 28-35 kg/m^2.

Methods: Sixty four T2DM patients with Glycated hemoglobin A1c (HbA1c) ≧ 7.0 % were randomly assigned to receive laparoscopic sleeve gastrectomy (SG) or Roux-en-Y gastric bypass (RYGB) procedure. Weight, percentage of excess weight loss (%EWL), BMI, waist circumference, HbA1c, fasting blood glucose (FBG), and C-peptide were measured. Serum lipid levels were also measured during three-year postoperative follow-up visits.

Results: Fifty five patients completed the 36-month follow-up. Both groups had similar baseline anthropometric and biochemical measures. At the end point, 22 patients (78.6 %) in SG group and 23 patients (85.2 %) in RYGB group achieved complete remission of diabetes mellitus with HbA1c < 6.0 % ($P = 0.525$) and without taking diabetic medications, and 25 patients in each group (89.3 % vs. 92.6 %) gained successful treatment of diabetes with HbA1c≦6.5 % ($P = 0.100$). Change in HbA1c, FBG and C peptide were comparable in the two groups. The RYGB group had significantly greater weight loss than the SG group [percentage of total weight loss (%TWL) of 31.0 % vs. 27.1 % ($P = 0.049$), %EWL of 92.3 % vs. 81.9 % ($P = 0.003$), and change in BMI of 11.0 vs. 9.1 kg/m^2 ($P = 0.017$), respectively]. Serum lipids in each group were also greatly improved.

Conclusion: In this three-year study, SG had similar positive effects on diabetes and dyslipidemia compared to RYGB in Chinese T2DM patients with BMI of 28-35 kg/m^2. Longer term follow-ups and larger sample studies are needed to confirm these outcomes, however.

Keywords: Bariatric surgery, Roux-en-Y gastric bypass, Sleeve gastrectomy, Type 2 diabetes, Mild obesity

Background

Obesity and type 2 diabetes mellitus (T2DM) are two of the most common metabolic disorders in the world. Both have significantly increased during the last decades [1, 2]. In China, the prevalence of obesity and T2DM is similar to the worldwide statistics. In China it is estimated that the number of people with diabetes was 98.4 million 2013 and will reach 142.7 million by 2035 [2].

Bariatric procedures are superior to conservative therapies in managing T2DM [3, 4]. Roux-en-Y gastric bypass (RYGB) is the most commonly supported procedure that can cure most T2DM in morbidly obese patients [3, 5, 6]. Sleeve gastrectomy (SG), a novel technique, is highly effective in the treatment of severe or morbid obesity [7, 8]. It is still controversial, however, whether SG has the same positive outcomes on T2DM in mild obese patients compared to RYGB [9, 10]. Importantly, most of the Chinese T2DM patients that have been studied have BMI less than 35 kg/m^2 and are newly detected diabetes cases with short

* Correspondence: twcc@jnu.edu.cn
Department of General Surgery, First Affiliated Hospital of Jinan University, Guangzhou 510630, China

disease durations [11]. Other relevant reports about long term effects of SG on Chinese diabetes with BMI of 28-35 kg/m^2 are scarce.

The aim of this study was to compare the long term efficacy of SG and RYGB in Chinese T2DM patients with BMI of 28-35 kg/m^2 using a prospective randomized trial over 36 months post-operatively.

Methods

We designed a prospective randomized study to determine whether SG is as effective as RYGB for T2DM remission in Chinese patients with BMI of 28-35 kg/m^2 and a short history of disease. The study was conducted in Department of Gastrointestinal Surgery of the 1st affiliated hospital and Jihua hospital of Jinan University, Guangzhou, China. The trial was conducted from July 1, 2009 through July 30, 2014. The human ethics committee of Jinan University approved and supervised the whole study.

Patients

Sixty-four patients enrolled in this study. Inclusion criteria included: (a) diagnosis of poorly controlled T2DM after 6 months medicine therapy [glycated hemoglobin A1c (HbA1c) level ≥7.0 %], (b) measured BMI of ≥28 and ≤ 35 kg/m2, (c) aged 25 to 60 years old, (d) diabetes duration of less than ten years, and (e) patients were excluded if they had undergone previous bariatric surgery or other complex abdominal surgery or if they had poorly controlled medical problems. Patients were also excluded if they had C-peptide levels below 0.8 ng/ml. In addition to the assessments for inclusion, each patient was assessed for their general condition and mental status, complications of obesity and diabetes mellitus, risk factors, and motivations for surgery (Fig.1). A computer-generated variable block schedule was used for randomization. Allocation to treatments was not concealed and patients knew which procedure they were to undergo.

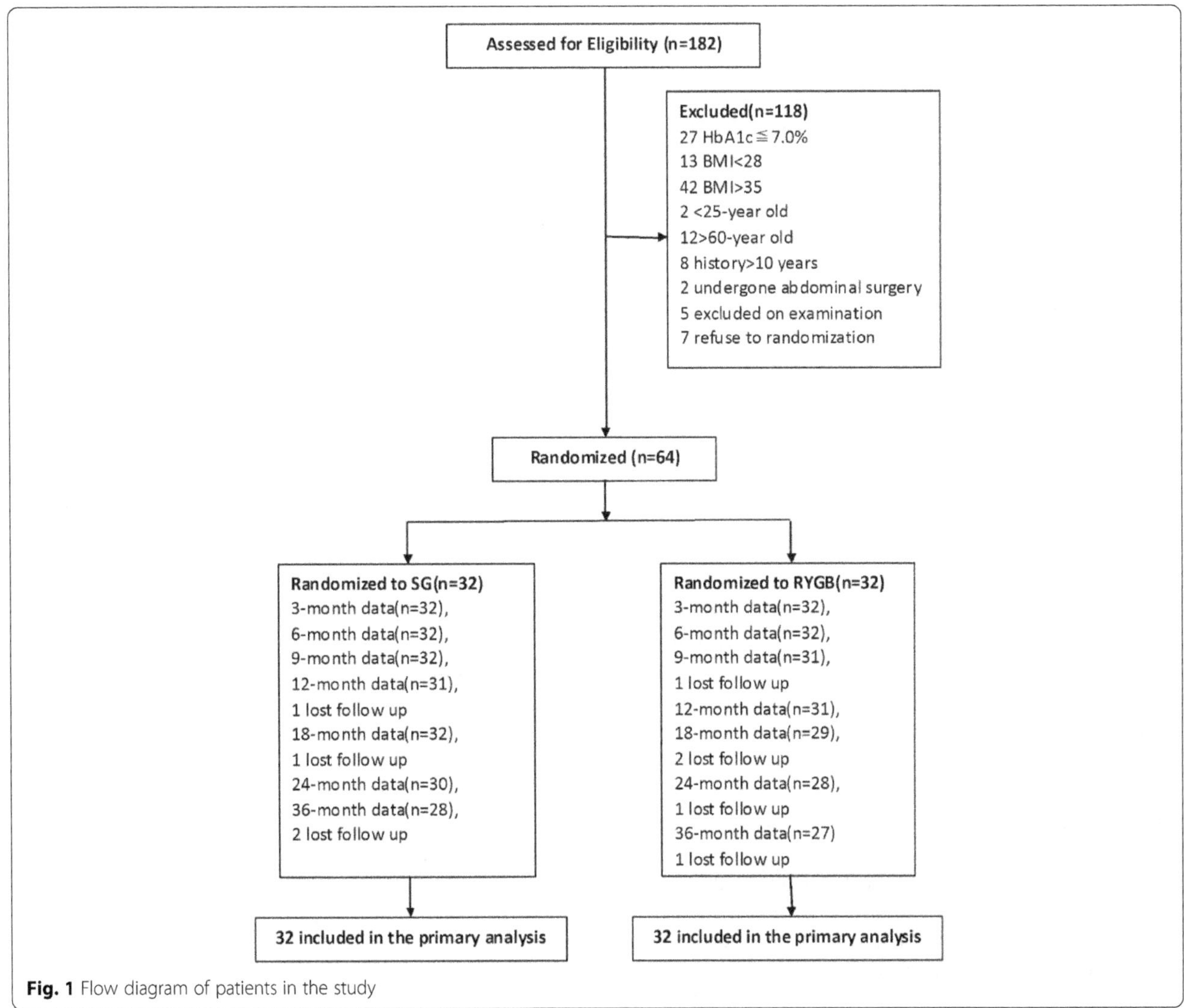

Fig. 1 Flow diagram of patients in the study

Surgical interventions

In order to reduce the differences in surgical techniques, the same team and the same physician (Cunchuan Wang) carried out the operations for both groups. Described briefly, the surgical methods were as follows: For laparoscopic SG, four trocars were placed and 38 Fr. Bougie was used to calibrate the sleeve. The greater curvature was cut out 4 cm from the pylorus using a linear stapler towards His angle to completely remove the fundus of the stomach. The remnant gastric cutting edge was 2 cm from the lesser curvature of stomach. Then, the cutting edge was continuously sutured with 3-0 absorbable sutures, which are good for hemostasis. For laparoscopic RYGB, 5 trocars were used. The volume of gastric pouch was approximate 10-20 ml. The length of the biliopancreatic limb was 25 cm, and the Roux limb was 125 cm. The anastomotic stoma between stomach and jejunum was 1.5 cm and 6 cm between jejuna.

During the operation, no routine stomach and drainage tubes were placed. Patients fasted the first day post-operation and followed a complete liquid and a soft diet for one month. Subsequently, patients followed a half liquid diet for three months and gradually arrived at a general diet. The patients received follow-up examinations in an outpatient clinic, Patients took a proton pump inhibitor and gastric mucosa protective agent for six weeks post-operation. In addition, the patients routinely took multi-vitamin supplementation and calcium tablet for a long period. The vitamin status was not checked regularly.

Follow up and data collection

In one year post operation, the patients attended the visit every three months, and half-yearly thereafter. We collected the patients' height, body weight, BMI, waist circumference, usage of medication and adverse events. The laboratory test included HbA1c, FBG, C-peptide, and serum lipid profiles.

Study end points

The primary outcome was glycemic control with HbA1c values less than 6.0 % in addition to fasting plasma glucose levels less than 7.0 mmol/L without glycemic agents at the 36-month visit. Secondary outcome measures included the percentage of weight loss and improvement of dyslipidemia. Any adverse events were also recorded.

Statistical analysis

As previous study has shown a remission rate in RYGB group of 80 % [12], we assumed that SG would lead to a lower remission rate of 40 % in the lower BMI patients. Using a sample size of 64 patients (32 per group), we would have had the power to detect this difference with an α level of 0.05 and power of 90 %.

All analyses were performed using SPSS 17.0 (SPSS Inc., Chicago, Illinois). Chi-square and t-tests were used to compare differences between two groups. Continuous variables were reported as means with standard deviation. A 2-sided P value of <0.05 was considered statistically significant.

Results

Patient characteristics

Nine (14.1 %) patients failed to finish the whole 36 months follow-up, and this included four from SG group and five from RYGB group. The patients' characteristics at baseline are summarized in Table 1. Both groups had similar baseline anthropometric measurements, including age, gender, weight, height, BMI, waist circumference, duration of diabetes, and medication usage conditions (Table 1). Baseline values of HbA1c (8.5 % vs. 8.9 %, $P = 0.321$), FBG (10.2 vs. 10.4 mmol/L, $P = 0.700$), and C-peptide (2.2 vs. 2.6 ng/ml, $P = 0.062$) in the SG group were comparable to the RYGB group. The two groups also had similar baseline serum lipid levels that included cholesterol, triglyceride, HDL, and LDL.

Table 1 Baseline patients characteristics

Characteristic	SG (n = 32)	RYGB (n = 32)	P value
Demographic, mean (SD)			
Age (yrs)	40.4 ± 9.4	41.4 ± 9.3	0.681
Sex, female-no.(%)	23 (71.9)	19 (59.4)	0.292
Height (cm)	166.8 ± 6.8	170.3 ± 8.6	0.077
Weight (kg)	88.4 ± 6.8	94.3 ± 13.3	0.055
Body mass index (kg/m^2)	31.8 ± 3.0	32.3 ± 2.4	0.374
Waist circumference (cm)	103.0 ± 7.7	104.5 ± 6.8	0.404
Duration of diabetes (yrs)	4.0 ± 1.7	4.2 ± 1.9	0.710
Glycemia, mean (SD)			
HbA1c (%)	8.5 ± 1.2	8.9 ± 1.3	0.321
FBG (mmol/L)	10.2 ± 2.7	10.4 ± 2.2	0.700
C-peptide (ng/ml)	2.2 ± 0.7	2.6 ± 1.0	0.062
Serum lipids, mean (SD)			
Cholesterol (mmol/L)	5.0 ± 1.1	4.6 ± 0.9	0.092
Triglyceride (mmol/L)	3.2 ± 1.7	3.0 ± 2.0	0.545
HDL (mmol/L)	1.1 ± 0.2	1.0 ± 0.1	0.067
LDL (mmol/L)	3.8 ± 1.1	3.9 ± 0.9	0.702
Medication usage-no.(%)			
Oral hypoglycemic	31 (96.9)	30 (93.8)	0.554
Insulin usage	15 (46.9)	18 (56.2)	0.453
Antihypertension	10 (31.2)	12 (37.5)	0.599
Lipid-lowering drug	21 (65.6)	18 (56.2)	0.442

Surgical treatments and complications

All procedures were successfully performed by laparoscopic techniques. The surgical time was shorter for the SG group than the RYGB group (58.0 vs.103.8 mins, $P = 0.000$). The mean post-operative hospital stay was 5.2 days for the SG group and 6.6 days for the RYGB group ($P = 0.000$). There were no deaths or major complications in either group. Minor complications occurred in 3 of 55 patients (5.5 %), including 2 gastroesophageal reflux cases in the SG group and 1 case of anemia in the RYGB group. All cases with complications were resolved with medications. The case with anemia was cured with ferralia and vitamin B12 for a long term.

Table 2 Outcomes at 36 months

Variable	SG (28)	RYGB (27)	*P* Value
Primary outcome-no.(%)			
HbA1c ≤ 6.5 % without medications	25 (89.3)	25 (92.6)	1.000
HbA1c ≤ 6.5 % with medication	2 (7.1)	1 (3.7)	1.000
HbA1c < 6.0 % without medications	22 (78.6)	23 (85.2)	0.525
HbA1c < 6.0 % with medications	1 (3.6)	0 (0)	1.000
Glycemia, mean (SD)			
HbA1c (%)	5.9 ± 0.7	5.7 ± 0.7	0.334
Change from baseline (%)	2.7 ± 1.1	3.1 ± 1.3	0.175
FBG (mmol/L)	5.9 ± 0.7	5.8 ± 0.7	0.371
Change from baseline (mmol/L)	4.3 ± 2.7	4.8 ± 2.0	0.448
C-peptide (ng/mL)	1.7 ± 0.5	1.8 ± 0.6	0.285
Change from baseline (ng/mL)	0.5 ± 0.5	0.7 ± 0.4	0.060
Weight, mean (SD)			
%TWL	27.1 ± 7.1	31.0 ± 7.1	0.049
%EWL	81.9 ± 14.0	92.3 ± 10.5	0.003
Weight (kg)	63.3 ± 7.9	64.4 ± 8.9	0.610
Change from baseline (kg)	24.3 ± 6.5	29.5 ± 8.9	0.017
BMI (kg/m^2)	22.8 ± 1.7	22.0 ± 1.1	0.032
Change from baseline (kg/m^2)	9.1 ± 2.7	11.0 ± 3.2	0.017
Waist circumference (cm)	81.2 ± 3.6	79.2 ± 3.1	0.029
Change from baseline (cm)	21.6 ± 10.8	25.0 ± 6.3	0.166
Serum lipids, mean (SD)			
Cholesterol (mmol/L)	3.9 ± 0.7	3.8 ± 0.8	0.674
Triglyceride (mmol/L)	1.5 ± 0.6	1.4 ± 0.6	0.310
HDL (mmol/L)	1.5 ± 0.3	1.7 ± 0.4	0.105
LDL (mmol/L)	2.2 ± 0.7	1.9 ± 0.7	0.120
Medication usage-no.(%)			
Oral hypoglycemic agents	4 (14.3)	2 (7.4)	0.700
Insulin usage	2 (7.1)	0	0.488
Antihypertension agent	5 (17.9)	3 (11.1)	0.744
Lipid-lowering drug	3 (10.7)	1 (3.7)	0.630

Treatment effects

Primary and secondary outcomes at 36 months are shown in Table 2. 22 patients (78.6 %) in SG group and 23 patients (85.2 %) in RYGB group achieved complete remission of diabetes mellitus with HbA1c < 6.0 % ($P = 0.525$) and without taking antidiabetic medications, and 25 patients in each group (89.3 % vs. 92.6 %) gained successful treatment of diabetes with HbA1c ≤ 6.5 % ($P = 0.100$). Meanwhile, at study end point, 27 patients in SG group and 28 in RYGB group stopped receiving oral hypoglycemic agents, and 13 patients in the SG group and 18 patients in the RYGB group no longer needed insulin injections.

Each group had significant weight loss compared to baseline in the follow-up. At each visit time, percentage of total weight loss (%TWL), %EWL and change in BMI were greater in the RYGB group compared to the SG group. The most weight loss time point was two-year post operation in both groups, and after that maintained the weight reduction outcomes (Fig. 2).

At three-year post operation, HbA1c were similar in the two study groups (5.9 vs. 5.7 mmol/L, $P = 0.334$). At 3-month and 6-month visiting post operation, HbA1c values were much lower for RYGB group than SG group, and meanwhile reductions of HbA1c were more significant for RYGB group ($P < 0.01$). After that, the values of HbA1c and changes of HbA1c were similar in the two groups ($P > 0.05$) (Fig. 3a b). FBG levels were comparable for the SG and RYGB groups at all-time points (Fig. 3c). In both groups, HbA1c and FBG levels were significantly improved after 3 months ($P < 0.05$), and the improvements were maintained through the 36-month evaluation.

Compared to the baseline, post-operative serum lipid levels in each group were significantly improved. The serum levels of cholesterol, triglyceride, HDL, and LDL were similar at each time point for the SG group compared to the RYGB group. 35 patients (18 from SG group, and 17 from RYGB group) no longer needed lipid-lowering medications and 14 patients (5 from SG and 9 from RYGB group) no longer needed antihypertensive medications at the 36-month follow-up.

Discussion

Bariatric surgery has favorable effects on obesity and related metabolic problems. Of available procedures, Roux-en-Y gastric bypass is a common choice. For T2DM patients with severe obesity and BMI over 35 kg/m^2, a large number of studies have shown that both sleeve gastrectomy and RYGB procedures have favorable effects [5, 6, 13, 14]. As for T2DM patients with mild obesity, gastric bypass surgery has also shown to be effective. However, it is still controversial whether sleeve gastrectomy has the same effect for the lower BMI patients [10, 15, 16].

In Asian and Chinese populations, obesity related health risks are observed in people with BMI as low as

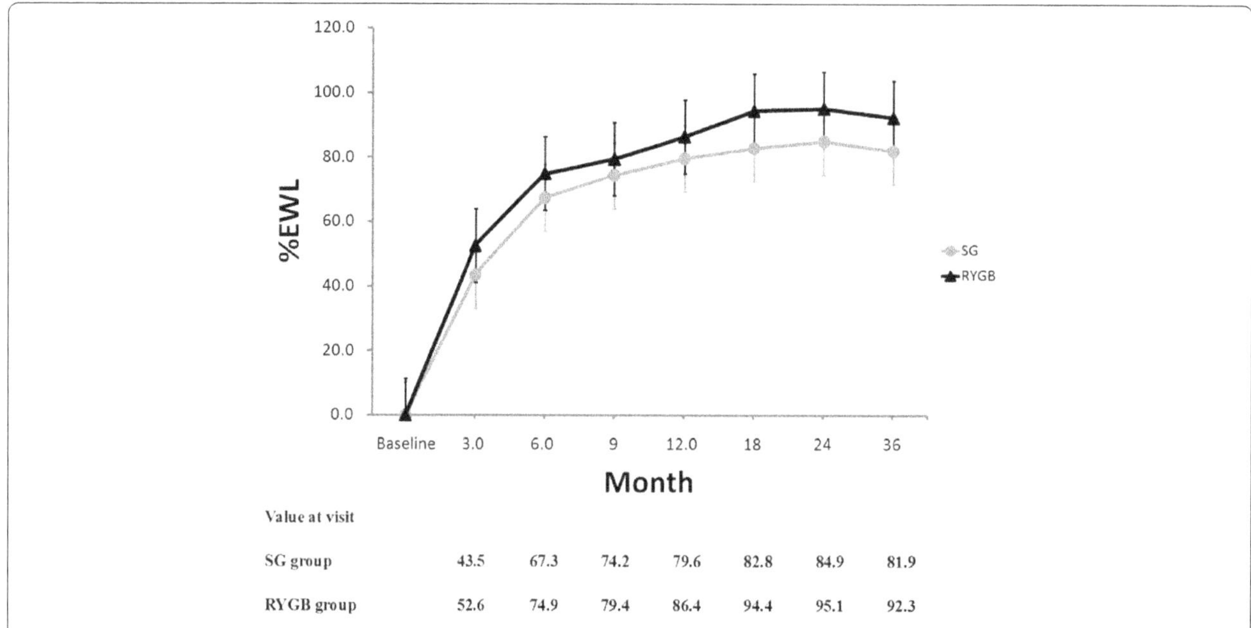

Fig. 2 Percentage of excess weight loss are plotted for the 3, 6, 9, 12, 18, 24 and 36 month time points. Error bars indicate 95 % CIs; *P* values for differences are all <0.05

22 to 23 [17]. Compared to Caucasians with the same BMI, Chinese populations have significantly higher levels of subcutaneous and visceral fat, which corresponds to higher risk of cardiovascular and metabolic diseases. Thus, BMI used for diagnosing obesity in Asian and Chinese populations should be lower than in western populations [18, 19]. The Asian branch of ASMBS suggests that when treating T2DM patients with bariatric surgery, BMI should be lowered appropriately, and T2DM patients with BMI over 28 kg/m^2 should be enrolled in clinical studies [20]. To our knowledge, there are rare studies onT2DM patients with BMI of 28-35 kg/m^2 in the Chinese mainland. At the same time, more studies have shown that early bariatric surgical intervention can enhance the remission rates of T2DM [21, 22]. Therefore, the subjects in this study are mildly obese T2DM patients with BMI of 28-35 kg/m^2 and disease histories of less than 10 years.

The results of this study show that three years after operation, both SG and RYGB procedures were effective in weight reduction and remission of T2DM. RYGB had significantly better effects on %TWL, %EWL, and BMI change when compared with SG, which is consistent with previous studies [23, 24]. Moreover, patients in both groups had normal BMI and achieved ideal weights one year after operation without major complications. Three years after operation, the complete T2DM remission rates (HbA1c < 6.0 % without taking anti-diabetic medicines) were 78.6 % in the SG group and 85.2 % in the RYGB group. The average HbA1c and FBG levels in both groups reached normal levels, indicating that the effects of SG were equivalent to RYGB in mildly obese T2DM patients. This is consistent with the previous prospective study from Andrei Keidar and the retrospective study from Sylvie Pham with the patients of BMI > 35 kg/m^2 [13, 14]. However, a research outcomes from Lee et al. suggested that RYGB achieved better blood glucose control compared to SG at one and five years post-operation for the T2DM patients with BMI 25-35 kg/m^2 [10, 16]. In Lee's study, BMI of the patients was relatively lower and the diabetic history was longer (RYGB 5.8 years vs. SG 6.9 years). These factors may have caused the patients to be more pancreatic insufficient than peripheral insulin resistance, and that may cause the lower remission rate of T2DM.

Additionally, our study showed that in both groups, all blood lipid indexes were significantly decreased after operation in the patients with dyslipidemia. Three years after operation, the blood lipid indexes, including total cholesterol, triglyceride, LDL, and HDL, stayed at normal levels with similar degrees of decline. Meanwhile, the percentages of patients that stopped taking lipid-lowering drugs and antihypertensive drugs were the same, illustrating that both SG and RYGB have similar effects on obesity relevant metabolic disturbances.

Even now, the mechanism through which bariatric surgery treats T2DM is unclear. This study investigates clinical effects but not the underling mechanism. We can see from this study, RYGB gained more significant HbA1c reduction than SG in the first 6 months after operation, and

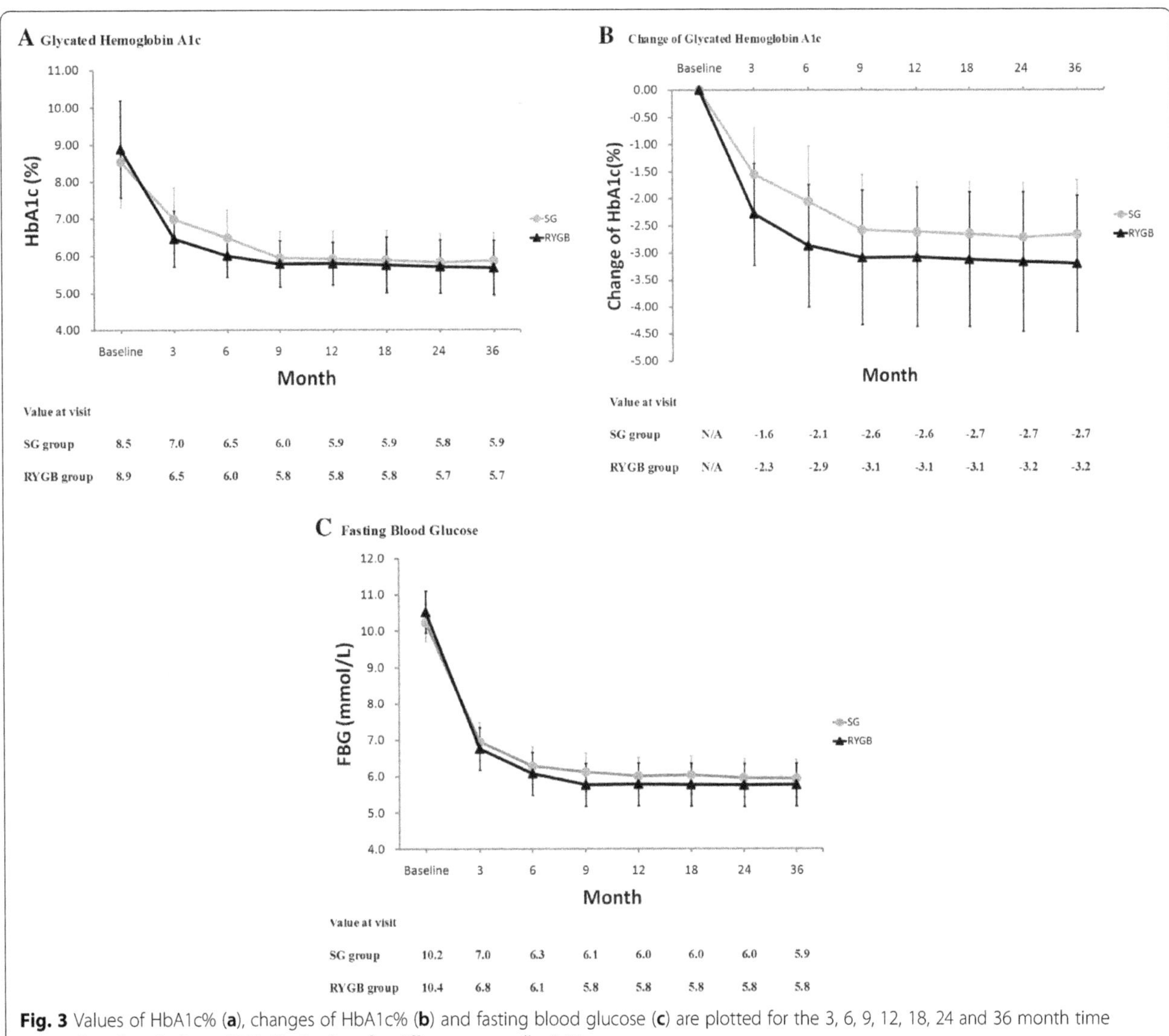

Fig. 3 Values of HbA1c% (**a**), changes of HbA1c% (**b**) and fasting blood glucose (**c**) are plotted for the 3, 6, 9, 12, 18, 24 and 36 month time points. Error bars indicate 95 % CIs; *P* values for differences are all < 0.05

that implied RYGB improves more rapidly for T2DM. Because the RYGB operation bypasses the proximal intestine, hypotheses of its mechanism include the Ghrelin hypothesis, hindgut hypothesis, and foregut hypothesis [25, 26]. After the SG operation, insulin resistance was obviously alleviated, while the incretin hormones level was significantly increased [26–29]. Peterli et al. found that one year after surgery, RYGB ghrelin levels approached preoperative values while SG ghrelin levels were still markedly attenuated. Meanwhile cholecystokinin concentrations after test meals increased less in the RYGB group than in the SG group. They suggested that bypassing the foregut is not the only mechanism responsible for improved glucose homeostasis [30]. Schauer PR et al. concluded that weight loss and a shorter duration of diabetes were the main predictors of having a glycated hemoglobin level of 6.0 % or less after surgery [31]. Our study suggests that both groups obtained similar diabetic remission rate but different weight loss effects 3 years after operation. The relationship between glycemic control and weight loss needs to be further investigated.

This comparative study on clinical effects has some limitations that include lack of data collection on insulin resistance alleviation degree and lack of gastrointestinal GLP-1, GIP, and PYY hormones data collection. These data would help to determine the surgical mechanism for T2DM resolution in Chinese patients with BMI of 28-35 kg/m^2. In addition, three-year follow-up is not long enough to assure that RYGB or SG can completely alleviate T2DM. Therefore, a longer period of follow-up is required.

Conclusion

Through three-year clinical data analysis, it can be concluded that for Chinese mildly obese T2DM patients with BMI of 28-35 kg/m^2, SG had similar effects to RYGB in remission of T2DM and metabolic disorders, but a longer follow-up period is still required to confirm the long-term effects.

Abbreviations

SG: Sleeve gastrectomy; RYGB: Roux-en-Y gastric bypass; T2DM: Type 2 diabetes mellitus; BMI: Body mass index; HbA1c: Hemoglobin A1c; %EWL: Percentage of excess weight loss; FBG: Fasting blood glucose; %TWL: Percentage of total weight loss; HDL: high density lipoprotein; LDL: low density lipoprotein; GLP-1: Glucagon-like peptide 1; GIP: Gastric inhibitory polypeptide; PYY: Peptide YY.

Competing interests

The authors declare that they have no competing interests.

Authors' contributions

YJJ and WCC designed the study. WCC, YJJ, CG and YW performed the surgeries and conducted the study. YSQ and ZHN collected the data and performed the statistical analysis. PYL helped to draft the manuscript. All authors approved the final manuscript.

Acknowledgement

The authors thank the patients and their families and all the investigators, including the physicians, nurses, and laboratory technicians in this study.

References

1 Wadden TA, Brownell KD, Foster GD. Obesity: responding to the global epidemic. J Consult Clin Psychol. 2002;70(3):510–25. PMID:12090366.
2. Guariguata L, Whiting DR, Hambleton I, Beagley J, Linnenkamp U, Shaw JE. Global estimates of diabetes prevalence for 2013 and projections for 2035. Diabetes Res Clin Pract. 2014;103(2):137–49.
3. Mingrone G, Panunzi S, De Gaetano A, Guidone C, Iaconelli A, Leccesi L, et al. Bariatric surgery versus conventional medical therapy for type 2 diabetes. N Engl J Med. 2012;366(17):1577–85.
4. Rajendra Raghow. Bariatric surgery-mediated weight loss and its metabolic consequences for type-2 diabetes. World J Diabetes. 2013;4(3):47–50.
5. Still CD, Wood GC, Benotti P, Petrick AT, Gabrielsen J, Strodel WE, et al. Preoperative prediction of type 2 diabetes remission after Roux-en-Y gastric bypass surgery: a retrospective cohort study. Lancet Diabetes Endocrinol. 2014;2(1):38–45.
6. Zimmet P, Alberti KG. Surgery or medical therapy for obese patients with type 2 diabetes? New England journal of medicine. N Engl J Med. 2012;366(17):1635–6.
7. Alexandrou A, Athanasiou A, Michalinos A, Felekouras E, Tsigris C, Diamantis T. Laparoscopic sleeve gastrectomy for morbid obesity: 5-year results. Am J Surg. 2014 Jun 20. pii: S0002-9610 (14) 00262-1. doi:10.1016/j.amjsurg.2014.04.006. [Epub ahead of print]
8. Van Rutte PW, Smulders JF, De Zoete JP, Nienhuijs SW. Outcome of sleeve gastrectomy as a primary bariatric procedure. Br J Surg. 2014;101(6):661–8.
9. De Gordejuela AG, Pujol Gebelli J, García NV, Alsina EF, Medayo LS, Masdevall NC. Is sleeve gastrectomy as effective as gastric bypass for remission of type 2 diabetes in morbidly obese patients? Surg Obes Relat Dis. 2011;7(4):506–9.
10. Lee WJ, Chong K, Ser KH, Lee YC, Chen SC, Chen JC, et al. Gastric bypass vs sleeve gastrectomy for type 2 diabetes mellitus: a randomized controlled trial. Arch Surg. 2011;146(2):143–8.
11. Xu Y, Wang L, He J, Bi Y, Li M, Wang T, et al. Prevalence and control of diabetes in Chinese adults. JAMA. 2010;310(9):948–59.
12. Abbatini F, Rizzello M, Casella G, Alessandri G, Capoccia D, Leonetti F, et al. Long-term effects of laparoscopic sleeve gastrectomy, gastric bypass, and adjustable gastric banding on type 2 diabetes. Surg Endosc. 2010;24(5):1005–10. doi:10.1007/s00464-009-0715-9. Epub 2009 Oct 29
13. Keidar A, Hershkop KJ, Marko L, Schweiger C, Hecht L, Bartov N, et al. Roux-en-Y gastric bypass vs sleeve gastrectomy for obese patients with type 2 diabetes: a randomized trial. Diabetologia. 2013;56(9):1914–8.
14. Pham S, Gancel A, Scotte M, Houivet E, Huet E, Lefebvre H, et al. Comparison of the effectiveness of four bariatric surgery procedures in obese patients With type 2 diabetes: a retrospective study. J Obes. 2014;2014:638203. doi:10.1155/2014/638203. Epub 2014 May 22.
15. Al SJ. STAMPEDE: Bariatric surgery gains more evidence based support. Glob Cardiol Sci Pract. 2014;2014(1):45–8.
16. Lee WJ, Chong K, Lin YH, Wei JH, Chen SC. Laparoscopic sleeve gastrectomy versus Single anastomosis (mini-) gastric bypass for the treatment of type 2 diabetes mellitus: 5-year results of a randomized trial and study of incretin effect. Obes Surg. 2014;24(9):1552–62.
17. Ko GT, Tang JS. Waist circumference and BMI cut-off based on 10-year cardiovascular risk: evidence for central pre-obesity. Obesity. 2007;15(11):2832–9.
18. Wang J, Thornton JC, Russell M, Burastero S, Heymsfield S, Pierson Jr RN. Asians have lower body mass index (BMI) but higher percent body fat than do whites: comparisons of anthropometric measurements. Am J Clin Nutr. 1994;60(1):23–8.
19. Chang CJ, Wu CH, Chang CS, Yao WJ, Yang YC, Wu JS, et al. Low body mass index but high percent body fat in Taiwanese subjects: implications of obesity cutoffs. Int J Obes Relat Metab Disord. 2003;27(2):253–9.
20. Lakdawala M, Bhasker A. Asian consensus meeting on metabolic surgery (ACMOMS).Asian consensus meeting on metabolic surgery (ACMOMS).report: Asian consensus meeting on metabolic surgery. Recommendations for the use of bariatric and gastrointestinal metabolic surgery for treatment of obesity and type 2 diabetes mellitus in the Asian population: august 9th and 10th, 2008, Trivandrum, India. Obes Surg. 2010;20(7):929–36.
21. Dixon JB, Zimmet P, Alberti KG, Rubino F. International diabetes federation taskforce on epidemiology and prevention. Bariatric surgery: an IDF statement for obese type2 diabetes. Diabet Med. 2011;28(6):628–42.
22. Campos GM1, Rabl C, Roll GR, Peeva S, Prado K, Smith J, et al. Better weight loss, resolution of diabetes, and quality of life for laparoscopic gastric bypass versus banding results of a 2-cohort pair-matched study. Arch Surg. 2011;146(2):149–55.
23. Li K, Gao F, Xue H, Jiang Q, Wang Y, Shen Q, et al. Comparative study on laparoscopic sleeve gastrectomy and laparoscopic gastric bypass for treatment of morbid obesity patients. Hepatogastroenterol. 2014;61(130):319–22.
24. Zerrweck C, Sepúlveda EM, Maydón HG, Campos F, Spaventa AG, Pratti V, et al. Laparoscopic gastric bypass vs. sleeve gastrectomy in the super obese patient: early outcomes of an observational study. Obes Surg. 2014;24(5):712–7.
25. Samat A, Malin SK, Huang H, Schauer PR, Kirwan JP, Kashyap SR. Ghrelin suppression is associated with weight loss and insulin action following gastric bypass surgery at 12 months in obese adults with type 2 diabetes. Diabetes Obes Metab. 2013;15(10):963–6.
26. Allen RE, Hughes TD, Ng JL, Ortiz RD, Ghantous MA, Bouhali O, et al. Mechanisms behind the immediate effects of Roux-en-Y gastric bypass surgery on type 2 diabetes. Theor Biol Med Model. 2013;10:45.
27. Anderson B, Switzer NJ, Almamar A, Shi X, Birch DW, Karmali S. The impact of laparoscopic sleeve gastrectomy on plasma ghrelin levels: a systematic review. Obes Surg. 2013;23(9):1476–80.
28. Mallipedhi A, Prior SL, Barry JD, Caplin S, Baxter JN, Stephens JW. Temporal changes in glucose homeostasis and incretin hormone response at 1 and 6 months after laparoscopic sleeve gastrectomy. Surg Obes Relat Dis. 2014;10(5):860–9.
29. Eickhoff H, Guimarães A, Louro TM, Seiça RM, Castro E Sousa F. Insulin resistance and beta cell function before and after sleeve Gastrectomy in obese patients with impaired fasting glucose or type 2 diabetes. Surg Endosc. 2014 Jul 4. [Epub ahead of print].
30. Peterli R, Steinert RE, Woelnerhanssen B, Peters T, Christoffel-Courtin C, Gass M, et al. Metabolic and hormonal changes after laparoscopic Roux-en-Y gastric bypass and sleeve gastrectomy: arandomized, prospective trial. Obes Surg. 2012;22(5):740–8.
31. Schauer PR, Bhatt DL, Kirwan JP, Wolski K, Brethauer SA, Navaneethan SD, et al. STAMPEDE Investigators. Bariatric surgery versus intensive medical therapy for diabetes–3-year outcomes. N Engl J Med. 2014;370(21):2002–13.

18

Predictive factors for major postoperative complications related to gastric conduit reconstruction in thoracoscopic esophagectomy for esophageal cancer: a case control study

Shinichiro Kobayashi[1], Kengo Kanetaka[1], Yasuhiro Nagata[1,2], Masahiko Nakayama[1], Ryo Matsumoto[1], Mitsuhisa Takatsuki[1] and Susumu Eguchi[1*]

Abstract

Background: Regardless of developments in thoracoscopic esophagectomy (TE), postoperative complications relative to gastric conduit reconstruction are common after esophagectomy. The aim of the present study was to evaluate the predictive factors of major complications related to gastric conduit after TE.

Methods: From 2006 to 2015, 75 patients with esophageal cancer who underwent TE were evaluated to explore the predictive factors of major postoperative complications related to gastric conduit.

Results: Patients with major complications related to gastric conduit had a significantly longer postoperative hospital stay than patients without these complications ($P < 0.01$). Multivariate analysis demonstrated that three-field lymph node dissection (3FLND) and high serum levels of creatine phosphokinase (CPK) and C-reactive protein (CRP) at 1 postoperative day (1POD) after TE were significant predictive factors of major complications related to gastric conduit [odds ratio (OR) 5.37, 95% confidence interval (CI) 1.41–24.33, $P = 0.02$; OR 5.40, 95% CI 1.60–20.20, $P < 0.01$; OR 5.07, 95% CI 1.47–20.25, $P = 0.01$, respectively]. The incidence rates of major complications related to gastric conduit for 0, 1, 2, and 3 predictive factors were 5.3%, 18.8%, 58.8%, and 85.7%, respectively ($P < 0.01$).

Conclusions: Two or more factors in 3FLND and the high levels of CPK and CRP at 1POD after TE were identified as the risk model for major complications related to gastric conduit after TE.

Keywords: Esophageal cancer, Thoracoscopic surgery, Esophagectomy

Background

Although esophagectomy remains the curative treatment for patients with esophageal cancer, this procedure is accompanied by high incidences of complications [1, 2]. The rates of morbidity and mortality after esophagectomy in large national databases were reported to be from 42% to 50% and 2.85% to 4.3%, respectively [3–7]. Recent developments and improvements in thoracoscopic esophagectomy (TE) have reduced severe pulmonary complications after esophagectomy [8]. However, postoperative complications related to gastric conduit reconstruction are still common after esophagectomy [9]. Regarding cervical anastomotic complications after esophagectomy, leak and stricture formation are major issues [10, 11]. In particular, ischemia of the proximal portion of the graft predisposes these patients to a high incidence of anastomotic complications after esophagectomy [12]. Less commonly, severe graft ischemia can lead to transmural necrosis. Thus, early diagnosis of an ischemic reaction may facilitate appropriate

* Correspondence: sueguchi@nagasaki-u.ac.jp
[1]Department of Surgery, Nagasaki University Graduate School of Biomedical Sciences, Sakamoto 1-7-1, Nagasaki 8528102, Japan
Full list of author information is available at the end of the article

postoperative management and therapeutic intervention to prevent leakage, strictures and necrosis. The aim of the present study was to determine the predictive factors of severe gastric conduit-related postoperative complications.

Methods

Patient population and operations

From 2006 to 2015, 105 patients with esophageal cancer underwent esophagectomy and lymph node dissection at the Department of Surgery at Nagasaki University Hospital. Treatment plans for each patient were provided according to the clinical guidelines edited by the Japan Esophageal Society [13]. We chose open esophagectomy for the patients with severe adhesions in the chest or invasive neoplasia with lymph node involvement. Thirty patients were excluded because they required open esophagectomy with lymph node dissection. Seventy-five consecutive patients with esophageal cancer who underwent TE were retrospectively studied to evaluate the predictive factors for major complications related to gastric conduit after TE. The rules for classification and staging corresponded to the 7th edition of the International Union Against Cancer (UICC)/ American Joint Committee on Cancer (AJCC) Tumor Node Metastasis (TNM) staging system [14].

TE was performed from the right side in the left lateral position. Esophagectomy with lymphadenectomy in the mediastinum and around both recurrent nerves were performed. In the abdominal section, hand-assisted laparoscopic gastrectomy was performed to remove the mobilized esophagus with lymphadenectomy around the left gastric artery and aorta. After mobilization of the full stomach and esophagus, a gastric conduit was created by dividing the lesser curve of the stomach. The right gastric and right gastroepiploic artery provided the vascular supply to the created gastric conduit. In 73 patients, the gastric conduit was pulled up in the post-sternal route; in 2 patients, it was pulled up in the post-mediastinal route. The esophagogastrostomy was performed in the neck by end-to-side anastomosis. A 21-mm or 25-mm intraluminal stapler was used as the stapling device (CDH21, CDH25, Ethicon Ltd., Edinburgh, United Kingdom). The inserted part of the gastric conduit was crossed by linear stapling. All staple lines were oversewn.

Three-field lymph node dissection (3FLND) was performed in patients who had upper thoracic esophageal cancer or middle or lower thoracic esophageal cancer with lymph node metastasis in the neck region or around the right recurrent nerve [15].

This study was approved by the Ethics Committee of Nagasaki University Hospital (16082215). The written informed consent from the patients was waved from the Ethics Committee because the information on the opportunity to opt out was presented on the web site (http://www.mh.nagasaki-u.ac.jp/research/rinsho/patients/open_surgery2.html). This study was registered in the UMIN Clinical Trials Registry as UMIN000024436.

Postoperative management

The nasogastric tube was removed before anastomosis. On the first postoperative day (1POD), transintestinal nutrition was started from a jejunostomy feeding tube to prevent postoperative complications [16]. In the first three postoperative days, the patients without hoarseness and aspiration pneumonia started to drink fluids, followed by a soft diet.

Definition of major postoperative complications related to gastric conduit reconstruction

Major complications related to gastric conduit after TE were defined as anastomotic leakage, refractory anastomotic strictures, and gastric conduit necrosis. Anastomotic leakage was defined as fistula formation that required any invasive treatment (Clavien-Dindo classification of grade III or more). Anastomotic strictures were defined as the presence of a lumen requiring endoscopic balloon dilatation for the passage of a normal endoscope (9.2 mm diameter) with symptomatic dysphagia. Refractory esophageal strictures were defined as more than 5 sessions of balloon dilation 6 months after the operation [17, 18]. Gastric conduit necrosis was defined as a severe ischemic condition that required resection of the gastric graft.

Statistical analysis

The data are expressed as the means ± standard deviation (SD) or medians and interquartile ranges (IQR). The relationships among major complications related to gastric conduit and age, body mass index (BMI), total operation time, operation time of thoracic surgery, and C-reactive protein (CRP) at 1POD were evaluated using Student's t-tests. The relationships between major postoperative complications related to gastric conduit reconstruction and other values were evaluated using Wilcoxon's tests. The relationships among anastomotic leakage and age, body mass index (BMI), total operation time, operation time of thoracic surgery, and C-reactive protein (CRP) at 1POD were evaluated using Student's t-tests. The relationships between anastomotic leakage and other values were evaluated using Wilcoxon's tests. The relationships among refractory anastomotic strictures and age, body mass index (BMI), total operation time, operation time of thoracic surgery, and C-reactive protein (CRP) at 1POD were evaluated using Student's t-tests. The relationships between refractory anastomotic strictures and other values were evaluated using Wilcoxon's tests. Receiver operating characteristic (ROC) curves and the area under the ROC curve (AUC) were used to assess the feasibility of using CRP and creatine phosphokinase (CPK) at 1POD as diagnostic tools for major complications related to gastric conduit [19]. The 95% CI values greater than 0.5 for AUC indicated that prediction was better than chance [20]. The patients were divided into two groups according to the cut-off values of CRP and CPK at 1POD. The relationships of categorical clinical factors between the groups were analyzed using chi-square tests or Fisher's exact tests. A Fisher's exact test was applied if the theoretical frequency was less than five. Probability values (P) less than 0.05 were considered statistically significant. Multiple logistic regression (stepwise) models were developed, and odds ratios (OR) were used to evaluate predictive factors associated with major complications related to gastric conduit. The Cochrane-Armitage trend test was used to test for a linear trend in the proportion of patients who developed major postoperative complications related to gastric conduit reconstruction according to numbers of predictive factors. All statistical analyses were performed using SAS-JMP programs for Windows (SAS Institute Inc., Cary, NC).

Results

Patient characteristics

The clinical characteristics of the 75 patients, which included 18 females and 57 males, are summarized in Table 1. The average age of all patients was 61.3 ± 8.1 years. The average BMI of all patients was 21.3 ± 2.7. Preoperative chemotherapy was performed in 51 patients (68.0%). Three patients (4.0%) were diagnosed with adenocarcinoma, and 72 patients (96.0%) were diagnosed with squamous cell carcinoma. According to the TNM classification, 47 patients (62.7%) had tumors more advanced than stage I. 3FLND was performed in 23 patients (30.7%). The average operating time was 605 ± 114 min. The median estimated blood loss was 370 g (IQR 270–600). Blood transfusion was performed in 7 patients (9.3%). The median length of the postoperative hospital stay was 27 days (IQR 20–39).

Table 1 Patients' characteristics

Characteristic	Values
Age (year)	61.3 ± 8.1
Gender (Male, Female)	57, 18
BMI	21.3 ± 2.7
Preoperative chemotherapy	51 (68.0%)
TNM Stage (I, II(IIA, IIB), III(IIIA, IIIB, IIIC), IV)	28, 19 (7, 12), 24 (13, 7, 4), 4
Total operating time (min)	605 ± 114
Operation time of thoracic surgery (min)	331 ± 73
Blood loss (g)	370 (270–600)
Blood transfusions	7 (9.3%)
3-field lymph node dissection	23 (30.7%)
Paroxysmal atrial fibrillation	13 (17.3%)
Vasopressor agents	8 (10.7%)
WBC (10^3/μl) at 1POD	9.4 (7.7–12.3)
CRP (10^4 μg/L) at 1POD	9.2 ± 2.4
Lactic acid (mmol/L) at 1POD	1.8 ± 1.2
CPK (IU/L) at 1POD	961 (670–1504)
Postoperative hospital stay (days)	27 (20, 39)

Major complications related to gastric conduit reconstruction after TE

The major complications related to gastric conduit after TE are summarized in Fig. 1. Twenty-three patients (30.7%) developed major complications related to gastric conduit reconstruction after TE. Anastomotic leakage occurred in 17 patients who required drainage to manage infectious conditions. No patients died within 30 days after the operation due to anastomotic leakage. A stricture occurred in 33 patients who required endoscopic balloon dilation. Twenty patients developed simple esophageal strictures without other gastric conduit-related complications. Seven patients developed anastomotic leakage followed by simple esophageal strictures. Six patients developed refractory esophageal strictures. All patient with refractory strictures developed symptomatic strictures within 2 months after TE (28.0 ± 7.0 days). Two patients developed anastomotic leakage followed by refractory esophageal strictures. Two patients had gastric conduit necrosis, and one of these two patients died due to non-occlusive mesenteric ischemia after resection of the necrotic gastric conduit. The length of postoperative hospital stay after TE in the patients with major complications related to gastric conduit (39 days, IQR 28–47) was significantly longer than in those without these complications (22 days, IQR 19–28) ($P < 0.01$).

Predictive factors for the development of major complications related to gastric conduit after TE

The predictive factors for developing major complications related to gastric conduit are shown in Table 2. In a univariate analysis, the predictive factors for developing major complications related to gastric conduit included age, 3FLND and levels of CRP and CPK at 1POD. The AUC for CRP and CPK at 1POD was 0.684 (95%CI; 0.546–0.796) and 0.670 (95%CI; 0.514–0.796). ROC curve analysis also identified the following cut-off values for CRP and CPK at 1POD: 9.6 × 10^4 μg/L and 1164 IU/L, respectively (Fig. 2). At a threshold of 9.6 × 10^4 μg/L for CRP at 1POD, the optimal sensitivity and specificity were 73.9% and 65.4%, respectively, in patients developing major complications related to gastric conduit. At a threshold of 1164 IU/L for CPK at

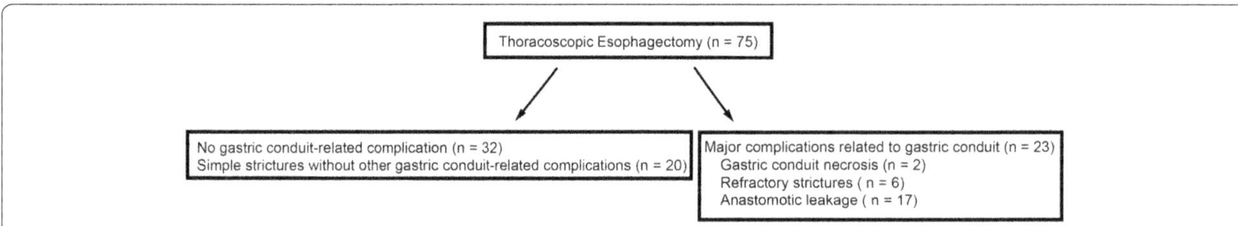

Fig. 1 Major complications related to gastric conduit reconstruction in 75 patients who underwent thoracoscopic esophagectomy. Seventeen patients developed anastomotic leakage. Refractory esophageal strictures were defined as more than 5 sessions of balloon dilation 6 months after the operation. Six patients developed refractory esophageal strictures. Two patients who had developed anastomotic leakage developed refractory esophageal strictures

1POD, the sensitivity and the specificity were 69.6% and 75.0%, respectively.

The predictive factors for developing major complications related to gastric conduit are shown in Tables 3 and 4. In a univariate analysis, the predictive factors for developing anastomotic leakage related to gastric conduit included levels of CRP and CPK at 1POD.

When a multiple logistic regression analysis was performed to evaluate confounding factors, 3FLND and the levels of CPK and CRP at 1POD were found to be significantly associated with developing major complications related to gastric conduit (Table 5). The incidence rates of these complications for 0, 1, 2, and 3 predictive factors were 5.3% (1/19), 18.8% (6/32), 58.8% (10/17), and 85.7% (6/7), respectively (Fig. 3). There was a strong trend toward increasing the prevalence of major complications related to gastric conduit based on the number of predictive factors ($P < 0.01$). The accuracy of 2 or more factors for major complications related to gastric conduit after TE was 0.800.

Discussion

Our results showed that major postoperative complications related to gastric conduit were frequently present after TE and significantly prolonged the length of the postoperative hospital stay. We first evaluated the predictive factors for major complications related to gastric conduit after TE. Our study investigated the number of factors that could predict these complications after TE.

TE has been shown to reduce pulmonary complications and the length of postoperative hospital stay [8, 21, 22]. These results indicate a faster postoperative recovery in patients after TE than in patients after open esophagectomy. However, the morbidity after TE remains high

Table 2 Univariate analysis for factors predicting major complications related to gastric conduit after TE

	Postoperative complications related to gastric conduit reconstruction		*P*-value
	Negative (*n* = 52)	Positive (*n* = 23)	
Age (years)	62.9 ± 7.2	57.5 ± 8.7	< 0.01
Gender (Male, Female)	37, 15	20, 3	N.S.
BMI	21.4 ± 2.7	21.1 ± 2.7	N.S.
Preoperative chemotherapy	21 (40.4%)	13 (56.5%)	N.S.
TNM Stage (I, II, III, IV)	22, 10, 18, 2	6, 9, 6, 2	N.S.
Total operation time (min)	604 ± 113	606 ± 116	N.S.
Operation time of thoracic surgery (min)	337 ± 77	318 ± 64	N.S.
Blood loss (g)	380 (303–623)	340 (200–500)	N.S.
Blood Transfusion	5 (9.6%)	2 (5.2%)	N.S.
3-field lymph node dissection	12 (23.1%)	11 (47.8%)	0.03
Paroxysmal atrial fibrillation	10 (19.2%)	3 (13.0%)	N.S.
Vasopressor agents	5 (9.6%)	3 (13.0%)	N.S.
WBC (10^3/μl) at 1POD	9.7 (8.2–12.8)	8.9 (7.0–11.5)	N.S.
CRP (10^4 μg/L) at 1POD	8.7 ± 0.3	10.3 ± 0.5	< 0.01
Lactic acid (mmol/L) at 1POD	1.4 (1.1–1,8)	2.1 (1.2–2.7)	N.S.
CPK (IU/L) at 1POD	890 (620–1309)	1277 (675–2041)	0.02
Postoperative hospital stay (days)	22 (19–28)	39 (28–47)	< 0.01

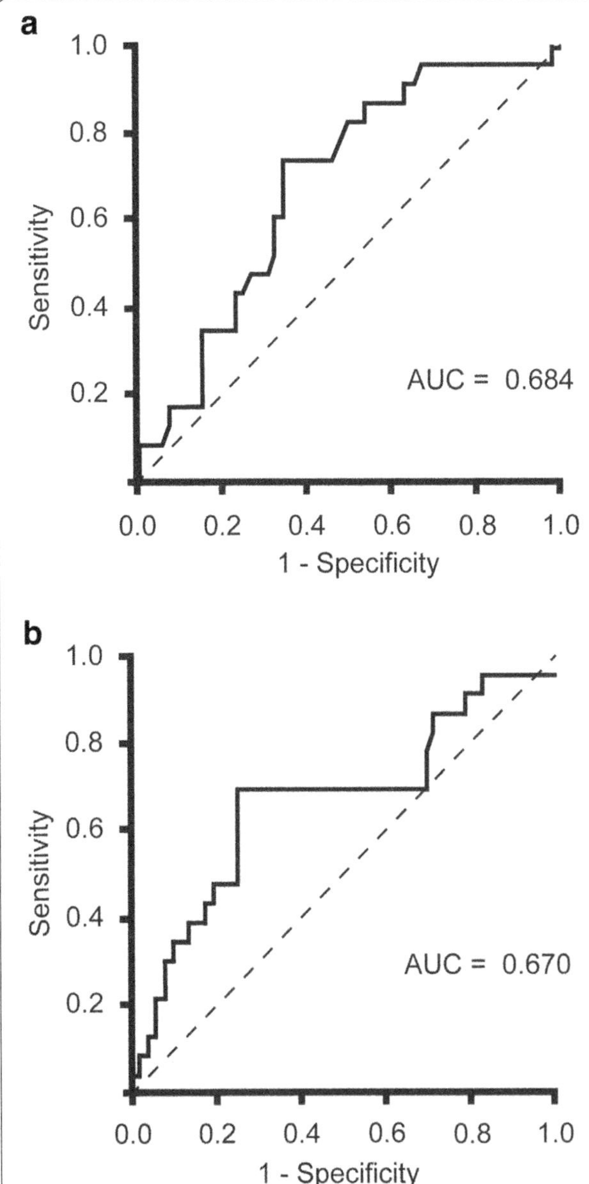

Fig. 2 ROC curve analysis of CRP (**a**) and CPK (**b**) at the first postoperative day after thoracoscopic esophagectomy. At a threshold of 9.6 x 10^4μg/L CRP at 1POD, the optimal sensitivity and specificity were 73.9% and 65.4%, respectively, in patients developing major postoperative complications related to gastric conduit reconstruction. At a threshold of 1164 IU/L CPK at 1POD, the sensitivity and the specificity were 69.6% and 75.0%, respectively, in patients developing major postoperative complications related to gastric conduit reconstruction. ROC, receiver operating characteristic; CRP, C-reactive protein; POD, postoperative days; CPK, creatine phosphokinase. AUC, area under the ROC curve; CI, confidence interval

(approximately 30–40%) [1, 2, 23], and preventing gastric conduit-related complications after TE remains difficult. Our data are similar to the Japanese nationwide web--based database and other articles regarding BMI, operation time, the rate of anastomotic leakage, and postoperative days [5, 7, 24, 25]. There is a therapeutic benefit in predicting the postoperative complications of gastric conduit reconstruction after TE. The 3 predictive factors identified in this study may facilitate the decision to delay oral intake and perform early interventional treatments, such as re-operation, drainage and dilation, after TE.

Our study showed that 3FLND led to major complications related to gastric conduit. Lymph node dissection for thoracic esophageal cancer is controversial, and whether 3FLND or 2-field lymph node dissection (2FLND) is better remains a subject of debate [26–29]. The advantages and disadvantages of 3FLND remain controversial when compared to 2FLND of esophagectomy [30, 31]. One meta-analysis showed that 3FLND improves the overall survival rate but leads to more major complications than 2FLND [32, 33]. Anastomotic leakage is likely linked to cervical lymph node dissection due to inflammation and reduced angiogenesis around the anastomotic area [34], which strongly supports our results. However, future studies should determine whether 3FLND or 2FLND is better according to the patient's physical condition and tumor staging.

The retrosternal route in almost all cases was applied to the gastric conduit of reconstruction after esophagectomy. There are several advantages of this method for the management of local recurrence, including fewer complications in gastric conduit and a short route in the retrosternal route of reconstruction [13, 35, 36]. In RCT studies, both posterior and anterior mediastinal routes of reconstruction were associated with similar surgical outcomes after esophagectomy for cancer [37]. In the Japanese registry, the retrosternal route of reconstruction was selected in 34% of patients, although the posterior mediastinal route was used for reconstruction in 41.3% of patients [38]. Thus, the route of reconstruction remains controversial.

High CRP levels after esophagectomy are reported to precede the clinical diagnosis of postoperative infectious complications [39, 40]. With regard to postoperative infectious complications, there is no difference between patients with and without postoperative infectious complications on 1POD [39, 40]. Consistent with previous reports, our results showed that some infectious complications developed but hardly affected the serum CRP levels on 1POD after TE. Moreover, TE minimizes lung injury and severe pulmonary complications after esophagostomy. Thus, high CRP levels on 1POD may be induced in response to surgical trauma and gastric conduit ischemic conditions after TE. We also identified high CPK levels as a predictive factor for major complications related to gastric conduit after TE. CPK was also reported as a biomarker of ischemic small bowel disease in animal models [41, 42]. CPK may reflect not only

Table 3 Univariate analysis for factors predicting anastomotic leakage after TE

	Anastomotic leakage		*P*-value
	Negative (*n* = 58)	Positive (*n* = 17)	
Age (years)	62.3 ± 7.8	57.8 ± 8.3	N.S.
Gender (Male, Female)	43, 15	14, 3	N.S.
BMI	21.3 ± 2.7	21.1 ± 2.8	N.S.
Preoperative chemotherapy	25 (43.1%)	9 (52.9%)	N.S.
TNM Stage (I, II, III, IV)	22, 13, 20, 3	6, 6, 4, 1	N.S.
Total operation time (min)	608 ± 112	594 ± 122	N.S.
Operation time of thoracic surgery (min)	338 ± 76	305 ± 60	N.S.
Blood loss (g)	380 (290–608)	350 (235–615)	N.S.
Blood Transfusion	6 (10.3%)	1 (5.9%)	N.S.
3-field lymph node dissection	15 (25.9%)	8 (47.1%)	N.S.
Paroxysmal atrial fibrillation	10 (17.2%)	3 (17.7%)	N.S.
Vasopressor agents	7 (12.1%)	1 (5.9%)	N.S.
WBC (10^3/μl) at 1POD	9.7 (8.2–12.8)	8.9 (7.0–11.5)	N.S.
CRP (10^4 μg/L) at 1POD	8.7 ± 2.4	10.5 ± 2.0	< 0.01
Lactic acid (mmol/L) at 1POD	1.5 (1.1–2.0)	2.0 (0.7–2.6)	N.S.
CPK (IU/L) at 1POD	919.5 (629–1400)	1232 (683–2177)	< 0.05
Postoperative hospital stay (days)	22 (19–28)	42 (30–47)	< 0.01

Table 4 Univariate analysis for factors predicting refractory anastomotic strictures after TE

	Refractory anastomotic strictures		*P*-value
	Negative (*n* = 69)	Positive (n = 6)	
Age (years)	61.4 ± 8.2	59.0 ± 6.4	N.S.
Gender (Male, Female)	51, 18	6, 0	N.S.
BMI	21.4 ± 2.7	21.1 ± 2.7	N.S.
Preoperative chemotherapy	39 (56.5%)	2 (33.3%)	N.S.
TNM Stage (I, II, III, IV)	27, 16, 22, 4	1, 4, 1, 0	N.S.
Total operation time (min)	604 ± 113	606 ± 116	N.S.
Operation time of thoracic surgery (min)	331 ± 75	329 ± 55	N.S.
Blood loss (g)	380 (303–623)	340 (200–500)	N.S.
Blood Transfusion	6 (8.7%)	1 (16.7%)	N.S.
3-field lymph node dissection	22 (29.3%)	1 (16.7%)	N.S.
Paroxysmal atrial fibrillation	12 (17.4%)	1 (16.7%)	N.S.
Vasopressor agents	7 (10.1%)	1 (16.7%)	N.S.
WBC (10^3/μl) at 1POD	9.7 (8.2–12.8)	8.9 (7.0–11.5)	N.S.
CRP (10^4 μg/L) at 1POD	9.0 ± 2.3	10.9 ± 3.6	N.S.
Lactic acid (mmol/L) at 1POD	1.4 (1.1–1,8)	2.1 (1.2–2.7)	N.S.
CPK (IU/L) at 1POD	890 (620–1309)	1214 (675–2041)	N.S.
Postoperative hospital stay (days)	20 (20–35)	41 (25–61)	N.S.

Table 5 Multivariate analysis for factors predicting major complications related to gastric conduit after TE

	Odds ratio	*P*-value	95% CI
Age (years)	0.92	0.06	(0.85–1.00)
3-field lymph node dissection	5.37	0.02	(1.41–24.33)
CRP at 1POD (high / low)	5.07	0.01	(1.47–20.25)
CPK at 1POD (high / low)	5.40	< 0.01	(1.60–20.20)

ischemic changes in the muscle layer of the gastric conduit but also inflammation around the muscle layers of the neck, as the CPK level is not generally a good biomarker for bowel ischemia [43]. In open esophagectomy, high CPK levels may be observed in patients without major complications related to gastric conduit because of the large incision in the thoracic field.

Postoperative endoscopic examination is a highly accurate method to evaluate reconstruction of the gastric conduit after esophagectomy [12, 44–46]. However, endoscopic examination is complex and invasive after esophagectomy. Thus, these predictive factors after TE are useful to select patients who may benefit from endoscopic examination.

Published results have been inconclusive as to which anastomotic technique is ideal for esophagectomy [9, 47–51]. Thus, surgeons base their choice of anastomotic technique on personal preference. We applied end-to-side anastomosis with an intraluminal stapler in this study. Cervical anastomosis using a stapler more frequently causes anastomotic strictures than other techniques [9, 52]. However, almost all patients show improved anastomotic strictures after three or fewer dilatations within several months [52]. Thus, the ischemic condition of the gastric conduit may influence anastomotic healing in patients who develop refractory strictures [49, 52].

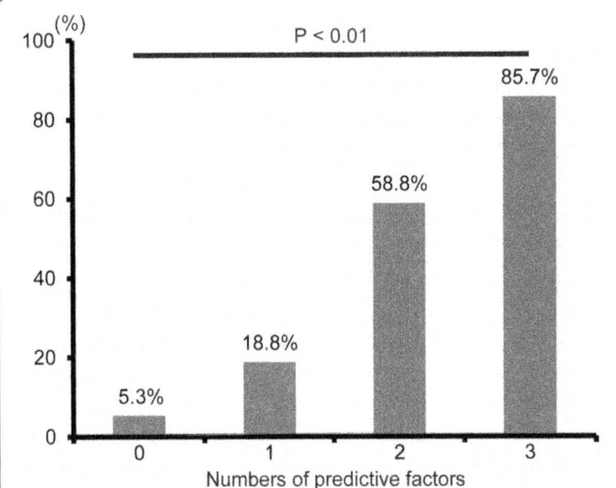

Fig. 3 Prevalence of major complications related to gastric conduit reconstruction compared according to the number of predictive factors after thoracoscopic esophagectomy. *P*-value based on the Cochrane-Armitage trend test

Our study has several limitations. First, our study was performed at a single institution, and further prospective studies are needed at multiple institutions. Second, the accuracy of the predictive factors is somewhat low. Third, almost all patients were diagnosed with squamous cell carcinoma. Thus, transthoracic extended radical esophagectomy with 3-field lymph node dissection is included in our data. The invasive procedure caused delayed recovery of the patients and resulted in a relatively long postoperative stay. 2-field lymphadenectomy using the Ivor Lewis procedure or trans-hiatal esophagectomy is more commonly performed for esophageal adenocarcinoma in Western countries [5]. Because differences in oncological features and health insurance systems may result in differences in surgical procedures and postoperative stay, it remains unclear whether the predictive factors are applicable to assess patients in Western countries [7, 53]. Fourth, delayed emptying of the gastric conduit was eliminated because there were no patients with endoscopic pyloric dilation and surgical intervention [54, 55]. Despite these limitations, this study is the first to address major complications related to gastric conduit after TE.

Conclusions

In conclusion, 3FLND and the levels of CPK and CRP at 1POD after TE were predictive factors for major complications related to gastric conduit. Two or more factors in 3FLND and the high levels of CPK and CRP at 1POD after TE were identified as the risk model for major complications related to gastric conduit after TE.

Abbreviations

3FLND: Three-field lymph node dissection; AUC: The area under the ROC curve; BMI: Body mass index; CI: Confidence interval; CPK: Creatine phosphokinase; CRP: C-reactive protein; IQR: Interquartile ranges; OR: Odds ratio; POD: Postoperative day; ROC: Receiver operating characteristic; SD: Standard deviation; TE: Thoracoscopic esophagectomy

Acknowledgements

The authors thank Shuntaro Sato, who helped with the statistical analysis.

Funding

This study was partially supported in writing and editing the manuscript by a Grant-in-Aid for Scientific Research from the Japan Society for the Promotion of Science (15H06503 and 17 K16569 Shinichiro Kobayashi).

Authors' contributions

SK. designed the study, analyzed data, and wrote the initial draft of the manuscript. KK. and YN. especially contributed to interpretation of data and supervised the patient treatments. MN., RM., and MT. especially participated in the discussion and assisted in the preparation of the manuscript. SE. supervised the patient treatments, and especially assisted in editing the manuscript. All other authors have contributed to data collection and interpretation, and critically reviewed the manuscript. All authors approved the final version of the manuscript, and agree to be accountable for all aspects of the work in ensuring that questions related to the accuracy or integrity of any part of the work are appropriately investigated and resolved.

Competing interests

Shinichiro Kobayashi, Kengo Kanetaka, Yasuhiro Nagata, Masahiko Nakayama, Ryo Matsumoto, Mitsuhisa Takatsuki, and Susumu Eguchi do not have any financial relationships relevant to this publication to disclose.

Author details

[1]Department of Surgery, Nagasaki University Graduate School of Biomedical Sciences, Sakamoto 1-7-1, Nagasaki 8528102, Japan. [2]Center for Comprehensive Community Care Education, Nagasaki University Graduate School of Biomedical Sciences, Sakamoto 1-12-4, Nagasaki, Japan.

References

1. Verhage RJ, Hazebroek EJ, Boone J, Van Hillegersberg R. Minimally invasive surgery compared to open procedures in esophagectomy for cancer: a systematic review of the literature. Minerva Chir. 2009;64(2):135–46.
2. Blencowe NS, Strong S, McNair AG, Brookes ST, Crosby T, Griffin SM, Blazeby JM. Reporting of short-term clinical outcomes after esophagectomy: a systematic review. Ann Surg. 2012;255(4):658–66.
3. Dhungel B, Diggs BS, Hunter JG, Sheppard BC, Vetto JT, Dolan JP. Patient and peri-operative predictors of morbidity and mortality after esophagectomy: American College of Surgeons National Surgical Quality Improvement Program (ACS-NSQIP), 2005-2008. J Gastrointest Surg. 2010; 14(10):1492–501.
4. Mamidanna R, Bottle A, Aylin P, Faiz O, Hanna GB. Short-term outcomes following open versus minimally invasive esophagectomy for cancer in England: a population-based national study. Ann Surg. 2012;255(2):197–203.
5. Takeuchi H, Miyata H, Gotoh M, Kitagawa Y, Baba H, Kimura W, Tomita N, Nakagoe T, Shimada M, Sugihara K, et al. A risk model for esophagectomy using data of 5354 patients included in a Japanese nationwide web-based database. Ann Surg. 2014;260(2):259–66.
6. Yerokun BA, Sun Z, Yang CJ, Gulack BC, Speicher PJ, Adam MA, D'Amico TA, Onaitis MW, Harpole DH, Berry MF, et al. Minimally invasive versus open Esophagectomy for esophageal cancer: a population-based analysis. Ann Thorac Surg. 2016;102(2):416–23.
7. Takeuchi H, Miyata H, Ozawa S, Udagawa H, Osugi H, Matsubara H, Konno H, Seto Y, Kitagawa Y. Comparison of short-term outcomes between open and minimally invasive Esophagectomy for esophageal cancer using a Nationwide database in Japan. Ann Surg Oncol. 2017;24(7):1821–7.
8. Findlay JM, Gillies RS, Millo J, Sgromo B, Marshall RE, Maynard ND. Enhanced recovery for esophagectomy: a systematic review and evidence-based guidelines. Ann Surg. 2014;259(3):413–31.
9. Honda M, Kuriyama A, Noma H, Nunobe S, Furukawa TA. Hand-sewn versus mechanical esophagogastric anastomosis after esophagectomy: a systematic review and meta-analysis. Ann Surg. 2013;257(2):238–48.
10. Cassivi SD. Leaks, strictures, and necrosis: a review of anastomotic complications following esophagectomy. Semin Thorac Cardiovasc Surg. 2004;16(2):124–32.
11. Nishikawa K, Fujita T, Yuda M, Yamamoto S, Tanaka Y, Matsumoto A, Tanishima Y, Yano F, Mitsumori N, Yanaga K. Early postoperative endoscopy for targeted management of patients at risks of anastomotic complications after esophagectomy. Surgery. 2016;160(5):1294–301.
12. Fujiwara H, Nakajima Y, Kawada K, Tokairin Y, Miyawaki Y, Okada T, Nagai K, Kawano T. Endoscopic assessment 1 day after esophagectomy for predicting cervical esophagogastric anastomosis-relating complications. Surg Endosc. 2016;30(4):1564–71.
13. Kuwano H, Nishimura Y, Oyama T, Kato H, Kitagawa Y, Kusano M, Shimada H, Takiuchi H, Toh Y, Doki Y, et al. Guidelines for diagnosis and treatment of carcinoma of the esophagus April 2012 edited by the Japan esophageal society. Esophagus. 2015;12(1):1–30.
14. Edge SB BD, Compton CC, Fritz AG, Greene FL, Trotti A. AJCC cancer staging manual. 7th ed. New York: Springer-Verlag; 2009. p.103–15.
15. Li H, Yang S, Zhang Y, Xiang J, Chen H. Thoracic recurrent laryngeal lymph node metastases predict cervical node metastases and benefit from three-field dissection in selected patients with thoracic esophageal squamous cell carcinoma. J Surg Oncol. 2012;105(6):548–52.
16. Lewis SJ, Andersen HK, Thomas S. Early enteral nutrition within 24 h of intestinal surgery versus later commencement of feeding: a systematic review and meta-analysis. J Gastrointest Surg. 2009;13(3):569–75.
17. Kochman ML, McClave SA, Boyce HW. The refractory and the recurrent esophageal stricture: a definition. Gastrointest Endosc. 2005;62(3):474–5.
18. Yano T, Yoda Y, Nomura S, Toyosaki K, Hasegawa H, Ono H, Tanaka M, Morimoto H, Horimatsu T, Nonaka S, et al. Prospective trial of biodegradable stents for refractory benign esophageal strictures after curative treatment of esophageal cancer. Gastrointest Endosc. 2017;86(3):492–9.
19. Hanley JA, McNeil BJ. The meaning and use of the area under a receiver operating characteristic (ROC) curve. Radiology. 1982;143(1):29–36.
20. Lasko TA, Bhagwat JG, Zou KH, Ohno-Machado L. The use of receiver operating characteristic curves in biomedical informatics. J Biomed Inform. 2005;38(5):404–15.
21. Biere SS, van Berge Henegouwen MI, Maas KW, Bonavina L, Rosman C, Garcia JR, Gisbertz SS, Klinkenbijl JH, Hollmann MW, de Lange ES, et al. Minimally invasive versus open oesophagectomy for patients with oesophageal cancer: a multicentre, open-label, randomised controlled trial. Lancet. 2012;379(9829):1887–92.
22. Straatman J, van der Wielen N, Cuesta MA, Daams F, Roig Garcia J, Bonavina L, Rosman C, van Berge Henegouwen MI, Gisbertz SS, van der Peet DL. Minimally invasive versus open esophageal resection: three-year follow-up of the previously reported randomized controlled trial: the TIME trial. Ann Surg. 2017;266(2):232–6.
23. Decker G, Coosemans W, De Leyn P, Decaluwe H, Nafteux P, Van Raemdonck D, Lerut T. Minimally invasive esophagectomy for cancer. Eur J Cardiothorac Surg. 2009;35(1):13–21.
24. Hirahara N, Matsubara T, Mizota Y, Ishibashi S, Tajima Y. Prognostic value of preoperative inflammatory response biomarkers in patients with esophageal cancer who undergo a curative thoracoscopic esophagectomy. BMC Surg. 2016;16(1):66.
25. Baba Y, Yoshida N, Shigaki H, Iwatsuki M, Miyamoto Y, Sakamoto Y, Watanabe M, Baba H. Prognostic impact of postoperative complications in 502 patients with surgically resected esophageal squamous cell carcinoma: a retrospective single-institution study. Ann Surg. 2016;264(2):305–11.
26. Tsurumaru M, Kajiyama Y, Udagawa H, Akiyama H. Outcomes of extended lymph node dissection for squamous cell carcinoma of the thoracic esophagus. Ann Thorac Cardiovasc Surg. 2001;7(6):325–9.
27. Tachibana M, Kinugasa S, Yoshimura H, Shibakita M, Tonomoto Y, Dhar DK, Nagasue N. Clinical outcomes of extended esophagectomy with three-field lymph node dissection for esophageal squamous cell carcinoma. Am J Surg. 2005;189(1):98–109.
28. Hsu WH, Hsu PK, Hsieh CC, Huang CS, Wu YC. The metastatic lymph node number and ratio are independent prognostic factors in esophageal cancer. J Gastrointest Surg. 2009;13(11):1913–20.
29. Japan Esophageal Society. Japanese classification of esophageal cancer. 11th edition, part I. Esophagus. 2017;17(1):1–36.
30. Lerut T, Nafteux P, Moons J, Coosemans W, Decker G, De Leyn P, Van Raemdonck D, Ectors N. Three-field lymphadenectomy for carcinoma of the esophagus and gastroesophageal junction in 174 R0 resections: impact on staging, disease-free survival, and outcome: a plea for adaptation of TNM classification in upper-half esophageal carcinoma. Ann Surg. 2004;240(6): 962–74.
31. Chen J, Wu S, Zheng X, Pan J, Zhu K, Chen Y, Li J, Liao L, Lin Y, Liao Z. Cervical lymph node metastasis classified as regional nodal staging in thoracic esophageal squamous cell carcinoma after radical esophagectomy and three-field lymph node dissection. BMC Surg. 2014;14:110.
32. Ye T, Sun Y, Zhang Y, Chen H. Three-field or two-field resection for thoracic esophageal cancer: a meta-analysis. Ann Thorac Surg. 2013;96(6):1933–41.
33. Ma GW, Situ DR, Ma QL, Long H, Zhang LJ, Lin P, Rong TH. Three-field vs two-field lymph node dissection for esophageal cancer: a meta-analysis. World J Gastroenterol. 2014;20(47):18022–30.
34. Zheng QF, Wang JJ, Ying MG, Liu SY. Omentoplasty in preventing anastomotic leakage of oesophagogastrostomy following radical oesophagectomy with three-field lymphadenectomy. Eur J Cardiothorac Surg. 2013;43(2):274–8.

35. Chen H, Lu JJ, Zhou J, Zhou X, Luo X, Liu Q, Tam J. Anterior versus posterior routes of reconstruction after esophagectomy: a comparative anatomic study. Ann Thorac Surg. 2009;87(2):400–4.
36. Hu H, Ye T, Tan D, Li H, Chen H. Is anterior mediastinum route a shorter choice for esophageal reconstruction? A comparative anatomic study. Eur J Cardiothorac Surg. 2011;40(6):1466–9.
37. Urschel JD, Urschel DM, Miller JD, Bennett WF, Young JE. A meta-analysis of randomized controlled trials of route of reconstruction after esophagectomy for cancer. Am J Surg. 2001;182(5):470–5.
38. Tachimori Y, Ozawa S, Numasaki H, Ishihara R, Matsubara H, Muro K, Oyama T, Toh Y, Udagawa H, Uno T. Comprehensive registry of esophageal cancer in Japan, 2010. Esophagus. 2017;14(3):189–214.
39. Miki Y, Toyokawa T, Kubo N, Tamura T, Sakurai K, Tanaka H, Muguruma K, Yashiro M, Hirakawa K, Ohira M. C-reactive protein indicates early stage of postoperative infectious complications in patients following minimally invasive Esophagectomy. World J Surg. 2017;41(3):796–803.
40. Hoeboer SH, Groeneveld AB, Engels N, van Genderen M, Wijnhoven BP, van Bommel J. Rising C-reactive protein and procalcitonin levels precede early complications after esophagectomy. J Gastrointest Surg. 2015;19(4):613–24.
41. Kanda T, Nakatomi Y, Ishikawa H, Hitomi M, Matsubara Y, Ono T, Muto T. Intestinal fatty acid-binding protein as a sensitive marker of intestinal ischemia. Dig Dis Sci. 1992;37(9):1362–7.
42. Kanda T, Tsukahara A, Ueki K, Sakai Y, Tani T, Nishimura A, Yamazaki T, Tamiya Y, Tada T, Hirota M, et al. Diagnosis of ischemic small bowel disease by measurement of serum intestinal fatty acid-binding protein in patients with acute abdomen: a multicenter, observer-blinded validation study. J Gastroenterol. 2011;46(4):492–500.
43. van der Voort PH, Westra B, Wester JP, Bosman RJ, van Stijn I, Haagen IA, Loupatty FJ, Rijkenberg S. Can serum L-lactate, D-lactate, creatine kinase and I-FABP be used as diagnostic markers in critically ill patients suspected for bowel ischemia. BMC Anesthesiol. 2014;14:111.
44. Oezcelik A, Banki F, Ayazi S, Abate E, Zehetner J, Sohn HJ, Hagen JA, DeMeester SR, Lipham JC, Palmer SL, et al. Detection of gastric conduit ischemia or anastomotic breakdown after cervical esophagogastrostomy: the use of computed tomography scan versus early endoscopy. Surg Endosc. 2010;24(8):1948–51.
45. Page RD, Asmat A, McShane J, Russell GN, Pennefather SH. Routine endoscopy to detect anastomotic leakage after esophagectomy. Ann Thorac Surg. 2013;95(1):292–8.
46. Schaible A, Sauer P, Hartwig W, Hackert T, Hinz U, Radeleff B, Büchler MW, Werner J. Radiologic versus endoscopic evaluation of the conduit after esophageal resection: a prospective, blinded, intraindividually controlled diagnostic study. Surg Endosc. 2014;28(7):2078–85.
47. Dewar L, Gelfand G, Finley RJ, Evans K, Inculet R, Nelems B. Factors affecting cervical anastomotic leak and stricture formation following esophagogastrectomy and gastric tube interposition. Am J Surg. 1992; 163(5):484–9.
48. Walther B, Johansson J, Johnsson F, Von Holstein CS, Zilling T. Cervical or thoracic anastomosis after esophageal resection and gastric tube reconstruction: a prospective randomized trial comparing sutured neck anastomosis with stapled intrathoracic anastomosis. Ann Surg. 2003;238(6): 803–14.
49. Zhang YS, Gao BR, Wang HJ, Su YF, Yang YZ, Zhang JH, Wang C. Comparison of anastomotic leakage and stricture formation following layered and stapler oesophagogastric anastomosis for cancer: a prospective randomized controlled trial. J Int Med Res. 2010;38(1):227–33.
50. Kim RH, Takabe K. Methods of esophagogastric anastomoses following esophagectomy for cancer: a systematic review. J Surg Oncol. 2010; 101(6):527–33.
51. Xu QR, Wang KN, Wang WP, Zhang K, Chen LQ. Linear stapled esophagogastrostomy is more effective than hand-sewn or circular stapler in prevention of anastomotic stricture: a comparative clinical study. J Gastrointest Surg. 2011;15(6):915–21.
52. Law S, Fok M, Chu KM, Wong J. Comparison of hand-sewn and stapled esophagogastric anastomosis after esophageal resection for cancer: a prospective randomized controlled trial. Ann Surg. 1997;226(2):169–73.
53. Muramatsu N, Liang J. Hospital length of stay in the United States and Japan: a case study of myocardial infarction patients. Int J Health Serv. 1999;29(1):189–209.
54. Akkerman RD, Haverkamp L, van Hillegersberg R, Ruurda JP. Surgical techniques to prevent delayed gastric emptying after esophagectomy with gastric interposition: a systematic review. Ann Thorac Surg. 2014;98(4):1512–9.
55. Poghosyan T, Gaujoux S, Chirica M, Munoz-Bongrand N, Sarfati E, Cattan P. Functional disorders and quality of life after esophagectomy and gastric tube reconstruction for cancer. J Visc Surg. 2011;148(5):e327–35.

19

Laparoscopic resection of gastric duplication cysts in newborns: a report of five cases

Hong-Xia Ren*, Li-Qiong Duan, Xiao-Xia Wu, Bao-Hong Zhao and Yuan-Yuan Jin

Abstract

Background: Gastric duplication cysts are rare congenital alimentary tract anomalies and most cases are recognized during childhood. There were few reports about gastric duplication cysts in newborns and even fewer reports about laparoscopic resection of gastric duplication cysts in newborns.

Case presentation: We report a series of five newborns with gastric duplication cysts which were successfully resected by laparoscopy between January 2010 and April 2015. Case 1, a male newborn was admitted because of severe salivation, choking cough and dyspnea for 30 min after birth. Case 2, a male, was suspected of duodenal ileus by antenatal examination. Case 3, a female was admitted because of vomiting for 5 days. Case 4,a female without significant symptoms simply visited us for the abdominal cyst detected by antenatal examination. Case 5, a male was admitted because of vomiting for 4 days. All patients were performed with a surgery after assistant examinations. Case 1 was died of respiratory failure and the other patients recovered uneventfully.

Conclusion: Gastric duplication cysts in newborns are very rare. Laparoscopic surgery play an important role on the diagnosis and treatment. Our experience and practice indicate that laparoscopic resection of gastric duplication cysts in newborns is viable and there is also a need to increase sample size to prove its safety and effectiveness.

Keywords: Gastric duplication cyst, Laparoscopic resection, Newborns

Background

Gastric duplication cysts (GDCs) are rare congenital alimentary tract anomalies and most cases are recognized during childhood. Nowadays, an increased number of cases of GDCs have been reported in newborns because of the accessibility of antenatal examination. Advancements in laparoscopic techniques and skills have made it possible to treat gastric duplication cysts in an earlier phase and with a minimal incision. We report five cases with gastric duplication cysts treated by laparoscopic surgery in newborns.

Case presentation

Included in this report, two male and three female newborns aged between 1 h and 28 days with a mean of 14 days, weighing between 2.3 and 4.4 kg with a mean of 3.45 kg. Details of the five cases are shown in Table 1. Case 1, a male newborn was admitted as an emergency because of severe salivation, choking cough and dyspnea for 30 min after birth, and preoperative examination suspected him of esophageal atresia (Gross A) complicated with an abdominal mass. Case 2 was a male newborn who was suspected as having duodenal ileus by antenatal examination, and admitted because of double bubble sign detected by postpartum X-ray radiography. Case 3, a 26-day-old female was admitted to the hospital because of vomiting for 5 days. Case 4,a 28-day female without significant symptoms simply visited us for the abdominal cyst detected by antenatal examination. Case 5, a 14-day-old male newborn was admitted because of vomiting for 4 days. All patients underwent transabdominal color Doppler ultrasonography and upper digestive tract radiography. In Case 3 and 4, the patients also underwent computed tomography (CT) and magnetic resonance imaging (MRI) before a surgery. The Case 3 was originally suspected as common bile duct cyst,

* Correspondence: renhongxia100@sina.com; renhongxia100@126.com
Department of Pediatric Surgery, Shanxi Children's Hospital, 13 New People Avenue, Taiyuan 030013, Shanxi, China

Table 1 Clinical data of the four neonates with gastric duplication cyst

NO.	1	2	3	4	5
Gender	male	female	female	female	male
Age	1 h	1 day	26 d	28 d	14 d
Weight (kg)	2.8	2.7	4.2	4.3	3.9
Presentation	saliva bucking	emesis	Emesis	asymptomatic	emesis
Preoperative diagnosis	esophageal atresia, abdominal mass	gastric duplication?	choledochal cyst?	abdominal mass	gastric duplication?
Surgical procedures	Laparoscopic resection and gastrostomy	laparoscopic resection and repair stomach	Cholangiography and laparoscopic resection	laparoscopic resection	laparoscopic resection
size of mass (cm^3)	2 × 3 × 3.5	2 × 3 × 2	5 × 4 × 3	2 × 3 × 4	2 × 2.5 × 2
Location of the mass	middle of greater curvature	near cardia	pylorus	antrum of pylorus	near cardia
Accompanied malformation	EA(Gross A), PDA, ASD	PDA, PDA	PFO	PFO	PFO
Prognosis	abandoned	cured	cured	cured	cured

EA esophageal atresia, *PDA* ventricular septa defect patent ductus arteriosus, *ASD* atrial septal defect, *PFO* patent foramen ovale

which was excluded by intraoperative cholangiography. Therefore, the diagnosis of GDCs was only confirmed pre-operative in Case 4 and 5. The ultrasound, CT, and upper gastroenterograpic images of the five patients are shown in Fig. 1.

Laparoscopic resection of the gastric duplication cysts was performed with a 5-mm, 30° or 0° camera and three ports, including a 5-mm port near the umbilicus and two 3-mm ports. Using a 4-0 needle, the ligamentum teres hepatis was pushed upward to expose the surgical filed. Among the five cases, Case 3 was preoperatively misdiagnosed by cholangiography and intraoperatively diagnosed as gastric duplication cyst, with was excised subsequently. As described previously, the patient in Case 3 was originally suspected as having common bile duct cyst, but intraoperative cholangiography did not find significant abnormality in the common bile duct. Further laparoscopic exploration revealed the existence of GDC, which was resected thereafter. As it was very difficult to expose the cyst in the cardia with a surgical forceps in the left upper abdomen in case 2 (Fig. 2a), laparoscopy was performed to confirm the diagnosis, location, adhesion and relationship of the cyst with the adjacent organs. Fluid in the duplication cyst was aspirated by percutaneous puncture using a syringe to decrease the tension and volume of the mass before excising the

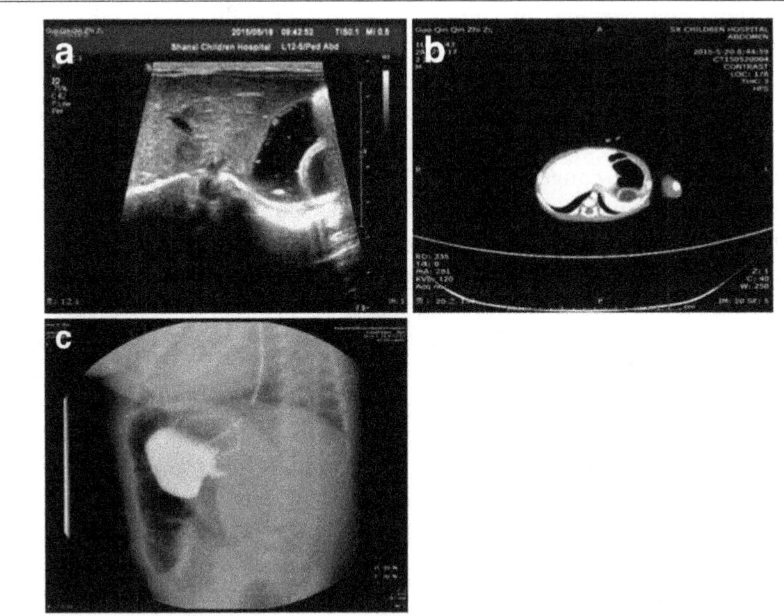

Fig. 1 Ultrasound image (**a**), CT image (**b**);Pyloric obstruction by radiography (**c**)

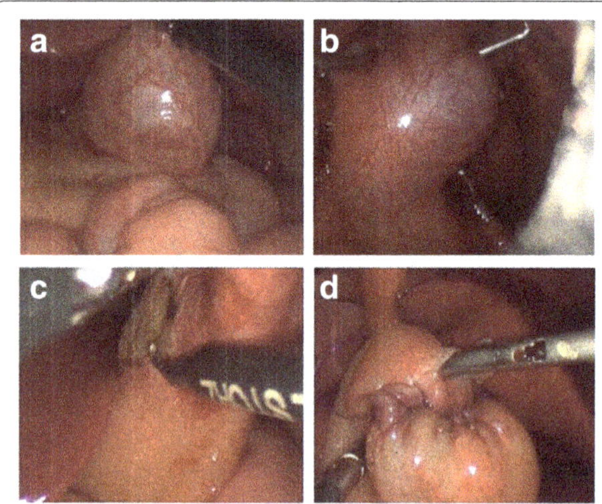

Fig. 2 Mass located in the cardia (**a**); Percutaneous puncture (**b**); Mass resection (**c**); Suturing of the wall of stomach (**d**)

cyst (Fig. 2b). During the operation, complete dissociation and excision of the cyst was performed along the serous membrane in Cases 1, 2 and 5 (Fig. 2c). In Case 2 the gastral cavity was exposed, and the wall of stomach was repaired with a 5-0 Coated Vicryl *Plus Antibacterial (ETHICON) (Fig. 2d). In Case 1, the wall of stomach was repaired by pouch suture and then raised to the abdominal wall for a gastric fistula because of the associated type I esophageal atresia. In cases 3 and 4, the cyst was mostly excised and the mucosa of the residual wall was cauterized. All the surgical procedures were completed successfully by laparoscopy. The patient in Case 1 was discharged three days after surgery because of the economic reason. Recoveries of the other four cases were uneventful without significant postoperative complications such as ileus, bleeding, anastomotic leakage, infection of incision or relapse.

Discussion

Gastric duplication is a relatively rare congenital malformation, accounting for about 9% of all gastrointestinal duplications. Numerous theories have been proposed about the etiology of foregut duplication, including the segmental twinning theory, recanalization barrier of the alimentary tract, persistence of fetal gut diverticula, and separation barrier of the notochord and archenteron. Gastric duplication cysts can be found at any part of the stomach. The typical ones are usually located along the greater gastric curvature, and some others may be along the anterior or posterior wall of stomach, or located in the cardia or pylorus. Most cysts are single, elliptical, spherical, cystic, and linked with gastric muscular layers. Rowling et al. [1] suggested the pathological diagnostic criteria of gastric duplications as follows: lining with the gastrointestinal mucosa, attachment to the gastrointestinal tract, the presence of a smooth muscle coat, communicating with gastric lumen or not, and sharing blood with the stomach.

Symptoms of gastric duplications are atypical and often present with gastrectasia, an abdominal mass and vomiting. Larger cysts can cause abdominal pain and discomfort; larger tension may cause stomach mucosa bleeding and vomiting; and those located in the cardia or pylorus may present with obstruction. Patients with gastric duplications were usually diagnosed because of abdominal pain, vomiting and abdominal swelling before 2 years old [2], while some cases were found in adulthood [3, 4]. Diagnostic work-up includes x-ray, ultrasound, CT and MRI. Hlouschek [5] reported a case of gastric duplication in an adult by endoscopic ultrasonography. Gastric duplication is so rare that it is often misdiagnosed as pancreatic cyst, adrenal cyst, or stomach muscle adenoma for that the muscle layer will be shared by the cyst and stomach . There was a reported case which the cyst located in the posterior gastric wall was preoperatively misdiagnosed as renal cyst [6]. In our series, Case 3 was misdiagnosed as choledochal cyst by MRI and later intraoperatively confirmed as a gastric duplication cyst, which reminded us of the possibility of a gastric duplication cyst located in the pylorus. To establish a definitive diagnosis, abdominal X-ray radiography and/or CT is often necessary for newborns or infants who present with vomiting, hematemesis in particular, bloody stools, and a palpable abdominal mass, although the definite diagnosis of gastric duplication cysts finally depends on surgery and pathology. In addition, The cyst lining may undergo ulceration, erosions, regenerative and increased fluid production pressure-induced in non-communicating cysts may result in necrosis of the mucosa, which may cause bleeding into the cyst or perforation into the peritoneal cavity. Besides duplication cysts have the potential for neoplastic transformation.

Machado et al. [7] first reported laparoscopic resection of gastric duplication, followed by Tayar et al. [8–11]. However, laparoscopic resection of gastric duplication cysts in newbrons is rarely reported. At present, laparoscopy has been used in newborns with choledochal cyst, duodenal obstruction and esophageal atresia. For gastric duplication cysts, laparoscopy can not only confirm the diagnosis but also avoid abdominal laparotomy, thus decreasing possible traumatic injury. All the five newborn patients in our series underwent gastric duplication cyst resection by laparoscopy, including one who even underwent a gastrostomy. Technically, all the five cases achieved satisfactory outcomes. So we believe that laparoscopy is quite safe, effective, and feasible in the diagnosis and treatment of gastric duplication cysts, and should also be applicable to detect other gastrointestinal multiple malformations. Compared with conventional surgery, laparoscopy is characterized by less trauma, more acceptability on the part of both the patient and the doctor, and quicker postoperative recovery. The Case 1 gave up treatment and died of respiratory failure. The other four patients recovered uneventfully without significant postoperative complications and grew up well with no significant difference as compared with average children of the same age during the follow-up period.

Conclusions

Gastric duplication cysts in newborns are very rare. Laparoscopic surgery play an important role on the diagnosis and treatment. Our experience and practice indicate that laparoscopic resection of gastric duplication cysts in newborns is viable and there is also a need to increase sample size to prove its safety and effectiveness.

Abbreviations

CT: Computed tomography; GDCs: Gastric duplication cysts; MRI: Magnetic resonance imaging

Acknowledgements

This work was partly supported by Children's Hospital of Shanxi Province, China. We would like to acknowledge with gratitude the contribution of the colleagues of the department of Pediatrics.

Funding

None.

Authors' contributions

HR and BZ designed the study; HR and LD drafted the manuscript and made the final revision; XW and YJ collected and analysis the data as well as neaten illustrations in the manuscript. All authors read and approved the final manuscript.

Competing interests

The authors declare that they have no competing interests.

References

1. Rowling JT. Some observations on gastric cysts. Br J Surg. 1959;46:441–5.
2. Bonacci JL, Schlatter MG. Gastric duplication cyst: a unique presentation. J Pediatr Surg. 2008;43:1203–5.
3. Blinder G, Hiller N, Adler SN. A Double Stomach in an Adult. Am J Gastroenterol. 1999;94(4):1100–2.
4. Jiang W, Zhang B, Fu YB, Wang JW, Gao SJ, Zhang SZ. Gastric duplication cyst lined by pseudo stratified columnar ciliated epithelium: a case report and Literature review. J Zhejiang Univ Sci B. 2011;12:28–31.
5. Hlouschek V, Domagk D, Naehrig J, Siewert JR, Domschke W. Gastric Duplication cyst: a rare endosonographic finding in an adult. Scand J Gastroenterol. 2005;40:1129–31.
6. Chen PH, Lee JY, Yang SF, Wang JY, Lin JY, Chang YT. A retroperitoneal gastric duplication Cyst mimicking a simple exophytic renal cyst in an adolescent. J Pediatr Surg. 2010;45:e5–8.
7. Machado MA, Makdissi FF, Surjan RC. Single-port for laparoscopia paroscopic gastric resection witha novel platform. Arq Bras Cir Dig. 2014;27:157–9.
8. Tayar C, Brunetti F, Tantawi B, Fagniez PL. Laparoscopic treatment of an adult gastric duplication cyst. Hospital Henri-Mondor, University Paris XII, Creteil, France. Ann Chir. 2003;128:105–8.
9. Sasaki T, Shimura H, Ryu S, Matsuo K, Ikeda S. Laparoscopic treatment of a gastric duplication cyst: report of a case. Int Surg. 2003;88:68–71.
10. Singh JP, Rajdeo H, Bhuta K. Gastric Duplication Cyst: Two Case Reports and Review of the Literature. Case Rep Surg. 2013;2013:605059.
11. Ford WD, Guelfand M, López PJ, Furness ME. Laparoscopic excision of a gastric duplication cyst detected on antenatal ultrasound scan. Women's & Children's Hospital, Adelaide, South Australia, Australia. J Pediatr Surg. 2004; 39:e8–10.

20

Robotic versus laparoscopic Gastrectomy for gastric cancer: a systematic review and updated meta-analysis

Ke Chen[1], Yu Pan[1], Bin Zhang[1], Hendi Maher[2], Xian-fa Wang[1] and Xiu-jun Cai[1*]

Abstract

Background: Advanced minimally invasive techniques including robotic surgery are being employed with increasing frequency around the world, primarily in order to improve the surgical outcomes of laparoscopic gastrectomy (LG). We conducted a systematic review and meta-analysis to evaluate the feasibility, safety and efficacy of robotic gastrectomy (RG).

Methods: Studies, which compared surgical outcomes between LG and RG, were retrieved from medical databases before May 2017. Outcomes of interest were estimated as weighted mean difference (WMD) or risk ratio (RR) using the random-effects model. The software Review Manage version 5.1 was used for all calculations.

Results: Nineteen comparative studies with 5953 patients were included in this analysis. Compared with LG, RG was associated with longer operation time (WMD = −49.05 min; 95% CI: -58.18 ~ −39.91, $P < 0.01$), less intraoperative blood loss (WMD = 24.38 ml; 95% CI: 12.32 ~ 36.43, $P < 0.01$), earlier time to oral intake (WMD = 0.23 days; 95% CI: 0.13 ~ 0.34, $P < 0.01$), and a higher expense (WMD = −3944.8 USD; 95% CI: -4943.5 ~ −2946.2, $P < 0.01$). There was no significant difference between RG and LG regarding time to flatus, hospitalization, morbidity, mortality, harvested lymph nodes, and cancer recurrence.

Conclusions: RG can be performed as safely as LG. However, it will take more effort to decrease operation time and expense.

Keywords: Laparoscopy, Robot, Gastrectomy, Stomach neoplasms, Morbidity, Meta-analysis

Background

Laparoscopic gastrectomy (LG) has been widely used for the treatment of gastric cancer and a number of other different minimally invasive procedures have been developed to date [1, 2]. There are several benefits for patients; including better cosmesis, reduced pain, early recovery of intestinal function, and shorter hospital stay, while maintaining comparable oncologic safety [1–4].

Robotic surgery was first put into practice in 2000, after being approved by the US Food and Drug Administration (FDA). It plays an essential role in ergonomics and offers advantages such as motion scaling, less fatigue, tremor filtering, seven degrees of wrist-like motion, and three-dimensional vision [5, 6]. Surgeons hoped that such innovative technology could overcome some limitations innate to traditional laparoscopic surgery. Thus, experienced laparoscopic surgeons are increasingly trying to develop new procedures that best exploit the capabilities of robotic surgery in the treatment of gastric cancer [7].

Nonetheless, the present status of robotic gastrectomy (RG) is, as of the writing of this paper, still restricted and this is in part to due to the lack of randomized controlled trials (RCTs). Several previous studies including meta-analyses have argued that RG can be a more effective and safer operation in comparison with conventional LG. In spite of these studies, many questions still need to be answered, most notably, RG's efficacy with regard to oncologic, long-term survival outcomes and its cost-effectiveness. Moreover, a series of studies on RG for the treatments of gastric cancer have been recently published. These studies are meaningful in highlighting the

* Correspondence: caixiujunzju@163.com
[1]Department of General Surgery, Sir Run Run Shaw Hospital, School of Medicine, Zhejiang University, 3 East Qingchun Road, Hangzhou, Zhejiang Province 310016, China
Full list of author information is available at the end of the article

status of RG in the treatment of gastric cancer. Therefore, this paper's current research is intended to conduct a comprehensive systematic review of all the currently available literature and a meta-analysis of RG in comparison to LG in order to assess the feasibility, security and efficacy of RG.

Methods

Search strategy

A systematic search of Web of Science, Cochrane Library, Embase, and PubMed was conducted to find studies comparing RG and LG for gastric cancer treatment published up until May 2017. Search terms included "gastric carcinoma", "gastric cancer", "laparoscopic", "robotic", and "gastrectomy". The links in search results and references were also reviewed to find the additional literature. Based on the language competencies of the reviewers, English and Chinese were the only languages of searched papers.

Eligibility criteria

The standards for research were comparative, using peer-reviewed studies of RG versus LG in gastric cancer for which the full texts were available. The most recent study or the study with the most subjects was chosen if overlapping research studies were found. Articles including any of the following were excluded: (1) Non-comparative studies such as letters, reviews, comments, posters, protocols, et al. (2) Studies including non-gastric carcinoma cases such as gastrointestinal stromal tumors, or benign gastric diseases; (3) Studies in which less than 2 of the interesting indices were reported.

Data extraction and quality assessment

Two reviewers (Chen K and Pan Y) reviewed the publications thoroughly and independently. Data extracted included the following items: author, region, operation time, intraoperative estimated blood loss (EBL), time to flatus, time to oral intake, length of hospital stay (LOS), morbidity, mortality, costs, retrieved lymph nodes (RLN), proximal and distal margin distance, and long-term oncologic outcomes. In accordance with the morbidity reporting system of Memorial Sloan-Kettering Cancer Center [8], postoperative complications were categorized into medical complications (respiratory, cardiovascular, metabolic events, deep venous thrombosis, phlebitis, et al.) or surgical complications (bleeding, any complication required reoperation, anastomotic leakage or stricture, delayed gastric emptying, et al.). The means and standard deviations (SDs) were estimated as described by Hozo et al. [9] if the research offered medians and ranges. The choice of the articles included in this review adhered to the Preferred Reporting Items for Systematic Reviews and Meta-Analyses statement (PRISMA). The Newcastle-Ottawa Quality Assessment Scale (NOS) was utilized to evaluate the research quality (http://www.ohri.ca/programs/clinical_epidemiology/oxford.asp). The scale ranges from 0 to 9 stars: research with a score higher than or equal to 6 could be deemed as methodologically sound.

Subgroup analysis

The uneven distribution of the surgical extension between the groups could affect the outcomes. Therefore, to eliminate the bias, a subgroup analysis of total or distal gastrectomy was conducted. It has been reported that robotic surgery may benefit obese patients, because of improved visualization, instrumentation, and ergonomics [10]. Therefore, we conducted a subgroup analysis to analyze the impact of operation-related factors on body mass index (BMI).

Statistical analysis

The risk ratio (RR) was utilized to analyze the dichotomous variables and the weighted mean difference (WMD) was utilized to assess the continuous variables. Based on DerSimonian and Laird's approach, the random-effects model was utilized to account for clinical heterogeneity, which refers to diversity in a sense that is relevant for clinical situations. According to the overall complication, the potential publication bias was determined by carrying out an informal visual inspection of funnel plots. The software of Review Manager version 5.1 (RevMan 5.1) was used to conduct data analysis. $P < 0.05$ was considered statistically significant.

Results

Studies selected

A total of 378 potential articles, which were published from 1996 to 2017, were found. 37 articles were chosen based on the titles and abstracts, and then a thorough check of each text was conducted. Seven of them failed to meet our standards and were excluded. A further eleven papers were excluded due to overlapping patient cohorts (one from Hospital Niguarda Ca Granda, Italy [11]; one from Fujita Health University, Japan [12]; one from Taipei Veterans General Hospital, Taiwan [13]; four from Yonsei University, Korea [14–17]; four from National Cancer Center, Korea [18–21]). Finally, a total of nineteen studies were included for final meta-analysis [22–40]. A flow chart of the search strategies, which contains reasons for the exclusion of studies, is elucidated in Fig. 1.

Study characteristics and quality

A total of 5953 patients were included in the analysis with 4123 undergoing LG (69.3%) and 1830 undergoing RG (30.7%). Most of the studies came from East Asia (10 Korea, 2 Japan, 4 China, 1 Taiwan) and 2 research studies came from Italy. The baseline features of the included studies are shown in Table 1; the evaluation of

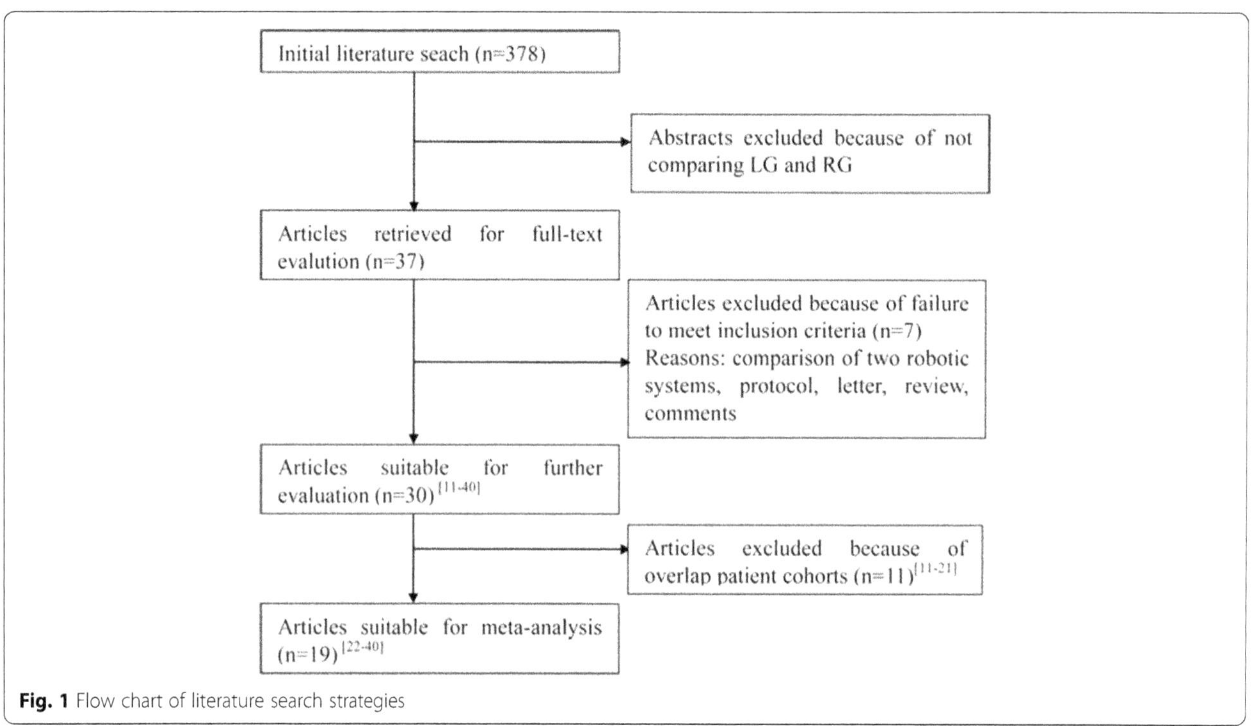

Fig. 1 Flow chart of literature search strategies

Table 1 Summary of studies included in the meta-analysis

Author	Region	Study design	Year	Study period	Sample size		Level of lymphadenectomy	Surgical extension	Reconstruction	Conversion (%)	
					LG	RG				LG	RG
Pugliese	Italy	OCS (R)	2010	2000–2009	48	16	D2	D	R-Y	3(6)	2(12)
Kim MC	Korea	OCS (P)	2010	2007–2008	11	16	D1 + β, D2	D	B-I, B-II	0	0
Kim KM	Korea	OCS (P)	2012	2005–2010	861	436	D1 + α/β, D2	D, T	B-I, B-II, R-Y	NR	NR
Son SY	Korea	OCS (R)	2012	2007–2011	42	21	D1 + β, D2	D, P, T	B-I, B-II, R-Y	NR	NR
Kang	Korea	OCS (P)	2012	2008–2011	282	100	D1 + α/β, D2	D, T	B-I, B-II, R-Y	E	0
Zhang	China	OCS (R)	2012	2009–2011	70	97	D2	D, P, T	B-I, B-II, R-Y	0	0
Hyun	Korea	OCS (P)	2013	2009–2010	83	38	D1 + α/β, D2	D, T	B-I, B-II, R-Y	0	0
Son T	Korea	OCS (R)	2014	2003–2010	58	51	D2	T	R-Y	0	0
Noshiro	Japan	OCS (P)	2014	2010–2012	160	21	D1 + α/β, D2	D	B-I, B-II, R-Y	0	0
Huang	Taiwan	OCS (P)	2014	2008–2014	73	72	D1 + α/β, D2	D, T	B-I, R-Y	NR	NR
Zhou	China	OCS (R)	2014	2010–2013	394	120	D1 + α/β, D2	D, P, T	B-I, B-II, R-Y	E	E
Liu	China	OCS (R)	2014	2012–2013	100	100	D2	D, P, T	B-I, B-II, R-Y	1(1)	0
Lee	Korea	OCS (P)	2015	2003–2010	267	133	D2	D	B-I, B-II, R-Y	NR	NR
Han	Korea	OCS (R)	2015	2008–2013	68	68	D1 + β	PPG	GG	0	0
Park	Korea	OCS (P)	2015	2009–2011	612	145	D1 + α/β	D, T	B-I, B-II, R-Y	10(1.6)	3(2.0)
Suda	Japan	OCS (R)	2015	2009–2012	438	88	D1 + α/β, D2	D, T	B-I, B-II, R-Y	0	0
Kim HI	Korea	OCS (P)	2016	2011–2012	185	185	D1 + α/β, D2	D, T	B-I, B-II, R-Y	2(1.1)	1(0.5)
Shen	China	OCS (R)	2016	2011–2014	330	93	D1 + α/β, D2	D, T	B-I, B-II, R-Y	0	0
Cianchi	Italy	OCS (R)	2016	2008–2015	41	30	D1 + α/β, D2	D	B-II, R-Y	0	0

OCS observational clinical study, *P* prospectively collected data, *R* retrospectively collected data, *D* distal gastrectomy, *P* proximal gastrectomy, *T* total gastrectomy, *PPG* pylorus-preserving gastrectomy, *B-I* Billroth-I, *B-II* Billroth-II, *R-Y* Roux-en-Y, *GG* gastro-gastro anastomosis, *E* exclude, *NR* not reported quality according to the NOS is shown in Table 2. NOS shows that four out of the 19 studies observed had 9 stars, one had 8 stars, seven had 7 stars and the remaining seven had 6 stars.

Intraoperative effects and postoperative recovery

As shown in Table 1, three studies did not report the information of conversion; two studies excluded the conversion cases, whereas another nine research studies had no conversion. The pooled data based on four studies, which reported conversion cases, showed similar conversion rates between groups (RR = 0.88, 95% CI: 0.36 ~ 2.17, $P = 0.78$). A longer operation time for RG than for LG was reported in the majority of research and meta-analysis revealed that the average operation time of LG was 49.05 min shorter than RG (WMD = −49.05 min; 95% CI: -58.18 ~ −39.91, $P < 0.01$) (Fig. 2a). Intraoperative EBL was reported in eighteen of the research studies, which was lower in RG than LG (WMD = 24.38 ml; 95% CI: 12.32 ~ 36.43, $P < 0.01$) (Fig. 2b).

The pooled mean time to first flatus indicated no significant difference between the two groups (WMD = 0.09 days; 95% CI: -0.10 ~ 0.27, $P = 0.36$) (Fig. 2c). Nonetheless, according to the meta-analysis, the mean time to restart oral intake was longer in LG than in RG (WMD = 0.23 days; 95% CI: 0.13 ~ 0.34, $P < 0.01$) (Fig. 2d). All studies reported the LOS. According to the pooled data, a significant difference did not exist between the two groups with regard to LOS (WMD = 0.35 days; 95% CI: -0.25 ~ 0.95, $P = 0.25$) (Fig. 2e). All intraoperative effects and postoperative recovery outcomes are summarized in Table 3.

Morbidity and mortality

All studies reported adverse incidents ranging from 0% to 47.4% in RG and from 4.3% to 38.6% in LG. No significant difference in the rate of overall postoperative complications was identified between the groups of RG and LG (RR = 0.96, 95% CI: 0.82 ~ 1.13, $P = 0.65$) (Fig. 3a). Symmetry was shown in the visual inspection of the funnel plot, showing no severe publication bias (Fig. 4). After further analysis, surgical complications were similar between groups (RR = 0.87, 95% CI: 0.72 ~ 1.05, $P = 0.15$) (Fig. 3b), as were the medical complications (RR = 1.34, 95% CI: 0.75 ~ 2.40, $P = 0.32$) (Fig. 3c).

Table 2 Quality assessment based on the NOS for observational studies

Author	Selection (Out of 4)				Comparability (Out of 2)	Outcomes (Out of 3)			Total (Out of 9)
	①	②	③	④		⑤	⑥	⑦	
Pugliese	*	*	*	*	**	*	*	*	9
Kim MC	*	*	*	*	*	*			6
Kim KM	*	*	*	*	*	*			6
Son SY	*	*	*	*	**	*			7
Kang	*	*	*	*	*	*			6
Zhang	*	*	*	*	**	*			7
Hyun	*	*	*	*	*	*			6
Son T	*	*	*	*	**	*	*	*	9
Noshiro	*	*	*	*	**	*			7
Huang	*	*	*	*	**	*			7
Zhou	*	*	*	*	**	*	*	*	9
Liu	*	*	*	*	**	*			7
Lee	*	*	*	*	*	*	*	*	8
Han	*	*	*	*	**	*	*	*	9
Park	*	*	*	*	*	*			6
Suda	*	*	*	*	*	*		*	7
Kim HI	*	*	*	*	*	*			6
Shen	*	*	*	*	**	*			7
Cianchi	*	*	*	*	*	*			6

①representativeness of exposed cohort
②selection of nonexposed cohort
③ascertainment of exposure
④outcome not present at the start of the study
⑤assessment of outcomes
⑥length of follow-up
⑦adequacy of follow-up

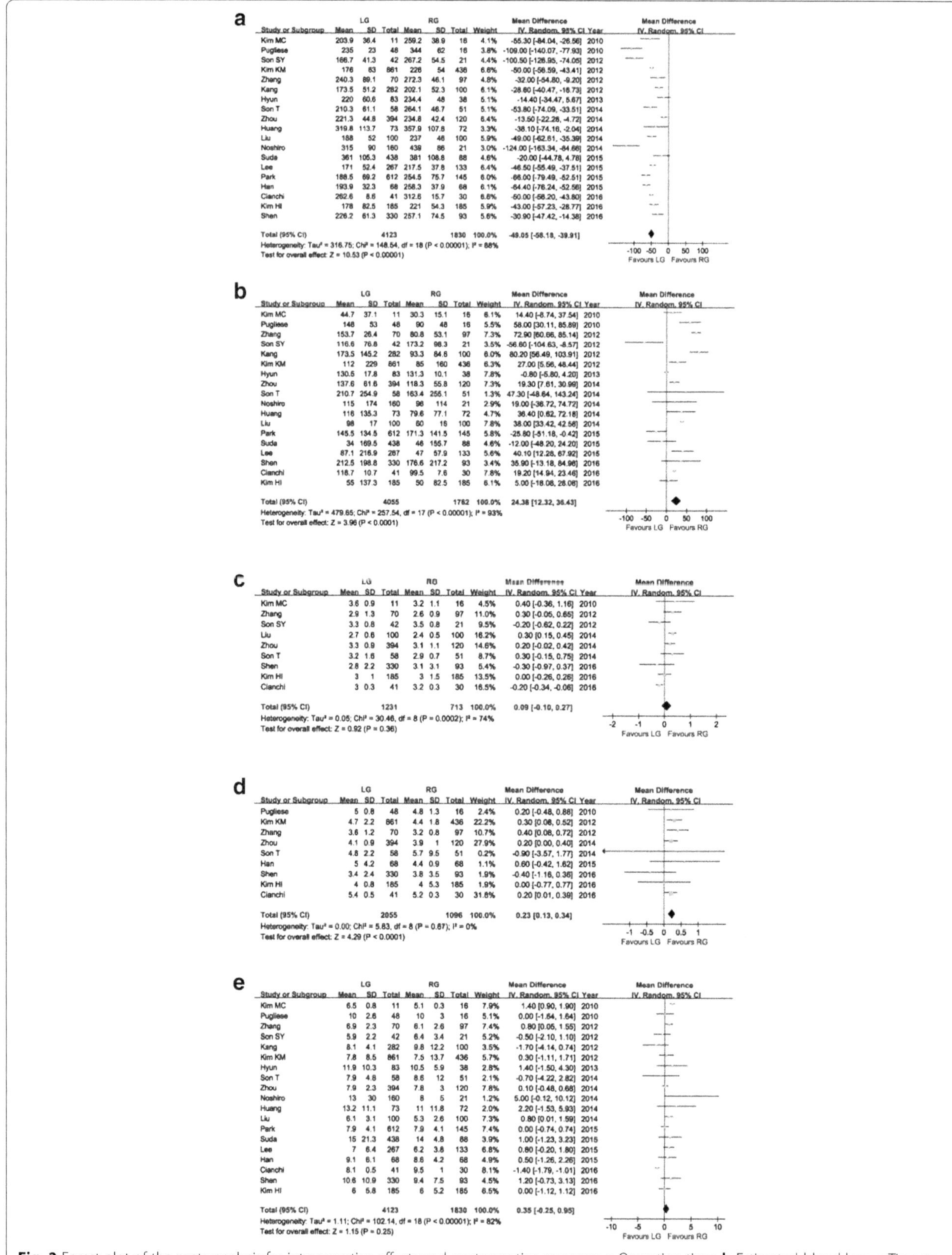

Fig. 2 Forest plot of the meta-analysis for intraoperative effects and postoperative recovery. **a** Operation time. **b** Estimated blood loss. **c** Time to first flatus. **d** Time to restart oral intake. **e** Length of postoperative hospital stay

Table 3 Results of the meta-analysis

Outcomes	No. of studies	Sample size		Heterogeneity (P, I^2)	Overall effect size	95% CI of overall effect	P
		LG	RG				
Conversion	4	16	6	0.68, 0%	RR =0.88	0.36 ~ 2.17	0.78
Operation time (min)	19	4123	1830	<0.001, 88%	WMD = −49.05	-58.18 ~ −39.91	<0.01
Blood loss (mL)	18	4055	1762	<0.001, 93%	WMD =24.38	12.32 ~ 36.43	<0.01
Time to first flatus (days)	9	1231	713	<0.001, 74%	WMD =0.09	-0.10 ~ 0.27	0.36
Time to oral intake (days)	9	2055	1096	0.67, 0%	WMD =0.23	0.13 ~ 0.34	<0.01
Hospital stay (days)	19	4123	1830	<0.001, 82%	WMD =0.35	-0.25 ~ 0.95	0.25
Overall complications	19	4123	1830	0.82, 0%	RR =0.96	0.82 ~ 1.13	0.65
Surgical complications	17	3234	1552	0.52, 0%	RR =0.87	0.72 ~ 1.05	0.15
Medical complications	12	2137	907	0.82, 0%	RR =1.34	0.75 ~ 2.40	0.32
Reoperation	7	1796	789	0.35, 11%	RR =0.69	0.29 ~ 1.62	0.39
Mortality	7	2131	838	0.91, 0%	RR =0.67	0.26 ~ 1.74	0.41
Retrieved lymph nodes	17	3229	1585	<0.001, 86%	WMD = −1.44	-3.26 ~ 0.37	0.12
Proximal margin (cm)	9	2006	1024	0.21, 26%	WMD = −0.14	-0.36 ~ 0.07	0.18
Distal margin (cm)	8	1948	973	<0.001, 81%	WMD =0.09	-0.46 ~ 0.65	0.74
Recurrence	3	500	187	0.39, 0%	RR =1.09	0.57 ~ 2.05	0.80
Cost (USD)	4	390	384	<0.001, 93%	WMD = −3944.8	-4943.5 ~ −2946.2	<0.01

Reoperation cases were reported in seven studies, and there was no significant difference in the reoperation rates (RR = 0.69, 95% CI: 0.29 ~ 1.62, P = 0.39) (Fig. 3d). Also, seven studies reported mortality and no significant difference could be found in postoperative mortality (RR = 0.67, 95% CI: 0.26 ~ 1.74, P = 0.41) (Fig. 3e). The specific reoperation and causes of mortality reported in the studies are summarized in Table 4. The meta-analysis results on morbidity and mortality are outlined in Table 3.

Oncologic outcomes and long-term survival

The differences in the average number of RLNs were not considerable in the pooled statistics with a tendency towards a reduction in the LG group when compared to the RG group (WMD = −1.44; 95% CI: -3.26 ~ 0.37, P = 0.12) (Fig. 5a). The distal or proximal margin distances were described in nine studies. Meta-analysis of the proximal margin distances showed no significant difference between the two groups (WMD = −0.14 cm; 95% CI: -0.36 ~ 0.07, P = 0.18) (Fig. 5b), the same applies to the distal margin distance (WMD = 0.09 cm; 95% CI: -0.46 ~ 0.65, P = 0.74) (Fig. 5c). Cancer recurrence was reported in three research studies and the pooled data indicated that the difference between RG and LG was not significant (RR = 1.09, 95% CI: 0.57 ~ 2.05, P = 0.80). Long-term survival rates were reported in three research studies, and no considerable difference in the survival rates between the LG group and RG group could be found. In addition, during the follow-up time, no significant difference in the survival rates between both of the groups could be found in the studies of Lee et al. [34] and Han et al. [35] though they failed to report the particular survival rates. The meta-analysis of survival rates cannot be done due to the limited data. The systematic review outcomes of follow-up time, recurrence patterns and sites, and long-term survival rates are summarized in Table 5.

Total cost

Only four studies recorded their total cost and they all reported a higher cost for RG than LG. The meta-analysis demonstrated that the total cost of RG groups was significantly higher than LG groups (WMD = −3944.8 USD; 95% CI: -4943.5 ~ −2946.2, P < 0.01) (Fig. 6).

Subgroup analysis of distal or total gastrectomy

For the subgroup analysis of distal gastrectomy (DG), the RG group still holds the longer operation time (P < 0.01), lower EBL (P < 0.05) and with similar LOS, overall complications, mortality as well as RLN (P > 0.05). However, there was a reduced time to oral intake for RG, but with only a marginal difference compared to the LG group (P = 0.05). As for total gastrectomy (TG), there is no large difference between the outcomes of operation time, EBL, time to oral intake, LOS, overall complications and mortality against DG subgroup analysis, the number of RLNs of RG was more than that of LG with a significant difference (P = 0.03). The subgroup analysis results of surgical extension are summarized in Table 6. Generally speaking, the difference in surgical extension had little effect on the overall meta-analysis results.

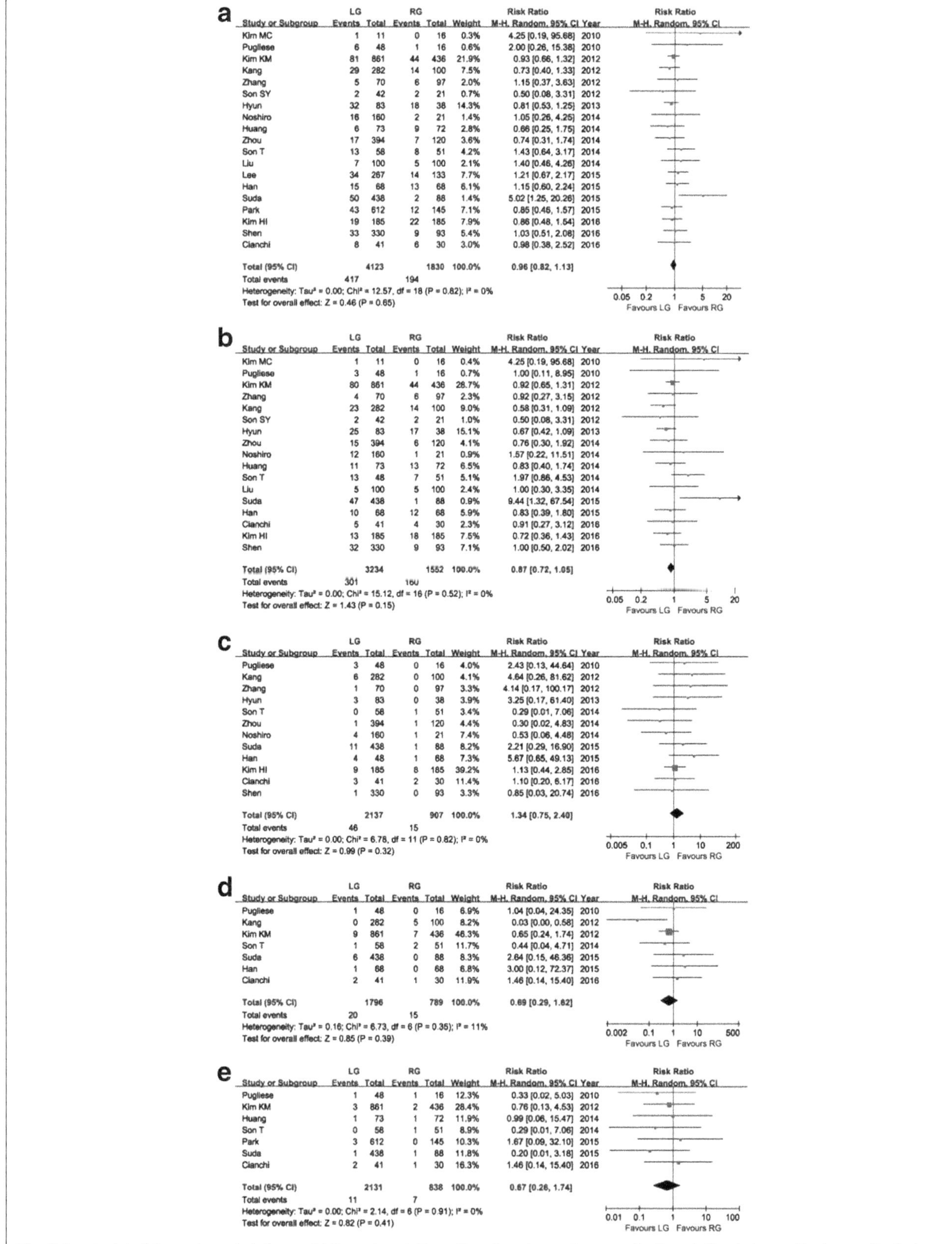

Fig. 3 Forest plot of the meta-analysis for morbidity and mortality. **a** Overall postoperative complications. **b** Surgical complications. **c** Medical complications. **d** Reoperation. **e** Mortality

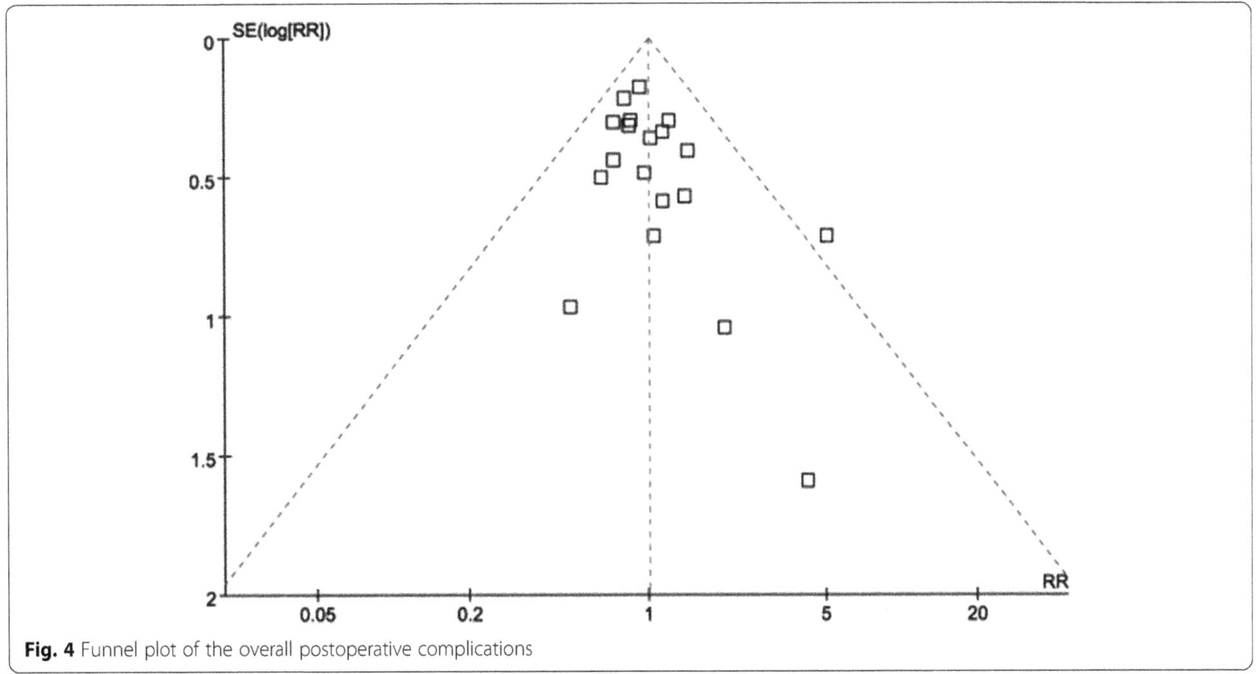

Fig. 4 Funnel plot of the overall postoperative complications

Subgroup analysis of weight influence

Only two studies had data for subgroup analysis based on weight [28, 34]. The patients were divided based on preoperative BMI into non-overweight (BMI < 25 kg/m^2) and overweight (BMI >25 kg/m^2) groups. In the non-overweight subgroup, the RG group still had a longer operation time ($P < 0.01$), while in the overweight subgroup; the operation time was similar between groups ($P = 0.27$). In addition, there was no significant difference between LG and RG for the outcomes of EBL and RLNs regardless of overweight or non-overweight subgroup. Other perioperative outcomes cannot be analyzed due to the limited data. The subgroup analysis results based on weight are summarized in Table 7.

Table 4 Systematic review of the specific reoperation and death reasons

Author	Group	Reoperation	Death
Pugliese	LG	Enterocutaneous leak (*n* = 1)	Severe bleeding due to hepatic failure (*n* = 1)
	RG	NC	Hemorrhagic stroke (*n* = 1)
Kim KM	LG	Leak-related (*n* = 4)[a]	Leak-related (*n* = 2)[a]
	RG	Leak-related (*n* = 6)[a]	NC
	RG	Leakage and obstruction (*n* = 5)	NC
Lee	LG	Anastomotic leakage (*n* = 1)	NC
	RG	Anastomotic leakage (*n* = 1), anastomotic bleeding (*n* = 1)	Anastomotic bleeding (*n* = 1)
Huang	LG	NC	Duodenal stump leakage (*n* = 1)
	RG	NC	Gastrojejunostomy leakage (*n* = 1)
Han	LG	Intra-abdominal bleeding due to liver capsular injury (*n* = 1)	NC
Park	LG	NC	Immediate postoperative bleeding (*n* = 1), mesenteric infarction (*n* = 1), septic shock caused by afferent loop syndrome (*n* = 1)
Cianchi	LG	NC	Duodenal stump leakage with peritonitis and sepsis (*n* = 1), acute myocardial infarction (*n* = 1)
	RG	Intestinal occlusion (*n* = 1)	Cerebral vascular accident (*n* = 1)

NC no case

[a]: included anastomotic leakage and duodenal stump leakage

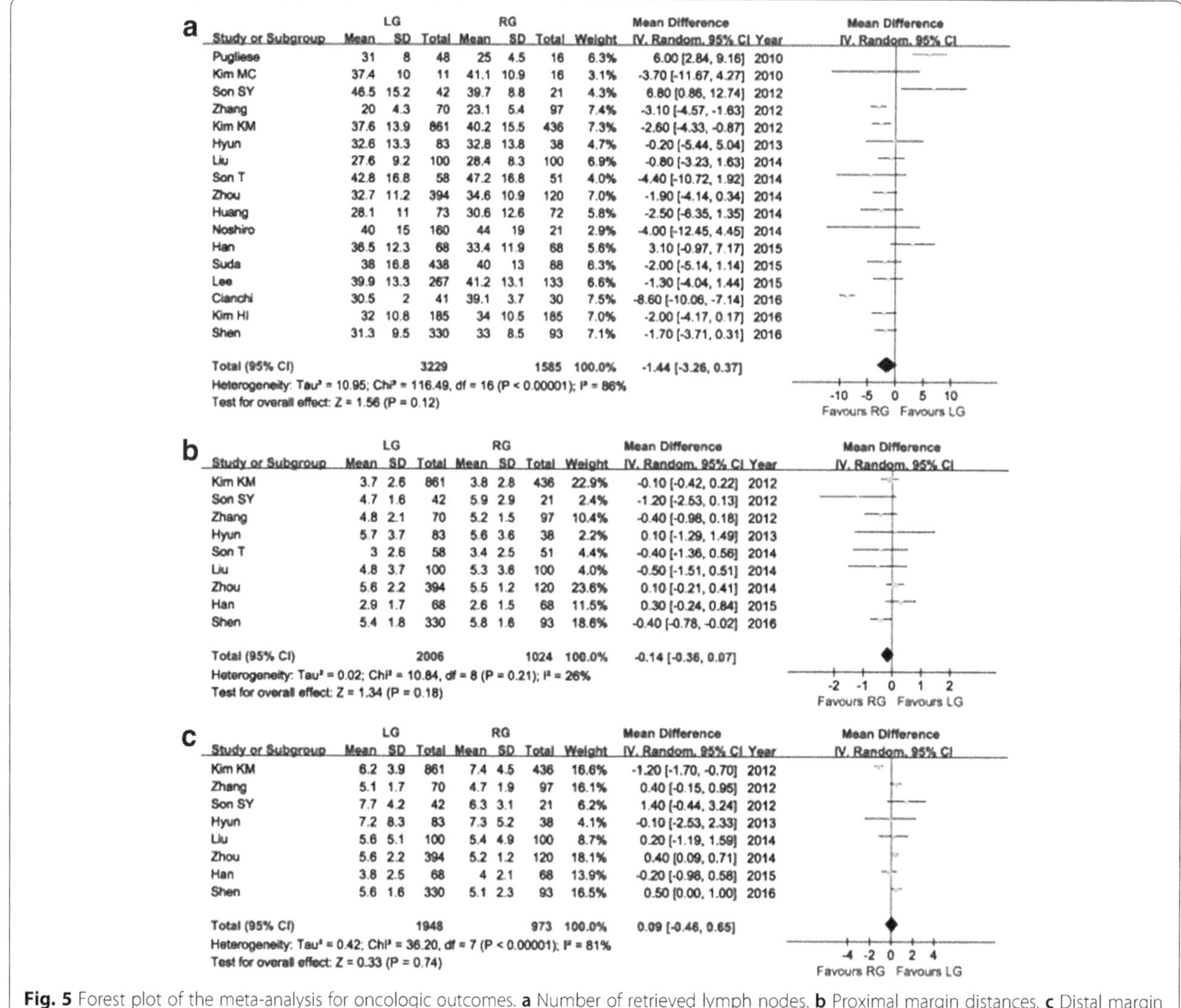

Fig. 5 Forest plot of the meta-analysis for oncologic outcomes. **a** Number of retrieved lymph nodes. **b** Proximal margin distances. **c** Distal margin distance. **d** Cancer recurrence

Discussion

The cost-effectiveness and definite advantages of RG have not been well documented, which is different when compared to the evolution of LG versus conventional open surgery [20]. However, the number of publications on RG has gradually increased in recent years. The oncologic outcomes, postoperative outcome, intraoperative effects and costs of a total of 1830 patients who underwent RG for gastric cancer treatment in 19 studies were reviewed as we believe such research would contribute to a more objective and comprehensive assessment of the current RG surgical status.

In spite of the considerable heterogeneity, the prolonged operating time in RG was shown in almost all the included research studies. The prolonged exposure time to pneumoperitoneum and the associated increased time of anesthesia is a major concern. Few publications describe the effect of longer operation times during RG. However, previous research of LG in senior patients has shown that longer operation time did not result in detrimental effects with regard to surgical results [41]. Therefore, a prolonged operating time should not affect surgeons directly on conducting research on RG's new utility. Inevitably, the docking time was considered as an essential factor, which enhanced the operating time. The docking time was between 20 min to 60 min as reported in our study [7, 13, 15, 31], We found RG had longer operation times than LG by 49 min, which suggested the 'true' time spent on operations was similar or even shorter than LG. Furthermore, with the increased utilization of the new robotic surgical system, operation times are expected to shorten. Several studies have reported that the da Vinci Xi robotic platform is more user-friendly and is easier to install in rectal and nephritic surgery [42, 43]. As a result, we believed that RG is technically feasible with regard to operation time.

Table 5 Systematic Review of Recurrence and Long-term Survivals

Author	Group	Stage	Chemotherapy	Follow-up (mo)	Recurrence	Survival (%)
Pugliese	LG	Any TNM_0	T_3 or any TN_+	53 (3–112)	8[a]	3y–OS: 85; 5y–OS: 83[&]
	RG			28 (2–44)	4[a]	3y–OS: 78[&]
Son T	LG	Any TNM_0	NR	70	3[b]	5y–DFS: 91.2; 5y–OS: 91.1
	RG				3[b]	5y–DFS: 90.2; 5y–OS: 89.5
Zhou	LG	Any TNM_0	Routinely[#]	17(3–41)	28	1, 2, 3-OS: 87.3, 77.1, 69.9 3y–OS N_-:82.6, 3y–OS N_+:60.3
	RG				5	1, 2, 3-OS: 90.2, 78.1, 67.8 3y–OS N_-: 84.4, 3y–OS N_+: 57.5
Lee	LG	Any TNM_0	NR	75	NR	NSD
	RG					
Han	LG	$cT_{1\text{-}2}N_0M_0$	3 cases (4.4%)[$]	19.3	0	NSD
	RG		3 cases (4.4%)[$]	22.7	0	

Follow-up time were shown as median (range) or median only

DFS disease-free survival, *OS* overall survival, *y* year, N_- negative nodal metastasis, N_+ positive nodal metastasis, *NR* not report, *NSD* only reported no significant difference between two groups without specific survival rate

[a]some patients had mixed tumor recurrence, identified recurrence in LG: local (*n* = 2), peritoneum (*n* = 2), liver (*n* = 1), lung (*n* = 2), bone (*n* = 1); identified recurrence in RG: peritoneum (*n* = 1), liver (*n* = 1), bone (*n* = 1). &: for overall patients, 5y–OS N_-: 97%, 5y–OS N_+: 52%

[b]LG, peritoneum (*n* = 2), lung (*n* = 1); RG, breast (*n* = 1), splenic hilum (*n* = 1), ovary (*n* = 1). #: 5-fluorouracil + oxaliplatin intravenous chemotherapy. $: because of advanced disease status after surgery

Surgeons have to go through a learning curve to master a technique. The surgical results, such as operation time, oncological outcomes and postoperative complications can be affected by surgeon's familiarity with the instrument, experience and assistant compliance. In general, before stabilization, LG should be conducted on around 40 to 60 cases [44]. The learning curve for RG was shorter for experienced surgeon who had performed LG, which is forecasted to be only 10 to 20 cases [12, 13, 18, 26]. A surgeon experienced in laparoscopic surgery can conduct robotic surgery securely even in their first case [16]. Several studies investigated in this meta-analysis compared the initial and later experiences of robotic surgery [12, 13, 18, 26]. The later cases performed by the same surgical team could progress toward shortening operation times.

Postoperative morbidity is the main indicator for assessing the safety and feasibility of one procedure. It is widely accepted that laparoscopic surgery for gastric cancer is safer and could have fewer complications than open surgery [45]. Our meta-analysis demonstrated a comparable complication rate in RG versus LG group, and the low heterogeneity regardless of overall, surgical or medical complications encourages us to believe that RG indeed is as safe as LG. Improvements such as three-dimension images and tremor filtering could theoretically contribute to safer implementations of the robotic system for gastrectomy and lymphadenectomy. According to the multivariate analyses in the Suda study, the application of RG was an important independent protective factor in regards to the postoperative complication [37]. Tokunaga et al. [46, 47] reported the incidences of overall adverse events after RG which were 14.2% and 22.2% based on their two-phase II studies, which are comparable to the rates of 19–27% in previous studies of LG [48, 49].

Obesity is one of the most significant health problems today and rates are still increasing around the world. Some studies claim obesity causes increased blood loss, operation time, and wound infection rate et al. [50, 51], whereas others did not observe any negative effect on surgical outcomes [52]. Recently, Harr et al. [10] showed

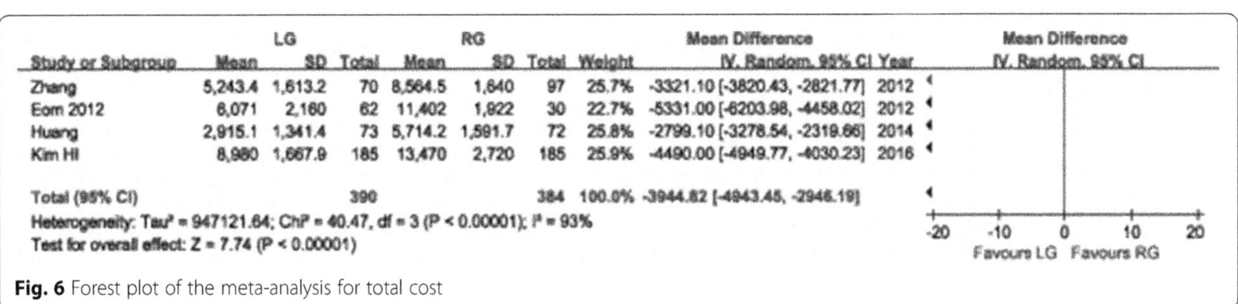

Fig. 6 Forest plot of the meta-analysis for total cost

Table 6 Results of the subgroup analysis of distal or total gastrectomy

Outcomes	No. of studies	Sample size		Heterogeneity (P, I^2)	Overall effect size	95% CI of overall effect	P
		LG	RG				
Operation time (min)							
DG	8	1635	453	<0.001, 78%	WMD = −57.08	−68.62 ~ −45.54	<0.01
TG	5	448	166	0.004, 74%	WMD = −42.62	−66.72 ~ −18.52	<0.01
Blood loss (mL)							
DG	8	1635	453	<0.001, 77%	WMD =19.27	3.86 ~ 34.68	0.01
TG	5	448	166	0.54, 0%	WMD =23.77	1.97 ~ 45.56	0.03
Time to oral intake (days)							
DG	3	344	116	0.49, 0%	WMD =0.18	0.00 ~ 0.36	0.05
TG	3	251	100	0.71, 0%	WMD = −0.18	−0.55 ~ 0.20	0.36
Hospital stay (days)							
DG	8	1635	453	<0.001, 92%	WMD =0.52	−0.69 ~ 1.74	0.40
TG	5	448	166	0.75, 0%	WMD =0.28	−0.80 ~ 1.36	0.61
Overall complications							
DG	8	1635	453	0.86, 0%	RR =1.19	0.83 ~ 1.71	0.34
TG	4	330	140	0.49, 0%	RR =1.32	0.80 ~ 2.18	0.27
Mortality							
DG	4	942	213	0.84, 0%	RR =0.84	0.21 ~ 3.30	0.80
TG	2	194	81	0.55, 0%	RR =0.15	0.02 ~ 1.41	0.10
Retrieved lymph nodes							
DG	8	1635	453	<0.001, 92%	WMD = −2.10	−5.90 ~ 1.70	0.28
TG	5	448	166	0.63, 0%	WMD = −2.51	−4.83 ~ −0.19	0.03

DG distal gastrectomy, *TG* total gastrectomy

that the benefits of robotic methods were more evident in high versus normal BMI patients when performing a colostomy. The authors concluded that robotic surgery might overcome the difficulties associated with thick abdominal walls and excessive intra-abdominal fat, thanks to improved visualization, instrumentation, and ergonomics [10]. However, compared to other operations such as the colorectal or prostatic surgeries, which are in relatively narrow regions, the superiority of da Vinci over the laparoscopy may not be obvious, in that gastric surgery is conducted in the upper abdomen of a relatively spacious location. In our study, the overall mean operation time of RG and LG were similar in the overweight subgroups, contrasting with those in the non-overweight subgroups, which implied RG to be superior to LG when used on overweight patients. However, the sample size of the overweight subgroups was not large enough to be conclusive.

Table 7 Results of the subgroup analysis of weight

Outcomes	No. of studies	Sample size		Heterogeneity (P, I^2)	Overall effect size	95% CI of overall effect	P
		LG	RG				
Operation time (min)							
non-overweight	2	232	127	0.06, 72%	WMD = −37.63	−62.82 ~ −12.43	<0.01
overweight	2	118	44	0.008, 86%	WMD = −28.58	−79.11 ~ 21.94	0.27
Blood loss (mL)							
non-overweight	2	232	127	0.11, 60%	WMD =0.90	−13.44 ~ 15.25	0.90
overweight	2	118	44	0.03, 80%	WMD =39.84	−41.71 ~ 121.39	0.34
Retrieved lymph nodes							
non-overweight	2	232	127	0.34, 0%	WMD = −1.88	−4.78 ~ 1.01	0.20
overweight	2	118	44	0.03, 79%	WMD =4.32	−4.10 ~ 12.74	0.31

The traditional straight forceps in LG fail to enable surgeons to reach deep-seated vessels and other areas, like the supra pancreatic one, in which the dissection of lymph nodes around the splenic hilum, splenic artery, and hepatic artery areas is deemed extremely hard. The tremor filtering, wristed instruments, as well as stable exposure and high-solution image can help surgeons thoroughly retrieve the lymph nodes around the delicate areas [21]. According to one included study, the amount of RLNs was considerably higher with robotic surgery in the splenic hilum and splenic artery areas [29]. Our meta-analysis shows adequate RLNs with means of 35.4 and 36.1 in the LG and RG groups, respectively. The mean number of RLNs of RG was more than that of LG with a marginal difference observed in the pooled data, even though most studies had been done during initial implementation of the robotic technique. Therefore, we believe that robotic technique could be superior to the conventional laparoscopic technique for lymphadenectomy. Since the history of the clinical application of RG is a short one, few reports have compared long-term survival outcomes with other methods. Coratti et al. [53] demonstrated that the 5-year survival rate after RG stratified with Stage IA, IB, II, and III was 100%, 84.6%, 76.9%, and 21.5%, respectively. Pugliese et al. [11] reported a cumulative overall 5-year survival rate of 78% with a mean follow up of 30 months (range 2–86) after RG for gastric cancer.

The application of robotic surgery remains controversial, mainly due to the considerable expense. The total difference in cost between the LG and RG groups has been predicted to be around 3900 USD [18, 31, 38], which is mainly derived from the robotic system itself. According to the opinions of some investigators, the higher cost of robotic surgery is not enough to justify the theoretical advantages of this technology [54]. If RG can reduce complications and shorten hospital stay, the higher costs of the robotic system would be partially offset. Based on this, it is essential for robotic operators to inspect whether the potential advantages of the robotic approach justifies its high cost in the treatment of gastric cancer.

Our research has the following limitations: (1) Selection bias: As no RCT was available to be included in the meta-analysis due to the higher cost of robotic surgery, selection biases are inevitable in surgical abstention which should be carefully interpreted. (2) Clinical heterogeneity: The homogeneity test for the continuous variables exhibited substantial heterogeneity due to the inherent flaws of a retrospective study, the uneven surgical skills of the different surgeons, as well as regional differences, etc. More importantly, for surgeons in the East, radical distal gastrectomy for middle and distal gastric cancer is popular [55], while the distal subtotal is preferred in the West [56]. Thus we cataloged distal gastrectomy and subtotal gastrectomy as a subgroup. Though it brings some interesting results due to the expansion of sample size, such a combination would result in clinical heterogeneity. (3) Regional difference: The majority of the included studies came from East Asia, because East Asia has the highest prevalence of gastric cancer, while gastric cancer is relatively uncommon in Western countries. Besides, in East Asia, particularly Korea, Japan and some areas of China, the proportion of early gastric cancer has increased as a result of the improved surveillance of gastric cancer in these regions [57, 58]. On the other hand, although increasing evidence continues to show no difference between patients undergoing open or laparoscopic surgery for oncologic outcomes, the Japanese Gastric Cancer Association still classifies minimal invasive surgery as investigational treatment and only recommends minimal invasive surgery for early stage gastric cancer patients [55]. Therefore, the cases in our studies, especially those from East Asia, were mainly early stage cases. All of the above limitations must be kept in mind when interpreting the results of our study.

Conclusions

Except for the longer operation time and higher costs, RG for the patients with gastric cancer was not inferior to LG. Besides; RG holds the potential benefits for larger numbers of lymph node dissection and reduced intraoperative blood loss. Further prospective studies are needed in order to confirm these advantages. In addition, long-term results are needed, particularly for the oncological adequacy of robotic gastric cancer resections.

Abbreviations

BMI: body mass index; EBL: estimated blood loss; LG: laparocopic gastrectomy; LOS: length of hospital stay; NOS: Newcastle-Ottawa Quality Assessment Scale; RCT: randomized controlled trial; RG: robotic gastrectomy; RLN: retrieved lymph nodes; RR: risk ratio; SD: standard deviation; WMD: weighted mean difference

Acknowledgments

Not applicable.

Funding

Not applicable.

Authors' contributions

KC and YP designed the study; BZ and XFW collected literatures and conducted the analysis of pooled data; HM helped to draft the manuscript; KC and YP wrote the manuscript; XJC proofread and revised the manuscript. All authors have approved the version to be published.

Competing interest

The authors declare that they have no competing interests.

Author details
[1]Department of General Surgery, Sir Run Run Shaw Hospital, School of Medicine, Zhejiang University, 3 East Qingchun Road, Hangzhou, Zhejiang Province 310016, China. [2]School of Medicine, Zhejiang University, 866 Yuhangtang Road, Hangzhou, Zhejiang Province 310058, China.

References

1. Chen K, Mou YP, Xu XW, Pan Y, Zhou YC, Cai JQ, et al. Comparison of short-term surgical outcomes between totally laparoscopic and laparoscopic-assisted distal gastrectomy for gastric cancer: a 10-y single-center experience with meta-analysis. J Surg Res. 2015;194:367–74.
2. Chen K, Wu D, Pan Y, Cai JQ, Yan JF, Chen DW, et al. Totally laparoscopic gastrectomy using intracorporeally stapler or hand-sewn anastomosis for gastric cancer: a single-center experience of 478 consecutive cases and outcomes. World J Surg Oncol. 2016;14:115.
3. Chen K, He Y, Cai JQ, Pan Y, Wu D, Chen DW, et al. Comparing the short-term outcomes of intracorporeal esophagojejunostomy with extracorporeal esophagojejunostomy after laparoscopic total gastrectomy for gastric cancer. BMC Surg. 2016;16:13.
4. Chen K, Xu XW, Zhang RC, Pan Y, Wu D, Mou YP. Systematic review and meta-analysis of laparoscopy-assisted and open total gastrectomy for gastric cancer. World J Gastroenterol. 2013;19:5365–76.
5. Rockall TA, Darzi A. Robot-assisted laparoscopic colorectal surgery. Surg Clin North Am. 2003;83:1463–8. xi
6. Gutt CN, Oniu T, Mehrabi A, Kashfi A, Schemmer P, Buchler MW. Robot-assisted abdominal surgery. Br J Surg. 2004;91:1390–7.
7. Song J, Oh SJ, Kang WH, Hyung WJ, Choi SH, Noh SH. Robot-assisted gastrectomy with lymph node dissection for gastric cancer: lessons learned from an initial 100 consecutive procedures. Ann Surg. 2009;249:927–32.
8. Grobmyer SR, Pieracci FM, Allen PJ, Brennan MF, Jaques DP. Defining morbidity after pancreaticoduodenectomy: use of a prospective complication grading system. J Am Coll Surg. 2007;204:356–64.
9. Hozo SP, Djulbegovic B, Hozo I. Estimating the mean and variance from the median, range, and the size of a sample. BMC Med Res Methodol. 2005;5:13.
10. Harr JN, Luka S, Kankaria A, Juo YY, Agarwal S, Obias V. Robotic-assisted colorectal surgery in obese patients: a case-matched series. Surg Endosc. 2017;31:2813–9.
11. Pugliese R, Maggioni D, Sansonna F, Ferrari GC, Forgione A, Costanzi A, et al. Outcomes and survival after laparoscopic gastrectomy for adenocarcinoma. Analysis on 65 patients operated on by conventional or robot-assisted minimal access procedures. Eur J Surg Oncol. 2009;35:281–8.
12. Uyama I, Kanaya S, Ishida Y, Inaba K, Suda K, Satoh S. Novel integrated robotic approach for suprapancreatic D_2 nodal dissection for treating gastric cancer: technique and initial experience. World J Surg. 2012;36:331–7.
13. Huang KH, Lan YT, Fang WL, Chen JH, Lo SS, Hsieh MC, et al. Initial experience of robotic gastrectomy and comparison with open and laparoscopic gastrectomy for gastric cancer. J Gastrointest Surg. 2012;16:1303–10.
14. Song J, Kang WH, Oh SJ, Hyung WJ, Choi SH, Noh SH. Role of robotic gastrectomy using da Vinci system compared with laparoscopic gastrectomy: initial experience of 20 consecutive cases. Surg Endosc. 2009; 23:1204–11.
15. Woo Y, Hyung WJ, Pak KH, Inaba K, Obama K, Choi SH, et al. Robotic gastrectomy as an oncologically sound alternative to laparoscopic resections for the treatment of early-stage gastric cancers. Arch Surg. 2011; 146(9):1086–92.
16. Kim HI, Park MS, Song KJ, Woo Y, Hyung WJ. Rapid and safe learning of robotic gastrectomy for gastric cancer: multidimensional analysis in a comparison with laparoscopic gastrectomy. Eur J Surg Oncol. 2014;40:1346–54.
17. Okumura N, Son T, Kim YM, Kim HI, An JY, Noh SH, et al. Robotic gastrectomy for elderly gastric cancer patients: comparisons with robotic gastrectomy in younger patients and laparoscopic gastrectomy in the elderly. Gastric Cancer. 2016;19:1125–34.
18. Eom BW, Yoon HM, Ryu KW, Lee JH, Cho SJ, Lee JY, et al. Comparison of surgical performance and short-term clinical outcomes between laparoscopic and robotic surgery in distal gastric cancer. Eur J Surg Oncol. 2012;38:57–63.
19. Yoon HM, Kim YW, Lee JH, Ryu KW, Eom BW, Park JY, et al. Robot-assisted total gastrectomy is comparable with laparoscopically assisted total gastrectomy for early gastric cancer. Surg Endosc. 2012;26:1377–81.
20. Park JY, Jo MJ, Nam BH, Kim Y, Eom BW, Yoon HM, et al. Surgical stress after robot-assisted distal gastrectomy and its economic implications. Br J Surg. 2012;99:1554–61.
21. Kim YW, Reim D, Park JY, Eom BW, Kook MC, Ryu KW, et al. Role of robot-assisted distal gastrectomy compared to laparoscopy-assisted distal gastrectomy in suprapancreatic nodal dissection for gastric cancer. Surg Endosc. 2016;30:1547–52.
22. Pugliese R, Maggioni D, Sansonna F, Costanzi A, Ferrari GC, Di Lernia S, et al. Subtotal gastrectomy with D_2 dissection by minimally invasive surgery for distal adenocarcinoma of the stomach: results and 5-year survival. Surg Endosc. 2010;24:2594–602.
23. Kim MC, Heo GU, Jung GJ. Robotic gastrectomy for gastric cancer: surgical techniques and clinical merits. Surg Endosc. 2010;24:610–5.
24. Kim KM, An JY, Kim HI, Cheong JH, Hyung WJ, Noh SH. Major early complications following open, laparoscopic and robotic gastrectomy. Br J Surg. 2012;99:1681–7.
25. Son SY, Lee CM, Ahn SH, Lee JH, Park DJ, Kim HH. Clinical outcome of robotic Gastrectomy in gastric cancer in comparison with laparoscopic Gastrectomy: a case-control study. Journal of Minimally Invasive Surgery. 2012;15:27–31.
26. Kang BH, Xuan Y, Hur H, Ahn CW, Cho YK, Han SU. Comparison of surgical outcomes between robotic and laparoscopic Gastrectomy for gastric cancer: the learning curve of robotic surgery. J Gastric Cancer. 2012;12:156–63.
27. Zhang XL, Jiang ZW, Zhao K. Comparative study on clinical efficacy of robot-assisted and laparoscopic gastrectomy for gastric cancer. Zhonghua Wei Chang Wai Ke Za Zhi. 2012;15:804–6.
28. Hyun MH, Lee CH, Kwon YJ, Cho SI, Jang YJ, Kim DH, et al. Robot versus laparoscopic gastrectomy for cancer by an experienced surgeon: comparisons of surgery, complications, and surgical stress. Ann Surg Oncol. 2013;20:1258–65.
29. Son T, Lee JH, Kim YM, Kim HI, Noh SH, Hyung WJ. Robotic spleen-preserving total gastrectomy for gastric cancer: comparison with conventional laparoscopic procedure. Surg Endosc. 2014;28:2606–15.
30. Noshiro H, Ikeda O, Urata M. Robotically-enhanced surgical anatomy enables surgeons to perform distal gastrectomy for gastric cancer using electric cautery devices alone. Surg Endosc. 2014;28:1180–7.
31. Huang KH, Lan YT, Fang WL, Chen JH, Lo SS, Li AF, et al. Comparison of the operative outcomes and learning curves between laparoscopic and robotic gastrectomy for gastric cancer. PLoS One. 2014;9:e111499.
32. Junfeng Z, Yan S, Bo T, Yingxue H, Dongzhu Z, Yongliang Z, et al. Robotic gastrectomy versus laparoscopic gastrectomy for gastric cancer: comparison of surgical performance and short-term outcomes. Surg Endosc. 2014;28: 1779–87.
33. Liu J, Ruan H, Zhao K, Wang G, Li M, Jiang Z. Comparative study on da Vince robotic and laparoscopic radical gastrectomy for gastric cancer. Zhonghua Wei Chang Wai Ke Za Zhi. 2014;17:461–4.
34. Lee J, Kim YM, Woo Y, Obama K, Noh SH, Hyung WJ. Robotic distal subtotal gastrectomy with D_2 lymphadenectomy for gastric cancer patients with high body mass index: comparison with conventional laparoscopic distal subtotal gastrectomy with D_2 lymphadenectomy. Surg Endosc. 2015;29: 3251–60.
35. Han DS, Suh YS, Ahn HS, Kong SH, Lee HJ, Kim WH, et al. Comparison of surgical outcomes of robot-assisted and laparoscopy-assisted pylorus-preserving Gastrectomy for gastric cancer: a propensity score matching analysis. Ann Surg Oncol. 2015;22:2323–8.
36. Park JY, Ryu KW, Reim D, Eom BW, Yoon HM, Rho JY, et al. Robot-assisted gastrectomy for early gastric cancer: is it beneficial in viscerally obese patients compared to laparoscopic gastrectomy? World J Surg. 2015;39:1789–97.
37. Suda K, Man IM, Ishida Y, Kawamura Y, Satoh S, Uyama I. Potential advantages of robotic radical gastrectomy for gastric adenocarcinoma in comparison with conventional laparoscopic approach: a single institutional retrospective comparative cohort study. Surg Endosc. 2015;29:673–85.
38. Kim HI, Han SU, Yang HK, Kim YW, Lee HJ, Ryu KW, et al. Multicenter prospective comparative study of robotic versus laparoscopic Gastrectomy for gastric Adenocarcinoma. Ann Surg. 2016;263:103–9.
39. Shen W, Xi H, Wei B, Cui J, Bian S, Zhang K, et al. Robotic versus laparoscopic gastrectomy for gastric cancer: comparison of short-term surgical outcomes. Surg Endosc. 2016;30:574–80.

40. Cianchi F, Indennitate G, Trallori G, Ortolani M, Paoli B, Macri G, et al. Robotic vs laparoscopic distal gastrectomy with D_2 lymphadenectomy for gastric cancer: a retrospective comparative mono-institutional study. BMC Surg. 2016;16:65.
41. Hwang SH, Park DJ, Jee YS, Kim HH, Lee HJ, Yang HK, et al. Risk factors for operative complications in elderly patients during laparoscopy-assisted gastrectomy. J Am Coll Surg. 2009;208:186–92.
42. Patel MN, Aboumohamed A, Hemal A. Does transition from the da Vinci Si to xi robotic platform impact single-docking technique for robot-assisted laparoscopic nephroureterectomy? BJU Int. 2015;116:990–4.
43. Morelli L, Guadagni S, Di Franco G, Palmeri M, Caprili G, D'Isidoro C, et al. Use of the new da Vinci xi during robotic rectal resection for cancer: a pilot matched-case comparison with the da Vinci Si. Int J Med Robot. 2017;13:e1728.
44. Jin SH, Kim DY, Kim H, Jeong IH, Kim MW, Cho YK, et al. Multidimensional learning curve in laparoscopy-assisted gastrectomy for early gastric cancer. Surg Endosc. 2007;21:28–33.
45. Vinuela EF, Gonen M, Brennan MF, Coit DG, Strong VE. Laparoscopic versus open distal gastrectomy for gastric cancer: a meta-analysis of randomized controlled trials and high-quality nonrandomized studies. Ann Surg. 2012; 255:446–56.
46. Tokunaga M, Sugisawa N, Kondo J, Tanizawa Y, Bando E, Kawamura T, et al. Early phase II study of robot-assisted distal gastrectomy with nodal dissection for clinical stage IA gastric cancer. Gastric Cancer. 2014;17:542–7.
47. Tokunaga M, Makuuchi R, Miki Y, Tanizawa Y, Bando E, Kawamura T, et al. Late phase II study of robot-assisted gastrectomy with nodal dissection for clinical stage I gastric cancer. Surg Endosc. 2016;30:3362–7.
48. Kim HH, Han SU, Kim MC, Hyung WJ, Kim W, Lee HJ, et al. Long-term results of laparoscopic gastrectomy for gastric cancer: a large-scale case-control and case-matched Korean multicenter study. J Clin Oncol. 2014;32:627–33.
49. Chen K, Xu X, Mou Y, Pan Y, Zhang R, Zhou Y, et al. Totally laparoscopic distal gastrectomy with D_2 lymphadenectomy and Billroth II gastrojejunostomy for gastric cancer: short- and medium-term results of 139 consecutive cases from a single institution. Int J Med Sci. 2013;10:1462–70.
50. Sugimoto M, Kinoshita T, Shibasaki H, Kato Y, Gotohda N, Takahashi S, et al. Short-term outcome of total laparoscopic distal gastrectomy for overweight and obese patients with gastric cancer. Surg Endosc. 2013;27:4291–6.
51. Chen K, Pan Y, Zhai ST, Cai JQ, Chen QL, Chen DW, et al. Laparoscopic gastrectomy in obese gastric cancer patients: a comparative study with non-obese patients and evaluation of difference in laparoscopic methods. BMC Gastroenterol. 2017;17:78.
52. Wang Z, Zhang X, Liang J, Hu J, Zeng W, Zhou Z. Short-term outcomes for laparoscopy-assisted distal gastrectomy for body mass index >/=30 patients with gastric cancer. J Surg Res. 2015;195:83–8.
53. Coratti A, Fernandes E, Lombardi A, Di Marino M, Annecchiarico M, Felicioni L, et al. Robot-assisted surgery for gastric carcinoma: five years follow-up and beyond: a single western center experience and long-term oncological outcomes. Eur J Surg Oncol. 2015;41:1106–13.
54. Park JS, Choi GS, Park SY, Kim HJ, Ryuk JP. Randomized clinical trial of robot-assisted versus standard laparoscopic right colectomy. Br J Surg. 2012;99: 1219–26.
55. Japanese Gastric Cancer Association. Japanese gastric cancer treatment guidelines 2014 (ver. 4). Gastric Cancer. 2017;20:1–19.
56. De Manzoni G, Marrelli D, Baiocchi GL, Morgagni P, Saragoni L, Degiuli M, et al. The Italian research Group for Gastric Cancer (GIRCG) guidelines for gastric cancer staging and treatment: 2015. Gastric Cancer. 2017;20:20–30.
57. Inoue M, Tsugane S. Epidemiology of gastric cancer in Japan. Postgrad Med J. 2005;81:419–24.
58. Jeong O, Park YK. Clinicopathological features and surgical treatment of gastric cancer in South Korea: the results of 2009 nationwide survey on surgically treated gastric cancer patients. J Gastric Cancer. 2011;11:69–77.

21

Primary malignant melanoma of the esophagus treated with subtotal esophagectomy: a case report

Shota Kuwabara, Yuma Ebihara*, Yoshitsugu Nakanishi, Toshimichi Asano, Takehiro Noji, Yo Kurashima, Soichi Murakami, Toru Nakamura, Takahiro Tsuchikawa, Keisuke Okamura, Toshiaki Shichinohe and Satoshi Hirano

Abstract

Background: Primary malignant melanoma of the esophagus (PMME) is a rare disease with a poor prognosis. There are few reports of early-stage cases in which tumor invasion reached the lamina propria or muscularis mucosae, as in the present case. A standard treatment for early-stage PMME has not yet been established. The present study aimed to summarize previous reports and to discuss the indications for surgical treatment of early-stage primary malignant melanoma of the esophagus.

Case presentation: A 70-year-old woman with PMME was referred to our hospital. She underwent thoracoscopic and laparoscopic subtotal esophagectomy with lymphadenectomy. The resected specimen showed melanocytosis and junctional activity. Melanoma-specific antigens melan-A, S-100, and HMB45 were detected by immunohistochemical staining. The pathological diagnosis was pT1a-MM, pN0, pM0, and pStage IA. She remains alive without evidence of recurrence 39 months later.

Conclusion: Subtotal esophagectomy with regional radical lymphadenectomy could be recommended to patients with early-stage primary malignant melanoma of the esophagus, and curative surgical resection could improve their prognosis.

Keywords: Esophagus, Melanoma, Pathology, Treatment, Prognosis

Background

Primary malignant melanoma of the esophagus (PMME) is a rare disease. The incidence of PMME in all esophageal malignancies is low at 0.1%–0.2% [1]. The prognosis of PMME is poor because of its highly malignant biological behavior and its tendency to frequently disseminate even at the time of diagnosis. The recently reported 5-year survival rate after surgical resection is 37.5% [2], which is lower than that of esophageal cancer. Given that PMME is a rare disease with a poor prognosis, an appropriate treatment of choice for PMME is still under investigation. Here, we present a case of early-stage PMME in which tumor invasion reached the muscularis mucosae that followed a favorable course after subtotal esophagectomy.

* Correspondence: yuma-ebi@wc4.so-net.ne.jp
Department of Gastroenterological Surgery II, Hokkaido University Graduate School of Medicine, North 15 West 7, Kita-ku, Sapporo, Hokkaido 0608638, Japan

Case presentation

A 70-year-old woman presented at her local hospital with a sticky sensation in her throat and a weight loss of 2 kg over 10 months.

Esophagogastroduodenoscopy (EGD) revealed an elevated lesion 35 cm from the incisors that was diagnosed as malignant melanoma by biopsy. She was referred to our institution for further examination and treatment. Her blood examination was normal, including tumor markers such as CEA and CA19–9, except for a slightly elevated HbA1c level.

A barium swallow test was arranged and showed a filling defect in the lower esophagus (Fig. 1). EGD showed a pigmented and elevated lesion 7 mm in diameter, associated with a hemi-circumferential, irregular-shaped, pigmented, and flat lesion in the lower esophagus. The flat lesion ranged from dark

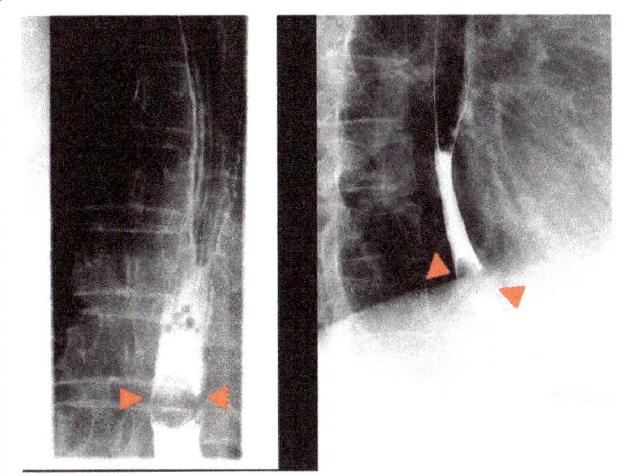

Fig. 1 Findings of a barium swallow test. A barium swallow test shows a filling defect in the lower esophagus (arrows)

brown to black in color, and the black area contained a well-demarcated mucosal abnormality (Fig. 2).

A biopsy specimen showed malignant melanoma cells in the esophageal mucosa, which were strongly positive for melanoma-specific antigens S-100 and HMB45 by immunohistochemical staining. A computed tomography (CT) scan also showed an intraluminal mass in the lower esophagus, which was well-defined without infiltration into the surrounding tissues (Fig. 3a). There was no enlargement of mediastinal lymph nodes or any visible metastatic lesion. 18F–fluorodeoxyglucose (18F–FDG) positron-emission tomography (PET) combined with CT showed abnormal 18F–FDG uptake in the same part of the esophagus identified on EGD and barium swallow as the site of the lesion with a maximum standardized uptake value (SUV max) of 3.1 (Fig. 3b). Detailed clinical examination of the eyes, oral cavity, nose, and skin did not indicate any malignant melanoma lesions.

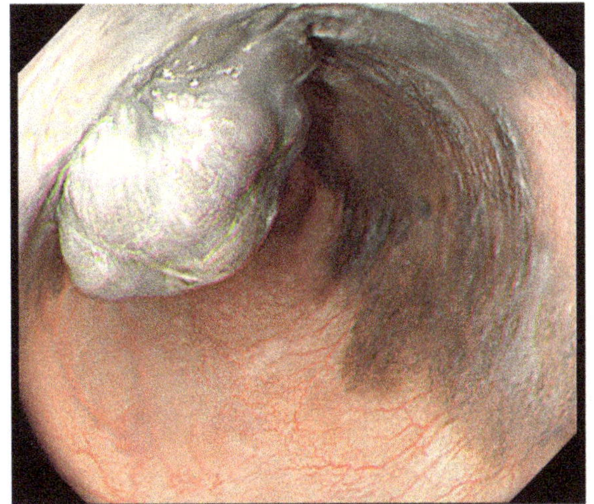

Fig. 2 Findings of esophagogastroduodenoscopy (EGD). EGD shows a pigmented, elevated 7-mm lesion, indicating an almost circumferential, irregular-shaped pigmentation in the lower esophagus, ranging from dark brown to black. The black area contains a well-demarcated mucosal abnormality

Based on these findings, the preoperative diagnosis of the lesion was PMME without metastasis (cT2N0M0, cStage II) according to the UICC TNM classification of esophageal cancer [3]. Then, thoracoscopic and laparoscopic subtotal thoracic esophagectomy with lymphadenectomy of the neck, mediastinum, and abdomen was performed. The cervical esophagus and the elevated gastric tube were anastomosed via the posterior mediastinal approach. The operation time was 536 min, and blood loss was 95 mL.

The resected specimen showed an elevated, black, and pigmented polyp-like lesion (15 mm × 13 mm × 9 mm) in a flat and pigmented area (57 mm × 38 mm) (Fig. 4a). A faintly marked depression that was partly tinged with white on the surface of the polyp-like lesion was found (Fig. 4b). Microscopic examination showed that most of the polyp-like lesion was composed of solid growth, with pseudocircular and spindle-shaped atypical cells containing melanin pigmentation and irregularly demarcated nucleoli. Many melanophages were present in the intervening interstitial stroma (Fig. 5). The lesion was immunohistochemically stained strongly for melanoma-specific antigens melan-A, S-100, and HMB45 (Fig. 6a–c). Around the polyp-like lesion, the same characteristic cells were spread laterally in the epithelium. Melanophages were also present in the lamina propria beneath the polyp-like lesion. The tumor cells were thought to invade the muscularis mucosae directly and then spread horizontally in the basal layer of the esophageal epithelium, which is called "junctional activity" [4] (Fig. 7a–c). The proximal and distal margins were considered safe. No lymph node metastases were detected. Pathologically, a diagnosis of pT1a-MM, pN0, pM0, pStage IA [3] was rendered.

Her postoperative course was uneventful and favorable. Adjuvant chemotherapy was not administered, and she has survived 39 months so far without any evidence of recurrence. She has been followed up once a half year and underwent blood tests and contrast-enhanced CT to search for metastasis or recurrence.

Discussion and conclusions

PMME is a rare disease with an extremely low incidence, comprising 0.1%–0.2% of all esophageal malignant tumors [1]. Over 70% of patients with PMME visit the hospital with chief complaints of dysphagia and epigastralgia [5]. Because the tumor is softer than other esophageal carcinomas, and wall extensibility of the

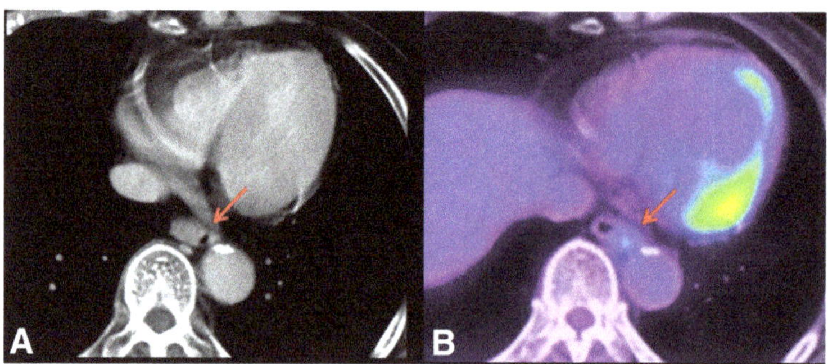

Fig. 3 Findings of computed tomography (CT) and 18F–fluorodeoxyglucose (18F–FDG) positron-emission tomography/computed tomography (PET-CT). **a** A transverse plane of an enhanced CT scan shows an intraluminal mass in the lower esophagus, which is well-defined without infiltration of the surrounding tissue (arrows). **b** 18F–FDG PET-CT scan shows 18F–FDG uptake at the same lesion of the lower esophagus; the SUV max of the lesion is 3.1 (arrows)

esophagus is maintained, the onset of symptoms is slow despite the size of the tumor. Therefore, more than 90% of the tumors are found to be larger than 2 cm at the initial diagnosis [5], and the detection of PMME at an early stage is rare.

Generally, PMME tends to originate in the lower to middle esophagus with endoscopic findings of a well-circumscribed, elevated, and pigmented tumor that is partially covered by normal mucosa and rarely accompanied by ulcers. A black tone is well known as a characteristic of PMME, but various colors such as purple and brown are often present in 10%–25% of PMMEs depending on the melanin quantity [1, 6]. The diagnosis of PMME should be suspected when a black or dark brown mass is observed [7]; however, it is important to be aware of amelanotic melanoma without white melanin pigmentation. Therefore, careful assessment is necessary for an accurate diagnosis [6] by endoscopy.

Esophageal melanocytosis is characterized by the presence of an increased number of pigment-laden melanocytes in the basal layer of the esophageal squamous epithelium, and the transfer of melanin granules to the epithelium around the melanocytes [8]. It has been described as a premalignant lesion of PMME; therefore, differentiation from melanoma in situ is important [9]. A biopsy can be conducted on patients for definitive diagnosis, but its accuracy is only approximately 80% [5]. Moreover, 20%–50% of patients are misdiagnosed with a poorly differentiated carcinoma [5], especially in cases of amelanotic melanoma. Immunohistochemical investigations are supportive for definitive diagnosis [10].

Diagnostic criteria are defined by Allen and Spitz [4] as follows: (1) a typical histological pattern of melanoma, with melanin granules inside the tumor cells, and an (2) origin in an area of junctional activity in the squamous epithelium. Junctional activity is defined as some nests of melanocytes with varying degrees of atypia found at the mucosal-submucosal junction adjacent to the tumor mass [4]. In other words, the tumor cells are spread horizontally in the basal layer of the esophageal epithelium. These findings and the presence of in situ melanoma without previous history of cutaneous melanoma lead to the absolute diagnosis of PMME [10]. In the present case, melanocytosis and junctional activity were surrounding the main tumor, and positive results of melan-A, S-100, and HMB45 were revealed by immunohistochemical staining, which led to a definitive diagnosis of PMME.

The prognosis of PMME seems to be improving because of the advances in endoscopic technology. In 1989,

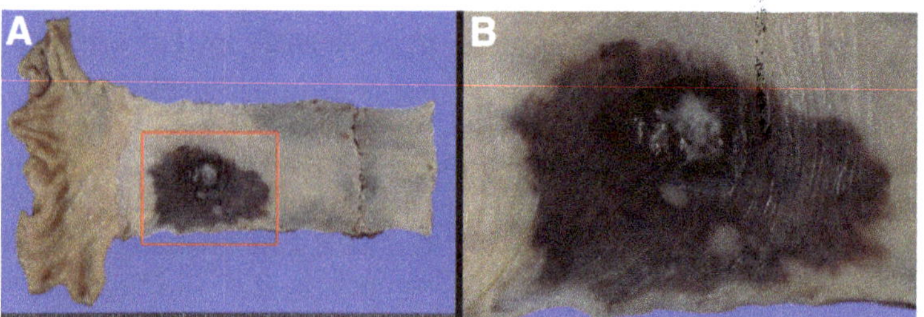

Fig. 4 Macroscopic findings. **a** The resected specimen showed an elevated, black-pigmented polyp-like lesion (15 mm × 13 mm × 9 mm) on a flat, black-pigmented area (57 mm × 38 mm) in the lower esophagus. **b** A magnified image of the lesion (the part surrounded by a red square in Fig. 4a). There is a faintly marked depression partly tinged with white on the surface of the polyp-like lesion

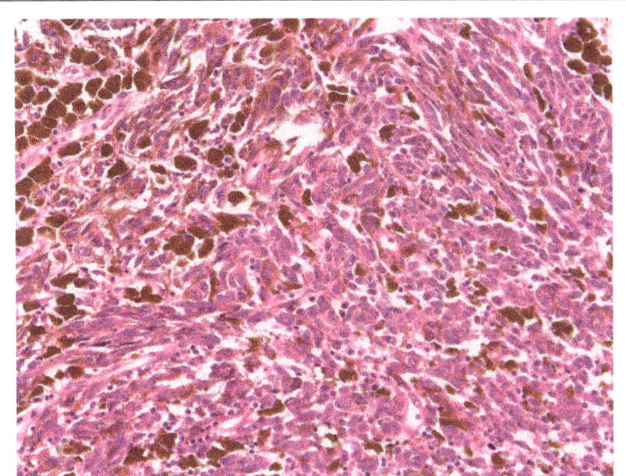

Fig. 5 Histopathological findings (hematoxylin and eosin (HE) staining). Most of the polyp-like lesion is composed of solid growth, pseudocircular, and spindle-shaped atypical cells containing melanin pigmentation and irregularly demarcated nucleoli. Many melanophages are present in the intervening interstitial stroma (HE ×200)

Sabanathan [5] reported that 5-year survival rate of PMME after surgery was 4.2%, whereas Volpin et al. reported it was up to 37% in 2002 [11]. The increasing number of cases with early detection is one of the contributing factors of improving the prognosis [12]. However, the overall 5-year survival rate of advanced squamous esophageal carcinoma was reported to be 40%–50% [13], which is higher than PMME; therefore, the biological behavior of PMME appears to be aggressive. Invasion deeper than T2 (hazard ratio: 2.288, $p = 0.0327$, 95% CI: 1.071–4.878) [14] and lymph node metastasis (hazard ratio: 15.05, $p = 0.013$, 95% CI: 1.757–128.795) [15] have been reported as predictive factors for worse survival. On the contrary, Takahashi et al. [16] reviewed 33 patients with invasion depth of T1b, pointed out the poor prognosis of T1b patients because of a high recurrence rate (20 of 33 patients), and reported that the 5-year survival rate was only 29.4%.

Detection of the lesion in early stages seems to be relatively rare because of the characteristic delay in symptoms' appearance. We identified 10 previous T1a cases [12, 15, 17–22] finally diagnosed by pathological tests, and their tumor location, size, depth of tumor, treatment, and outcomes were well-described. These cases were recorded from 1985 to 2015 and were found through literature search using the PubMed online database with "malignant melanoma" and "esophagus" as keywords (Table 1). In addition, no patients diagnosed in the early stage were reported in 1985–2000.

Among the 10 cases, subtotal esophagectomy with lymphadenectomy of the neck, mediastinal, and abdomen was performed in eight patients, and endoscopic mucosal resection (EMR) was performed in two patients because of the small tumor size. None of the cases received adjuvant therapy or had any signs of metastasis at diagnosis. Median disease-free survival time was 33 months and ranged from 15 to 94.7 months.

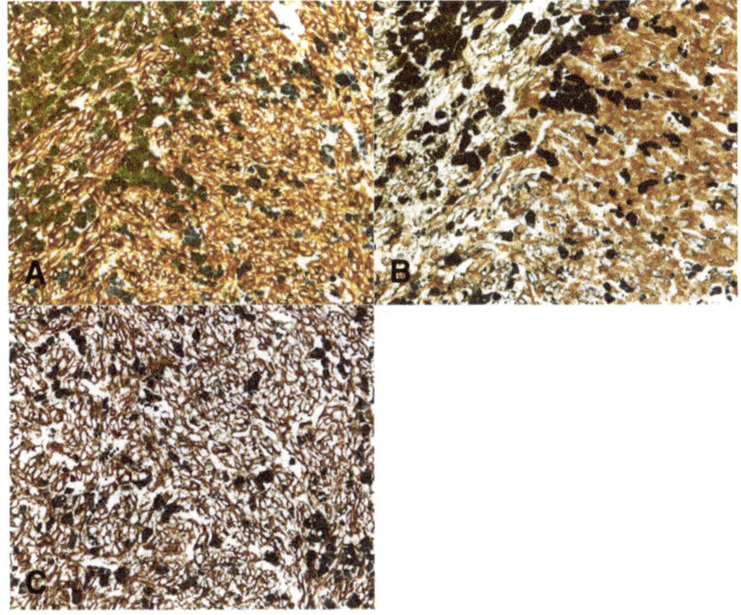

Fig. 6 Histopathological findings (immunohistochemical staining). Melanoma-specific antigens melan-A, S-100, and HMB45 are shown by immunohistochemical staining. **a** Melan-A × 200, **b** S-100 × 200, **c** HMB45 × 200. The tumor cells are presented as brown pigment, and melanin is presented as green pigment

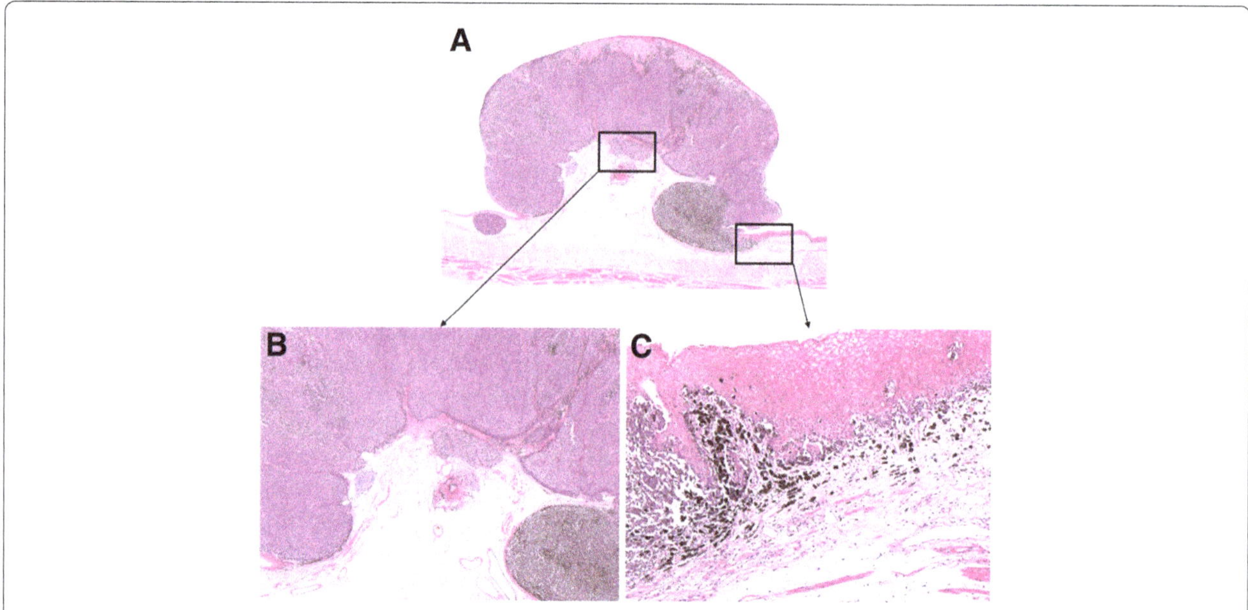

Fig. 7 Histopathological characteristics of the PMME (hematoxylin and eosin (HE) staining). **a** The PMME shows a polyp-like intraluminal mass (HE ×10). **b** The tumor cell invasion directly involves the muscularis mucosae (HE ×25). **c** The tumor cells are spread horizontally in the basal layer of the esophageal epithelium, which is considered junctional activity (HE ×100)

Treatment of PMME should be individualized for each patient. The choice should be based on tumor size and location, presence or absence of metastases, age, and comorbidities of the patients [23]. Kimura et al. [19] reported the first case of PMME treated by EMR and discussed the indications for EMR of superficial-type PMME. Miyatani et al. [12] reported that when the lesion was very small and a biopsy could not be obtained, EMR could be performed to obtain a definite diagnosis and to treat the patient. However, there have been few reports of PMME treated by EMR, and the indications for performing EMR should be evaluated cautiously after a detailed examination because of the risk of lymph node metastasis. Diagnosing PMME as T1a accurately is very difficult; therefore, we recommend subtotal esophagectomy with radical lymphadenectomy of the neck, mediastinum, and abdomen for treatment of PMME [D2]. Conversely, for patients with PMME at T1a, curative surgical resection could improve their prognosis. Although there is probably no absolute indication of adjuvant therapy for T1a and negative lymphoid metastatic cases because of low risk of metastasis and recurrence, as with esophageal cancer, careful follow-up such as blood tests including tumor marker and image inspection using contrast-enhanced CT would be necessary. On the contrary, systemic chemotherapy based on

Table 1 Case reports of early primary malignant melanoma of the esophagus stage T1a (1985–2015)

Author	Year	Age	Sex	Location	Size (cm)	Depth*[a]	Treatment	Course*[b]
Kido [16]	2000	60	M	Lt	4.0 × 2.0	T1a	CR	33 months
Mikami [17]	2001	41	F	Mt	0.8 × 0.6	T1a	CR	31 months
Kimura [18]	2005	73	M	Lt	1.8 × 1.3	T1a-LPM	EMR	15 months
Suzuki [19]	2008	62	M	Mt	7.0 × 4.5	T1a-EP	CR	33 months
Suzuki [19]	2008	67	M	Lt	5.5 × 5.5	T1a-LPM	CR	53 months
Miyatani [11]	2009	64	F	Lt	0.5	T1a-LPM	EMR	20 months
Minami [20]	2010	72	M	Lt	unknown	T1a-EP	CR	25 months
Wang [14]	2013	62	M	Mt	7.0 × 4.5	T1a	CR	93.7 months
Yamamoto [21]	2015	75	M	Lt	1.5 × 1.0	T1a-MM	CR	83 months
Our case	2015	78	F	Lt	5.7 × 3.8	T1a-MM	CR	39 months

*[a]: According to the Japanese Classification of Esophageal Cancer, 11th Edition. Japan Esophageal Society Esophagus (2017). *[b]: All reported cases are still alive after the treatment, and none have had any symptoms of relapse or distant metastasis

Mt middle of the esophagus, *Lt* lower esophagus, *EMR* endoscopic mucosal resection, *CR* curative resection (subtotal esophagectomy and radical lymphadenectomy of the neck, mediastinum, and abdomen)

cutaneous malignant melanoma should be considered for deeper than T1b and positive lymphoid metastatic cases, but its efficacy in increasing overall survival of patients with PMME is still unknown. Meanwhile, neoadjuvant therapy for PMME has not been reported. Therefore, if the lesion was evaluated to be resectable at the time of diagnosis, curative surgical resection with radical lymphadenectomy of the neck, mediastinum, and abdomen [D2] could be performed.

We presented a rare case of early-stage PMME. A standard treatment for early-stage PMME has not yet been established, but subtotal esophagectomy with regional radical lymphadenectomy could be recommended for patients with PMME at T1a, and curative surgical resection could improve their prognosis. Further accumulation of cases is necessary to evaluate the relationship between treatment strategy and long-term prognosis.

Abbreviations

CA19-9: Carbohydrate antigen 19-9; CEA: Carcinoembryonic antigen; EGD: Esophagogastroduodenoscopy; EMR: Endoscopic mucosal resection; PMME: Primary malignant melanoma of the esophagus

Acknowledgements

We would like to thank Editage (www.editage.jp) for English language editing.

Funding

None

Authors' contributions

SK and YE wrote the manuscript; TS and SH revised the manuscript; YE, YK, SM, and TS performed the surgery; YN, TA, TNa, TNo, TT, and KO acquired the data. All authors read and approved the final manuscript.

Competing interests

The authors declare that they have no competing interests relevant to this article.

References

1. Joob AW, Haines GK 3rd, Kies MS, Shields TW. Primary malignant melanoma of the esophagus. Ann Thorac Surg. 1995;60:217–22.
2. Yu H, Huang X, Li Y, et al. Primary malignant melanoma of the esophagus: a study of clinical features, pathology, management and prognosis. Dis Esophagus. 2011;24:109–13.
3. Sobin L, Gospodarowicz MK, Wittekind C. TMN classification of malignant Tumors, 7th ed. Hoboken: Wiley-Blackwell; 2010.
4. Allen AC, Spitz S. Malignant melanoma; a clinicopathological analysis of the criteria for diagnosis and prognosis. Cancer. 1953;6:1–45.
5. Sabanathan S, Eng J, Pradhan GN. Primary malignant of the esophagus. Am J Gastroenterol. 1989;84:1475–81.
6. Taniyama K, Suzuki H, Sakuramachi S, Toyoda T, Matsuda M, Tahara E. Amelanotic malignant melanoma of the esophagus: case report and review of the literature. Jpn J Clin Oncol. 1990;20:286–95.
7. Li Y-H, Xu L, Zou X-P. Primary malignant melanoma of the esophagus: a case report. World J Gastroenterol. 2014;20(10):2731–4.
8. Yamazaki K, Ohmori T, Kumagai Y, et al. Ultrastructure of oesophageal melanocytosis. Virchows Arch A Pathol Anat Histopathol. 1991;418:515–22.
9. Walter A, van Rees BP, Heijnen BH, van Lanschot JJ, Offerhaus GJ. Atypical melanocytic proliferation associated with squamous cell carcinoma in situ of the esophagus. Virchows Arch. 2000;437:203–7.
10. Iwanuma Y, Tomita N, Amano T, Isayama F, Tsurumaru M, Hayashi T, Kajiyama Y. Current status of primary malignant melanoma of the esophagus: clinical features, pathology, management and prognosis. J Gastroenterol. 2012;47:21–8.
11. Volpin E, Sauvanet A, Couvelard A, Belghiti J. Primary malignant melanoma of the esophagus: a case report and review of the literature. Dis Esophagus. 2002;15:244–9.
12. Miyatani H, Yoshida Y, Ushimaru S, Sagihara N, Yamada S. Slow growing flat-type primary malignant melanoma of the esophagus treated with cap-assisted EMR. Dig Endosc. 2009;21:255–7.
13. Ando N, Ozawa S, Kitajima Y. Improvement in the results of surgical treatment of advanced squamous esophageal carcinoma during 15 consecutive years. Ann Surg 2000;232:225-32.
14. Yamaguchi T, Shioaki Y, Koide K, et al. A case of primary malignant melanoma of the esophagus and analysis of 193 patients in Japan (in Japanese). Nihon Shokakibyo Gakkai Zassi. 2004;101:1087–94.
15. Wang S, Tachimori Y, Hokamura N, Igaki H, Kishino T, Kushima R. Diagnosis and surgical outcomes for primary malignant melanoma of the Esophagus: a single-Center experience. Ann Thorac Surg. 2013;96:1002–7.
16. Takahashi H, Ichikawa N, Takahashi S, Hirose K. Primary malignant of the esophagus of submucosal invasion: a case report. (in Japanese). Nihon Rinsyogeka Gakkai Zassi. 2013;74(6):1473–8.
17. Kido T, Morishima H, Nakahara M, Nakao K, Tanimura H, Nishimura R, Tsujimoto M. Early stage primary malignant melanoma of the esophagus. Gastrointest Endosc. 2000;51(1):90–1.
18. Mikami T, Fukuda S, Shimoyama T, Yamagata R, Nishiya D, Sasaki Y, Uno Y, Saito H, Takaya S, Kamata Y, Munataka A. A case of early-stage primary malignant melanoma of the esophagus. Gastrointest Endosc. 2001;53(3):365–7.
19. Kimura H, Kato H, Sohda M, Nakajima M, Fukai Y, Miyazaki T, Masuda N, Manda R, Fukuchi M, Ojima H, Tsukada K, Kuwano H. Flat-type primary malignant melanoma of the esophagus treated by EMR: case report. Gastrointest Endosc. 2005;61(6):787–9.
20. Suzuki H, Nakanishi Y, Taniguchi H, Shimoda T, Yamaguchi H, Igaki H, Tachimori Y, Kato H. Two cases of early-stage esophageal malignant melanoma with long-term survival. Pathol Int. 2008;58:432–5.
21. Minami H, Inoue H, Satodate H, Hamatani S, Kudo S. A case of primary malignant melanoma *in situ* in the esophagus. Gastrointest Endosc. 2011; 73(4):814–5.
22. Yamamoto S, Makuuchi H, Kumaki N, Ozawa S, Shimada H, Chino O, Kazuno A, Yasuda S, Tamayama T, Sakai I. A long surviving case of multiple early stage primary malignant melanoma of the esophagus and a review of the literature. Tokai J Exp Clin Med. 2015;40(3):90–5.
23. Machado J, Ministro P, Araujo R, Cancela E, Castanheira A, Silva A. Primary malignant melanoma of the esophagus: a case report. World J Gastroenterol. 2011;17(42):4734–8.

22

Impact of ABO blood group on the prognosis of patients undergoing surgery for esophageal cancer

Wei Wang[1†], Lei Liu[1†], Zhiwei Wang[2,3*], Min Wei[2], Qi He[2], Tianlong Ling[3], Ziang Cao[3], Yixin Zhang[1], Qiang Wang[1] and Minxin Shi[1*]

Abstract

Background: ABO blood type is an established prognostic factor in several malignancies, but its role in esophageal cancer (EC) is largely unknown. The aim of this study is to determine whether ABO blood group is associated with survival after esophagectomy for EC.

Methods: A total of 406 patients who underwent surgery for EC were enrolled. The associations of ABO blood group with clinical and pathological variables were assessed using chi-square test. Associations of ABO blood group with the survival were estimated using univariable and multivariable Cox proportional hazards regression models.

Results: The ABO blood group proportionally associated with the grade of EC tumor ($P = 0.049$). The ABO blood group status did not correlate with disease-free survival (DFS) in univariable analysis or multivariable analysis ($P > 0.05$) And there was no significant relationship between the ABO blood group and overall survival (OS) in univariable analysis or multivariable analysis ($P > 0.05$).

Conclusions: Our results suggested that no association between ABO blood group and the survival was observed in patients undergoing surgery for EC.

Keywords: Esophageal cancer, ABO blood group, Prognosis

Background

Esophageal cancer (EC) was ranked as the eighth most common cancer worldwide, with 482,300 new cases estimated in 2008, and the sixth most common cause of death from cancer with 406,800 deaths [1]. At present, surgery is still the mainstay of treatment for patients with EC. Despite that the surgical techniques have been improved over the past decades, the prognosis of this disease remains poor. One of the reasons is that many cases are at the advanced stage on diagnosis. It is well known that cancer can be caused by the interaction between environmental factors and genetic variations. Up to now, several risk factors related to EC have been previously evaluated, including cigarette smoking, alcohol consumption, low vegetable intake and family history of cancer, BMI and ABO blood group [2–6].

The ABO blood group system was one of the most widely used blood types in clinical practice, which has been discovered over a century. During the past years, several studies have investigated the possible relationship between ABO blood group and the risk of cancer. Individuals with blood group A with an increased incidence were observed in gastric cancer, hepatocellular cancer, pancreatic cancer, ovary cancer and nasopharyngeal cancer [7–11]. These findings indeed reminded us that ABO blood group played an important role in the development of the various human cancers. Therefore, the hypothesis that ABO blood group may also be seen as a candidate prognostic factor of these diseases comes to us. However, no significant association was found between ABO blood group and the survival of gastric cancer or pancreatic cancer [12, 13]. To date,

* Correspondence: docwang@yeah.net; Doczhangyx@126.com
†Equal contributors
[2]Department of Breast, International Peace Maternity and Child Health Hospital, Shanghai Jiao Tong University, Shanghai, China
[1]Department of Surgery, The Affiliated Tumor Hospital of Nantong University, Nantong, Jiangsu Province, China
Full list of author information is available at the end of the article

little information about whether the ABO blood group is associated with the survival of EC patients can be obtained.

As a result, the aim of this study was to determine whether ABO blood group system has an effect on clinicopathologic characteristics and prognosis of EC patients.

Methods

Patient selection

During the period of patient enrollment, among of 429 cases with symptom, 397 cases were diagnosed as EC, and among of 647 cases without symptom, 24 cases were diagnosed as EC. Fifteen EC cases with symptom were excluded from our study because of the following reasons, received chemotherapy and/or radiotherapy before surgery, with more than one primary cancer, with R1 or R2 resection. Finally, in this retrospective cohort study, we retrieved a total of 406 patients who have undergone esophagectomy for EC at Nantong tumor hospital (between January 2007 and July 2008) and Renji hospital, Shanghai (between January 2006 and September 2008). The cohort consisted of 275 males and 131 females with the median age of 60 years old (from 25 to 86 years old). EC was confirmed by post-operative histologic pathology in all cases. Tumor stage was classified by the routine histopathologic assessment according to the 7th edition of UICC TNM staging system [14], including 175, 124 and 107 patients with stage I, II, III, respectively. This study was approved by the institutional review board and ethics committee at Nantong tumor hospital (Institutional Review Board of Nantong Cancer Center) and Renji hospital (Specialty Committee on Ethics of Biomedicine Research, Renji, Shanghai). The written informed consents were obtained from all the patients.

Treatment and information collection

Preoperative evaluation was performed before the decision for surgery. These preoperative risk assessments included a complete medical history and physical examination, complete blood count and serum biochemistry tests, arterial blood gas analysis, ABO and Rh blood group, x-ray, electrocardiogram (ECG), pulmonary function tests, and computed tomography scans of the thorax and the upper abdomen.

For tumors of the upper-third esophagus, the cervico-thoraco-abdominal (right thoracotomy) procedure was performed. For lesions in the mid and lower third, esophagectomy was carried out by the left thoracotomy. Two or three-fielded lymph nodes dissection was performed for each patient. One hundred and twenty-two patients received adjuvant chemotherapy and eighty-four patients received adjuvant radiotherapy after surgery. And the most common chemotherapy regimen consists of 5-FU plus cisplatin for a mean of 3 cycles after surgery, depending on clinical response or the occurrence of adverse effect.

Clinical information was obtained from the medical records. Clinicopathologic features evaluated for each case included the diagnosed age, sex, ABO and Rh blood group status, tumor size, tumor location, clinical stage, tumor grade, histological type, margin status and perioperative blood transfusion.

Follow up

All the patients remained alive at least 30 days after the surgery, and were followed-up using a standard protocol after discharge from the hospital. The patients received follow up examinations every 3 months for the first 2 years after the operation, every 6 months for the following 3 years, and yearly examinations thereafter. Recording of medical history, physical examination, and CT of the chest were performed during the follow-up time. Endoscopic and whole-body examination was obtained in cases of recurrence or metastasis.

The endpoints were disease-free survival (DFS) and overall survival (OS). DFS was defined as the interval from the date of surgery to the date of local or regional disease recurrence, distant metastasis, or to the last follow-up date. OS was calculated from the time of surgery to the time of death from any cause, or to the time of last follow-up, at which point the data were censored.

The follow-up was performed until the end of September 2013. The median follow-up time was 29 months (range 2 to 92 months). In this cohort, the follow-up information was obtained for 390 cases (96.06 %). And the characteristic of the patients with loss to follow up was displayed in Additional file 1: Table S1. In the current study, there were 251 deaths regardless of the causes. Only 2 of them were due to causes not related to the EC. There were 287 patients who had recurrence or metastasis during the follow-up.

Statistical analysis

Categorical data were presented as counts and group comparisons were made with the chi-squared test or the Fisher's exact test. The Kaplan-Meier method was used to construct OS and DFS curves, and the two-side log-rank test was used to determine the statistical significance of differences. The prognostic significance of clinical and pathologic characteristics was determined using univariate Cox regression analysis. Only the factors with significant association in the univariate analysis ($P < 0.20$) and ABO blood group status were included in the multivariate analysis. The outcomes of Cox regression analysis was measured by hazard ratio

(HR) and its 95 % confidence intervals (CI). All data were processed using SPSS 15.0 software package. The P values less than 0.05 were considered as significant.

Results

ABO blood group and clinicopathologic characteristics

Clinicopathologic characteristics of all subjects stratified by ABO blood group were displayed in Table 1. Among the 406 subjects, 152 (37.4 %) were blood group A, 113 (27.8 %) were blood group B, 114 (28.1 %) were blood group O, and the remaining 27 (6.7 %) were blood group AB. The proportion of poorly-differentiated EC among patients with blood group AB was significantly lower than those with other blood groups ($P = 0.049$). However, no significant difference was observed with regard to age ($P = 0.669$), sex ($P = 0.511$), tumor location ($P = 0.174$), tumor size ($P = 0.218$), T stage ($P = 0.276$), N stage ($P = 0.924$), TNM stage ($P = 0.367$), histopathological type ($P = 0.218$), postoperative adjuvant treatments ($P = 0.839$), vascular invasion ($P = 0.344$) or perioperative blood transfusion ($P = 0.238$).

ABO blood group and disease-free survival

A total of 287 patients had recurrence or distant metastasis before the last follow-up. The 5-year DFS rate for EC patients with blood groups A, B, O and AB was 38.8 %, 31.4 %, 32.8 % and 23.8 %, respectively (Table 2). The Kaplan-Meier curves for DFS among different ABO blood group were presented in Fig. 1a. And no significant difference was observed between ABO blood groups and DFS rate for the EC patients ($P = 0.121$). In addition, we divided the whole cases into two subgroups, blood group O in one group, and blood group A, B and AB in the other group. However, there was still no significant difference. And the 5-year DFS rates was 32.8 % and 33.2 % for blood group O and non-O, respectively ($P = 0.812$) (Fig. 1b) (Table 2).

The relationship between clinicopathologic factors and DFS was assessed by univariate analyses (Table 3). The factors including depth of tumor infiltration, lymph nodes status, TNM stage, tumor grading, adjuvant treatment, vascular invasion, perioperative blood transfusion were significantly correlated with DFS ($P < 0.05$). However, the factor ABO blood group was not significantly associated with DFS ($P = 0.121$). Then the multivariate analysis containing the correlated factors with significant difference and ABO blood group was performed. The result showed that ABO blood group was not a significant prognostic factor for DFS ($P = 0.215$) (Table 3).

ABO blood group and overall survival

The median follow-up period for the entire study population was 29 months (range, 2-92 months). Death disregarding the causes occurred in 251 of 402 enrolled patients at the time of the final analysis. There were only two patients who died due to causes not related to cancer (one from suicide and the other from cerebral hemorrhage). The 5-year OS rate for blood group A, B, O, and AB was 46.9 %, 38.6 %, 42.9 % and 30.3 %, respectively (Table 2). As reflected in Fig. 2a, there was no significant difference in survival among the diversified blood groups ($P = 0.254$). Moreover, we compared the OS for blood group O with non-O groups (A, B and AB). And the 5-year OS rate for blood group O and non-O was 42.9 % and 43.2 %, respectively. Significant difference was still not found between the groups ($P = 0.846$) (Fig. 2b) (Table 2).

The univarite analysis suggested that the factors of T stage, lymph nodes metastasis, TNM stage, grade, postoperative adjuvant treatment, vascular invasion, perioperative blood transfusion were strong predictors of long-term OS ($P < 0.20$), whereas the factor ABO blood group was not significantly correlated with the OS ($P = 0.254$) (Table 4). The multivariate analyses contained those factors with significant difference in univarite analysis and ABO blood group. The multivariate analyses showed that ABO blood group was not significantly associated with OS ($P = 0.065$) (Table 4).

Sensitivity analysis

To evaluate the stability of our findings, sensitivity analysis was carried out by excluding those 24 EC cases without symptom. Among the 382 cases, 143 (37.4 %) were blood group A, 106 (27.7 %) were blood group B, 108 (28.3 %) were blood group O, and the remaining 25 (6.5 %) were blood group AB. With regard to disease-free survival, neither the univariate analyses nor the multivariate analyses showed that ABO blood group was a significant prognostic factor ($P = 0.138$ and $P = 0.241$). As for overall survival, neither the univariate analyses nor the multivariate analyses showed that ABO blood group was significantly associated with OS ($P = 0.276$ and $P = 0.068$). The results were not materially altered, indicating the robust stability of the current findings.

Discussion

ABO blood group has played an important role in transfusion medicine, which is widely used during clinical practice. Recently, much attention has been given to the connection between ABO blood group and the prognosis of cancer. Previously published studies have confirmed that ABO blood group was significantly associated with the prognosis and could be considered as one of the predictive factors in pancreatic cancer, bladder cancer and renal cell cancer [15–18]. However, there was little information regarding the relationship between ABO blood group and the outcomes of patients with EC.

Table 1 Associations of ABO blood group with clinical and pathological variables in 406 patients with EC

Variables	A (%)	B (%)	O (%)	AB (%)	Total (%)	*P*-value
Age (years)	59.2 ± 5.4	60.6 ± 7.5	60.3 ± 7.1	60.1 ± 7.0		0.669
Gender						0.511
Male	105(69.1 %)	66(58.4 %)	84(73.7 %)	20(74.1 %)	275(67.7 %)	
Female	47(30.9 %)	47(41.6 %)	30(26.3 %)	7(25.9 %)	131(32.3 %)	
Location of tumor						0.174
Upper	5(3.3 %)	10(8.8 %)	4(3.5 %)	2(7.4 %)	21(5.2 %)	
Middle	111(73.0 %)	85(75.2 %)	80(70.2 %)	17(63.0 %)	293(72.2 %)	
Lower	36(23.7 %)	18(15.9 %)	30(26.3 %)	8(29.6 %)	92(22.7 %)	
Tumor size						0.218
<5 cm	79(52.0 %)	52(46.0 %)	66(57.9 %)	17(63.0 %)	214(52.7 %)	
≥5 cm	73(48.0 %)	61(54.0 %)	48(42.1 %)	10(37.0 %)	192(47.3 %)	
T stage						0.276
pT1	33(21.7 %)	19(16.8 %)	20(17.5 %)	9(33.3 %)	81(20.0 %)	
pT2	46(30.3 %)	38(33.6 %)	30(26.3 %)	8(29.6 %)	122(30.0 %)	
pT3	67(44.1 %)	44(38.9 %)	54(47.4 %)	8(29.6 %)	173(42.6 %)	
pT4	6(3.9 %)	12(10.6 %)	10(8.8 %)	2(7.4 %)	30(7.4 %)	
N stage						0.924
N0	107(70.4 %)	78(69.0 %)	78(68.4 %)	19(70.4 %)	282(69.5 %)	
N1	27(17.8 %)	19(16.8 %)	21(18.4 %)	5(18.5 %)	72(17.7 %)	
N2	12(7.9 %)	8(7.1 %)	12(10.5 %)	2(7.4 %)	34(8.4 %)	
N3	6(3.9 %)	8(7.1 %)	3(2.6 %)	1(3.5 %)	18(4.4 %)	
TNM stage						0.367
I	71(48.7 %)	45(39.8 %)	46(40.4 %)	13(48.1 %)	175(43.1 %)	
II	44(28.9 %)	42(37.2 %)	30(26.3 %)	8(29.6 %)	124(30.5 %)	
III	37(24.3 %)	36(23.0 %)	38(33.3 %)	6(22.2 %)	107(26.4 %)	
Grade						0.049
Well-differentiated	28(18.4 %)	16(14.2 %)	17(14.9 %)	6(22.2 %)	67(16.5 %)	
Moderately-differentiated	20(58.4 %)	69(61.1 %)	52(45.6 %)	17(63.0 %)	208(51.2 %)	
Poorly-differentiated	54(35.5 %)	28(24.8 %)	45(39.5 %)	4(14.8 %)	131(32.3 %)	
Histopathological type						0.170
Squamous cell carcinoma	140(92.1 %)	105(92.9 %)	100(87.7 %)	27(100.0 %)	372(91.6 %)	
Others※	12(7.9 %)	8(7.1 %)	14(12.3 %)	0(0 %)	34(8.4 %)	
Adjuvant treatment						0.839
Yes	54(35.5 %)	40(35.4 %)	44(38.6 %)	8(29.6 %)	146(36.0 %)	
No	98(64.5 %)	73(64.6 %)	70(61.4 %)	19(70.4 %)	260(64.0 %)	
Vascular invasion						
Positive	14(9.2 %)	7(6.2 %)	14(12.3 %)	4(14.8 %)	39(9.6 %)	0.344
Negative	138(90.8 %)	106(93.8 %)	100(87.7 %)	23(85.2 %)	367(90.4 %)	
Blood transfusion						0.212
Yes	8(5.2 %)	6(5.2 %)	12(10.5 %)	2(7.1 %)	32(7.9 %)	
No	144(94.8 %)	107(94.8 %)	102(89.5 %)	25(92.9 %)	374(92.1 %)	

※Others included adenocarcinoma, adenosqumaous carcinoma and mucoepdermoid carcinoma

Table 2 Distribution of patients and 5-year survival rates by blood group

Blood group	n (%)	5-year DFS (%)	5-year OS (%)
A	146 (37.4)	38.1	46.9
B	108 (27.7)	31.4	38.6
O	109 (27.9)	32.8	42.9
AB	27 (6.9)	23.8	30.3
Non-O	281 (72.1)	33.2	43.2

To our best knowledge, it is the first for us to assess the possible association between ABO blood group and the DFS and OS for EC in China. In the current study, we retrospectively analyzed the data from 406 patients undergoing surgical therapy for EC in two centers. Except for the grade of tumor, we found no statistically significant association with clinical or pathological parameters. We did not observe significant associations between ABO blood type and DFS of EC. And no significant difference of OS was detected among different ABO blood groups in univariate analyses. However, in the multivariate analyses, our findings showed that patients with blood group B or AB had a worse OS compared with those with blood group A. The reasons why this difference in survival is not evident in univariate analyses remain unclear at this stage. Our findings were not consistent with a few previously published studies. In a sample of 496 patients who underwent esophagectomy, Yang and his colleagues found that patients with blood group O had a significantly worse overall survival than non-O blood groups [19]. However, the findings obtained in our study agreed with the results from other malignances, such as breast cancer and lung cancer [20–22], which also suggested that ABO blood group had no significant effect on the outcomes. It could be seen that the outcomes among diversified studies were indeed conflicting. The discrepancies might be due to various genetic backgrounds, retrospective data collection and inconsistent evaluation of endpoints. Due to only one patient with negative Rh blood type among the study population, any correlation of Rh blood group with biological behaviors of EC could not be evaluated in our study.

Direct biologic mechanisms underlying the association between ABO blood group and cancer are inconclusive. However, there are several hypotheses which may explain the relationships observed. The ABO gene is located on the Chromosome 9q and consists of 7 exons. It encodes a glycosyltranferase catalyzing the transfer of carbohydrates to the H antigen, thus forming the antigenic structure of the ABO blood groups [23–25]. Blood group antigens are expressed not only on the surface of red blood cells, but also on numerous other tissues, including esophageal epithelium [26]. Notably, previous report indicated that the loss of blood group H antigen occurred during carcinogenesis of the esophageal mucosa [27]. It has been shown that the modified expression of blood group antigens on the surface of tumor cells may alter cell motility, resistance to apoptosis and immune escape [28]. Additionally, recent studies have revealed the relationship between ABO group genotype and circulating levels of soluble intercellular adhesion molecule-1 (sICAM-1) [29, 30]. Increased levels of sICAM-1 are known to be correlated with a number of human malignancies and may play a role in escape from immune surveillance by tumor cells [31].

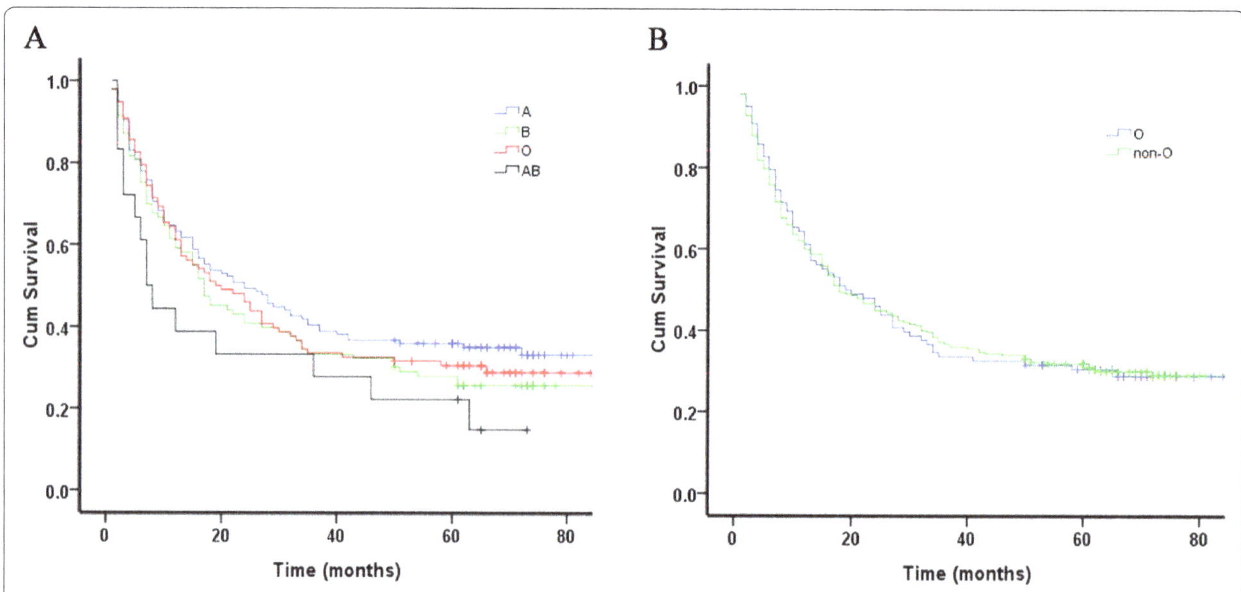

Fig. 1 Disease-free survival in 390 patients with esophageal cancer according to ABO blood group. **a** Survival rates of patients with each blood group. **b** Survival rates of patients with blood group O compared with patients with non-O (A, B, and AB) blood groups

Table 3 Univariate and multivariate Cox proportional hazards regression for disease-free survival

Variables	Category	Univariate analysis			Multivariate analysis		
		HR	95 % CI	*P*-value	HR	95 % CI	*P*-value
T stage	pT1+ pT2	1.00			1.00		
	pT3+ pT4	2.24	1.72–2.90	<0.001	1.79	1.21–2.64	0.004
N stage	N0	1.00			1.00		
	N1-3	2.38	1.83–3.09	<0.001	1.66	0.82–3.34	0.156
TNM stage	I + II	1.00			1.00		
	III	2.67	2.04–3.49	<0.001	1.72	1.17–2.53	0.006
Grade	G1	0.73	0.49–1.08		0.80	0.54–1.20	
	G2	1.00			1.00		
	G3	1.44	1.10–1.88	0.001	1.32	0.95–1.71	0.121
Vascular invasion	Negative	1.00			1.00		
	Positive	1.50	1.01–2.22	0.045	1.47	0.79–2.76	0.221
Adjuvant treatment	No	1.00			1.00		
	Yes	2.65	1.83–3.82	<0.001	2.19	1.49–3.22	<0.001
Blood transfusion	No	1.00			1.00		
	Yes	1.92	1.03–3.57	0.037	2.33	1.21–4.51	0.012
ABO blood group	A	1.00			1.00		
	B	0.97	0.71–1.34		0.94	0.60–1.47	
	O	1.07	0.79–1.47		1.06	0.67–1.68	
	AB	1.78	1.08–2.99	0.121	2.10	1.00–4.41	0.215
ABO blood group	O	1.00			-		
	A/B/AB	1.04	0.78–1.37	0.812	-		

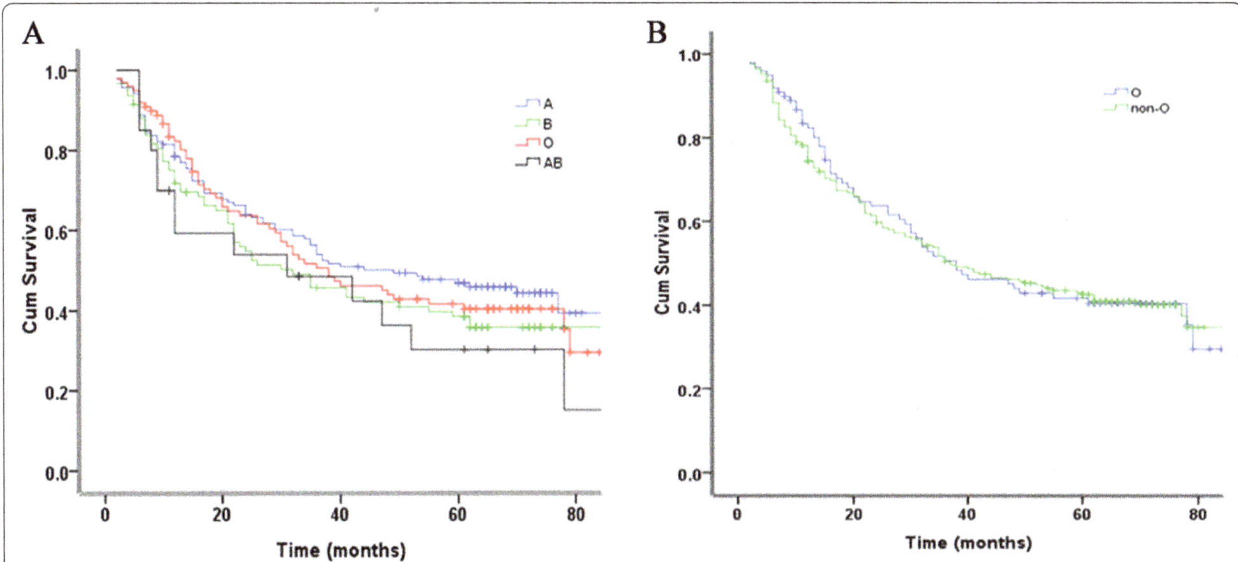

Fig. 2 Overall survival in 390 patients with esophageal cancer according to ABO blood group. **a** Survival rates of patients with each blood group. **b** Survival rates of patients with blood group O compared with patients with non-O (A, B, and AB) blood groups

Table 4 Univariate and multivariate Cox proportional hazards regression for overall survival

Variables	Category	Univariate analysis			Multivariate analysis		
		HR	95 % CI	*P*-value	HR	95 % CI	*P*-value
T stage	pT1+ pT2	1.00			1.00		
	pT3+ pT4	2.64	1.91–3.65	<0.001	1.82	1.23–2.70	0.002
N stage	N0	1.00			1.00		
	N1-3	2.35	1.71–3.23	<0.001	1.62	0.80–3.29	0.161
TNM stage	I + II	1.00			1.00		
	III	2.61	1.88–3.61	<0.001	1.65	1.13–2.42	0.011
Grade	G1	0.75	0.50–1.05		0.82	0.56–1.22	
	G2	1.00			1.00		
	G3	1.37	1.02–1.81	0.058	1.31	0.96–1.70	0.134
Vascular invasion	Negative	1.00			1.00		
	Positive	2.71	1.66–3.86	<0.001	1.47	0.79–2.76	0.221
Adjuvant treatment	No	1.00			1.00		
	Yes	2.76	2.02–3.78	<0.001	2.30	1.67–3.17	<0.001
Blood transfusion	No	1.00			1.00		
	Yes	2.40	1.47–3.94	<0.001	2.51	1.50–3.88	<0.001
ABO blood group	A	1.00			1.00		
	B	1.25	0.89–1.77		1.43	1.01–2.06	
	O	1.10	0.78–1.55		1.14	0.80–1.62	
	AB	1.72	0.95–3.10	0.254	1.96	0.98–3.52	0.065
ABO blood group	O	1.00			-		
	A/B/AB	1.03	0.76–1.40	0.846	-		

Several limitations should be noted in the current study. Firstly, the sample size of the entire cohort was relatively small. There were only 390 patients with complete information allowing for the multivariable analysis, although a majority of the patients in our study had follow-up information available. Secondly, similar to any retrospective study, there was the possibility of selection bias. Those uninvolved population during the study period were noted to have a worse outcome. There was no chance for those who with distant metastasis to have a radical operation, thus resulting in selection bias. Thus, prospective studies focused on this topic should be further investigated. Thirdly, some cases without symptom may be omitted from our study, which biases our results. During the period of cases enrollment, those who were diagnosed as precancerous lesion for EC were followed up. Finally, a few of such cases were also included in the study, because of developing into EC. To some extent, this could decrease the rate of missed diagnosis. Last but not least, it is difficult for us to control the various adjuvant treatment regimens administered, although the chemotherapy regiment for most patients was 5-FU plus cisplatin. Hence, this needs to be kept in mind when interpreting our results.

Conclusion

In summary, our results failed to suggest an association between ABO blood group and disease-free or overall survival in patients with EC.

Competing interests

The authors declare that they have no competing interests.

Authors' contributions

WW, LL, and ZWW were responsible for data collection and analysis, experiment job, interpretation of the results, and writing the manuscript. MW, QH, ZAC, YXZ and QW, were responsible for conducting the data analysis, reviewing and follow-up. WW and MXS were responsible for experimental design, analysis, and interpretation. All authors have read and approved the final manuscript.

Acknowledgments

This study was supported in part by grant funding of NSFC (Natural Science Foundation of China, 81101847), Doctoral Fund of Ministry of Education of China (20110073120089), project supported by the Shanghai Committee of Science and Technology, China (124119a4801), directory project from Nantong Science and Technology Commission (grant no.: HS149127). We gratefully acknowledge the assistance of Wenjing Wang and Chunxiao Wu from Department of Cancer Control & Prevention, Shanghai Municipal Center for Disease Control & Prevention, for their skillful technical assistance.

Author details
[1]Department of Surgery, The Affiliated Tumor Hospital of Nantong University, Nantong, Jiangsu Province, China. [2]Department of Breast, International Peace Maternity and Child Health Hospital, Shanghai Jiao Tong University, Shanghai, China. [3]Department of Thoracic Surgery, Shanghai Renji Hospital Affiliated to Shanghai Jiao Tong University School of Medicine, Shanghai, China.

References

1. Jemal A, Bray F, Center MM, Ferlay J, Ward E, Forman D. Global cancer statistics. CA Cancer J Clin. 2011;61:69–90.
2. Wang JB, Fan JH, Liang H, Li J, Xiao HJ, Wei WQ, et al. Attributable causes of esophageal cancer incidence and mortality in China. PLoS ONE. 2012;7, e42281.
3. Merry AH, Schouten LJ, Goldbohm RA, van den Brandt PA. Body mass index, height and risk of adenocarcinoma of the oesophagus and gastric cardia: a prospective cohort study. Gut. 2007;56:1503–11.
4. Turati F, Edefonti V, Bosetti C, Ferraroni M, Malvezzi M, Franceschi S, et al. Family history of cancer and the risk of cancer: a network of case-control studies. Ann Oncol. 2013;24:2651–6.
5. O'Doherty MG, Freedman ND, Hollenbeck AR, Schatzkin A, Abnet CC. A prospective cohort study of obesity and risk of oesophageal and gastric adenocarcinoma in the NIH-AARP Diet and Health Study. Gut. 2012;61:1261–8.
6. Gong Y, Yang YS, Zhang XM, Su M, Wang J, Han JD, et al. ABO blood type, diabetes and risk of gastrointestinal cancer in northern China. World J Gastroenterol. 2012;18:563–9.
7. Wang Z, Liu L, Ji J, Zhang J, Yan M, Liu B, et al. ABO blood group system and gastric cancer: a case-control study and meta-analysis. Int J Mol Sci. 2012;13:13308–21.
8. Li Q, Yu CH, Yu JH, Liu L, Xie SS, Li WW, et al. ABO blood group and the risk of hepatocellular carcinoma: a case-control study in patients with chronic hepatitis B. PLoS ONE. 2012;7, e29928.
9. Wang DS, Chen DL, Ren C, Wang ZQ, Qiu MZ, Luo HY, et al. ABO blood group, hepatitis B viral infection and risk of pancreatic cancer. Int J Cancer. 2012;131:461–8.
10. Poole EM, Gates MA, High BA, Chanock SJ, Cramer DW, Cunningham JM, et al. ABO blood group and risk of epithelial ovarian cancer within the Ovarian Cancer Association Consortium. Cancer Causes Control. 2012;23:1805–10.
11. Sheng L, Sun X, Zhang L, Su D. ABO blood group and nasopharyngeal carcinoma risk in a population of Southeast China. Int J Cancer. 2013;133:893–7.
12. Qiu MZ, Zhang DS, Ruan DY, Luo HY, Wang ZQ, Zhou ZW, et al. A relationship between ABO blood groups and clinicopathologic characteristics of patients with gastric adenocarcinoma in China. Med Oncol. 2011;28 Suppl 1:S268–73.
13. Wang DS, Wang ZQ, Zhang L, Qiu MZ, Luo HY, Ren C, et al. Are risk factors associated with outcomes in pancreatic cancer? PLoS ONE. 2012;7, e41984.
14. LH S, MK G, C W. International Union AgainstCancer (UICC):TNM Classification of Malignant Tumours. 7th edition. New York: Wiley-Liss. 2010.
15. Rahbari NN, Bork U, Hinz U, Leo A, Kirchberg J, Koch M, et al. AB0 blood group and prognosis in patients with pancreatic cancer. BMC Cancer. 2012;12:319.
16. Ben Q, Wang K, Yuan Y, Li Z. Pancreatic cancer incidence and outcome in relation to ABO blood groups among Han Chinese patients: a case-control study. Int J Cancer. 2011;128:1179–86.
17. Klatte T, Xylinas E, Rieken M, Kluth LA, Roupret M, Pycha A, et al. Impact of ABO blood type on outcomes of patients with primary non-muscle-invasive bladder cancer. J Urol 2013.
18. Kaffenberger SD, Morgan TM, Stratton KL, Boachie AM, Barocas DA, Chang SS, et al. ABO blood group is a predictor of survival in patients undergoing surgery for renal cell carcinoma. BJU Int. 2012;110:E641–6.
19. Yang X, Huang Y, Feng JF. Is there an association between ABO blood group and overall survival in patients with esophageal squamous cell carcinoma? Int J Clin Exp Med. 2014;7:2214–8.
20. Gates MA, Xu M, Chen WY, Kraft P, Hankinson SE, Wolpin BM. ABO blood group and breast cancer incidence and survival. Int J Cancer. 2012;130:2129–37.
21. Yu J, Gao F, Klimberg VS, Margenthaler JA. ABO blood type/Rh factor and the incidence and outcomes for patients with triple-negative breast cancer. Ann Surg Oncol. 2012;19:3159–64.
22. Unal D, Eroglu C, Kurtul N, Oguz A, Tasdemir A, Kaplan B. ABO blood groups are not associated with treatment response and prognosis in patients with local advanced non- small cell lung cancer. Asian Pac J Cancer Prev. 2013;14:3945–8.
23. Yamamoto F, Clausen H, White T, Marken J, Hakomori S. Molecular genetic basis of the histo-blood group ABO system. Nature. 1990;345:229–33.
24. Yamamoto F. Cloning the ABH genes. Transfusion. 1990;30:671–2.
25. Larsen RD, Ernst LK, Nair RP, Lowe JB. Molecular cloning, sequence, and expression of a human GDP-L-fucose:beta-D-galactoside 2-alpha-L-fucosyltransferase cDNA that can form the H blood group antigen. Proc Natl Acad Sci U S A. 1990;87:6674–8.
26. Yazer MH. What a difference 2 nucleotides make: a short review of ABO genetics. Transfus Med Rev. 2005;19:200–9.
27. Kayser K, Hauck E, Andre S, Bovin NV, Kaltner H, Banach L, et al. Expression of endogenous lectins (galectins, receptors for ABH-epitopes) and the MIB-1 antigen in esophageal carcinomas and their syntactic structure analysis in relation to post-surgical tumor stage and lymph node involvement. Anticancer Res. 2001;21:1439–44.
28. Le Pendu J, Marionneau S, Cailleau-Thomas A, Rocher J, Le Moullac-Vaidye B, Clement M. ABH and Lewis histo-blood group antigens in cancer. APMIS. 2001;109:9–31.
29. Pare G, Chasman DI, Kellogg M, Zee RY, Rifai N, Badola S, et al. Novel association of ABO histo-blood group antigen with soluble ICAM-1: results of a genome-wide association study of 6,578 women. PLoS Genet. 2008;4, e1000118.
30. Barbalic M, Dupuis J, Dehghan A, Bis JC, Hoogeveen RC, Schnabel RB, et al. Large-scale genomic studies reveal central role of ABO in sP-selectin and sICAM-1 levels. Hum Mol Genet. 2010;19:1863–72.
31. Banks RE, Gearing AJ, Hemingway IK, Norfolk DR, Perren TJ, Selby PJ. Circulating intercellular adhesion molecule-1 (ICAM-1), E-selectin and vascular cell adhesion molecule-1 (VCAM-1) in human malignancies. Br J Cancer. 1993;68:122–4.

A dissonance-based intervention for women post roux-en-Y gastric bypass surgery aiming at improving quality of life and physical activity 24 months after surgery: study protocol for a randomized controlled trial

Fanny Sellberg[1*], Sofie Possmark[1], Ata Ghaderi[2], Erik Näslund[3], Mikaela Willmer[4], Per Tynelius[1,5], Anders Thorell[6,7], Magnus Sundbom[8], Joanna Uddén[9,10], Eva Szabo[11] and Daniel Berglind[1]

Abstract

Background: Roux-en-Y gastric bypass (RYGB) surgery is the most common bariatric procedure in Sweden and results in substantial weight loss. Approximately one year post-surgery weight regain for these patient are common, followed by a decrease in health related quality of life (HRQoL) and physical activity (PA). Our aim is to investigate the effects of a dissonance-based intervention on HRQoL, PA and other health-related behaviors in female RYGB patients 24 months after surgery. We are not aware of any previous RCT that has investigated the effects of a similar intervention targeting health behaviors after RYGB.

Methods: The ongoing RCT, the "WELL-GBP"-trial (wellbeing after gastric bypass), is a dissonance-based intervention for female RYGB patients conducted at five hospitals in Sweden. The participants are randomized to either control group receiving usual follow-up care, or to receive an intervention consisting of four group sessions three months post-surgery during which a modified version of the Stice dissonance-based intervention model is used. The sessions are held at the hospitals, and topics discussed are PA, eating behavior, social and intimate relationships. All participants are asked to complete questionnaires measuring HRQoL and other health-related behaviors and wear an accelerometer for seven days before surgery and at six months, one year and two years after surgery. The intention to treat and per protocol analysis will focus on differences between the intervention and control group from pre-surgery assessments to follow-up assessments at 24 months after RYGB. Patients' baseline characteristics are presented in this protocol paper.

Discussion: A total of 259 RYGB female patients has been enrolled in the "WELL-GBP"-trial, of which 156 women have been randomized to receive the intervention and 103 women to control group. The trial is conducted within a Swedish health care setting where female RYGB patients from diverse geographical areas are represented. Our results may, therefore, be representative for female RYGB patients in the country as a whole. If the intervention is effective, implementation within the Swedish health care system is possible within the near future.

Keywords: Bariatric surgery, Roux-en-Y gastric bypass, Dissonance-based, Intervention, RCT, Quality of life, Physical activity,

* Correspondence: fanny.sellberg@ki.se
[1]Department of Public Health Sciences, Karolinska Institutet, K9, Social Medicin, SE-171 77 Stockholm, Sweden
Full list of author information is available at the end of the article

Background

Obesity with its health-related co-morbidities is a major public health problem world-wide [1]. However, lifestyle interventions, such as dietary restriction and increased physical activity (PA), have limited effect on weight loss and maintenance [2, 3]. On the other hand, Roux-en-Y Gastric Bypass (RYGB) surgery results in marked and sustained weight loss as well as improvements in obesity-related comorbidities, compared with lifestyle interventions [4]. In 2014, laparoscopic RYGB accounted for more than 80% of all approximately 7000 bariatric procedures performed in Sweden, of which 75% were women [5]. With the increased use of laparoscopic sleeve gastrectomy, the proportion of laparoscopic RYGB decreased to 64% of the bariatric procedures performed in Sweden 2016 [6].

Weight regain and reoccurrence of obesity related comorbidities after RYGB are not uncommon [7, 8]. In most cases, this is not caused by surgical issues [9], but rather by difficulties with adaptations to the psychosocial life changes brought about by the procedure [10], or by the patient's inability to adhere to the prescribed lifestyle recommendations [9]. Patient's health-related quality of life (HRQoL) and body esteem tend to improve, and is closely associated with weight loss, following RYGB [11, 12]. The improvement in HRQoL typically peaks during the first year after surgery, when the weight loss is most rapid, and then declines as gradual weight regain starts to occur at one to six years after surgery [11]. It is easy to imagine a negative spiral experienced by RYGB patients as their weight loss slows down or weight is regained. Shame and stigmatization lead to increased sedentary behaviors and avoidance of PA, which in its turn might induce even greater problems with body esteem and weight regain. It is therefore important to create efficient preventive measures to avoid this vicious circle.

There is a growing interest in the role of PA and sedentary behavior in achieving optimal weight loss and improving health outcomes after RYGB [13]. Participation in moderate to vigorous intensity PA and reduced sedentary time play an important role in body weight regulation and may contribute to improvements of surgical outcomes after RYGB [14, 15]. In addition, achieving sufficient amounts of PA after surgery is of importance for long-term all-cause and cardiovascular mortality [16] as well as weight maintenance [17].

Although previous research suggests that dysfunctional eating behaviors, issues with body esteem and becoming habitually physically active represents a major challenge for many RYGB patients [10, 12, 18], few interventions to assist patients in meeting these challenges have been conducted. A 2015 systematic review and meta-analysis on interventions before and/or after bariatric surgery stated that the strength of evidence is limited by few trials, low methodological quality and short follow-up duration. The authors concluded that well-designed randomized controlled trials (RCTs) with at least two years follow-up are required. Previous RCTs evaluate weight-loss as the main outcome, with little focus on HRQoL and healthy levels of PA and sedentary behavior. This is of special concern as barriers to engage in PA and exercise, such as feeling too fat, is more common among obese adults [19]. In particular, RYGB patients frequently feel too overweight to exercise, or have fear of exercise-related injuries [15]. Hence, it may be appropriate to aim at reducing sedentary behavior after RYGB surgery, since reduced time spent sedentary may have beneficial effects on health and weight stability in populations with obesity, beyond the effects of light and moderate to vigorous PA (MVPA) [20, 21].

The need for an adequately powered RCT targeting patients undergoing bariatric surgery is justified for several reasons. Firstly, we are not aware of any theory-based counselling intervention for obese female patients after RYGB with appropriate statistical power. Secondly, as RYGB has been the most dominant bariatric procedure performed annually in Sweden during several years [6], it is timely to evaluate the effects of a novel theory-based post-bariatric intervention aimed at facilitating female patients' psychosocial adjustment to daily life, including HRQoL, eating behavior, mood, body esteem, PA and sedentary behaviors. Such an intervention might also prevent further weight re-gain. Finally, a RCT is needed to evaluate the effects of an intervention, where the attainment of unbiased estimates is crucial and almost impossible to attain by observational studies.

The intervention framework was based on cognitive dissonance theory, which states that psychological distress is created when a person attempts to hold inconsistent sets of cognitions at the same time. People experience dissonance when they are encouraged to act in a way that is contrary to their cognitions, and they are prone to change their cognitions to create consistency [22]. People are also prone to change their future behavior to reduce dissonance [23]. In the current intervention, a modified version of Stice's dissonance-based prevention model for eating disorders was adapted to RYGB patients. Apart from prevention of eating disorders, the model has been used for smoking cessation, prevention of unhealthy weight gain [24] and for promoting healthy PA behaviors [25].

Aim

This paper presents the study design and methodology of the "WELL-GBP" intervention (wellbeing after gastric bypass) and describes the baseline characteristics of the participating women. The "WELL-GBP" trial is targeting female RYGB patients in a health care setting to improve HRQoL and health related behaviors after RYGB. The overreaching goal of the current study is to find ways of optimizing the outcome for the RYGB patient, not only in terms of maintained weight loss but also in terms of HRQoL, eating behavior, body esteem, social adjustment, PA and sedentary behavior. The specific aims of the "WELL-GBP" trial are to answer the following questions within a randomized controlled trial:

- What are the effects of a dissonance-based intervention on HRQoL (primary outcome), eating behavior, body esteem and social adjustment of female RYGB patients 24 months after surgery?
- What are the effects of a dissonance-based intervention on objectively measured levels of physical activity and sedentary behavior of female RYGB patients 24 months after surgery?

Methods and design

This randomized controlled intervention study started in January 2015 in Sweden and is still ongoing: all baseline data has been collected and follow up measurements are going to be collected until end of 2019. The trial operates in three counties (Uppland, Närke and Södermanland counties), where participants are recruited from five hospitals: Uppsala University hospital, Danderyd hospital, St Görans hospital, Örebro University hospital and Ersta hospital. The trial has been approved by the Ethical Review Board Stockholm, Dnr 2013/1847–31/2. The trial has also been registered: ISRCTN16417174.

Participants

As stated previously, approximately 75% of all bariatric surgery patients in Sweden are women [5]. To avoid lack of power associated with stratification of sex and limited number of male patients, we included only women in the current trial. Participants were recruited at each hospital approximately one to three months before RYGB surgery. The inclusion criteria were severe obesity (BMI $\geq$ 35 kg/m^2), being able to understand and speak Swedish and the absence of any serious chronic disease such as stroke or myocardial infarction. All women who fulfilled the inclusion criteria and were accepted for primary RYGB surgery were asked to participate in the study. In general, patients are not eligible for surgery if they are under 18 years old, have not made previous serious attempts to lose weight or alcohol/substance abuse, recent heart disease or stroke or certain kinds of cancer, although the guidelines may to some extent differ between counties.

Setting and recruitment

The study is conducted by Karolinska Institutet (KI) in collaboration with the five previously mentioned hospitals for recruitment. Altogether, the five hospitals account for approximately 25% of all bariatric surgery procedures performed in Sweden [6]. The recruitment procedure differed across the hospitals. At Uppsala University hospital and Örebro University hospital, the eligible RYGB patients were sent an information sheet together with a form for declaration of interest to participate in the study approximately three months before surgery. Thereafter the participants filled in the declaration of interest to the hospital, from which it was forwarded to KI. Ersta, Danderyd and St Görans hospitals had group information meetings, led by dietitians and specialized obesity nurses approximately one to three months before surgery. These group meetings occurred weekly and were visited by research staff from the current trial who informed patients about the trial and handed out declarations of interest forms for patients to fill in on-site. For all participants, research staff from KI then contacted the interested patients by telephone for consultation regarding participation in the study (n = 600). Participants were excluded if they failed to meet the inclusion criteria (n = 57), declined participation (n = 67), or if the research staff were unable to reach them by telephone, mail or e-mail (n = 73). The eligible participants received an accelerometer (Actigraph GT3X+) and questionnaires together with a form for informed consent, all sent by mail to their homes (n = 403). Once the participants sent back baseline assessments they were defined as a participant in the study (n = 304) (See Fig. 1). Participants who returned the baseline assessments received the results from their accelerometer measurement together with either a movie ticket voucher or a gift card (value 100 SEK) to promote participant retention. They received the same gift for all follow-up measures. Participant questionnaire were stored in numerical order in a secure and accessible place and manner. Data from questionnaires were entered manually twice by two different researchers to minimize bias. All personal data is handled in a confidential way according to KIs rules and the Swedish law.

Eligible participants who sent back the material (n = 304) were excluded from the study if they did not speak Swedish (n = 3), did not undergo the planned surgery (n = 9), changed their minds about wanting to participate (n = 2), died (n = 1), or if they underwent a sleeve gastrectomy instead of RYGB (n = 30) (see Fig. 1).

Participants were randomized to either intervention group (60%, n = 153) or control group (40%, n = 103) after surgery. Participants in the intervention group received a telephone call from the research staff

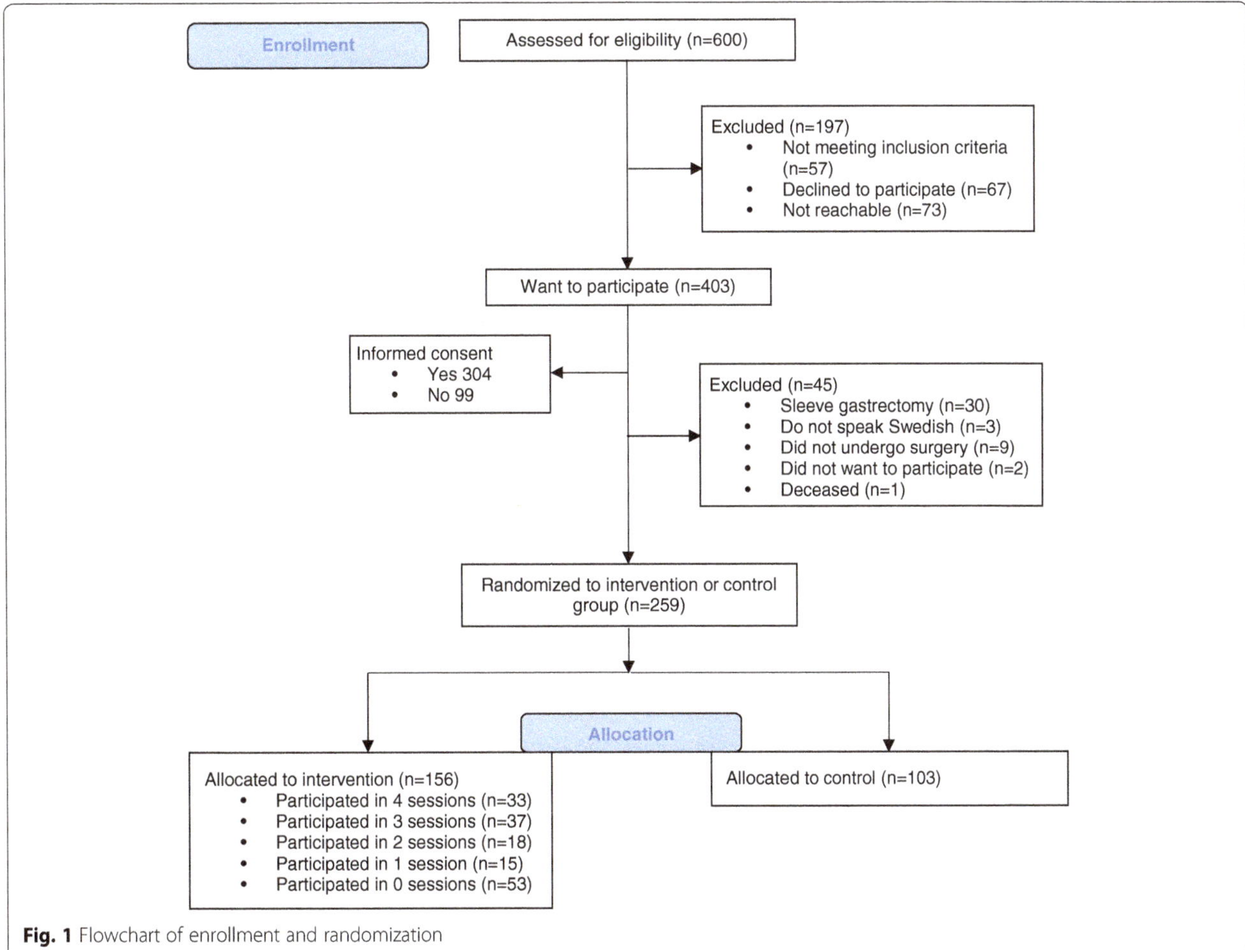

Fig. 1 Flowchart of enrollment and randomization

approximately two months after RYGB where they obtained more detailed information about the group sessions. The dates for the four sessions were decided by the moderator in an attempt to fit the schedule of all group members. The control group participants were informed by mail.

Pilot study

The first eight post-surgical patients at Ersta hospital in March and April 2015, were invited to participate in a pilot study (pilots are not included in the flow-chart). The aim was to test the intervention manual to see if it was understandable and acceptable for both the participants and the moderator. The participants provided feedback after each session, and small adjustments to the manual were made. The pilot intervention was conducted in June 2015 and five of the eight participants attended at least one of the sessions.

Intervention description

The intervention started approximately two to three months after RYGB, and consisted of four group sessions during which a modified version of the Stice dissonance-based intervention model was used [24, 26]. See Table 1 for an overview of the intervention sessions. The sessions were offered once per week during four weeks, at the clinic where the women had surgery. Each session lasted for approximately 1,5 h and preferred group size was approximately five women per group. One of the research staff acted as a moderator and followed an intervention manual. As mentioned above, the intervention was based on the principle of cognitive dissonance theory [27] and the moderator encouraged the participants to talk to each other about how they wanted to act and behave to certain situations in the future, and in that way create the dissonance in relation to how they had been acting before their surgery. The group sessions aimed to provide the participants with strategies for coping with future difficulties with eating and PA behaviors, feelings of shame and other negative emotions, as well as to give them the opportunity to actively engage in thinking about their own and others' current standpoints and perspectives in these areas. The sessions were not focused on teaching or informing the participants about appropriate eating or PA behaviors, but rather on eliciting active engagement and discussion

Table 1 Overview of the 4 intervention sessions in groups post RYGB Surgery

Topic for group sessions	Duration (mins)	Time after RYGB (weeks)	Content
1. Physical activity	90	12	-Sedentary behavior and motivation to minimize it -PA, how to avoid failure and make it a routine -How to overcome fears/difficulties with PA for RYGB patients
2. Eating Behaviors	90	13	-How to deal with cravings, powerlessness, feelings of emptiness and shame in relation to eating behavior -Different interpretations of health and appearance -Expectations and relation to food
3. Social relationships	90	14	How to handle different difficult social scenarios after RYGB, for example: -Comments from one's surroundings about foods -Comments from one's surroundings about weight loss -Eating at restaurants, buffets, parties
4. Intimate relationships	90	15	-Intimate and sexual relations, sexuality, avoidance and lust -Self-esteem and shame, how to improve it -Summarizing all sessions

and to take a stand on preferred ways of handling the discussed difficulties. Each of the four sessions focused on a different aspect of difficulties that might occur following RYGB. The manual for this project was developed by three researchers included in the development of the intervention, of whom two had previous experiences with RYGB patients, and one of whom is professor in clinical psychology.

The first session included PA and sedentary behavior. The participants were asked to suggest and discuss behaviors that may decrease sedentary behaviors throughout the day. For example, to think about what makes them not carry out planned PA, and to reflect on their own attitudes and approaches to PA. They were also asked to complete a home exercise, which entailed to write down what it meant for them to be physically active, what their long-term goal was in this area, how they were planning to realize their plans, what obstacles they expected to encounter, and how they would cope with them.

The second session addressed eating behavior and problems that are relatively common post- RYGB. The session focused on two (fictional) letters from women who had undergone RYGB two years earlier, and were now facing eating-related problems. The first woman reported extreme cravings for sweet, followed by uncontrolled eating, shame and feelings of loss of control. The second woman described a sense of loss and grief as she could no longer eat the types and amounts of food that she used to, including the foods she used to bake and cook for her family. Additionally, this session included expectations from the participants themselves and their surroundings, and different interpretations of health and appearance. The homework exercise was to write a reply to one of the letters, entailing support, understanding and suggestions for action that marked a clear stance toward the problem and obstacles.

The third session focused on social relations, including family, friends and colleagues. The participants were given the opportunity to reflect on and to role play different scenarios they often experienced themselves. For example, people around them tried to get them to eat foods that are unsuitable after RYGB, gave unhelpful comments or criticisms, or they found themselves at a restaurant with big portions and/or lack of suitable menu options. As a homework exercise each participant wrote a letter to herself to be sent back to her after six months, containing overall goals, mindset and strategies and at least one "lesson learned" from the group sessions.

The fourth session dealt with intimate relations and sexuality. The participants were asked to reflect on and to discuss possible expectations, from themselves and from their partners, as well issues related to lack of a partner, which might arise after surgery. In addition to this, this session also included (fictional) letters. These might have to do with experiencing or not experiencing sexual desire, feelings about one's own body following major weight loss, and to deal with desired or unwanted sexual attention from others.

During the four sessions, the majority of participants expressed a desire to have more group meetings approximately one year after the surgery, since they felt they wanted to discuss problems and strategies when they had recovered and started to get into their new habits post-surgery. Therefore, a booster session was added and was held approximately one year after surgery. The booster session was a compilation of the four previous sessions. The participants were asked to reflect on the previous topics: PA, eating behavior, social relations and intimate relations and sexuality for approximately ten minutes per topic. Lastly, participants were encouraged to share the experience of receiving the letter six months after they had written it to themselves and to further reflect on experienced problems and possible resolutions after surgery. To the best of our knowledge, none of the participants included in the "WELL-RYGB" Intervention study have suffered any adverse effects so far.

Measurements

At baseline, approximately one month before RYGB, and at clinical follow-up visits at 6, 12 and 24 months after RYGB, participants will be weighed and have their height measured. The women will, at baseline and at the follow-up visits, be asked to complete a number of questionnaires, sent to their home to fill in and return to KI by mail. The following questionnaires are used:

SF-36 [28] is measuring HRQoL (primary outcome) and is a widely-used instrument which measures health-related quality of life with 36 questions divided in eight dimensions: physical functioning, role limitations due to physical health problems, bodily pain, general health, vitality, social functioning, role limitations due to emotional problems and mental health. We also present data in a summary score for the physical components (PCS) and the mental components (MCS) including a cut off value of ≤42 for the MCS as having a risk for depression. The final scores for the different parts is made into a zero to 100 scale with higher numbers indicating better HRQoL.

Three-Factor Eating Questionnaire (TFEQ) [29] is a 21-item questionnaire measuring dietary restraint, emotional eating and uncontrolled eating. A higher score indicates higher restraint, uncontrolled eating and emotional eating [30, 31].

Body Esteem Scale (BES) [32] is a 23-item questionnaire measuring weight concerns, appearance and attribution. A lower score indicates worse body esteem.

Social Adjustment Scale (SAS) [33, 34] is a 45-item questionnaire measuring satisfaction with one's social life in the different dimensions: work role, social and leisure activities, relationships with extended family, role as marital partner, parental role and role within the family unit. Lower scores indicates better social adjustment.

Disordered Eating after Bariatric Surgery (DEBS) [35] is a 7-item questionnaire which specifically measures disordered eating after bariatric surgery over the last 28 days. A higher score indicates a higher rate of disordered eating.

Furthermore, women will be asked to wear the validated GT3X+ accelerometer [36, 37] during all waking hours, for seven consecutive days, to objectively measure levels, patterns and intensity of PA and sedentary behavior [38] according to the latest definition, including intensity and posture [39]. Minimal wear time to qualify as a valid measurement is three weekdays and one weekend day with a minimum of ten hours wear time per day.

To be able to compare the intervention to no intervention the control group will receive the usual follow-up care, including weight measures at six and 12 months after RYGB, at the clinic where they had surgery, and like the intervention group, will be asked to complete the questionnaires, to wear the GT3X+ before and six, 12 and 24 months after RYGB. The usual follow-up care differs slightly between hospitals. However, in general it contains consultation with a dietitian about food intake after surgery, and appointments with a nurse and/or the surgeons to measure weight loss, results of laboratory tests and to ensure that no complications have occurred.

Power calculations

Power calculations showed that 95 participants were needed in each group to attain a statistical power of at least 0.80 (based on HRQoL as the primary outcome), with an expected moderate effect size (Cohen's d = 50), and alpha set at 0.05. Based on previous similar studies [25, 40], we expect 20% drop-out of patients during two years of follow-up. Thus, a minimum of 240 patients was required, and at final total of 259 participants were recruited and randomized either to the intervention (60%) or to usual care (40%).

Randomization

Approximately two months after surgery 60% of the participants were block randomized to the intervention group (n = 163) and 40% to the control group (n = 103). One member of the research staff who was not currently working with the data collection was in charge of the randomization, which was computer generated randomization 60/40. The randomization was divided according to counties (Danderyd, Ersta and St Görans were randomized together, Uppsala and Örebro separately) in blocks of 5 participants and was carried out after date of surgery. Only RYGB participants with informed consent and baseline questionnaire data were randomized.

Statistical analyses

The statistical analyses will focus on differences between the intervention and the control group from pre-surgery assessment to follow-up assessments at 24 months after RYGB. The women's changes in weight will be taken into account in the analysis by stratification or adjustment. Primary analysis will be intention to treat analysis, including women who attended at least one session (n = 103). We will also conduct per protocol analysis including the women who have attended all four sessions (n = 33). We will also perform sensitivity analysis in order to detect any possible dose-response effects such as if the main outcomes will differ depending on if a woman have attended one, two three or all four sessions. Furthermore, individual factors, e.g. patient beliefs about causality of obesity, and contextual factors, e.g. variations in implementation of the intervention between centers for bariatric surgery, might moderate the effect of the intervention on health outcomes. These issues will be analyzed by mixed linear regression models or generalized estimation equations (GEE) to analyze repeated measurements over time. [41].

For the assessments of the baseline characteristics for the intervention and control group presented in this protocol, the analysis have been separated into women randomized to intervention group and women randomized to control. X^2-tests were performed for categorical variables and t-tests for continuous variables, and because the majority of the continuous variables were not linear distributed, the Kruskal-Wallis test was used.

Table 2 Baseline characteristics of women undergoing RYGB Surgery

Characteristics	Intervention (n = 156) % (n)/Mean (SD)	Control (n = 103) % (n)/Mean (SD)	p-value
Age (yrs)	43.6 (10.7)	45.1 (10.1)	0.218
Weight (kg)	110.8 (14.0)	111.0 (17.6)	0.784
Height (cm)	164.9 (6.6)	164.2 (6.7)	0.315
BMI (kg/m^2)	40.7 (4.3)	41.2 (5.2)	0.712
With diabetes type 2	20.5 (32)	22.3 (23)	0.726
Daily smokers	6.4 (10)	6.8 (7)	0.902
Education			0.535
Primary	12.3 (19)	8.7 (9)	
Secondary	56.1 (87)	54.4 (56)	
Post-secondary	31.6 (49)	36.9 (87)	
Born in Sweden	86.6 (97)	79.7 (59)	0.212

Baseline data

This intervention study includes a total of 259 women who have been treated with gastric bypass surgery, of which 156 were randomized to receive a dissonance based intervention consisting of four group sessions, and 103 women to receive usual follow-up care from the clinic where they had surgery. For all tests, there were no statistical significant differences between intervention and control group, which confirms that the randomization was successful. In total, 66% (n = 103) of the women in the intervention group attended at least one of the intervention sessions. Baseline characteristics are presented in Table 2. Pre-RYGB measures were: mean age of 44.2 ± 10.5 years (intervention: 43.6 ± 10.7; control: 45.1 ± 10.1), a mean BMI of 40.9 ± 4.7 (intervention: 40.7 ± 4.3; control: 41.2 ± 5.2), a mean weight of 110.9 ± 15.5 kg (intervention: 110.8 ± 14.0; control: 111.0 ± 17.6), and 21% (n = 32) in the intervention group and 22% (n = 23) in the control group had diabetes type 2.

The baseline HRQoL, measured by the SF-36, is shown in Table 3. In general the physical component summary score (PCS) was 42.2 ± 9.6 (intervention: 41.6 ± 9.5; control: 42.9 ± 9.6) and 35% (n = 54) in the intervention group and 31% (n = 31) in the control group showed an indication for risk of depression (mental component summary score (MCS) ≤42).

Baseline measurement of the women's levels of PA, sedentary behavior and wear time are presented in Table 4. The women in the intervention group wore the accelerometer for a mean of 6.6 ± 1.1 days, spent 28.8 ± 17.5 min/day in MVPA and 465.1 ± 98.0 min/day was spent sedentary. For the control group, the women wore the accelerometer for a mean of 6.9 ± 1.4 days, spent 28.8 ± 22.4 min/day in MVPA and were sedentary for 447.0 ± 104.2 min/day.

Discussion

The ongoing RCT with a dissonance-based intervention, "WELL-GBP", targeting female RYGB patients in a health care setting, aims to improve HRQoL and health-related behaviors after RYGB. The intervention is manual-based, free of charge, delivered in health care settings and could be delivered by health-care personnel such as nurses, dietitians, physiotherapists or counsellors, after some practice. We are not aware of any previous randomized controlled trial that has investigated the effects of a similar intervention on HRQoL and following RYGB.

Previous studies using dissonance-based interventions have had positive results on health outcomes and showed greater effect sizes compared to non-dissonance-based interventions or no intervention, regarding disordered eating, body dissatisfaction [24–26], and also increased PA at post-test, but not at 1–2 year follow-up [25, 26]. This trial uses a modified version of Stice's dissonance-based prevention model and has been adapted to RYGB patients.

The women participating in this trial could be representative of women who undergo RYGB surgery in Sweden, as they are from different geographical areas and are similar in age and BMI at the time of surgery to other RYGB patients in Sweden [42]. They are also comparable in this respect to other bariatric patients from other parts of the world, although they tend to be slightly older and have a higher BMI [43]. A previous study comparing levels of PA pre-bariatric surgery

Table 3 Baseline health-related quality of life, measured by the SF-36, in women undergoing RYGB Surgery

Characteristic	Intervention (n = 155[a]) Mean (SD)	Control (n = 102[a]) Mean (SD)	p-value
Physical Functioning (PF)	58.2 (22.4)	58.8 (24.4)	0.656
Role Physical (RP)	67.7 (28.4)	72.3 (30.1)	0.099
Bodily Pain (BP)	47.9 (28.0)	48.8 (28.8)	0.799
General Health (GH)	50.4 (23.9)	53.1 (22.7)	0.336
Vitality (VT)	37.9 (23.5)	40.1 (35.6)	0.453
Social Functioning (SF)	64.5 (27.9)	64.5 (29.2)	0.922
Role Emotional (RE)	77.2 (28.0)	77.3 (28.5)	0.912
Mental Health (MH)	64.9 (19.5)	64.9 (21.4)	0.770
Physical component summary score (PCS)	41.6 (9.5)	42.9 (9.6)	0.205
Mental component summary score (MCS)	45.8 (11.0)	45.9 (11.3)	0.848
Prevalence of risk of depression (MCS score ≤ 42), % (n)	35.1 (54)	30.7 (31)	0.469

[a]One participant in the intervention group and one participant in the control group did not answer the SF-36 questionnaire

measured by an accelerometer in Swedish women have similar characteristics in the different PA levels as the women in the "WELL-GBP" trial [44]. HRQoL in our sample was similar, although somewhat higher, than the general Swedish bariatric surgery patients [45]. HRQoL, especially PCS score, improves after bariatric surgery and is related to weight loss, gender and age, with lower PCS and MCS scores in women than men, and lower PCS but higher MCS with increased age [45].

The current "WELL-GBP" trial only includes Swedish-speaking women, as resources such as an interpreter at the group sessions were not feasible. This may affect the external validity as the future results will not be representative of women who live in Sweden but don't master the Swedish language. Also, because this current trial only includes women, any possible intervention effect on men who undergo RYGB will not be possible to predict.

To reduce the problems associated with drop-out, a larger proportion (60%) of the participants were randomized to intervention. Unfortunately, 34% (n = 53) of the women in the intervention group did not attend any of the intervention sessions, even though they agreed to participate when invited and had completed the baseline assessments. This may have a negative effect on the upcoming results, but in accordance with the power calculations (see above), a minimum of 95 participants was needed to attain a statistical power of at least 0.80. In this trial 103 women (66%) in the intervention group completed the baseline assessments and attended at least one of the intervention session. Even so, the results may not be representative to the general Swedish women who undergo RYGB surgery.

Conclusions

The "WELL-GBP" trial is conducted within a Swedish health care setting where female RYGB patients from diverse geographical areas are represented. Our results may, therefore, be representative for female RYGB patients in the country as a whole. If the intervention is effective, implementation within the Swedish health care system is possible within the near future.

Table 4 Baseline total and intensity-specific levels of accelerometer-measured physical activity (PA) and sedentary behavior (SB) of women undergoing RYGB Surgery

Characteristic	Intervention (n = 97[a]) Mean (SD)	Control (n = 58[a]) Mean (SD)	p-value
Wear time: nr of days (≥10 h/day)	6.6 (1.1)	6.9 (1.4)	0.169
Wear time: hours/day	14.4 (1.2)	14.3 (1.1)	0.369
Total PA (cpm)	576.6 (179.3)	621.2 (230.1)	0.342
Moderate to vigorous PA (min/day)	28.8 (17.4)	28.8 (22.4)	0.579
Light PA (min/day)	369.4 (88.1)	380.2 (78.1)	0.518
SB (min/day)	465.1 (98.0)	447.0 (104.1)	0.399

[a]59 participants in the intervention group and 45 participants in the control group declined to wear an accelerometer or the timing for wearing an accelerometer were too close to their surgery date

Abbreviations

BMI: Body mass index; HRQoL: Health related quality of life; KI: Karolinska Institutet; MVPA: Moderate to vigorous physical activity; PA: Physical activity; RYGB: Roux-en-Y gastric bypass; WELL-GBP: Wellbeing after gastric bypass

Acknowledgements

We would like to thank the staff involved in this study from the five hospitals Danderyd Hospital, Ersta Hospital, Uppsala University Hospital, Örebro University Hospital, and St. Görans Hospital, for their help in recruiting study participants and to the study participants that participated in the data collection.

Funding

This study was financially supported by the Swedish Scientific Council (Vetenskapsrådet), Erling-Persson Family Foundation and the Research School of Caring Sciences Karolinska Institutet.

Authors' contributions

FS: writing and data collection, SP: writing, data collection and analyzing data, AG: study design and writing, EN: study design and writing, MW: study design and writing, PT: statistics, AT: writing, MS: writing, JU: writing, ES: writing, DB: principal investigator, study design and writing. All authors read and approved the final manuscript.

Competing interests

The authors declare that they have no competing interests.

Author details

[1]Department of Public Health Sciences, Karolinska Institutet, K9, Social Medicin, SE-171 77 Stockholm, Sweden. [2]Department of Clinical Neuroscience, Karolinska Institutet, SE-171 77 Stockholm, Sweden. [3]Division of Clinical Sciences, Danderyd Hospital, Karolinska Institutet, SE-182 88 Stockholm, Sweden. [4]Department of Health and Caring Sciences, University of Gävle, SE-801 76 Gävle, Sweden. [5]Centre for Epidemiology and Community Medicine, Stockholm County Council, Box 45436, SE-104 31 Stockholm, Sweden. [6]Department of Clinical Science at Danderyd Hospital, Karolinska Institutet, SE-116 91 Stockholm, Sweden. [7]Department of Surgery, Ersta Hospital, SE-116 91 Stockholm, Sweden. [8]Department of Surgical Sciences, Uppsala University, SE-751 85 Uppsala, Sweden. [9]Department of Medicine, Karolinska Institutet, SE-141 86 Stockholm, Sweden. [10]Department of Endocrine and Obesity, Capio st Görans Hospital, SE-141 86 Stockholm, Sweden. [11]Department of Surgery, Faculty of Medicine and Health, Örebro University, SE-701 85 Örebro, Sweden.

References

1. Collaborators GBDO, Afshin A, Forouzanfar MH, Reitsma MB, Sur P, Estep K, Lee A, Marczak L, Mokdad AH, Moradi-Lakeh M, et al. Health effects of overweight and obesity in 195 countries over 25 years. N Engl J Med. 2017;377(1):13–27.
2. Danielsen KK, Svendsen M, Maehlum S, Sundgot-Borgen J. Changes in body composition, cardiovascular disease risk factors, and eating behavior after an intensive lifestyle intervention with high volume of physical activity in severely obese subjects: a prospective clinical controlled trial. J Obes. 2013; 2013:325464.
3. Unick JL, Beavers D, Jakicic JM, Kitabchi AE, Knowler WC, Wadden TA, Wing RR, Look ARG. Effectiveness of lifestyle interventions for individuals with severe obesity and type 2 diabetes: results from the look AHEAD trial. Diabetes Care. 2011;34(10):2152–7.
4. Colquitt JL, Pickett K, Loveman E, Frampton GK. Surgery for weight loss in adults. Cochrane Database Syst Rev. 2014;8(8):Cd003641.
5. (SOReg) SOSR. Årsrapport SOReg 2014. Del 1 – operationsstatistik, case mix och tidiga komplikationer, vol. 6; 2015. p. 1. www.ucr.uu.se/soreg/arsrapporter.
6. (SOReg) SOSR. Årsrapport SOReg 2016. Del 1-operationsstatistik och tidiga komplikationer, vol. 8; 2017. p. 1. www.ucr.uu.se/soreg/arsrapporter.
7. Higa K, Ho T, Tercero F, Yunus T, Boone KB. Laparoscopic roux-en-Y gastric bypass: 10-year follow-up. Surg Obes Relat Dis. 2011;7(4):516–25.
8. Nakamura KM, Haglind EG, Clowes JA, Achenbach SJ, Atkinson EJ, Melton LJ 3rd, Kennel KA. Fracture risk following bariatric surgery: a population-based study. Osteoporos Int. 2014;25(1):151–8.
9. Sarwer DB, Wadden TA, Moore RH, Eisenberg MH, Raper SE, Williams NN. Changes in quality of life and body image after gastric bypass surgery. Surg Obes Relat Dis. 2010;6(6):608–14.
10. van Hout GC, Verschure SK, van Heck GL. Psychosocial predictors of success following bariatric surgery. Obes Surg. 2005;15(4):552–60.
11. Karlsson J, Taft C, Ryden A, Sjostrom L, Sullivan M. Ten-year trends in health-related quality of life after surgical and conventional treatment for severe obesity: the SOS intervention study. Int J Obes (2005). 2007;31(8):1248–61.
12. Saunders R. "Grazing": a high-risk behavior. Obes Surg. 2004;14(1):98–102.
13. Welch G, Wesolowski C, Piepul B, Kuhn J, Romanelli J, Garb J. Physical activity predicts weight loss following gastric bypass surgery: findings from a support group survey. Obes Surg. 2008;18(5):517–24.
14. Jacobi D, Ciangura C, Couet C, Oppert JM. Physical activity and weight loss following bariatric surgery. Obes Rev. 2011;12(5):366–77.
15. King WC, Bond DS. The importance of preoperative and postoperative physical activity counseling in bariatric surgery. Exerc Sport Sci Rev. 2013; 41(1):26–35.
16. Fogelholm M. Physical activity, fitness and fatness: relations to mortality, morbidity and disease risk factors. A systematic review. Obes Rev. 2010; 11(3):202–21.
17. Donnelly JE, Blair SN, Jakicic JM, Manore MM, Rankin JW, Smith BK. American College of Sports Medicine position stand. Appropriate physical activity intervention strategies for weight loss and prevention of weight regain for adults. Med Sci Sports Exerc. 2009;41(2):459–71.
18. Berglind DWM, Eriksson U, Thorell A, Sundbom M, Uddén J, Raoof M, Hedberg J, Tynelius P, Näslund E, Rasmussen F. Longitudinal assessment of physical activity in women undergoing roux-en-Y gastric bypass. Obes Surg. 2015;25(1):119–25.
19. Ball K, Crawford D, Owen N. Too fat to exercise? Obesity as a barrier to physical activity. Aust N Z J Public Health. 2000;24(3):331–3.
20. Dunstan DW, Howard B, Healy GN, Owen N. Too much sitting–a health hazard. Diabetes Res Clin Pract. 2012;97(3):368–76.
21. de Rezende LF, Rodrigues Lopes M, Rey-Lopez JP, Matsudo VK, Luiz Odo C. Sedentary behavior and health outcomes: an overview of systematic reviews. PLoS One. 2014;9(8):e105620.
22. Stone J, Focella E. Hypocrisy, dissonance and the self-regulation processes that improve health. Self Identity. 2011;10(3):295–303.
23. Aronson E. Persuasion via self-justification: large commitments for small rewards. In: Festinger L, editor. Retrospection on social psychology. New York: Oxford University Press; 1980. p. 3–21.
24. Stice E, Shaw H, Becker CB, Rohde P. Dissonance-based interventions for the prevention of eating disorders: using persuasion principles to promote health. Prev Sci. 2008;9(2):114–28.
25. Stice E, Rohde P, Shaw H, Marti CN. Efficacy trial of a selective prevention program targeting both eating disorders and obesity among female college students: 1- and 2-year follow-up effects. J Consult Clin Psychol. 2013;81(1):183–9.
26. Stice E, Rohde P, Shaw H, Marti CN. Efficacy trial of a selective prevention program targeting both eating disorder symptoms and unhealthy weight gain among female college students. J Consult Clin Psychol. 2012;80(1):164–70.
27. Shapira Lots I, Stone L. Perception of musical consonance and dissonance: an outcome of neural synchronization. J R Soc Interface. 2008;5(29):1429–34.
28. Sullivan M, Karlsson J, Ware JE Jr. The Swedish SF-36 health survey–I. Evaluation of data quality, scaling assumptions, reliability and construct validity across general populations in Sweden. Soc Sci Med (1982). 1995; 41(10):1349–58.
29. Karlsson J, Persson LO, Sjostrom L, Sullivan M. Psychometric properties and factor structure of the three-factor eating questionnaire (TFEQ) in obese men and women. Results from the Swedish obese subjects (SOS) study. Int J Obes Relat Metab Disord. 2000;24(12):1715–25.

30. Laurenius A, Larsson I, Bueter M, Melanson KJ, Bosaeus I, Forslund HB, Lonroth H, Fandriks L, Olbers T. Changes in eating behaviour and meal pattern following roux-en-Y gastric bypass. Int J Obesity (2005). 2012;36(3):348–55.
31. Willmer M, Berglind D, Tynelius P, Ghaderi A, Naslund E, Rasmussen F. Changes in eating behaviour and food choices in families where the mother undergoes gastric bypass surgery for obesity. Eur J Clin Nutr. 2016;70(1):35–40.
32. Mendelson BK, Mendelson MJ, White DR. Body-esteem scale for adolescents and adults. J Pers Assess. 2001;76(1):90–106.
33. Achard S, Chignon JM, Poirier-Littre MF, Galinowski A, Pringuey D, Van Os J, Lemonnier F. Social adjustment and depression: value of the SAS-SR (social adjustment scale self-report). L'Encephale. 1995;21(2):107–16.
34. Gameroff MJ, Wickramaratne P, Weissman MM. Testing the short and screener versions of the social adjustment scale-self-report (SAS-SR). Int J Methods Psychiatr Res. 2012;21(1):52–65.
35. Weineland S, Alfonsson S, Dahl J, Ghaderi A. Development and validation of a new questionnaire measuring eating disordered behaviours post bariatric surgery. Clin Obesity. 2013;2:160–7.
36. Sasaki JE, John D, Freedson PS. Validation and comparison of ActiGraph activity monitors. J Sci Med Sport. 2011;14(5):411–6.
37. Santos-Lozano A, Santin-Medeiros F, Cardon G, Torres-Luque G, Bailon R, Bergmeir C, Ruiz JR, Lucia A, Garatachea N. Actigraph GT3X: validation and determination of physical activity intensity cut points. Int J Sports Med. 2013;34(11):975–82.
38. Santos-Lozano A, Marin PJ, Torres-Luque G, Ruiz JR, Lucia A, Garatachea N. Technical variability of the GT3X accelerometer. Med Eng Phys. 2012;34(6): 787–90.
39. Sedentary Behaviour Research N. Letter to the editor: standardized use of the terms "sedentary" and "sedentary behaviours". Appl Physiol Nutr Metab. 2012;37(3):540–2.
40. Stice E, Marti CN, Spoor S, Presnell K, Shaw H. Dissonance and healthy weight eating disorder prevention programs: long-term effects from a randomized efficacy trial. J Consult Clin Psychol. 2008;76(2):329–40.
41. VanderWeele TJ. A unification of mediation and interaction: a 4-way decomposition. Epidemiology. 2014;25(5):749–61.
42. (SOReg) Sosr. Årsrapport SOReg 2015. Del 2. Uppföljning, viktförändringar, förändring av samsjuklighet, långsiktiga komplikationer och kvalitetsindikatorer på kliniknivå, vol. 7; 2016. p. 2. http://www.ucr.uu.se/soreg/arsrapporter.
43. Welbourn R, Pournaras DJ, Dixon J, Higa K, Kinsman R, Ottosson J, Ramos A, van Wagensveld B, Walton P, Weiner R, et al. Bariatric surgery worldwide: baseline demographic description and one-year outcomes from the second IFSO global registry report 2013-2015. Obes Surg. 2018;28(2):313–22.
44. Berglind D, Willmer M, Tynelius P, Ghaderi A, Naslund E, Rasmussen F. Accelerometer-measured versus self-reported physical activity levels and sedentary behavior in women before and 9 months after roux-en-Y gastric bypass. Obes Surg. 2016;26(7):1463–70.
45. (SOReg) SOSR. Årsrapport SOReg 2016. Del 3. Livskvalitet, Mortalitet, Datakvalitet, Forskning, vol. 8; 2017. p. 3. http://www.ucr.uu.se/soreg/arsrapporter.

24

Obstruction in the third portion of the duodenum due to a diospyrobezoar: a case report

Yukinori Yamagata*, Kazuyuki Saito, Kosuke Hirano, Yawara Kubota, Ryuji Yoshioka, Takashi Okuyama, Emiko Takeshita, Nobumi Tagaya, Shinichi Sameshima, Tamaki Noie and Masatoshi Oya

Abstract

Background: Duodenal obstruction occurs mainly due to physical lesions such as duodenal ulcers or tumors. Obstruction due to bezoars is rare. We describe an extremely rare case of obstruction in the third portion of the duodenum caused by a diospyrobezoar 15 months after laparoscopic distal gastrectomy for early gastric cancer.

Case presentation: A 73-year-old man who underwent laparoscopic distal gastrectomy for early gastric cancer 15 months before admission experienced abdominal distension and occasional vomiting. The symptoms worsened and ingestion became difficult; therefore, he was admitted to our department. Computed tomography (CT) performed on admission revealed a solid mass in the third portion of the duodenum and dilatation of the oral side of the duodenum and remnant stomach. Esophagogastroduodenoscopy (EGD) revealed a bezoar deep in the third portion of the duodenum. We could neither remove nor crush the bezoar. At midnight on the day of EGD, he experienced sudden abdominal pain. Repeat CT revealed that the bezoar had vanished from the duodenum and was observed in the ileum. Moreover, small bowel dilatation was observed on the oral side of the bezoar. Although CT showed neither free air nor ascites, laboratory data showed the increase of leukocyte (8400/μL) and C-reactive protein (18.1 mg/dL), and abdominal pain was severe. Emergency surgery was performed because conservative treatment was considered ineffective. We tried advancing the bezoar into the colon, but the ileum was too narrow; therefore, we incised the ileum and removed the bezoar. The bezoar was ocher, elastic, and hard, and its cross-section was uniform and orange. The postsurgical interview revealed that the patient loved eating Japanese persimmons (*Diospyros kaki*); therefore, he was diagnosed with a diospyrobezoar. His postoperative progress was good and without complications. He left the hospital 10 days after surgery. EGD performed 4 weeks after surgery revealed no abnormal duodenal findings.

Conclusions: We describe a rare case of obstruction in the third portion of the duodenum caused by a diospyrobezoar 15 months after laparoscopic distal gastrectomy with Billroth I reconstruction for early gastric cancer.

Keywords: Duodenal obstruction, Diospyrobezoar, Gastrectomy

Background

Duodenal obstruction occurs mainly due to physical lesions such as duodenal ulcers or tumors [1]. Reports documented duodenal obstruction due to bezoars are relatively rare [2–11]. Furthermore, obstruction in the third portion of the duodenum due to a bezoar is extremely rare [2, 12, 13]. We describe a rare case of obstruction in the third portion of the duodenum caused by a diospyrobezoar 15 months after laparoscopic distal gastrectomy with Billroth I reconstruction for early gastric cancer.

* Correspondence: yamagay-tky@umin.ac.jp
Department of Surgery, Dokkyo Medical University Koshigaya Hospital, 2-1-50 Minami-Koshigaya, Koshigaya City, Saitama 343-8555, Japan

Case presentation

A 73-year-old man who had undergone laparoscopic distal gastrectomy with Billroth I reconstruction for early gastric cancer 15 months before experiencing abdominal distension and occasional vomiting was admitted to our hospital. The patient had undergone follow-up computed tomography (CT) and esophagogastroduodenoscopy (EGD) for 1 year after surgery (2 months before admission), during which time no abnormal findings, including the previously observed dilatation of the bile and pancreatic ducts, were found.

Symptoms worsened and ingestion became difficult. On admission, blood tests showed a slightly inflammatory reaction, and CT revealed a solid mass in the third portion of the duodenum and dilatation of the oral side of the duodenum and remnant stomach (Fig. 1). EGD revealed a bezoar deep in the third portion of the duodenum (Fig. 2). The bezoar collapsed while trying to grasp it with forceps. We then tried crushing the bezoar with the forceps, but it was too deep to crush completely. We were also unable to search the duodenum on the other side of the bezoar. At midnight on the day of the EGD, he experienced sudden abdominal pain. Blood tests performed the next morning showed a significant increase in inflammatory response. Therefore, CT was repeated. The bezoar had disappeared from the duodenum but was observed in the ileum (Figs. 3 and 4a). Moreover, small bowel dilatation was observed on the oral side of the bezoar. Although CT showed no free air or ascites, laboratory data showed the increase of leukocyte (8400/μL) and C-reactive protein (18.1 mg/dL), and abdominal pain was severe. Emergency surgery was performed because conservative treatment was considered ineffective. Although the small intestine was expanded and edematous

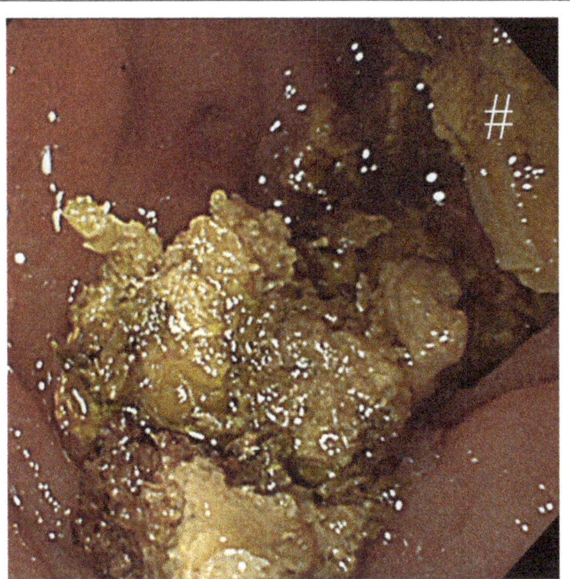

Fig. 2 Esophagogastroduodenoscopy (EGD) on admission. EGD revealed a bezoar deep in the third portion of the duodenum (#)

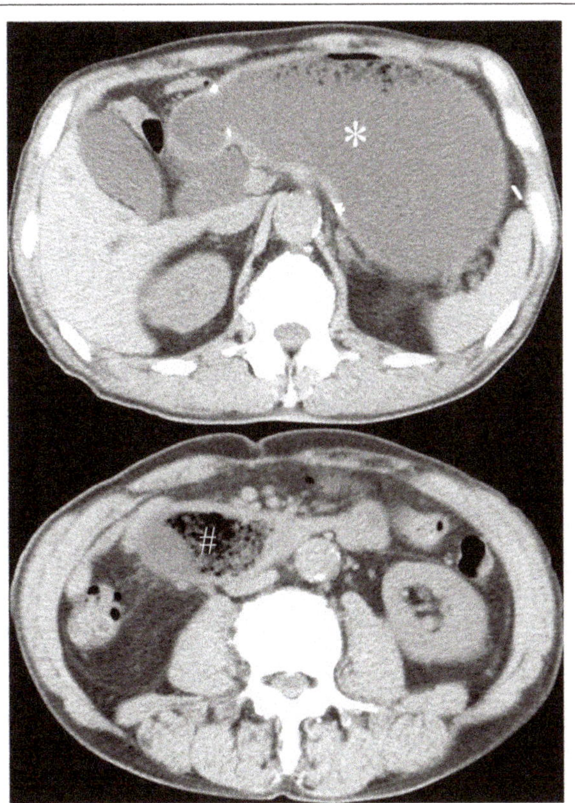

Fig. 1 Computed tomography (CT) on admission. CT revealed dilatation of the remnant stomach (*) and a bezoar in the third portion of the duodenum (#)

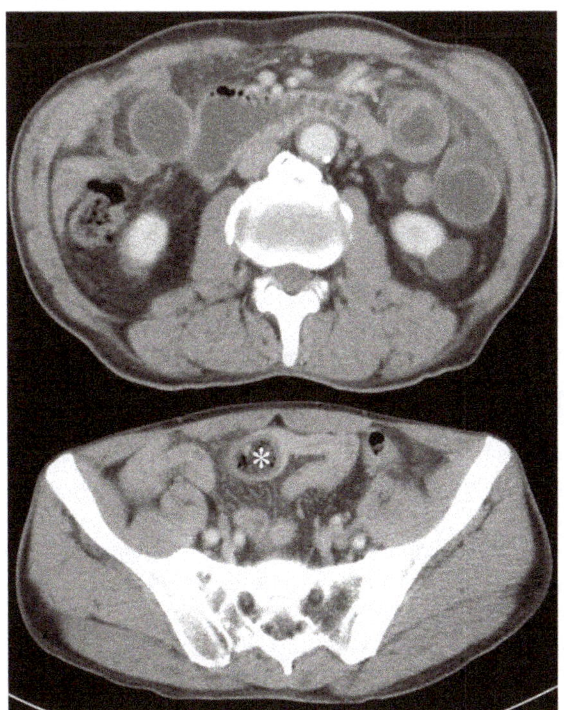

Fig. 3 Computed tomography performed the day after esophagogastroduodenoscopy. The bezoar had disappeared from the duodenum and moved through the ileum (*)

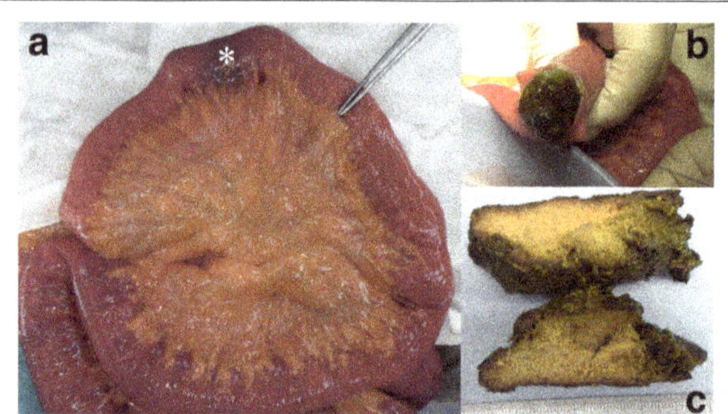

Fig. 4 Intraoperative findings and bezoar. **a** The bezoar (*) was observed in the ileum. **b** The ileum was incised and the bezoar was removed. **c** The bezoar was ocher, elastic, and hard, and its cross-section was uniform and orange

on the oral side of the bezoar, no perforation or necrosis was observed. We tried advancing the bezoar into the colon, but the ileum was too narrow; therefore, we incised the ileum and removed the bezoar (Fig. 4b). The bezoar was ocher, elastic, and hard, and its cross-section was uniform and orange (Fig. 4c). We found no abnormal duodenal findings on palpation. The postsurgical interview revealed that there was the tree of persimmon in the garden of his house and he loved eating Japanese persimmons (*Diospyros kaki*) and seemed to eat 30-40 persimmons in one season; therefore, a diospyrobezoar was diagnosed. His postoperative progress was good and without complications. He left the hospital 10 days after surgery. EGD performed 4 weeks after surgery revealed no abnormal duodenal findings.

Discussion and conclusions

Bezoars are solid masses of ingested foreign materials found in the lumen of the gastrointestinal tract and are named according to their composition, such as phytobezoars (food fibers), trichobezoars (hair), and pharmacobezoars (drugs) [14]. The diospyrobezoar is a type of phytobezoar caused by ingestion of persimmons (*Diospyros kaki*) [14]. Persimmons are rich in fiber and *shibuol*, which is a type of tannin [14]. When *shibuol* comes in contact with gastric juice, polymerization of the persimmon fiber occurs and contributes to the formation of diospyrobezoars [14].

Moreover, gastrectomy is associated with the formation of diospyrobezoars [14]. Gastrectomy may reduce the motion of the remnant stomach and delay gastric emptying, leading to easy formation of bezoars [14]. Our patient had a history of gastrectomy and loved to eat persimmons, and it was suggested that the diospyrobezoar formed in the remnant stomach or duodenum.

We searched for articles with 'duodenal obstruction' and 'bezoar' as keywords in PubMed, 93 articles were hit. Filtered 93 articles by the publication date (in this decade) and the language (English), 17 articles remained. In addition, excluded those of animals, duodenal obstruction due to trauma, other than duodenal obstruction and reviews, 10 articles remained [2–11]. In these 10 articles, there were 11 cases of duodenal obstruction caused by bezoar. Among these 11 cases, 2 cases were so-called Rapunzel Syndrome (caused by trichobezoar) [3, 4], 1 case was bezoar resulting from industrial material [8], and other 9 cases were phytobezoar [2, 5–7, 9–11]. The location of bezoars were as follows: 6 for first portion [3, 6, 7, 9–11], 2 for second portion [7, 8], 1 for third portion [2], 1 for diverticulum of the duodenum [5], and 1 for entire duodenum [4].

In our case, bezoar was located in the third portion of the duopdenum. Leanness due to gastrectomy causes superior mesenteric artery (SMA) syndrome, which involves compression of the third portion of the duodenum between the aorta and the SMA. The diospyrobezoar formed in the remnant stomach or in the duodenum, suggesting that it was caught in the third portion of the duodenum and suggesting SMA syndrome. Among previous 11 cases, only a case was similar to our case [2]. We searched furthermore articles for 'SMA syndrome' and 'bezoar', we could find only 2 articles [12, 13]. This case suggested to be rare.

As a treatment for trichobezoar, surgical methods, endoscopic methods (crushing, removal) and dissolution therapy by Coca-Cola are known. Dissolution therapy by Coca-Cola was introduced by Ladas et al. in 2002 [15]. Recent systematic review have shown that Coca-Cola therapy (alone or combined with endoscopic therapy) for trichobezoar was effective in 91.3% of the cases [16]. In our case, initially, the bezoar existed in the third portion of the duodenum, Coca-cola lavage therapy was considered to be difficult to implement. After the bezoar fell in the ileum, the patient had severe abdominal pain, and the conservative treatment considered ineffective. Hence we selected surgical treatment.

We describe an extremely rare case of obstruction in the third portion of the duodenum caused by a diospyrobezoar 15 months after laparoscopic distal gastrectomy with Billroth I reconstruction for early gastric cancer.

Abbreviations

CT: Computed tomography; D: Esophagogastroduodenoscopy; SMA: Superior mesenteric artery

Acknowledgments

Not applicable.

Funding

None.

Authors' contributions

All authors were involved in the management of the patient and in the conception of the manuscript. YY was involved in drafting the manuscript and its critical revision for important intellectual content. All authors have read and approved the final manuscript.

Competing interests

The authors declare that they have no competing interests.

References

1. Carbo AI, Sangster GP, Caraway J, Heldmann MG, Thomas J, Takalkar A. Acquired constricting and restricting lesions of the descending duodenum. Radiographics. 2014;34:1196–217.
2. Fan S, Wang J, Li Y. An unusual cause of duodenal obstruction: persimmon Phytobezoar. Indian J Surg. 2016;78:502–4.
3. Caiazzo P, Di Lascio P, Crocoli A, Del Prete I. The Rapunzel syndrome. Report of a case. G Chir. 2016;37:90–4.
4. Koushk Jalali B, Bingöl A, Reyad A. Laparoscopic Management of Acute Pancreatitis Secondary to Rapunzel syndrome. Case Rep Surg. 2016;2016:7638504.
5. Kim JH, Chang JH, Nam SM, Lee MJ, Maeng IH, Park JY, et al. Duodenal obstruction following acute pancreatitis caused by a large duodenal diverticular bezoar. World J Gastroenterol. 2012;18:5485–8.
6. Guner A, Kahraman I, Aktas A, Kece C, Reis E. Gastric outlet obstruction due to duodenal bezoar: a case report. Int J Surg Case Rep. 2012;3:523–5.
7. Chao HC, Chang KW, Wang CJ. Intestinal obstruction caused by potato bezoar in infancy: a report of three cases. Pediatr Neonatol. 2012;53:151–3.
8. Selcuk H, Unal H, Korkmaz M, Yilmaz U. Subacutely formed bezoar resulting from accidentally ingested industrial material. J Chin Med Assoc. 2009;72:202–3.
9. Hussain A, Mahmood H, Singhal T, El-Hasani S. An unusual cause of gastric outlet obstruction during percutaneous endogastric feeding: a case report. J Med Case Rep. 2008;2:199.
10. Singh SK, Marupaka SK. Duodenal date seed bezoar: a very unusual cause of partial gastric outlet obstruction. Australas Radiol. 2007;51:126–9.
11. Chiu HH, Li JH. Gastric outlet obstruction caused by a dumbbell-shaped phytobezoar impacted in a deformed duodenal bulb. Gastrointest Endosc. 2007;65:322–3.
12. Doski JJ, Priebe CJ Jr, Smith T, Chumas JC. Duodenal trichobezoar caused by compression of the superior mesenteric artery. J Pediatr Surg. 1995;30:1598–9.
13. Fuhrman MA, Felig DM, Tanchel ME. Superior mesenteric artery syndrome with obstructing duodenal bezoar. Gastrointest Endosc. 2003;57:387.
14. de Toledo AP, Rodrigues FH, Rodrigues MR, Sato DT, Nonose R, Nascimento EF, et al. Diospyrobezoar as a cause of small bowel obstruction. Case Rep Gastroenterol. 2012;6:596–603.
15. Ladas SD, Triantafyllou K, Tzathas C, Tassios P, Rokkas T, Raptis SA. Gastric phytobezoars may be treated by nasogastric Coca-Cola lavage. Eur J Gastroenterol Hepatol. 2002;14:801–3.
16. Ladas SD, Kamberoglou D, Karamanolis G, Vlachogiannakos J, Zouboulis-Vafiadis I. Systematic review: Coca-Cola can effectively dissolve gastric phytobezoars as a first-line treatment. Aliment Pharmacol Ther. 2013;37:169–73.

25

Gastrointestinal schwannomas: a rare but important differential diagnosis of mesenchymal tumors of gastrointestinal tract

Alexandros Mekras[2], Veit Krenn[3], Aristotelis Perrakis[1], Roland S Croner[1], Vasileios Kalles[2], Cem Atamer[2], Robert Grützmann[1] and Nikolaos Vassos[1*]

Abstract

Background: Schwannomas of gastrointestinal tract are rare, mostly benign and notably different neoplasms from conventional schwannomas that arise in soft tissue or the central nervous system. These tumors are of clinical importance since they should always be considered in the differential diagnosis of submucosal lesions of gastrointestinal tract.

Methods: Seven patients with a pathologically proven gastrointestinal schwannoma were identified in our series of mesenchymal tumors and reviewed retrospectively. Clinicopathological and immunohistochemical parameters along with the follow-up results were analysed.

Results: The series included two males and five females, with a mean age 69 years (range, 39–81). Most patients were asymptomatic on presentation, except for two patients with abdominal pain. In the other cases ($n = 5$), the tumor was an incidental finding during other medical, imaging or surgical procedures. The tumors were located in the stomach ($n = 4$) and in the small intestine ($n = 3$) with an average size of 29 mm (range, 12–70). A preoperative diagnosis was achieved only in one case with a CT-guided core biopsy. Otherwise the clinical, intraoperative, endoscopic or radiological findings were unspecific. Patients with gastric tumor underwent either laparoscopic ($n = 2$) or open ($n = 2$) gastric wedge resection of the tumor; in the cases of intestinal tumor ($n = 3$) a segmentectomy was performed. Pathological examination revealed solid homogenous tumors, which were highly cellular and composed of spindle cells with positive staining for S100 protein, and confirmed the diagnosis of schwannoma. All tumors were negative for c-Kit, smooth muscle actin, desmin and DOG-1 and showed very low proliferation index. There were negative resection margins and no malignant variants were recognized. At an average follow-up of 60 months (range, 24–185) all patients were free of disease with no signs of recurrence or metastases and acceptable gastrointestinal function.

Conclusions: Schwannomas are rare, slow-growing and mostly asymptomatic gastrointestinal mesenchymal tumors. They are difficult to be diagnosed preoperatively as endoscopic and radiological findings are nonspecific but histological and immunohistochemical features are of paramount importance to differentiate between benign and malignant schwannomas, or other spindle cell sarcomas. The treatment of choice is complete surgical excision without a conclusive preoperative diagnosis, and the long-term outcome is excellent as these lesions are mostly benign.

Keywords: Schwannoma, Gastrointestinal, Mesenchymal tumor

* Correspondence: nikolaos.vassos@uk-erlangen.de
[1]Department of Surgery, University Hospital Erlangen, Krankenhausstrasse 12, 91054 Erlangen, Germany
Full list of author information is available at the end of the article

Background

Schwannomas are slow-growing, homogeneous, mostly benign tumors arising from the schwann cells of the nerve sheath [1, 2]. They are most commonly found in the cranial vault including the myelin-forming cells of the 8th cranial nerve [1, 3]. They can rarely occur in the gastrointestinal (GI) tract, representing about 2–6% of all mesenchymal tumors [4]. The most common site (60–70% of all GI cases) is the stomach, followed by the colon and rectum (3%) [5–10]. Small-intestinal and esophageal schwannomas have been very rarely reported [7].

Schwannomas of the GI tract, firstly presented by Daimaru et al. in 1988 [11], are usually benign and notably different neoplasms from conventional schwannomas that arise in the soft tissue or the central nervous system [7]. They are classified under a heterogeneous group of mesenchymal or neuroectodermal neoplasms which arise from the wall of the gastrointestinal tract and include schwannomas, gastrointestinal stromal tumors (GIST), leiomyomas, leiomyosarcomas, neurofibromas, lipomas, ganglioneuromas, paragangliomas, granular cell tumors, and glomus tumors [7]. The GI schwannomas are most frequently asymptomatic presenting as submucosal lesions, usually detected incidentally during a laparoscopy / laparotomy, esophagogastroduodenoscopy (EGD), endoscopic ultrasonography (EUS) or at imaging [6, 7]. A preoperative diagnosis of schwannomas cannot always be carried out with high accuracy and the diagnosis is established by the pathological examination of the surgical specimen [5].

The purpose of our study was the description of clinical, histopathological and immunohistochemical features of GI schwannomas, providing long-term follow-up and confirming the benign nature of these tumors.

Methods

Seven patients with histologically identified GI schwannoma during a 10 year period, were involved in this retrospective study. Clinical, histopathological, immunohistochemical and surgical data were reviewed. A complete surgical excision of the tumors was performed in all patients. Specimens were obtained from all patients. The diagnosis of GI schwannomas was based on histopathological analysis accompanied by immunohistochemical staining performed for S-100 protein, glial fibrillary acidic protein (GFAP), c-kit (CD117), CD34, discovered on GIST-1 (DOG-1), smooth muscle actin (SMA) and desmin. The patients were regularly followed up on an outpatient basis. Follow-up included physical examination, blood counts, serum chemistries, endoscopy and computed tomography (CT)-scan. Median follow-up was 60 months (range, 24–185).

Results

Clinical features and preoperative evaluation

The demographic and clinicopathologic data of our patients are summarized in Table 1. Five women and two men, with a median age of 69 years (range, 39–81) were diagnosed with a schwannoma of the GI tract. The tumor was localized to the stomach in four patients ($n = 4$) and in the small intestine in three patients ($n = 3$), with a median tumor size of 29 mm (range, 12–70). Out of the four gastric schwannomas, two were localized in the gastric body and two in the antrum. Symptoms were reported in only one patient with gastric schwannoma who complained of persistent epigastric pain and nausea. In six cases the tumor was an incidental finding during imaging, endoscopic or surgical procedures for other reason. Particularly the tumors were incidentally discovered during surgery for colon carcinoma (case Nr. 1) and diverticulitis of sigmoid (case Nr. 3, 4), during an abdominal ultrasound as preventative measure (case Nr. 2) and during a upper GI gastroscopy performed as preventative measure as well (case Nr. 5). Furthermore, in the seventh patient, the tumor was an incidental finding on a thoracic CT scan performed for evaluation of hemoptysis. CT scan

Table 1 Demographical and clinicopathological data of our cases with GI schwannomas

Case	Age/ Sex	Presentation	Location	Operation	Size/ mm	Follow up
1	73/F	Incidental finding during operation	Gastric body	Gastric wedge resection	25	DF/ 185 m
2	70/F	Incidental finding during routine US	Duodenum	Local tumor resection	22	DF/ 90 m
3	72/F	Incidental fining during operation	Ileum	Small bowel segmentectomy	70	DF/ 42 m
4	81/M	Incidental finding during operation	Jejunum	Small bowel segmentectomy	12	DF/ 21 m
5	72/M	Incidental finding during upper GI endoscopy	Antrum	Gastric wedge resection	16	DF /21 m
6	77/F	Epigastric pain/ upper GI endoscopy	Antrum (greater curvature)	Laparoscopic gastric wedge resection	15	DF/ 20 m
7	39/F	Incidental finding during thoracic CT	Gastric body (lesser curvature)	Laparoscopic gastric wedge resection	25	DF/ 24 m

M Male, *F* Female, *DF* Disease Free, *m* months, *US* Ultrasound, GI Gastrointestinal revealed a round homogeneous mass with contrast enhancement and a predominantly exophytic pattern arising from the lesser curvature of stomach (Fig. 1a, b). None of the patients had a history of neurofibromatosis.

An upper gastrointestinal endoscopy was carried out in 3/4 of the cases with gastric schwannoma, which demonstrated submucosal gastric tumors with smooth overlying mucosa and without any ulceration (Fig. 1c), ranging from 12.5 mm to 25 mm. For further diagnostic evaluation, in two of the gastric cases an EUS was performed, in which a heterogeneous hypoechoic submucosal tumor arising from the muscularis propria of the stomach was demonstrated (Fig. 1d). Biopsy was attempted but it was nondiagnostic, suggesting mostly a stromal tumor with nonspecific spindle cells. A preoperative diagnosis of schwannoma was obtained only in one case (small intestine schwannoma) with a CT-guided needle biopsy, which was performed because of the adherence of tumor with the pancreas and its unclear entity (case Nr. 3).

Surgical, histopathological and immunochemical features

All patients underwent a tumor resection with negative resection margins (R0). Patients with gastric schwannomas ($n = 4$) underwent a gastric wedge resection by using either an open ($n = 2$) or a laparoscopic approach ($n = 2$) (Fig. 1e-g). In both laparoscopic cases the exophytic mass was located along the lesser and the greater curvature of the stomach and was easily detected and

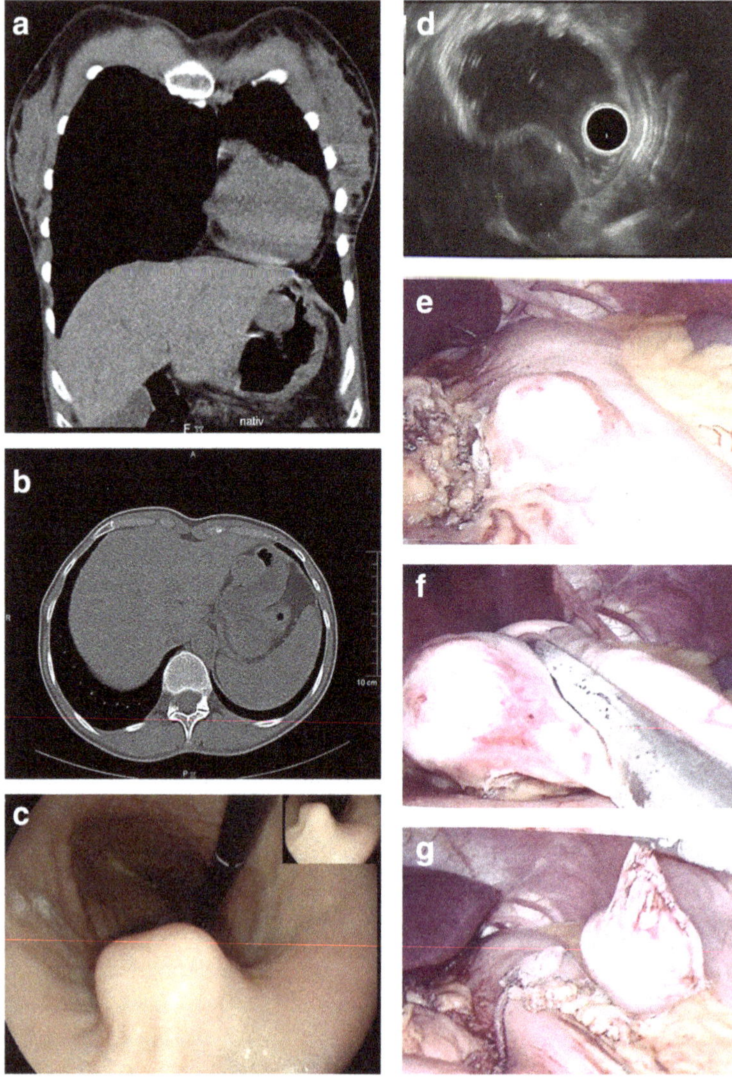

Fig. 1 a, b. Incidental contrast-enhanced computed tomography (CT) finding shows a round, exophytic, well-defined, homogeneous mass (30 mm) with contrast enhancement, arising from the lesser curvature of the gastric body. **c** GI endoscopy submucosal mass (26 mm × 22 mm) with smooth overlying normal mucosa in the lesser curvature of the gastric body. **d** EUS picture showing a hypoechoic lesion located within the muscularis propria. **e** Laparoscopic intraoperative picture of an exophytic mass along the lesser curvature of the body of the stomach. **f, g** Laparoscopic tumor wedge resection using mechanical laparoscopic sutures

clearly identified by the laparoscope. Patients with intestinal schwannomas ($n = 3$) received a small bowel segmentectomy (segmental resection). The median tumor size was 26.5 mm (range, 12–70 mm). Neither morbidity nor mortality was observed in our series.

The histopathologic diagnosis of schwannoma was confirmed in all patients. Pathological examination demonstrated the GI schwannomas to be solid homogenous tumors, which were highly cellular and composed of spindle cells. No areas of cystic change of gross necrosis were reported in any of the cases. Mitotic activity was very low (< 5/50 high power fields). All specimens demonstrated strong positive immunostaining for S-100 and GFAP proteins, whereas the tumor cells were not immunoreactive to DOG1, c-Kit (CD117), CD34, SMA and desmin (Fig. 2).

Follow-up

Median follow-up was 60 months (range, 24–185). During the follow-up period no recurrence was detected. Furthermore no excessive body weight loss and no gastrointestinal symptoms such as dyspepsia and bloating were observed.

Discussion

Gastrointestinal schwannomas are rare mesenchymal tumors [5–7], firstly reported by Daimaru, who identified a schwannoma as a primary GI tumor entity based on the positive S-100 immunostaining [11]. They represent ca. 2 to 6% of all mesenchymal tumours of the GI tract [4, 12, 13]. They are of clinical importance since GI schwannomas are notably different neoplasms from conventional soft-tissue and central nervous system schwannomas, some of which may be associated with neurofibromatosis 2.

In terms of pathologic evaluation, GI schwannomas are classified as non-epithelial tumours, and represent a separate, homogenous entity, distinct from leiomyomas, leiomyosarcomas, gastrointestinal autonomic nerve tumors (GANTs) and GISTs [12, 14, 15]. They can be identified in every part of the GI tract but they occur predominantly in stomach. The second most common site seems is colon, whereas schwannomas located to small intestine or esophagus are rare [5–9, 16, 17].

Our series shows a remarkable regularity regarding to the characteristics of GI-schwannomas. They occur more frequently in the sixth decade of life and there is a predominance of females [11, 12, 15, 17–21]. Our results showed that all of our patients except one woman (39 years-old), were over 70 years of age at the time of diagnosis. These tumors do not usually cause any symptoms and can be found out incidentally, as presented in our series. However, when symptomatic, they represent with unspecific clinical symptoms, and particularly

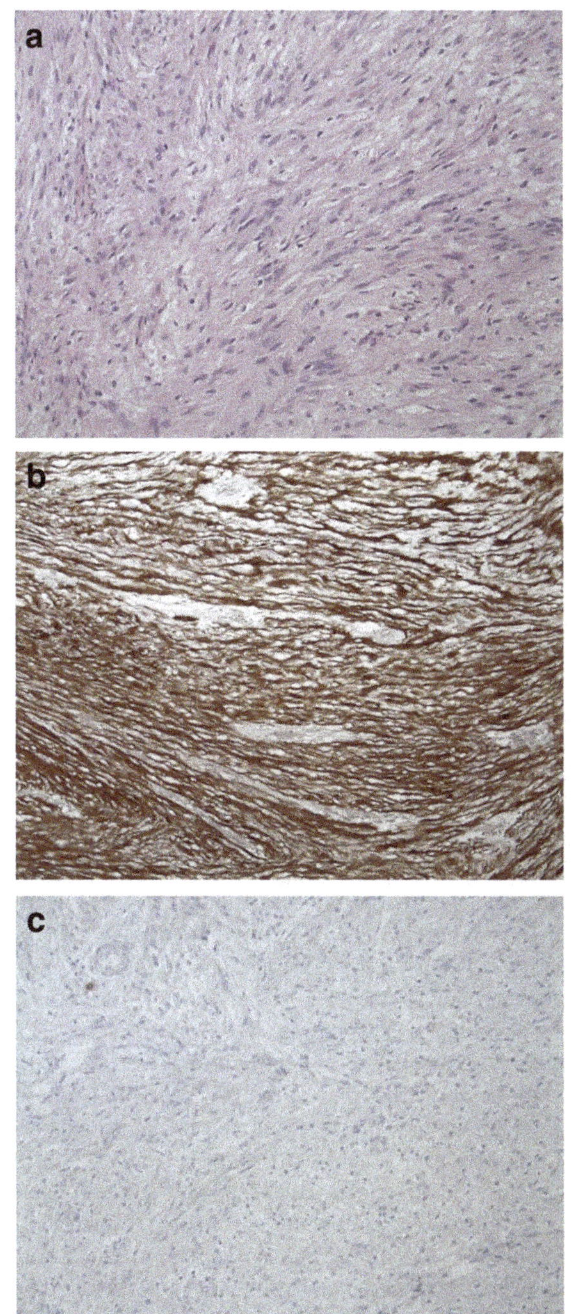

Fig. 2 Representative illustrations from GI schwannoma cases. **a** The tumor cells are spindle shaped with elongated nuclei and form loose interlacing fascicles or whorls (HE, original magnification × 250). **b** Intense expression of S100 immunostain in tumor cells (DAB magnification × 250). c CD117 absence of staining in tumor population (DAB magnification × 250)

Bruneton et al. reported that most common symptoms of these patients are bleeding and abdominal pain [22].

A preoperative diagnosis of GI schwannomas is generally difficult and challenging, if not impossible, since the tumor have no specific clinical symptoms and no diagnostic modality can show any pathognomonic features unique to this tumor [22]. On CT examination, these tumors mostly represent as exophytic masses displaying homogeneous enhancement in most cases whereas cystic change, cavity formation, necrosis or calcification are uncommon [7, 16, 24]. Our CT findings were comparable to previous reports in terms of enhancement patterns and growth patterns. On endoscopy, gastric schwannomas appear grossly as elevated submucosal lesions, and a central ulcer can be seen in 25–50% due to ischemic changes in the covering mucosa [16, 25]. It should be noted that there is an important false-negative rate of endoscopic biopsy diagnosis because of normal mucosa overlying a submucosal lesion [22]. Therefore, endoscopic biopsy is supposed to be not as effective as expected in the diagnosis of gastric schwannomas, since the results mostly demonstrate nonspecific spindle cells. EUS-guided fine needle aspiration (FNA) biopsies of submucosal lesions in the upper GI tract can be helpful in preoperative diagnosis of spindle cell tumors but are sometimes not representative of deeper submucosal tissue [25–29]. Two patients with gastric schwannomas underwent an EUS-guided FNA without representative findings. However, in one case (case Nr. 3) a CT-guided biopsy of a 2.2 cm mass of duodenum was performed and detected a GI schwannoma. Generally, the CT and endoscopic findings in our patients were similar to those from previous studies as far as the location and mucosal change.

GI-schwannomas are supposed to arise from the myenteric plexus of the GI wall because of their immunophenotypic similarities; both schwannomas and myenteric plexus cells express S-100 protein and GFAP [7, 11]. Pathologically, GI schwannomas are considered to be notably different tumors from conventional schwannomas, which arise from central nervous system and soft tissues [7, 21]. Macroscopically, these tumors are round or fusiform and their cut surface reveals smooth, glistening, grey-white appearance. Microscopically, unlike conventional schwannomas, GI schwannomas are not always encapsulated, but mostly well circumscribed. Cystic areas of hemorrhage and calcification may be present. These tumors are composed of uniformly spindled schwann cells arranged in a interlacing fascicles, often with germical centers [4, 21].

The pathologic findings of the GI schwannomas in the present analysis were consistent with the previously described findings. On immunohistochemistry, vimentin, GFAP and S100 protein are diffusely and strongly expressed by the cells of GI schwannomas [21]; the S100 immunostaining pattern is both in a nuclear and cytoplasmic distribution [4]. Expression of CD34 is rare, whereas there is lack of CD117, SMA and desmin positivity [30]. This immunohistochemical pattern is very important because it can differentiate GI schwannomas from other GI tract mesenchymal neoplasms.

The main differential diagnosis for an exophytic lesion arising in the wall of the GI tract is a GIST, as it is the most common mesenchymal tumor located in GI tract [7, 31, 32]. Voltaggio et al. estimated that the ratio of gastric GIST to gastric schwannoma is approximately 45 to 1 [33]. Some other smaller studies have shown lower gastric GIST frequencies (8-14 to 1) in relation to schwannoma [11, 19]. In these cases, immunohistochemistry is extremely helpful. Another tumor entity included in the differential diagnostic of GI schwannomas is the primary and secondary lymphomas because of their similar CT appearance to schwannomas. Both of them arise from the GI wall and tend to appear as a homogeneous mass in CT. However, the presence of adenopathy in most of lymphomas, in contrast to GI schwannomas, is an important distinguishing feature [7]. Other entities included in the differential diagnosis are GI variant of clear cell sarcoma, metastatic malignant melanoma and GI adenocarcinoma [7, 34].

Schwannomas of the GI tract are generally benign since previous follow-up studies have not identified any malignant variants [4, 9, 11, 19–21]. Therefore, pathologic parameters such as tumor size and mitotic rate seem not to have any prognostic significance. The complete surgical resection seems to be the treatment of choice because of the preoperative diagnostic uncertainty and the excellent long-term outcome, as these tumors are uniformly benign [23, 35]. Tumor recurrence is generally associated with an incomplete surgical margin. The outcome after surgical resection in our study was excellent with no malignant variant and no recurrences or metastases. However, a very few cases of gastric malignant schwannomas have been reported in the literature [25, 36, 37]. Malignant GI schwannomas are extremely rare and they cannot be distinguished from benign schwannomas only on the basis of the histopathological examination of the resected specimens. Furthermore, cases of "malignant schwannomas" also called malignant peripheral nerve sheath tumors have been reported [38]. These malignant tumors with neural differentiation are considered to be distinct tumors from GI schwannomas and are called gastrointestinal autonomic nerve tumors (GANTs) [38]. The usefulness of molecular therapy for gastric malignant schwannomas is not clearly established because only a few cases have been reported. Further molecular therapy studies will be useful in order to determine its role in the treatment of GI malignant schwannoma.

Conclusions

Schwannomas are rare, slow-growing and mostly asymptomatic gastrointestinal mesenchymal tumors, notably different from conventional soft-tissue and central nervous system schwannomas. They present a challenge in GI tract surgical oncology due to difficulty in the preoperative diagnosis, as the clinical, endoscopic and imaging findings are nonspecific. The definitive diagnosis can only be established through the histopathological and immunohistochemical examination, which is confirmatory. Complete surgical excision is the gold standard in the treatment of schwannomas and the prognosis of patients is excellent since these lesions are mostly benign.

Abbreviations

CT: Computed tomography; DOG-1: Discovered on GIST-1; EGD : Esophagogastroduodenoscopy; EUS : Endoscopic ultrasonography; FNA: Fine needle aspiration; GANT: Gastrointestinal autonomic nerve tumors; GFAP: Glial fibrillary acidic protein; GI: Gastrointestinal; GIST: Gastrointestinal stromal tumor; SMA: Smooth muscle actin

Authors' contributions

AM made the literature research, participated in the design of the study, collected and analysed the data, wrote the manuscript, and evaluated critically the manuscript. VKrenn participated in the design of the study, assisted in drafting the manuscript and evaluated critically the manuscript. AP participated in the design of the study and evaluated critically the manuscript. RSC participated in the design of the study and evaluated critically the manuscript. VKalles participated in the design of the study and evaluated critically the manuscript. CA participated in the design of the study and evaluated critically the manuscript. RG participated in the design of the study, assisted in drafting the manuscript and evaluated critically the manuscript. NV made the literature research, participated in the design of the study, collected and analysed the data, participated in the writing of the manuscript, and evaluated critically the manuscript. All authors read and approved the final manuscript.

Competing interests

The authors declare that they have no competing interests.

Author details

[1]Department of Surgery, University Hospital Erlangen, Krankenhausstrasse 12, 91054 Erlangen, Germany. [2]Department of Surgery, S. Elisabeth Hospital, Bernkastel/Wittlich, Germany. [3]MVZ-Zentrum für Histologie, Zytologie und Molekulare Diagnostik, Trier, Germany.

References

1. Mark X. Gastric schwannoma: a rare schwann cell tumour of the GI tract. Univ West Ont Med J. 2011;80(S1):14–6.
2. Raber MH, Ziedses d, Plantes CM, Vink R, et al. Gastric schwannoma presenting as an incidentaloma on CT-scan and MRI. Gastroenterology Res. 2010;3:276–80.
3. Darrouzet V, Martel J, Enee V, et al. Vestibular schwannoma surgery outcomes: our multidisciplinary experience in 400 cases over 17 years. Laryngoscope. 2004;114:681–8.
4. Hou YY, Tan YS, Xu JF, et al. Schwannoma of the gastrointestinal tract: a clinicopathological, immunohistochemical and ultrastructural study of 33 cases. Histopathology. 2006;48:536–45.
5. Oh SJ, Suh BJ, Park JK. Gastric schwannoma mimicking malignant gastrointestinal stromal tumor exhibiting increased fluorodeoxyglucose uptake. Case Rep Oncol. 2016;9:228–34.
6. Zheng L, Wu X, Kreis ME, et al. Clinicopathological and immunohistochemical characterisation of gastric schwannomas in 29 cases. Gastroenterol Res Pract. 2014;2014:202960.
7. Levy AD, Quiles AM, Miettinen M, et al. Gastrointestinal schwannomas: CT features with clinicopathologic correlation. AJR Am J Roentgenol. 2005;184:797–802.
8. Tashiro Y, Matsumoto F, Iwama K, et al. Laparoscopic resection of schwannoma of the ascending colon. Case Rep Gastroenterol. 2015;9:15–9.
9. Miettinen M, Shekitka KM, Sobin LH. Schwannomas in the colon and rectum: a clinicopathologic and immunohistochemical study of 20 cases. Am J Surg Pathol. 2001;25:846–55.
10. Zhang K, Qu S, Cheng Y, et al. A case report of rectal schwannoma treated with laparoscopic proctectomy. Medicine (Baltimore). 2018;97:e9866.
11. Daimaru Y, Kido H, Hashimoto H, et al. Benign schwannoma of the gastrointestinal tract: a clinicopathologic and immunohistochemical study. Hum Pathol. 1988;19:257–64.
12. Wilde BK, Senger JL, Kanthan R. Gastrointestinal schwannoma: an unusual colonic lesion mimicking adenocarcinoma. Can J Gastroenterol. 2010;24:233–6.
13. Inagawa S, Hori M, Shimazaki J, et al. Solitary schwannoma of the colon: report of two cases. Surg Today. 2001;31:833–8.
14. Yoon W, Paulson K, Mazzara P, et al. Gastric schwannoma: a rare but important differential diagnosis of a gastric submucosal mass. Case Rep Surg. 2012;2012:280–2.
15. Miettinen M, Blay JY, Sobin LH. Mesenchymal tumours of the stomach. In: Hamilton SR, Aaltonen LA, editors. Pathology and genetics Tumours of the digestive system. Lyon: IARC Press; 2000. p. 62–5.
16. Hong HS, Ha HK, Won HJ, et al. Gastric schwannomas: radiological features with endoscopic and pathological correlation. Clin Radiol. 2008;63:536–42.
17. Melvin WS, Wilkinson MG. Gastric schwannoma: clinical and pathological conditions. Am Surg. 1993;59:293–6.
18. Matsuki A, Kosugi S, Kanda T, et al. Schwannoma of the esophagus: a case exhibiting high 18F-fluorodeoxyglucose uptake in positron emission tomography imaging. Dis Esophagus. 2009;22:E6–E10.
19. Sarlomo-Rikala M, Miettinen M. Gastric schwannoma: a clinicopathological analysis of six cases. Histopathology. 1995;27:355–60.
20. Prevot S, Bienvenu L, Vaillant JC, et al. Benign schwannoma of the digestive tract: a clinicopathologic and immunohistochemical study of five cases, including a case of esophageal tumor. Am J Surg Pathol. 1999;23:431–6.
21. Kwon MS, Lee SS, Ahn GH. Schwannomas of the gastrointestinal tract: clinicopathological features of 12 cases including a case of esophageal tumor compared with those of gastrointestinal stromal tumors and leiomyomas of the gastrointestinal tract. Pathol Res Pract. 2002;198:605–13.
22. Bruneton JN, Drouillard J, Roux P, et al. Neurogenic tumors of the stomach. Report of 18 cases and review of the literature. Rofo. 1983;139:192–8.
23. Goh BK, Chow PK, Kesavan S, et al. Intraabdominal schwannomas: a single institution experience. J Gastrointest Surg. 2008;12:756–60.
24. He MY, Zhang R, Peng Z, et al. Differentiation between gastrointestinal schwannomas and gastrointestinal stromal tumors by computed tomography. Oncol Lett. 2017;13:3746–52.
25. Takemura M, Yoshida K, Takkii M, et al. Gastric malignant schwannoma presenting with upper gastrointestinal bleeding: a case report. J Med Case Rep. 2012;6:37.
26. Hoda KM, Rodriguez SA, Faigel DO. EUS-guided sampling of suspected GI stromal tumors. Gastrointest Endosc. 2009;69:1218–23.
27. Mekky MA, Yamao K, Sawaki A, et al. Diagnostic utility of EUS-guided FNA in patients with gastric submucosal tumors. Gastrointest Endosc. 2010;71:913–9.
28. Yoon JM, Kim GH, Park DY, et al. Endosonographic features of gastric schwannoma: a single center experience. Clin Endosc. 2016;49:548–54.
29. Takasumi M, Hikichi T, Takaqi T, et al. Efficacy of endoscopic ultrasound-guided fine-needle aspiration for schwannoma: six cases of a retrospective study. Fukushima J Med Sci. 2017;63:75–80.
30. Miettinen M, Virolainen M, Rikala MS. Gastrointestinal stromal tumors - value of CD34 antigen in their identification and separation from true leiomyomas and schwannomas. Am J Surg Pathol. 1995;19:207–16.
31. Hu BG, Wu FJ, Zhu J, et al. Gastric schwannoma: a tumor must be included in differential diagnosis of gastric submucosal tumors. Case Rep Gastrointest Med. 2017;2017:9615359.
32. Sunkara T, Then EO, Reddy M, et al. Gastric schwannoma - a rare benign mimic of gastrointestinal stromal tumor. Oxf Med Case Reports. 2018; 2018(3):omy002.

33. Voltaggio L, Murra R, Lasota J, et al. Gastric schwannoma: a clinicopathological study of 51 cases and critical review of the literature. Hum Pathol. 2012;43:650–9.
34. Stockman DL, Miettinen M, Spagnolo D, et al. Clinicopathological, immunohistochemical, ultrastructural and molecular analysis of clear cell sarcoma (CCS)-like tumor of the gastrointestinal tract. Abstract Mod Pathol. 2011;21A:23.
35. Hu J, Liu X, Ge N, et al. Role of endoscopic ultrasound and endoscopic resection for the treatment of gastric schwannoma. Medicine (Baltimore). 2017;96:e7175.
36. Loffeld RJ, Balk TG, Oomen JL, et al. Upper gastrointestinal bleeding due to a malignant schwannoma of the stomach. Eur J Gastroenterol Hepatol. 1998;10:159–62.
37. Bees NR, Ng CS, Dicks-Mireaux C, et al. Gastric malignant schwannoma in a child. Br J Radiol. 1997;70:952–5.
38. Agaimy A, Märkl B, Kitz J, et al. Peripheral nerve sheath tumors of the gastrointestinal tract: a multicenter study of 58 patients including NF-1 associated gastric schwannoma and unusual morphological variants. Virchows Arch. 2010;456:411–22.

Comparison of the surgical outcomes of minimally invasive and open surgery for octogenarian and older compared to younger gastric cancer patients: a retrospective cohort study

Chien-An Liu[1,5], Kuo-Hung Huang[2,5,6], Ming-Huang Chen[3,5], Su-Shun Lo[5,7], Anna Fen-Yau Li[4,5], Chew-Wun Wu[2,5], Yi-Ming Shyr[2,5] and Wen-Liang Fang[2,5*]

Abstract

Background: As life expectancy continues to increase around the world, the use of minimally invasive surgery (MIS) could be beneficial for octogenarian and older gastric cancer patients.

Methods: A total of 359 gastric cancer patients who underwent curative surgery between March 2011 and March 2015 were enrolled; 80 of these patients (22.2%) were octogenarians and older. Surgical approaches included MIS (50 laparoscopic and 65 robotic) and open surgery (n = 244). Surgical outcomes of MIS and open surgery in octogenarian and older patients were compared with younger patients.

Results: Among octogenarian and older patients, relative to open surgery (n = 53), MIS (n = 27) was associated with less operative blood loss, a shorter postoperative hospital stay and similar rates of surgical complications and mortality. For MIS (n = 115), octogenarian and older patients exhibited similar postoperative outcomes to those of younger patients. For open surgery (n = 244), relative to younger patients, octogenarian and older patients experienced longer postoperative hospital stays, a higher rate of wound infection and a higher incidence of pneumonia.

Conclusions: MIS for gastric cancer is beneficial and can be performed safely in octogenarian and older patients.

Keywords: Minimally invasive surgery, Open surgery, Octogenarian and older, Gastric cancer

Background

As life expectancy continues to increase around the world, the proportion of octogenarian and older patients who undergo gastrectomies for gastric cancer is also increasing. Advanced age is frequently associated with significant comorbidity and a limited functional reserve; given these characteristics, octogenarian and older patients generally exhibit higher rates of complications and longer hospital stays than younger patients.

Advantages of minimally invasive surgery (MIS) relative to open surgery include less wound pain, earlier functional recovery and shorter hospital stay [1–3]. Surgical treatment is the only known approach for curing gastric cancer. The advantages of MIS might cause octogenarian and older patients with high risks of operative morbidity and mortality to become more willing to receive surgery instead of strictly conservative treatment.

To date, only one study has compared MIS with open surgery for octogenarian and older gastric cancer patients [4]. In that series, relative to open surgery, MIS was associated with significantly less blood loss, lower analgesic consumption, faster time to first flatus and a soft diet, and a shorter postoperative hospital stay.

* Correspondence: s821094@hotmail.com
[2]Division of General Surgery, Department of Surgery, Taipei Veterans General Hospital, No. 201, Sec. 2, Shipai Rd., Beitou District, Taipei City 11217, Taiwan
[5]School of Medicine, National Yang-Ming University, Taipei City, Taiwan
Full list of author information is available at the end of the article

Therefore, MIS for gastric cancer may be performed safely in octogenarian and older patients; in this context, MIS continues to exhibit the advantages associated with minimal invasiveness.

The aim of this study was to compare the outcomes of MIS and open surgery for octogenarian and older compared to younger gastric cancer patients, in terms of mortality, complication rate, blood loss and hospital stay.

Methods

Between March 2011 and March 2015, a total of 359 gastric cancer patients were enrolled in this study. All consecutive patients were treated for gastric cancer in our institution. The current study was approved by the institutional review board of Taipei Veterans General Hospital. Pathological stages were determined in accordance with the 7th edition of the classification guidelines issued by the American Joint Committee on Cancer [5].

All the operations were performed by surgeons who specialized in gastric cancer. We retrospectively reviewed our gastric cancer database that was prospectively collected and regularly updated using a computer. Prior to surgery, all patients underwent chest radiography, abdominal sonography, or a CT scan for tumor staging. The patients were evaluated on the basis of their gender, age, tumor size, tumor location, operative methods, pathological tumor and lymph node stage, lymphovascular invasion, comorbidities, stromal reaction type and gross appearance.

Most of the patients received continuous intravenous or epidural injection of mixed analgesics for 3–4 days after surgery. Water was started on postoperative day 3 or day 4, and a soft diet was started on postoperative day 5 to day 7. The patient was discharged if no complication occurred.

Indication for open and minimally invasive (laparoscopic or robotic) gastrectomy

At our hospital, the indications for laparoscopic or robotic gastrectomy are the same, which is gastric cancer at a less advanced clinical stage than T3N1M0. Patients who had a history of gastric surgery or were referred to gastrointestinal endoscopists for endoscopic mucosal resection or endoscopic submucosal dissection were excluded from this study.

Compared with laparoscopic or robotic gastrectomy, the indication of open surgery is not limited to the clinical stage. No matter what stage the cancer is at, patients who are diagnosed as gastric cancer can choose open surgery of their own will.

The surgeons comprehensively explained the advantages and disadvantages of the three possible surgical approaches to each patient prior to surgery. After receiving this explanation, patients decided which surgical approach would be utilized and provided written informed consent.

A total or distal subtotal gastrectomy is performed, depending on the distance between the cardia and the tumor. A margin of 3 cm is needed for superficial and well defined tumors; a margin of 5 cm is needed for advanced or poorly defined tumors. A subtotal gastrectomy is the standard procedure for distal gastric cancer, whereas a total gastrectomy is the more common procedure for proximal gastric cancer.

All patients were subjected to gastrectomy with at least D1 + α (perigastric lymph nodes + No. 7 lymph nodes) or D1 + β (perigastric lymph nodes + Nos. 7, 8, 9 lymph nodes) for early gastric cancer and D2 lymphadenectomy for advanced gastric cancer.

Statistical analysis

Statistical analysis was conducted using IBM SPSS Statistics V22.0. The chi-square test was used to compare categorical variables between groups, while the independent Student's t-test was used to evaluate the difference in continuous variables between the minimally invasive surgery group and the open surgery group. The one-way analysis of variance (ANOVA) was used to determine whether there are any statistically significant differences in the continuous variables between the three different age groups. P values less than 0.05 were considered to be statistically significant.

Results

A total of 359 gastric cancer patients who received curative resection in our institution were enrolled in this study. In particular, 80 patients (22.3%) were octogenarian or older, 167 patients (46.5%) were 60–79 years of age, and 112 patients (31.2%) were younger than 60 years of age. Among the 359 patients, 115 patients (32%) underwent MIS and 244 patients (68%) underwent open surgery.

Surgical mortality occurred in two cases, both of which involved open surgery. In particular, an 81-year-old male patient who underwent total gastrectomy died of aspiration pneumonia. In addition, a 78-year old female patient who received total gastrectomy experienced esophagojejunostomy leakage and peritonitis. She underwent an exploratory laparotomy, multiple drainage procedures and esophageal stent implantation; but eventually died of sepsis and multiple organ failure.

Octogenarian and older patients

As indicated in Table 1, among the 80 octogenarian and older patients, a comparison of MIS and open surgery indicated that MIS was associated with higher BMI (24.4 ± 3.1 vs. 22.7 ± 3.5, P = 0.032), more subtotal

Table 1 Comparison of the clinicopathological differences between minimally invasive gastrectomy and open gastrectomy for octogenarian and older gastric cancer patients

	Minimally invasive gastrectomy *n* = 27	Open gastrectomy *n* = 53	*P* value
Age (years)	84.3 ± 3.3	84.1 ± 3.2	0.831
Gender (M/F)	19/8	41/12	0.587
Tumor size (cm)	3.9 ± 2.3	4.3 ± 2.5	0.478
BMI (kg/m^2)	24.4 ± 3.1	22.7 ± 3.5	0.032
Resection extent			0.015
Subtotal/total gastrectomy	26/1	39/14	
Reconstruction method			0.345
Billroth-I	6 (22.2)	7 (13.2)	
Roux-en-Y or uncut R-Y	21 (77.8)	46 (86.8)	
Extent of lymphadenectomy			
<D2/D2	2/25	6/47	0.710
Retrieved LN number	26.0 ± 10.1	28.4 ± 13.4	0.428
Pathological T category			0.017
T1/T2/T3/T4	17/3/6/1	17/12/17/7	
Pathological N category			0.058
N0/N1/N2/N3	20/2/4/1	29/4/12/8	
Pathological TNM stage			0.051
I/II/III	18/6/3	22/13/18	
Number of comorbidities			0.363
0	5 (18.5)	9 (17)	
1	6 (22.2)	22 (41.5)	
≧2	16 (59.3)	22 (41.5)	
Operative outcomes			
Operative time (min)	311.5 ± 106.6	313.2 ± 101.9	0.945
Operative blood loss (mL)	63.7 ± 59.2	372.3 ± 340.4	<0.001
Postoperative hospital stay (day)	10.7 ± 8.6	15.4 ± 9.7	0.036
Surgical complications	6 (22.2)	6 (11.3)	0.207
Anastomosis leakage	1 (3.7)	1 (1.9)	1.000
Anastomosis stenosis	1 (3.7)	0	0.337
Delayed gastric emptying	4 (14.8)	2 (3.8)	0.172
Intestinal obstruction	1 (3.7)	0	0.337
Pneumonia	0	2 (3.8)	0.547
Surgical Mortality	0	1 (1.9)	1.000

BMI: body mass index; LN: lymph node; comorbidities including cardiovascular disease, cerebrovascular accident, endocrine disease, pulmonary disease, liver cirrhosis, benign prostate hyperplasia, etc.
Some patients had more than one complication
Data were presented as mean ± SD or n (%)

gastrectomy (96.3% vs. 73.6%, P = 0.015), less advanced pathological T category (P = 0.017), less operative blood loss (63.7 ± 59.2 mL vs. 372.3 ± 340.4 mL, P < 0.001) and shorter hospital stay (10.7 ± 8.6 vs. 15.4 ± 9.7 days, P = 0.036). The surgical complication rates (22.2% vs. 11.3%, P = 0.207) and surgical mortality rates (0% vs 1.9%, P = 1.000) were not significantly different between MIS and open surgery in octogenarian and older patients.

Minimally invasive surgery

As indicated in Table 2, MIS was performed on 115 patients, including 62 females (53.9%) and 53 males (46.1%). The median age of these patients was 68 years (range, 35–91 years). Patients were classified into three groups according to their ages. Group 1 included 40 patients (34.8%) younger than 60 years of age (18 males and 22 females), with a median age of 51 years (range,

Table 2 Comparison of the clinicopathological differences and operative outcomes of minimally invasive gastrectomy according to age

	<60 yr n = 40	60–79 yr n = 48	≧80 yr n = 27	P value
Gender (M/F)	18/22	25/23	19/8	0.117
Tumor size (cm)	3.5 ± 1.5	3.5 ± 1.6	3.9 ± 2.3	0.574
BMI (kg/m^2)	23.7 ± 4.1	23.8 ± 3.2	24.4 ± 3.1	0.713
Resection extent				0.005
Subtotal/total gastrectomy	30/10	45/3	26/1	
Reconstruction method				0.012
Billroth-I	11 (27.5)	25 (52.1)	6 (22.2)	
Roux-en-Y or uncut R-Y	29 (72.5)	23 (47.9)	21 (77.8)	
Extent of lymphadenectomy				
<D2/D2	3/36	1/47	2/25	0.838
Retrieved LN number	35.0 ± 10.4	29.7 ± 12.0	26.0 ± 10.1	0.005
Pathological T category				0.820
T1/T2/T3/T4	25/5/6/4	30/4/12/2	17/3/6/1	
Pathological N category				0.271
N0/N1/N2/N3	26/4/4/6	31/7/8/2	20/2/4/1	
Pathological TNM stage				0.390
I/II/III	22/12/6	28/14/6	18/6/3	
Number of comorbidities				<0.001
0	28 (70)	18 (37.5)	5 (18.5)	
1	7 (17.5)	15 (31.3)	6 (22.2)	
≧2	5 (12.5)	15 (31.3)	16 (59.3)	
Operative outcomes				
Operative time (min)	344.9 ± 142.9	270.3 ± 109.9	311.5 ± 106.6	0.019
Operative blood loss (mL)	59.8 ± 59.9	71.3 ± 74.1	63.7 ± 59.2	0.710
Postoperative hospital stay (day)	9.5 ± 6.4	12.2 ± 14.0	10.7 ± 8.6	0.499
Surgical complications	3 (7.5)	8 (16.7)	6 (22.2)	0.088
Anastomosis leakage	0	1 (2.1)	1 (3.7)	0.249
Anastomosis stenosis	1 (2.5)	1 (2.1)	1 (3.7)	0.794
Chylous leakage	1 (2.5)	0	0	0.240
Intraabdominal abscess	0	1 (2.1)	0	0.881
Delayed gastric emptying	1 (2.5)	6 (12.5)	4 (14.8)	0.076
Intestinal obstruction	0	0	1 (3.7)	0.140
Surgical Mortality	0	0	0	1.000

BMI: body mass index; LN: lymph node; comorbidities including cardiovascular disease, cerebrovascular accident, endocrine disease, pulmonary disease, liver cirrhosis, benign prostate hyperplasia, etc.
Some patients had more than one complication
Data were presented as mean ± SD or n (%)

35–59 years). Group 2 included 48 patients (41.7%) of 65 to 79 years of age (25 males and 23 females), with a median age of 70.5 years (range, 60–79 years). Group 3 included 27 patients (24.5%) of at least 80 years of age (19 males and 8 females), with a median age of 84 years (range, 80–91 years).

Relative to patients in groups 2 and 3, patients in group 1 were more likely to receive total gastrectomy (25% vs. 6.3% vs. 3.7% for groups 1, 2 and 3, respectively, $P = 0.005$), had more retrieved lymph nodes (35.0 ± 10.4 vs. 29.7 ± 12.0 vs. 26.0 ± 10.1 for groups 1, 2 and 3, respectively, $P = 0.005$), exhibited fewer comorbidities ($P < 0.001$) and experienced longer operative time (344.9 ± 142.9 vs. 270.3 ± 109.9 vs. 311.5 ± 106.6 min for groups 1, 2 and 3, respectively, $P = 0.019$) compared to group 2 and group 3 patients. There were no differences among different age groups regarding postoperative hospital stay (9.5 ± 6.4 vs. 12.2 ± 14.0 vs. 10.7 ± 8.6 days, P = 0.499) and surgical complications (7.5% vs. 16.7% vs. 22.2%, P = 0.088).

According to an intention to treat method, one 55 y/o female patient in the MIS group was converted to open surgery. The reason for open conversion is a firm and fixed enlarged lymph node over the splenic hilum involving the pancreatic tail. Radical total gastrectomy with splenectomy, distal pancreatectomy and D2 lymphadenectomy was performed. She recovered well and was discharged 10 days after surgery.

Open surgery

As indicated in Table 3, 244 patients received open surgery including 170 females (70%) and 73 males (30%), the median age of these patients was 68 years (range, 24–94 years). Patients were classified into three groups according to their ages. Group 1 included 72 patients (29.5%) younger than 60 years of age (47 males and 25 females), with a median age of 52 years (range, 24–59 years). Group 2 included 119 patients (48.8%) of 60 to 79 years of age (82 males and 36 females), with a median age of 70 years (range, 60–79 years). Group 3 included 53 patients (21.7%) of at least 80 years of age (41 males and 12 females), with a median age of 84 years (range, 80–94 years).

Relative to patients in groups 1 and 2, patients in group 3 had fewer retrieved lymph nodes (36.3 ± 13.9 vs. 32.7 ± 13.0 vs. 28.2 ± 13.4 for groups 1, 2 and 3, respectively, P = 0.004), were less advanced with respect to pathological N category (P = 0.003) and TNM stage (P = 0.004), suffered from more comorbidities (P = 0.001), and experienced longer hospital stays (10.8 ± 5.6 vs. 14.1 ± 12.8 vs. 15.2 ± 9.7 for groups 1, 2 and 3, respectively, P = 0.041), a higher rate of wound infection (0% vs. 0%, vs. 3.8% for groups 1, 2 and 3, respectively, P = 0.032) and a higher incidence of pneumonia (0% vs. 0% vs. 3.8% for groups 1, 2 and 3, respectively, P = 0.032).

Discussion

In the present study, among octogenarian and older gastric cancer patients, a comparison of MIS and open surgery demonstrated that MIS was associated with less operative blood loss and a shorter postoperative hospital stay; however, there were no significant differences between MIS and open surgery with respect to the rates of surgical complications or mortality.

Our results indicated that following open surgery for gastric cancer, longer postoperative hospital stays, higher rates of wound infection rate and a higher incidence of pneumonia were observed among octogenarian and older patients than among younger patients. However, for gastric cancer patients treated using MIS, no differences were observed among different age groups with respect to postoperative hospital stay and surgical complications. Among aged patients, the use of MIS instead of open surgery might provide the benefits of fewer surgical complications and shorter postoperative hospital stays. One encouraging finding of this study is that octogenarian and older patients could recover from MIS as rapidly as younger patients.

A previous report [6] addressing the surgical outcomes of open surgery for gastric cancer indicated that even patients with early gastric cancer, older patients exhibited significantly worse overall survival rates than younger patients after curative surgery. In a series examined by Kwon et al. [4], among patients who were at least 80 years of age, MIS and open surgery produced comparable rates of 5-year overall survival and disease-free survival. As the global population ages, increasing numbers of octogenarian and older gastric cancer patients will require surgical treatment. Oncological outcomes would not be the primary concern for octogenarian and older patients after surgery. To achieve more rapid postoperative recoveries, the indications for MIS for octogenarian and older patients should be extended to include patients with advanced gastric cancer.

Although aged patients are considered to be at high surgical risk and have limited functional reserve, our results demonstrated that MIS is beneficial for octogenarian and older patients. For these patients, the use of MIS instead of open surgery was also associated with earlier recovery and no increase in surgical complications. Our future study will compare the long-term survival rates for open surgery and MIS among aged patients.

Our study had certain limitations. Because this investigation is a retrospective study, selection bias may exist. Besides, the surgeon is still a major part of choosing the surgical approach for each patient, and the patient would hardly make this decision on his own. Hence, the surgeon's selection strongly biases the results. In particular, patients who received MIS tended to be diagnosed at an earlier stage than patients who received open surgery. Furthermore, octogenarian and older patients who underwent surgery were screened for cardiopulmonary function prior to surgery; as a result, octogenarian and older patients with poor cardiopulmonary function were excluded as candidates for surgery.

Surgeons will undoubtedly select for patients in good overall condition, particularly when screening octogenarian and older patients. However, our results indicate that for selected octogenarian and older patients, MIS produced faster postoperative recovery than open surgery. To date, few reports regarding MIS for octogenarian and older patients have been published; thus only a limited number of cases involving these patients have been examined. A future meta-analysis involving a large number

Table 3 Comparison of the clinicopathological differences and operative outcomes of open gastrectomy according to age

	<60 yr n = 72	60–79 yr n = 119	≧80 yr n = 53	P value
Gender (M/F)	47/25	82/36	41/12	0.153
Tumor size (cm)	5.4 ± 2.8	6.8 ± 18.5	4.3 ± 2.5	0.471
BMI (kg/m^2)	23.6 ± 4.0	23.3 ± 4.0	22.6 ± 3.5	0.342
Resection extent				0.582
Subtotal/total gastrectomy	48/24	87/32	39/14	
Reconstruction method				0.185
Billroth-I	4 (5.6)	17 (14.3)	7 (13.2)	
Billroth-II	1 (1.4)	0	0	
Roux-en-Y or uncut R-Y	67 (93)	102 (85.7)	46 (86.8)	
Extent of lymphadenectomy				0.452
<D2/D2	5/64	5/109	6/47	
Retrieved LN number	36.3 ± 13.9	32.7 ± 13.0	28.2 ± 13.4	0.004
Pathological T category				0.114
T1/T2/T3/T4	15/11/30/16	28/12/45/34	17/12/17/7	
Pathological N category				0.003
N0/N1/N2/N3	22/17/16/17	43/10/26/40	29/4/12/8	
Pathological TNM stage				0.004
I/II/III	19/20/33	31/15/73	22/13/18	
Number of comorbidities				<0.001
0	46 (63.9)	22 (18.5)	9 (17)	
1	19 (26.4)	57 (47.9)	22 (41.5)	
≧2	7 (9.7)	40 (33.6)	22 (41.5)	
Operative outcomes				
Operative time	328.9 ± 101.1	312.0 ± 96.0	312.2 ± 101.2	0.475
Operative blood loss	294.1 ± 232.5	384.3 ± 457.7	366.9 ± 339.6	0.267
Postoperative hospital stay	10.8 ± 5.6	14.1 ± 12.8	15.2 ± 9.7	0.041
Surgical complications	3 (4.2)	10 (8.4)	6 (11.3)	0.317
Anastomosis leakage	2 (2.8)	2 (1.7)	1 (1.9)	0.699
Chylous leakage	0	2 (1.7)	0	0.877
Delayed gastric emptying	0	1 (0.8)	2 (3.8)	0.069
Intestinal obstruction	0	1 (0.8)	0	0.913
Wound infection	0	0	2 (3.8)	0.032
Intraabdominal abscess	0	4 (3.4)	0	0.826
Choledochofistula	0	1 (0.8)	0	0.913
Pancreatic fistula	1 (1.4)	0	0	0.195
Pneumonia	0	0	2 (3.8)	0.032
Surgical Mortality	0	1 (0.8)	1 (1.9)	0.250

BMI: body mass index; LN: lymph node; comorbidities including cardiovascular disease, cerebrovascular accident, endocrine disease, pulmonary disease, liver cirrhosis, benign prostate hyperplasia, etc.
Some patients had more than one complication
Data were presented as mean ± SD or n (%)

of octogenarian and older patients is necessary to compare the operative outcomes of open surgery and MIS for these patients.

Conclusion

In conclusion, MIS is an advantageous technique for octogenarian and older gastric cancer patients. Among these patients, relative to open surgery, MIS produced better postoperative recovery and comparable rates of surgical complications and mortality. MIS for gastric cancer can be performed safely in octogenarian and older patients and may be regarded as the preferred surgical approach for such patients.

Abbreviation
MIS: Minimally invasive surgery

Acknowledgments
This study was supported by Taipei Veterans General Hospital (V104C-071, V104B-005). The funders had no role in study design, data collection and analysis, decision to publish, or preparation of the manuscript.

Authors' contributions
CAL, KHH, MHC, SSL, AFYL, CWW, YMS and WLF participated in the design of the study. CAL, KHH and WLF performed the statistical analysis and wrote the manuscript. KHH and WLF conceived of the study, and participated in its design and coordination. All authors read and approved the final manuscript.

Competing interests
The authors declared that they have no competing interests.

Author details
[1]Department of Radiology, Taipei Veterans General Hospital, Taipei City, Taiwan. [2]Division of General Surgery, Department of Surgery, Taipei Veterans General Hospital, No. 201, Sec. 2, Shipai Rd., Beitou District, Taipei City 11217, Taiwan. [3]Division of Medical Oncology, Department of Oncology, Taipei Veterans General Hospital, Taipei City, Taiwan. [4]Department of Pathology, Taipei Veterans General Hospital, Taipei City, Taiwan. [5]School of Medicine, National Yang-Ming University, Taipei City, Taiwan. [6]Institute of Clinical Medicine, School of Medicine, National Yang-Ming University, Taipei City, Taiwan. [7]National Yang-Ming University Hospital, Yilan City, Taiwan.

References
1. Zeng Y, Yang Z, Peng J, Lin HS, Cai L. Laparoscopy assisted versus open distal gastrectomy for early gastric cancer: evidence from randomized and nonrandomized clinical trials. Ann Surg. 2012;256:39–52.
2. The Clinical Outcomes of Surgical Therapy Study Group. A comparison of laparoscopically assisted and open colectomy for colon cancer. N Engl J Med. 2004;350:2050–9.
3. Yasuda K, Sonoda K, Shiroshita H, Inomata M, Shiraishi N, Kitano S. Laparoscopically assisted distal gastrectomy for early gastric cancer in the elderly. Br J Surg. 2004;91:1061–5.
4. Kwon IG, Cho I, Guner A, Kim HI, Noh SH, Hyung WJ. Minimally invasive surgery as a treatment option for gastric cancer in the elderly: comparison with open surgery for patients 80 years and older. Surg Endosc. 2015;29:2321–30.
5. Sobin L, Gospodarowicz M, Wittekind C, eds. TNM classification of malignant tumours. In: 7th ed. International Union against Cancer (UICC). New York: Wiley, 2009.
6. Lo SS, Wu CW, Chen JH, Li AF, Hsieh MC, Shen KH, et al. Surgical results of early gastric cancer and proposing a treatment strategy. Ann Surg Oncol. 2007;14:340–7.

Duodenal gastrointestinal stromal tumors: clinicopathological characteristics, surgery, and long-term outcome

Chaoyong Shen[1†], Haining Chen[1†], Yuan Yin[1], Jiaju Chen[1], Luyin Han[2], Bo Zhang[1*], Zhixin Chen[1] and Jiaping Chen[1]

Abstract

Background: Duodenal gastrointestinal stromal tumors (DGIST) are rare, and data on their management is limited. We here report the clinicopathological characteristics, different surgical treatments, and long-term prognosis of DGIST.

Methods: Data of 74 consecutive patients with DGIST in a single institution from June 2000 to June 2014 were retrospectively analyzed. The overall survival (OS) and recurrence/metastasis-free survival rates of 74 cases were calculated using Kaplan–Meier method.

Results: Out of 74 cases, 42 cases were female (56.76 %) and 32 cases (43.24 %) were male. Approximately 22.97, 47.30, 16.22, and 13.51 % of the tumors originated in the first to fourth portion of the duodenum, respectively, with a tumor size of 5.08 ± 2.90 cm. Patients presented with gastrointestinal bleeding ($n = 37$, 50.00 %), abdominal pain ($n = 25$, 33.78 %), mass ($n = 5$, 6.76 %), and others ($n = 7$, 9.76 %). A total of 18 patients (24.3 %) underwent wedge resection (WR); 39 patients (52.7 %) underwent segmental resection (SR); and 17 cases (23 %) underwent pancreaticoduodenectomy (PD). The median follow-up was 56 months (1–159 months); 19 patients (25.68 %) experienced tumor recurrence or metastasis, and 14 cases (18.92 %) died. The 1-, 3-, and 5-year recurrence/metastasis-free survival rates were 93.9, 73.7, and 69 %, respectively. The 1-, 3- and 5-year OS were 100, 92.5, and 86 %, respectively. The recurrence/metastasis-free survival rate in the PD group within 5 years was lower than that in the WR group ($P = 0.047$), but was not different from that in the SR group ($P = 0.060$). No statistically significant difference was found among the three operation types ($P = 0.294$).

Conclusions: DGIST patients have favorable prognosis after complete tumor removal, and surgical procedures should be determined by the DGIST tumor location and size.

Keywords: Duodenum, Gastrointestinal stromal tumor, Clinicopathological Surgery, Prognosis

Background

Mazur and Clark re-evaluated the histogenesis of gastrointestinal stromal tumors (GIST) in 1983, and following research has confirmed that GIST are the most common mesenchymal tumors [1–4]. Although GIST can originate within the entire gastrointestinal tract, the most common location is the stomach (approximately 60 %), followed by the small intestine (about 20–30 %), and rarely in the duodenum (5 %) [5, 6]. Duodenal gastrointestinal stromal tumor (DGIST) accounted for 10–30 % of all malignant tumors of the duodenum, with a global incidence rate of approximately $10/10^6$–$20/10^6$. Nonspecific abdominal pain and gastrointestinal hemorrhage are the most frequent symptoms in GIST patients, and several emergency patients have been admitted to a hospital because of this disease [2, 7].

Primary GIST is categorized into very low, low, intermediate, and high risk based on a previous study of Fletcher [8]. However, subsequent studies have shown that GIST have different clinical, histological, and immunohistochemical features due to different tumor locations;

* Correspondence: hxwcwk@126.com
†Equal contributors
[1]Department of Gastrointestinal Surgery, West China Hospital, Sichuan University, Chengdu 610041 ,Sichuan, China
Full list of author information is available at the end of the article

this difference is also one of the independent risk factors for tumor recurrence [9, 10]. To date, surgery with histologically negative margins is mainstream treatment for primary resectable GIST. However, surgical operations for DGIST are often difficult because of anatomical and physiological specificities (the proximity of the head of pancreas, common bile duct, ampullary part, kidney, and mesenteric vessels). There is no consensus on the optimal operation procedures for DGIST at present [11, 12]. Operations vary from a mini-invasive approach to a pancreaticoduodenectomy, which are mainly determined by tumor location and size. Pancreaticoduodenectomy (PD) is considered a safe operation with low mortality; however, PD is highly complicated, and serious immediate and long-term complications occur to some patients [13]. Theoretically, wedge resection (WR) and segmental resection (SR) are simple and feasible. And the main concern on WR or SR is increased risk of tumor recurrence because of incomplete resection [7].

Currently, numerous studies involving DGIST have been published, but most of these studies have small samples or are retrospective case series [6, 14–18]. In the present study, we aimed to evaluate clinical and pathological characteristics, operation curative effects, and long-term prognosis of DGIST patients from a single medical institution.

Methods

Patient selection

Medical records of DGIST patients admitted in the Department of General Surgery of West China Hospital of Sichuan University from June 2000 to June 2014 were retrospectively analyzed. Inclusion criteria are as follows: (1)Patients who underwent laparotomy; (2)Patients with DGIST, as proven by pathological, immunohistochemical, and gene mutation detection examinations (spindle cells are observed under microscope; and CD117+ was analyzed through immunohistochemistry or detected through *KIT/PDGFRA* gene mutation, confirmed by senior pathologists); (3)The tumor was located in the duodenum, as confirmed by preoperative abdominal CT scan, ultrasound endoscopy, upper gastrointestinal barium swallow radioscopy, and operation; (4)Patients with GIST synchronous with other malignancies were excluded in this study. A total of 74 DGIST patients were included and examined in this study. The Institutional Review Board and Ethics Committee of the West China Hospital of Sichuan University informed that an ethical review was not needed for this retrospective study.

Surgery and medication treatment

All patients underwent laparotomy with general anesthesia, and surgical procedures were performed according to intraoperative exploratory results. Surgical procedures were considered to achieve R0 resection as much as possible. Frozen slices of incisal margin and surgical specimen were routinely collected during the surgery. Surgeries included WR (without duodenal transection or anastomosis, local resection with pure closure), SR (duodenal transaction with reconstruction by Roux-en-Y duodenojejunostomy, end-to-end duodenoduodenostomy, or gastrojejunostomy), and PD (operation with pancreaticogastrostomy or pancreatojejunostomy). WR with primary closure was mainly performed for small or abluminal lesions. Tumor risk categories were evaluated according to the modified National Institutes of Health (NIH) risk classification [19]. The patients with intermediate- and high-risk were recommended to take imatinib mesylate (IM) as adjuvant therapy. The recommended IM dosage was 400 mg/d. One patient who received preoperative IM therapy underwent endoscopic ultrasonography-guided fine needle aspiration to confirm the diagnosis, according to the National Comprehensive Cancer Network guideline [20]. All patients signed informed consents and voluntarily accepted the treatment.

Data collection and follow-up

Data on clinical symptoms, gender, age, hospital stay, surgical procedures (WR, SR, and PD), operation complications (including postoperative abdominal or wound infection, anastomotic fistula, and gastric emptying, etc.), emergency admission, tumor size (maximal tumor diameter, cm), tumor location (first, second, third, and fourth duodenum portion), NIH risk classification, mitotic count per 50 high power fields (HPF) of the microscope, medication before and after surgery (dosage and duration), tumor recurrence/metastasis time, and postoperative follow-up information were collected. All patients were followed up by office visit, telephone call, or outpatient clinic visit after being discharged from the hospital (once every 2–3 months in the first half of the year and then once every 6–12 months a year later). The censor date of the follow-up was July 2014.

Statistical analysis

Categorical variables were described in terms of frequency and percentages. The measurement data were expressed as mean ± SD. One-way ANOVA was used to compare the clinicopathological characteristics of the three surgical groups. Chi-square test was used to enumerate the data. Wilcoxon test was used to test rank the data. The recurrence/metastasis-free survival rate was measured from operation to tumor recurrence or metastasis (based on radiological findings or proven by biopsy). Overall survival (OS) time includes the period from surgery to death or until the last follow-up. Survival curves were performed using Kaplan–Meier method and compared using log-rank test. Statistical significance was defined as a two-tailed $P < 0.05$. All data analyses were performed using

SPSS version 18.0 statistical software package for Microsoft Windows.

Results

Patient characteristics

Table 1 shows the clinicopathological characteristics of the patients. One patient was diagnosed as DGIST preoperatively and had undergone complete tumor resection. However, liver metastasis had occurred at 44 months postoperatively (Fig. 1a–c). Two patients had distant metastasis at the time of diagnosis (a patient with left hepatic metastasis underwent complete resection; no recurrence or metastasis occurred after 25 months of follow-up; another patient had extensive abdominal metastasis and died at 26 months postoperatively). A total of 16 patients received tyrosine kinase inhibitor as adjuvant therapy and were treated for a median time of 28 months (1–52 months). Among them, 1 patient took SUTENT (sunitinib malate, because of intolerance of IM therapy) at 50 mg/d, and 15 patients took imatinib mesylate at 400 mg/day; 6 patients had mild eyelid edema, and 1 patient had mild abnormal liver function. However, these patients did not stop the medication. One patient underwent surgery with complete tumor resection after treatment with IM. However, liver metastasis occurred at 44 months postoperatively. The remaining cases refused to undergo adjuvant therapy mainly due to economic reasons.

Table 1 Clinicopathological characteristics and demographic data for patients with duodenal GIST

Variables	No. of patients ($n = 74$)	Percentage (%)
Gender		
Male	32	43.24
Female	42	56.76
Age (years)	54.36 ± 13.13	-
Hospital stay (days)	19.47 ± 10.19	-
Clinical presentation		
Gastrointestinal hemorrhage	37	50.00
Abdominal pain	25	33.78
Palpable mass	5	6.76
others[a]	7	9.46
Tumor location (portion)		
First	17	22.97
Second	35	47.30
Third	12	16.22
Forth	10	13.51
Tumor size (cm)	5.08 ± 2.90	-
No. of mitosis		
≤5/50 HPF	41	55.41
6–10/50 HPF	27	36.49
>10/50 HPF	6	8.10
Modified NIH risk classification		
Low	32	43.24
Intermediate	8	10.81
High	34	45.96
Mutational analysis		
KIT exon 11	9	12.16
KIT exon 9	3	4.05
NA	62	83.78
Preoperative imatinib therapy	1	1.35
Postoperative adjuvant therapy	16	21.62
Patients with emergency visit	5	6.76
Patients with metastases at diagnosis	2	2.70
Tumor recurrence or metastasis	19	25.68
Death case	14	18.92

GIST, gastrointestinal stromal tumors; [a]others include jaundice, incidentally found, abdominal distension, *et al.*; HPF, High power field; NIH, National Institutes of Health; NA, not available

Surgery and postoperative complications

Table 2 summarizes the clinicopathological characteristics of the three types of surgical procedures. Out of the 74 DGIST patients, 18 (24.3 %), 39 (52.7 %), and 17 underwent WR, SR, and PD, respectively. A total of 73 patients obtained R0 resection, and 1 patient in the SR group underwent palliative operation due to extensive abdominal metastasis. Of note, the tumor size in the PD group patients was larger than those in the WR ($P = 0.005$) and SR groups ($P = 0.011$). PDs were mainly chosen for patients with ampullary involvement or close proximity of the tumor to the second segment of the duodenum, whereas those with lesions in the other portion of the duodenum were treated with WR or SR. The hospital stay of patients in the PD group was longer than those in the WR group ($P = 0.011$), but was not significantly different from those in the SR group ($P = 0.194$). No statistically significant difference was noted regarding to gender, age, clinical manifestation, mitotic count (50HPF), and NIH risk classification among the three groups ($P > 0.05$). In addition, 5 patients in the SR and PD groups underwent multivisceral resection respectively; 8 patients underwent cholecystectomy; 1 patient underwent hepatic left lateral lobectomy; and 1 patient had combined right kidney and colon resection. Four patients (23.5 %) experienced postoperative complications in the PD group, such as wound infection ($n = 2$), delayed gastric emptying ($n = 1$), and anastomotic fistula ($n = 1$). In addition, 1 patient from the SR group had intraperitoneal infection, whereas 1 patient in the WR group had intestinal obstruction. The serious complications of reoperation and surgery-related death were not observed among the 3 groups. A total of 3 (16.7 %), 8 (20.5 %), and 4 patients

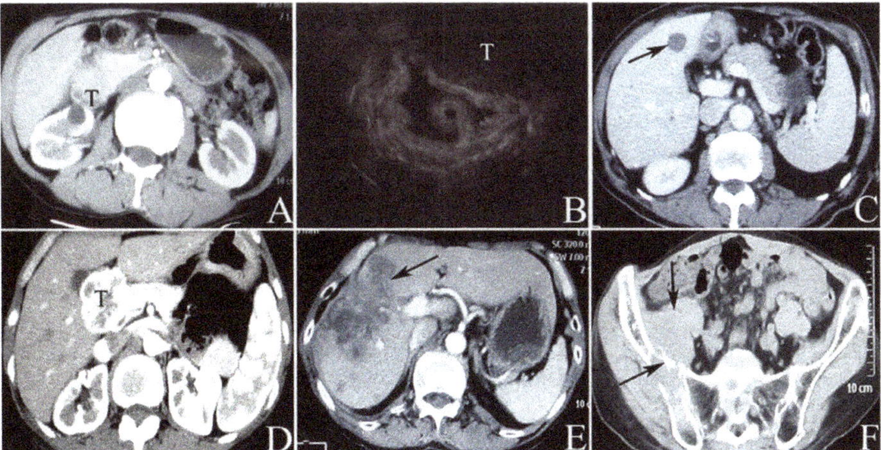

Fig. 1 a, b: The abdominal CT scan and endoscopic ultrasonography images reveal a soft tissue mass with size of 6.5 × 4.5 cm located in the second portion of the duodenum, and with an unclear boundary with head of pancreas, right liver, and kidney. **c** shows a metastasis in the liver at 44 months postoperatively. **d**: A lump with a size of 4.5 × 3.7 cm adjacent to pancreas. **e, f**: Liver (mainly in the right liver lobe) and bone (multiple bone destruction of ilium) metastasis occurred 12 years after operation

(23.5 %) in the WR, SR, and PD groups, respectively, underwent perioperative blood transfusions.

Overall and recurrence/metastasis-free survival

With a median follow-up of 56 months (1–159 months), 7 cases were lost to follow-up. A total of 19 patients (25.68 %) had tumor recurrence or metastasis and 1 patient experienced liver and multiple bone metastases (Fig. 1d–f). Fourteen patients (18.92 %) died. The 1-, 3-, and 5-year recurrence/metastasis-free survival rates were 93.9, 73.7, and 69 %, respectively. The 1-, 3- and 5-year OS were 100, 92.5, and 86 %, respectively. The recurrence/metastasis-free survival of the PD group within 5 years was lower than that of the WR group ($P = 0.047$) but was not significantly different compared with that of the SR group ($P = 0.060$, as shown in Fig. 2). Moreover, the median recurrence/metastasis-free survival in the PD group (22 months) was shorter than that in the SR group (35 months). However, this difference was not statistically significant ($P = 0.064$). Notably, the OS among the three surgical procedures was not statistically significant ($P = 0.294$). The 5-year recurrence/metastasis-free survival rate of patients with tumor size of <5 cm was higher than those with tumor size of ≥5 cm ($P < 0.001$). The 5-year recurrence/metastasis-free survival rate of patients with mitosis count of ≤5, 6–10, and >10 were 88.5 %, 56.7 % ($P = 0.012$), and 33.3 % ($P = 0.002$ for mitotic count ≤ 5, $P = 0.346$ for mitotic count 6–10), respectively. Patients with low-, intermediate-, and high-risk, the 5-year recurrence/metastasis-free survival rates were 94.7 %, 57.1 % ($P = 0.025$), and 53.1 % ($P = 0.001$ for low risk and $P = 0.364$ for intermediate risk), respectively. Patients with intermediate- or high-risk who took IM adjuvant therapy revealed a trend of higher recurrence/metastasis-free survival than that of patients without taking IM ($P = 0.326$).

Discussion

GIST has been misdiagnosed as smooth muscle or neurogenic tumor for decades because of the insufficient understanding of the GIST concept. However, GIST has been confirmed as an independently oriented differentiated mesenchymal tumor of the digestive tract along with the rapid development of immunohistochemical and molecular biological technologies. To date, most preliminary studies on DGIST are case reports or small sample studies, and only a limited number of studies have reported the operation and long-term prognosis of DGIST [14, 21, 22]. In the present study, the clinicopathological features and long-term prognosis of 74 DGIST patients from a single institution were retrospectively analyzed. This research is important because aside from summarizing the disease's clinical presentation, the long-term prognosis of the different surgical procedures, and OS and recurrence/metastasis-free survival rate were explored as well.

The clinical presentations of DGIST were non-specific, which were related with the tumor size, growth location, and ulcer in the mucous layer. Alimentary tract hemor rhage is the main clinical manifestation of DGIST, as previously reported in literature [23]. DGIST is mainly located in the duodenum muscle layer and may move inward to the submucosa and lamina propria, leading to mucosal ulceration and hemorrhage [24]. Similar to two recent reports [25, 26], the tumors were mainly located in the second portion of the duodenum (47.30 %), followed by the first portion (22.97 %). Furthermore, we have found that the PD ratio in the second portion of the duodenum was higher than that in other portions (76.5 %). The

Table 2 Main clinical characteristics and surgical information in three surgical procedures for duodenal GIST

Variables	WR ($n = 18$)	SR ($n = 39$)	PD ($n = 17$)
Gender			
Male (%)	5 (27.8)	19 (48.7)	8 (47.1)
Female (%)	13 (72.2)	20 (51.3)	9 (52.9)
Age (years)	51.50 ± 12.28	49.74 ± 14.60	50.59 ± 13.13
Hospital stay (days)	15.05 ± 2.71	19.36 ± 9.00	22.59 ± 10.88
Clinical presentation			
Gastrointestinal hemorrhage (%)	9 (50.0)	21 (53.8)	9 (52.9)
Abdominal pain (%)	6 (33.3)	9 (23.1)	4 (23.5)
Mass (%)	1 (5.6)	4 (10.3)	3 (17.6)
Others[a] (%)	2 (11.1)	5 (12.8)	0 (0.0)
Tumor location (portion)			
First (%)	2 (11.1)	14 (35.9)	1 (5.9)
Second (%)	11 (61.1)	11 (28.2)	13 (76.5)
Third (%)	3 (16.7)	7 (17.9)	2 (11.8)
Forth (%)	2 (11.1)	7 (17.9)	1 (5.9)
Tumor size (cm)	4.17 ± 2.83	4.74 ± 2.11	6.84 ± 3.82
No. of mitosis			
≤5/50 HPF (%)	11 (61.1)	23 (59.0)	7 (41.2)
6–10/50 HPF (%)	5 (27.8)	13 (33.3)	9 (52.9)
>10/50 HPF (%)	2 (11.1)	3 (7.7)	1 (5.9)
Modified NIH risk classification			
Low (%)	9 (50.0)	17 (43.6)	6 (35.3)
Intermediate (%)	2 (11.1)	6 (15.4)	0 (0.0)
High (%)	7 (38.9)	16 (41.0)	11 (64.7)
Mutational analysis			
KIT exon 11 (%)	0 (0.0)	6 (15.4)	3 (17.6)
KIT exon 9 (%)	2 (11.1)	1 (2.6)	0 (0.0)
NA (%)	16 (88.9)	32 (82.1)	14 (82.4)
Margins status			
R0 (%)	18 (100.0)	38 (97.4)	17 (100.0)
R1 (%)	0 (0.0)	1 (2.6)	0 (0.0)
Postoperative complication			
Wound infection (%)	0 (0.0)	0 (0.0)	2 (11.8)
Intra-abdominal infection (%)	0 (0.0)	1 (2.6)	0 (0.0)
Delayed gastric emptying (%)	0 (0.0)	0 (0.0)	1 (5.9)
Intestinal obstruction (%)	1 (5.6)	0 (0.0)	0 (0.0)
Death related surgery (%)	0 (0.0)	0 (0.0)	0 (0.0)
Anastomotic fistula (%)	0 (0.0)	0 (0.0)	1 (5.9)
Multivisceral resection (%)	0 (0.0)	5 (12.8)	5 (29.4)
Perioperative blood transfusion (%)	3 (16.7)	8 (20.5)	4 (23.5)
Tumor recurrence or metastasis (%)	1 (5.6)	11 (28.2)	7 (41.2)

GIST, gastrointestinal stromal tumors; WR, wedge resection; SR, segmental resection (SR); PD, pancreaticoduodenectomy; [a]others include jaundice, incidentally found, abdominal distension, *et al.*; HPF, High power field; NIH, National Institutes of Health; NA, not available

tumor around this site was often located in the inner or posteromedial side of the second portion of DGIST, and the ampulla of Vater and pancreatic head were involved. Our data showed that the low mitotic count proportion (≤5/50 HPF) in DGIST patients was higher (55.41 %) than patients with GIST in the stomach and small intestine; this result is similar with previous reports [12, 23, 26]. The tumor (4–5 cm) of DGIST patients at diagnosis was smaller than tumors in the stomach or other sites [23, 27]. The tumor size was 5.08 ± 2.90 cm in this cohort, which was agreement with their reports.

Currently, surgery is the only potential curative treatment of GIST if R0 is performed [7]. But surgical resection is difficult, and digestive tract reconstruction is not easy for DGIST. Generally, the choice of surgical approach depends on the tumor site, size, and invasion degree into adjacent organs. In this cohort, a total of 10 patients underwent combined organ resection, and all of them obtained R0 resection. Patients who had PD were more likely to experience a higher risk of postoperative complications. The present study also confirmed this finding (PD, SR, WR: 23.5, 2.6, 5.6 %). Patients with larger tumors or lesions located in the second portion of the duodenum, the probability of undergoing PD increased. Notably, no surgery-related death was noted in the three surgical procedures. Thus, we assumed that these three procedures for DGIST were safe and reliable. However, there were still disagreements over the optimal surgical procedures for DGIST [12, 23, 24]. Furthermore, WR or SR can also be safely performed by means of laparoscopic and robotic approaches for DGIST [28, 29]. GIST seldom occurs in lymph node metastasis or peritoneal metastasis; therefore, extensive lymphadenectomy was unnecessary. In this study, only one patient had distant multiple bone metastases.

In the current series, the 5-year OS and recurrence/metastasis-free survival rates were 86 and 69 %, respectively, which were similar to the results of other reports [23, 25]. By contrast, the 5-year disease-free survival rate of small intestine GIST in other parts was lower (about 40 %) compared with DGIST patients [30]. A favorable prognosis of DGIST patients may be related with the early clinical symptoms and small diameter tumor. We found

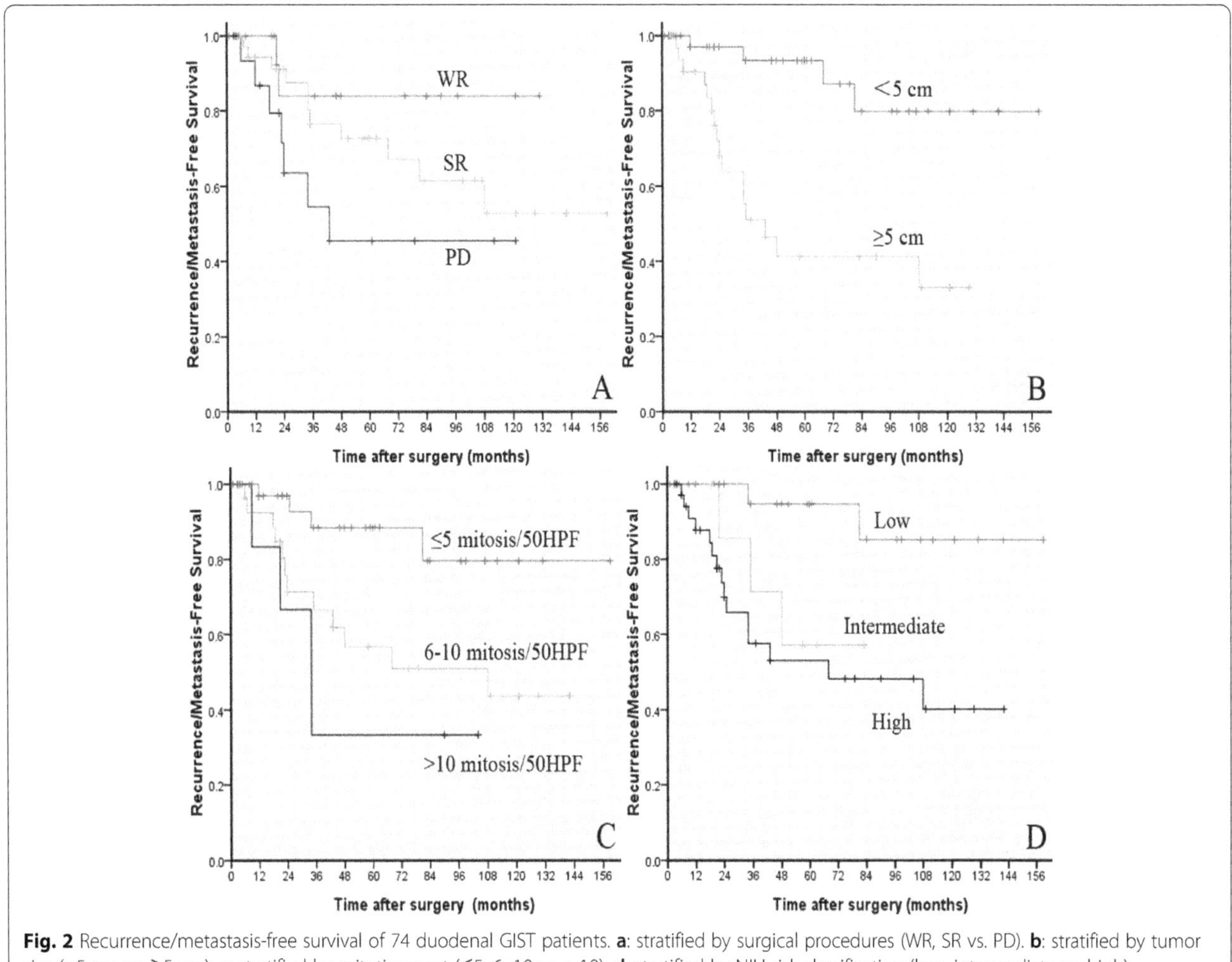

Fig. 2 Recurrence/metastasis-free survival of 74 duodenal GIST patients. **a**: stratified by surgical procedures (WR, SR vs. PD). **b**: stratified by tumor size (<5 cm vs. ≥5 cm). **c**: stratified by mitotic count (≤5, 6–10 vs. > 10). **d**: stratified by NIH risk classification (low, intermediate vs. high)

that the type of surgical procedure can affect outcomes of DGIST patients to a certain extent, and this finding is consistent with the results of Colombo et al. [25]. However, Johnston et al. showed that the DGIST recurrence depends on tumor biology, rather than the operation type or microscopic margins [26]. This phenomenon could be attributed to the fact that the tumor size in the PD group was often larger than that of the other two groups in this study. It is well known that tumor size was one of most important prognostic indicator for GIST.

Nowadays, IM played a key role in the management of GIST when used as adjuvant therapy. The intermediate-risk subgroup of GIST Patients should take IM at least 1 year, while patients with high risk should last for at least 3 years postoperatively [31, 32]. In this study, a total of 16 patients with intermediate- or high-risk underwent adjuvant therapy by using tyrosine kinase inhibitors with a median time of 28 months (1–52 months). We have observed that the recurrence/metastasis-free survival rate of patients with intermediate- or high-risk who underwent postoperative adjuvant therapy was higher than that of patients who did not undergo adjuvant therapy. But no significant difference was noted, thus preventing us from drawing any conclusions. This finding could be attributed to the fact that small number of patients underwent adjuvant therapy and short medication duration. The possibility of complete resection can be evaluated by auxiliary examination preoperatively. Preoperative IM treatment could reduce the proportion of multi-organ resection, downstage giant tumors and increase the opportunity of R0 resection [33, 34]. In this study, one patient underwent preoperative IM treatment and obtained complete resection, thus avoiding combined organ resection and PD.

Conclusion

In sum, patients with DGIST have a favorable prognosis after complete resection. The 5-year recurrence/metastasis-free survival and OS rates of DGIST were 69 and 86 %, respectively. The treatment of choice for DGIST should be selected according to the DGIST tumor site and size. This study showed that the PD group has a higher complication rate than the WD group, and patients of the former group experienced prolonged hospitalization. In addition, the recurrence/metastasis-free survival rate within 5 years was lower than that of the WR group, but had no significant difference with the SR group.

Competing interests

The authors declare that they have no competing interests.

Authors' contributions

ZB, CZX, and CJP conceived the study and participated in its design and coordination. CHN, SCY, YY, CJJ, and HLY helped collect data. CHN and SCY drafted the manuscript. ZB helped revise the paper critically for important intellectual content. All authors read and approved the final manuscript.

Acknowledgement

The authors sincerely acknowledge the entire staff of the Department of Gastrointestinal Surgery, West China Hospital, who offered assistance in the coursing of this study.

Author details

[1]Department of Gastrointestinal Surgery, West China Hospital, Sichuan University, Chengdu 610041 ,Sichuan, China. [2]Intensive Care Unit, West China Hospital, Sichuan University, Chengdu 610041, China.

References

1. Mazur MT, Clark HB. Gastric stromal tumors. Reappraisal of histogenesis. Am J Surg Pathol. 1983;7:507–19.
2. Liegl-Atzwanger B, Fletcher JA, Fletcher CD. Gastrointestinal stromal tumors. Virchows Arch. 2010;456:111–27.
3. Corless CL, Barnett CM, Heinrich MC. Gastrointestinal stromal tumours: origin and molecular oncology. Nat Rev Cancer. 2011;11:865–78.
4. Kiśluk J, Gryko M, Guzińska-Ustymowicz K, et al. Immunohistochemical diagnosis of gastrointestinal stromal tumors-an analysis of 80 cases from 2004 to 2010. Adv Clin Exp Med. 2013;22:33–9.
5. Grotz TE, Donohue JH. Surveillance strategies for gastrointestinal stromal tumors. J Surg Oncol. 2011;104:921–7.
6. Buchs NC, Bucher P, Gervaz P, Ostermann S, Pugin F, Morel P. Segmental duodenectomy for gastrointestinal stromal tumor of the duodenum. World J Gastroenterol. 2010;16:2788–92.
7. Gervaz P, Huber O, Morel P. Surgical management of gastrointestinal stromal tumours. Br J Surg. 2009;96:567–78.
8. Fletcher CD, Berman JJ, Corless C, Gorstein F, Lasota J, Longley BJ, et al. Diagnosis of gastrointestinal stromal tumors: A consensus approach. Hum Pathol. 2002;33:459–65.
9. Wasag B, Debiec-Rychter M, Pauwels P, Stul M, Vranckx H, Oosterom AV, et al. Differential expression of KIT/PDGFRA mutant isoforms in epithelioid and mixed variants of gastrointestinal stromal tumors depends predominantly on the tumor site. Mod Pathol. 2004;17:889–94.
10. Miettinen M, Lasota J. Gastrointestinal stromal tumors: pathology and prognosis at different sites. Semin Diagn Pathol. 2006;23:70–83.
11. Zhong Y, Deng M, Liu B, Chen C, Li M, Xu R. Primary gastrointestinal stromal tumors: Current advances in diagnostic biomarkers, prognostic factors and management of its duodenal location. Intractable Rare Dis Res. 2013;2:11-7.
12. Machado NO, Chopra PJ, Al-Haddabi IH, Al-Qadhi H. Large duodenal gastrointestinal stromal tumor presenting with acute bleeding managed by a whipple resection. A review of surgical options and the prognostic indicators of outcome. JOP. 2011;12:194–9.
13. Cameron JL, Riall TS, Coleman J, Belcher KA. One thousand consecutive pancreaticoduodenectomies. Ann Surg. 2006;244:10–5.
14. Bourgouin S, Hornez E, Guiramand J, Barbier L, Delpero JR, Le Treut YP, et al. Duodenal gastrointestinal stromal tumors (GISTS): arguments for conservative surgery. J Gastrointest Surg. 2013;17:482–7.
15. Liang X, Yu H, Zhu LH, Wang XF, Cai XJ. Gastrointestinal stromal tumors of the duodenum: surgical management and survival results. World J Gastroenterol. 2013;19:6000–10.
16. Cassier PA, Blay JY. Gastrointestinal stromal tumors of the stomach and duodenum. Curr Opin Gastroenterol. 2011;27:571–5.
17. Zhou B, Zhang M, Wu J, Yan S, Zhou J, Zheng S. Pancreaticoduodenectomy versus local resection in the treatment of gastrointestinal stromal tumors of the duodenum. World J Surg Oncol. 2013;11:196.
18. Hoeppner J, Kulemann B, Marjanovic G, Bronsert P, Hopt UT. Limited resection for duodenal gastrointestinal stromal tumors: Surgical management and clinical outcome. World J Gastrointest Surg. 2013;5:16–21.
19. Joensuu H. Risk stratification of patients diagnosed with gastrointestinal stromal tumor. Hum Pathol. 2008;39:1411–9.
20. Demetri GD, von Mehren M, Antonescu CR, DeMatteo RP, Ganjoo KN, Maki RG, et al. NCCN task force report: update on the management of patients with gastrointestinal stromal tumors. J Nat Compr Canc Netw. 2010;8:S1–S41.
21. Miki Y, Kurokawa Y, Hirao M, Fujitani K, Iwasa Y, Mano M, et al. Survival analysis of patients with duodenal gastrointestinal stromal tumors. J Clin Gastroenterol. 2010;44:97–101.
22. Sakata K, Nishimura T, Okada T, Nakamura M. Local resection and jejunal patch duodeno-plasty for the duodenal gastrointestinal stromal tumor–a case report. Gan To Kagaku Ryoho. 2009;36:2348–50.
23. Chung JC, Chu CW, Cho GS, Shin EJ, Lim CW, Kim HC, et al. Management and outcome of gastrointestinal stromal tumors of the duodenum. J Gastrointest Surg. 2010;14:880–3.
24. Miettinen M, Kopczynski J, Makhlouf HR, Sarlomo-Rikala M, Gyorffy H, Burke A, et al. Gastrointestinal stromal tumors, intramural leiomyomas, and leiomyosarcomas in the duodenum: a clinicopathologic, immunohistochemical, and molecular genetic study of 167 cases. Am J Surg Pathol. 2003;27:625–41.
25. Colombo C, Ronellenfitsch U, Yuxin Z, Rutkowski P, Miceli R, Bylina E, et al. Clinical, pathological and surgical characteristics of duodenal gastrointestinal stromal tumor and their influence on survival: a multi-center study. Ann Surg Oncol. 2012;19:3361–7.
26. Johnston FM, Kneuertz PJ, Cameron JL, Sanford D, Fisher S, Turley R, et al. Presentation and Management of Gastrointestinal Stromal Tumors of the Duodenum: A Multi-Institutional Analysis. Ann Surg Oncol. 2012;19:3351–60.
27. Yang WL, Yu JR, Wu YJ, Zhu KK, Ding W, Gao Y, et al. Duodenal gastrointestinal stromal tumor: clinical, pathologic, immunohistochemical characteristics, and surgical prognosis. J Surg Oncol. 2009;100:606–10.
28. Kato M, Nakajima K, Nishida T, Yamasaki M, Nishida T, Tsutsui S, et al. Local resection by combined laparoendoscopic surgery for duodenal gastrointestinal stromal tumor. Diagn Ther Endosc. 2011;2011:645609.
29. Downs-Canner S, Van der Vliet WJ, Thoolen SJ, Boone BA, Zureikat AH, Hogg ME, et al. Robotic Surgery for Benign Duodenal Tumors. J Gastrointest Surg. 2015;19:306–12.
30. Rutkowski P, Nowecki ZI, Michej W, Debiec-Rychter M, Woźniak A, Limon J, et al. Risk criteria and prognostic factors for predicting recurrences after resection of primary gastrointestinal stromal tumor. Ann Surg Oncol. 2007;14:2018–27.
31. Sjölund K, Andersson A, Nilsson E, Nilsson O, Ahlman H, Nilsson B, et al. Downsizing treatment with tyrosine kinase inhibitors in patients with advanced gastrointestinal stromal tumors improved resectablity. World J Surg. 2010;34:2090–7.
32. Joensuu H, Eriksson M, Sundby Hall K, Hartmann JT, Pink D, Schütte J, et al. One vs three years of adjuvant imatinib for operable gastrointestinal stromal tumor: a randomized trial. JAMA. 2012;307:1265–72.
33. Blesius A, Cassier PA, Bertucci F, et al. Neoadjuvant imatinib in patients with locally advanced GIST in the prospective BFR 14 trial. BMC Cancer. 2011;11:72.
34. Eisenberg BL, Trent JC. Adjuvant and neoadjuvant imatinib therapy: current role in the management of gastrointestinal stromal tumors. Int J Cancer. 2011;129:2533–42.

Jejunal pouch reconstruction after total gastrectomy is associated with better short-term absorption capacity and quality of life in early-stage gastric cancer patients

Wei Chen[1], Xumian Jiang[1*], Hui Huang[1], Zao Ding[2] and Chihua Li[3]

Abstract

Background: No consensus exists regarding the best reconstruction style after total gastrectomy (TG). Roux-en-Y oesophagojejunostomy is a simple option for gastrointestinal tract reconstruction. Recently, jejunal pouch reconstruction has been suggested as an appropriate approach. We compared the postoperative outcomes of the two surgical approaches using a well-characterized cohort of gastric carcinoma patients.

Methods: A total of 60 patients who underwent TG were divided into two groups according to the reconstruction style. Both groups were compared regarding patient characteristics, perioperative data and quality of life (QoL), which was assessed using the Spitzer QoL index (QLI) and Visick grade. The incidence of long-term surgery-related complications, including reflux oesophagitis, dumping syndrome, and retention syndrome, was also compared to evaluate postoperative restoration.

Results: Both study groups were comparable with respect to general patient characteristics. No mortality or no significant differences in surgery-related data were found except in the operation time. Compared to Orr Roux-en-Y reconstruction, pouch reconstruction was associated with a longer procedure time, a lower incidence of dumping/retention syndrome and better QoL parameters ($p < 0.05$).

Conclusion: In this study, jejunal pouch reconstruction after TG was superior to the traditional Roux-n-Y oesophagojejunostomy with respect to improved dietary intake and QoL.

Keywords: Total gastrectomy, Reconstruction, Jejunal pouch, Quality of life

Background

Gastric cancer is a common gastrointestinal (GI) tract malignant tumour disorder with high morbidity and mortality [1], and surgical intervention remains a cornerstone for treating gastric cancer. Radical total gastrectomy (TG) is one of the common procedures of choice and has provided relief for stomach cancer via wide use over more than 100 years [2]. Appropriate GI reconstruction is most likely associated with a better quality of life (QoL) [3], and various styles of GI reconstruction can be applied after TG. The preferred approach for reconstruction of the digestive tract following total stomach resection is oesophagojejunostomy with pouch formation and duodenal transit preservation [4]. However, the procedure is complex and difficult to promote in basic-level hospitals in China. In our hospital,pure jejunal pouch reconstruction with Roux-en-Y oesophagojejunostomy has been shown to be an alternative approach as it provides a reservoir for digestion and absorption and is easy to brand. However, studies in the literature describing this technique are scarce.The aim of the present study was to investigate the operation-related complication rate, nutritional status, prognosis and quality of daily life following TG with jejunal pouch reconstruction in three tertiary institutions. For this purpose, we have used defined and validated scoring systems to evaluate postoperative functional outcomes, as previously reported [5–7].

* Correspondence: jxm2015@sina.cn
[1]Department of Gastrointestinal Surgery, The Central Hospital of the Wuhan, Tongji Medical College, Huazhong University of Science and Technology, Wuhan 430000, People's Republic of China
Full list of author information is available at the end of the article

Methods

Reconstruction technique

In 1952, Hunt and Cope [8, 9] first reported a pouch or reservoir fashioned from a loop of the jejunum with the Roux-en-Y principle of oesophagojejunostomy. Ten years later, Lawrence [10] modified this procedure and successfully used it in several patients after gastrectomy. Here, we present a modified pouch reconstruction style using stapled anastomosis, which is safe and convenient.Abdominal radical gastrectomy for cancer was performed according to the routine procedure [11].After removal of the entire stomach, the ligament of Treitz was identified, and a pre-removal line approximately 30–40 cm from the ligament was marked. A loop of the jejunal bowel that was freely mobile was selected and

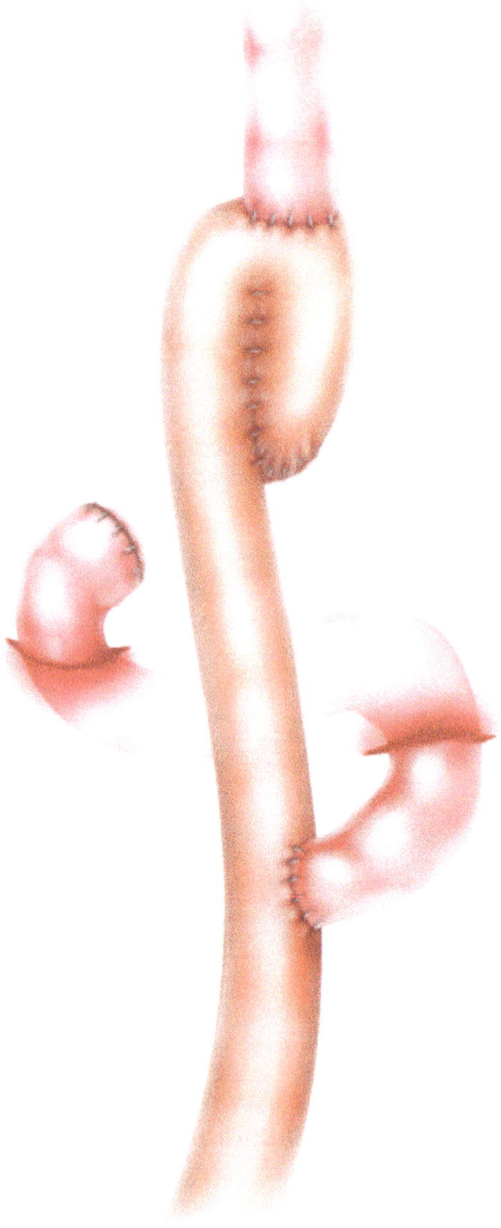

Fig. 1 Schematic illustration of the jejunal pouch after total gastrectomy, which was accomplished using a linearstapler: the jejunum was repositioned to allow anastomosis(using a 100-mm linear stapler) with no tension and a larger capacity

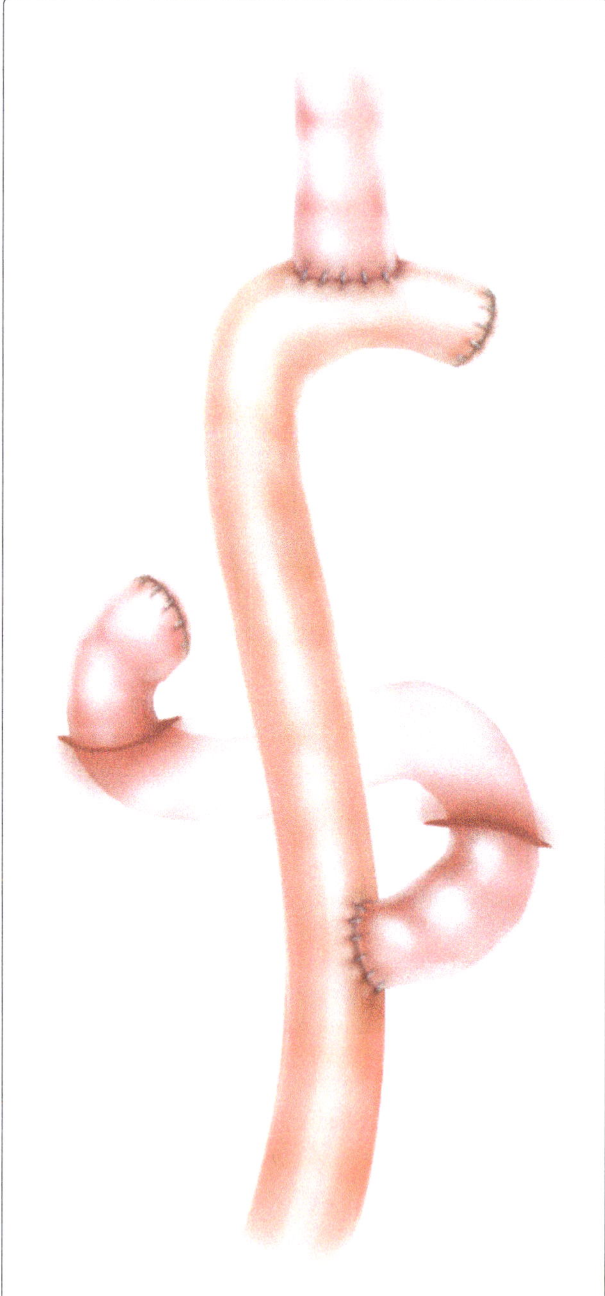

Fig. 2 Schematic illustration of the conventional OrrRoux-en-Y technique. Aftertotal gastrectomy, this type of reconstruction was performed using the double-staplingtechnique

Table 1 Patients' general information

Clinicopathologic feature	P-pouch group($n = 32$)	Orr-RYgroup ($n = 28$)	P
Age (<60y/≥60y)	12/20	10/18	0.886
Sexual (male/female)	21/9	18/10	0.643
Pathology grading			0.499
Well differentiated	12	7	
Moderate differentiated	19	19	
Poor differentiated	1	2	
TNM			0.577
IA	7	4	
IB	19	16	
IIA	6	8	
BMI	23.90 ± 2.3	23.2 ± 2.1	0.153
ALB	44.6 ± 6.2	42.9 ± 5.3	0.254
HB	124.4 ± 10.2	120.8 ± 8.3	0.137

divided before bringing the already divided distal jejunum up to the lower oesophagus to complete the future end for the pouch reconstruction. Before this key step, the divided distal jejunum was folded on itself in a form similar to a reservoir; pouch reconstruction was primarily performed using a 100-mm linear stapler(-Johnson linear stapler, TLC100 Proximate,USA),which provides the largest possible scale (Fig. 1). After creation of the jejunal pouch, the oesophagojejunostomy was finished using a circular stapler (Johnson columnar stapler, CDH25A/29A,USA)with the anvil inserted through the oesophagus and the stapler inserted through the enterotomy of the pouch. Then, the enterotomy was closed with 3–0 polydioxanone (PDS, Ethicon, Cincinnati, USA).Notably,after the anvil was inserted into the oesophageal stub, a purse-string suture was placed to secure it, preventing retraction of the oesophageal mucosa and increasing the possibility of obtaining complete loops during the anastomotic process. Next, the Roux-Y jejuno-jejunostomy was created viaside-to-side hand-sewn anastomosis 2 cm in diameter with continuous 3–0 PDS, approximately 50 cm from the site of the future oesophageal-jejunal anastomosis (EJA). For the conventional Roux-en-Y procedure, EJA was performed with a simple end-to-side technique (Fig. 2). Because all patients underwent typical abdominal TG with different digestive reconstruction methods, the surgical outcomes are sufficiently comparable for comparison.

Patients

Sixty patients who underwent abdominal TG with jejunal pouch reconstruction or simple Roux-en-Y anastomosis at three tertiary hospitals(the Central Hospital of Wuhan/Zhongnan Hospital of Wuhan University/Hubei Cancer Hospital) between January 2010 and December 2015 were reviewed. The clinicopathological data are shown in Table 1. Thirty-two patients underwent TG with jejunal pouch reconstruction, whileanother twenty-eight patients underwent single Roux-en-Y reconstruction after TG. All preoperative and postoperative data were reviewed using the institutional surgical databases involved in this research. The inclusion and exclusion criteria for patient selection are shown in a simple flow chart (Fig. 3).

Functional outcome assessment

To evaluate postoperative recovery, two validated and internationally accepted tools were employed in this research for data collection: the modified Spitzer quality of life index (QLI) and the Visick grade [12, 13]. These assessment tools are considered reliable and objective methods for assessing the outcomes of patients after GI surgery. The modified Spitzer QLI focuses on oral food intake and its influence on daily life, and the index ranges from 1 (poor) to 3 (fine).The maximum score is 52,with higher scores representing better outcomes. The Visick grade ranges from 1 (excellent) to 4 (poor) and focuses on disease-related mental states and relevant digestive tract symptoms. In general, lower Visick grades and higher Spitzer QLIs represent better postoperative recovery. Moreover, the prognostic nutritional index (PNI) was also used to evaluate the nutritional condition of patients in this research. The PNI was calculated according to the serum albumin concentration and peripheral blood lymphocyte count with the aim of evaluating the preoperative nutritional status, the risk of surgical infection and postoperative complications in the patients; the PNI is currently widely used in patients after GI and cardiac surgery [14].All assessments were carried out at three months, six months and one year after the

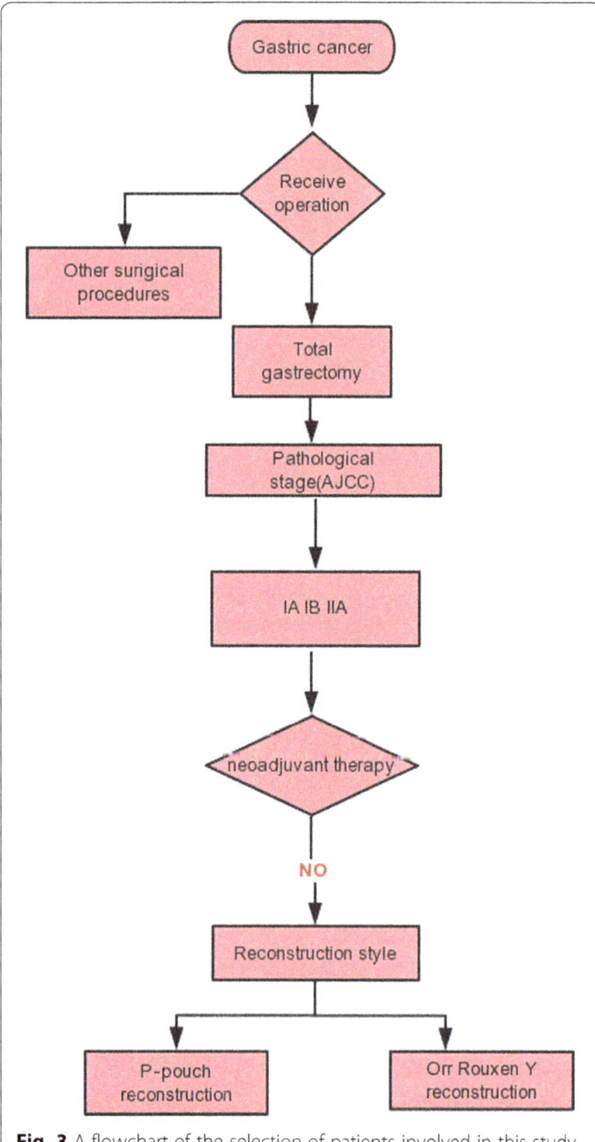

Fig. 3 A flowchart of the selection of patients involved in this study

Fig. 4 The Spitzerquality of life index (QLI)at different times after the two surgical procedures. Data collected from the first, second and third follow-up visits showed a higher QLI (represented by the mean ± SD) in the jejunalpouch group than in the Orr Roux-en-Y group ($p < 0.05$)

operation. Data were collected through the outpatient clinic as well as through a telephone interview.

Statistical analyses

Variables that fulfilled the criteria for a normal distribution were analysed using the Kolmogorov–Smirnov test.Normally distributed data are expressed as the mean ± SD and were analysed by two-tailed Student's t tests.The chi-square test was used to assess categorical data. Statistical analyses were performed using SPSS software, version 19.0(SPSS, Chicago, IL, USA).A difference between groups with a p-value of < 0.05 was considered statistically significant.

Results

No significant differences were found between the groups in demographic or clinical characteristics (Table 1). We considered the cohort suitable for comparing the outcomes of jejunal pouch reconstruction and simple Roux-en-Y. The surgery-related results and the patient satisfaction rate are shown in Table 2. No mortality was found during the early postoperative period. Anastomotic fistulae occurred in five patients after the operation. Anastomotic bleeding or stenosis was not

Table 2 Surgical results

Parameters	P-pouch group($n = 32$)	Orr-RY group($n = 28$)	P
Operative time(min)[a]	245.8 ± 27.6	222.7 ± 24.7	0.010
Blood loss in operation(ml)	301.3 ± 80.9	283.2 ± 60.7	0.339
Iincision infection	2/32	1/28	0.635
Small bowel obstruction	9/32	11/28	0.360
Pulmonary infection	10/32	9/28	0.941
Anastomotic fistula	3/32	2/28	0.755
Hospital stay(day)	12.6 ± 1.6	12.3 ± 1.7	0.589
Satisfaction rate	25/32	20/28	0.550

[a]Significant difference bewteen the P-pouch and Orr-RY group parameters

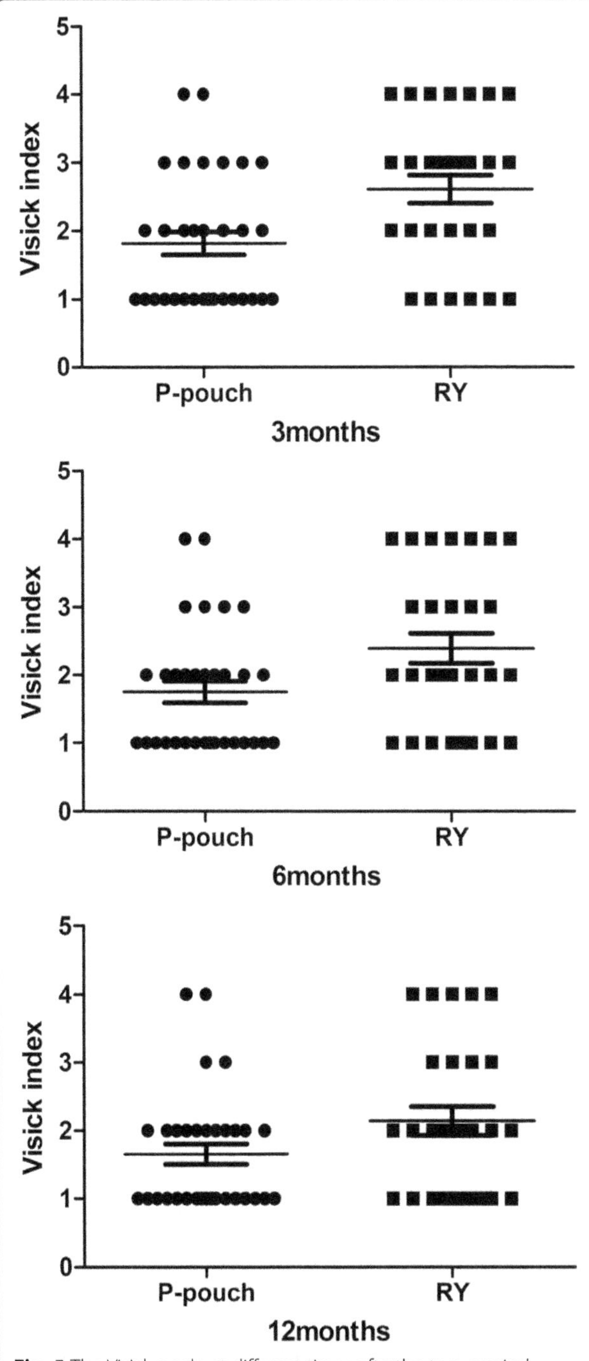

Fig. 5 The Visick grade at different times afterthe two surgical procedures. Data collected from the first two follow-up visits showed better performance (represented by a ratio) in the jejunalpouch group than in the Orr Roux-en-Y group ($p < 0.05$). The last follow-up visit showed no significant difference between the 2 groups ($p > 0.05$)

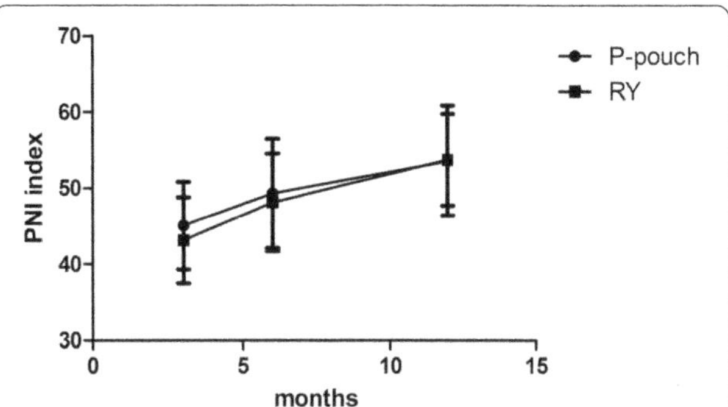

Fig. 6 The prognostic nutritional index (PNI) performed better in the jejunal pouch group; however, the difference was notsignificant ($p > 0.05$)

observed. The more common complications directly related to surgery were paralytic ileus (33.3%) and pulmonary infection (31.6%). No significant differences were found between the two digestive tract reconstruction styles in any of the factors that were directly linked to the expected operation time(245.8 ± 27.6 vs. 222.7 ± 24.7,$p = 0.01$).Other severe surgery-related complications, such as pancreatic fistula and abdominal abscess, were not found in our cohort. Patients were generally satisfied with the surgical outcomes, and the vast majority of patients reiterated that under the same circumstances, they would opt for pouch reconstruction again(78.1%).Up to 3 months after the operation, significantly less abdominal discomfort, appetite loss and weight loss were observed in the jejunal pouch group than in the conventional Orr-RY group(3-month Spitzer QLI:28.1 ± 4.0 vs. 24.3 ± 4.9, $p = 0.002$).Similar results were observed again during the follow-up period (6-month Spitzer QLI:31.3 ± 4.0 vs.26.3 ± 4.8, $p = 0.000$; 12-monthSpitzer QLI: 32.7 ± 3.4 vs. 27.8 ± 4.8, $p = 0.000$). Interestingly, both sets of data related to postoperative rehabilitation improved over time in these patients, probably due to general improvements in diet control and the adaptive capacity of body over the long term (Fig. 4). Similar outcomes were observed for the Visick grade in the two groups (Fig. 5). At the first two follow-up time points, a discernible difference between the jejunal pouch and Orr Roux-en-Y reconstruction groups was identified by univariate analysis (I/IIvs III/IV at 3 months:$p = 0.005$; I/IIvsIII/IV at 6 months: $p = 0.028$).However, at the last follow-up time point, the jejunal pouch procedure was no longer superior to Orr Roux-en-Y with respect to the Visick grade (I/IIIvsIII/IV at 12 months: $p = 0.137$).Regarding prognostic indicators, the PNI was better in the jejunal pouch group, although the difference was not significant (Fig. 6).To assess long-term complications, we conducted a survey 1 year after the operation.The incidence of reflux oesophagitis(-RE)was rare in the jejunal pouch group compared to that in the traditional OrrRoux-en-Y group, although the difference was not significant. Complaints about dumping syndrome and retention syndrome were significantly more commonly reported in the conventional OrrRoux-en-Y group during the follow-up phone calls (Table 3).

Table 3 Long term complication comparison 12 months after operation

Complication	P-pouch group(*n* = 32)		Orr-RY group(*n* = 28)		P
	Case number	ratio%	Case number	ratio%	
RE syndrome	11	34.3	16	57.1	0.006
Dumping syndrome[a]	2	6.2	8	21.0	0.021
Retention syndrome[a]	3	9.3	10	35.7	0.013

RE reflux esophagitis.[a]Significant difference bewteen the P-pouch and Orr-RY group parameters

Discussion

In 1897, George Schlatter performed TG in a female patient with gastric cancer in Zurich using simple EJA to rebuild the digestive tract;however,anaemia and diarrhoea were noticeable and insurmountable [15].Patients who undergo TG usually complain of diarrhoea, upper abdominal pain after dinner, RE, early or late dumping syndrome and refractory anaemia, collectively called postgastrectomy syndrome [16]. To resolve this outcome, continuous improvement in the reconstruction of the alimentary tract after TG has occurred over the past 100 years; more than 50 reconstruction types have been reported in the literature [2, 15].Unfortunately, no gold standard has been established due to a lack of clinical evidence. In China,the commonly used strategy is called the modified Orr Roux-en-Y style [17].This reconstruction method has the advantage of being easy to perform, less traumatic and associated with reduced surgery-related morbidity. However, a relatively higher incidence of bowel-related complications is a disadvantage of this technique due to the lack of physiological storage and rapid food emptying [18].

The currently increasing emphasis on the recovery of psychological and social parameters, coupled with changes in health conception and medical models, has drawn our attention.Both the Spitzer QLI questionnaire and Visick grade self-assessment form are widely used for assessing the QoL of GI tumour patients after surgery.Reconstruction of the GI tract not only involves a continuation of the anatomical structure but also aims to preserve as much of the physiological function as possible. Choosing an appropriate reconstruction method is intrinsic to achieving satisfactory postoperative outcomes, reducing complication rates and improving the QoL.

Little is known about the efficacy of jejunal pouch reconstruction after TG [19].It has been suggested that TG with Roux-en-Y reconstruction might lead to a poor QoL due to malnutrition and intractable dumping syndrome. Recently, several clinical studies have reported that the presence of a reservoir after TG is related to an increased body weight and better QoL [20–22].In contrast, Fujiwara Y demonstrated that the benefit of constructing are servoir after TG is limited [23].Miyoshi K also argued that pouch reconstruction after TG does not significantly contribute to weight gain [24].Accordingly, the desirability of reservoir reconstruction after TG remains unclear.

In this study, after analysing the postoperative follow-up data, we found that patients who underwent reservoir reconstruction showed an improved body mass and daily QoL, which may support the former view point. In general, both traditional OrrRoux-en-Y and jejunal pouch reconstruction strategies appear to work well. No surgery-related mortality occurred during our study. Furthermore, no significant differences were found in terms of the clinical data or surgery-related complications.However, it is worth noting that the operation time in the jejunal pouch group was longer than that in the OrrRoux-en-Y group, but the extended operation time did not seem to be harmful. This factor served to minimize the chances of any spurious differences influencing the long-term results, and it truly increased the ascription of the success(or otherwise) of the reconstruction style to the intrinsic properties of the particular surgical technique. Moreover, with the greater application of the reconstruction technique, surgeons will become more proficient, and the operation times will become shorter. In recent years, with the application of stapling, the reconstruction procedure has become rapid, safe and practical [25].With respect to postoperative reflux symptoms or related morbidities, although no significant difference was found during the follow-up period,the lower postoperative reflux rate in the jejunal pouch group was consistent with the notion that pouch reconstruction achieves better results. Compared to traditional reconstruction, this reconstruction resulted in a lower incidence of dumping syndrome and/or retention syndrome, better postoperative recovery and a better global health status.A noteworthy observation was the general occurrence of gastrointestinal dynamic disorders, nutrient deficiencies and anaemia during the initial postoperative period,which often necessitated pharmacological intervention due to absence of the stomach.However, for the majority of the patients, these symptoms eventually resolved over time.As documented during the follow-up examinations, the incidence of surgery-related complications, including RE,dumping syndrome,diarrhoea and retention syndrome, after EJA with Roux-en-Y reconstruction or pouch-style reconstruction can be controlled, as improvements would achieved in both two groups.This finding is in line with the results reported by Iivonen MK [26] andis possibly related to the adaptation capacity of the body and diet control. In their study, postoperative dumping and early satiety were more common in the Roux-en-Y group after 3 months. In the jejunal pouch group, better results were found in terms of intestinal motility and the nutritional status, demonstrating that the effect of the jejunal pouch reconstruction technique on GI symptoms was more pronounced than that of the traditional OrrRoux-en-Y reconstruction technique. Bracale U reported a lower rate of anastomosis leaks and more comfortable deglutition achieved with SS-stapled anastomosis after oesophagectomy [27]; these results are consistent with the gastrectomy results presented here.

In our opinion, jejunal pouch reconstruction has several advantages. It may alleviate postoperative gastric-related complications because the resulting curvature has valve-like characteristics that mitigate reflux disease and effectively change the direction of food,thereby giving the chyme more time to be assimilated.Additionally, this reconstruction style is not restricted by the intestinal diameter, thereby reducing the risk of strictures. Moreover, the OrrRoux-en-Y procedure produces a distal closed loop of jejunal bowel near the anastomotic site, easily leading to pouchitis. Thus, the pouch technique appears to be a more physiological reconstruction method for application in patients undergoing TG.

There were certain limitations in our research. First, the short follow-up period—just 12 months—was a limitation, and the data analysed were inferior to data more indicative of the dynamic state; additionally, the sample size was small. Second, a relatively simple questionnaire was involved in the data analysis, and other parameters might also influence the analysed outcomes. Clearly, the perceptions of the definition of functional recovery may also lead to an unconscious bias among participants completing the modified Spitzer QLI questionnaire and the Visick grade self-assessment form; thus, the data rely on the individual understanding of each patient. Finally, the exact mechanism mediating the reduced incidence of dumping syndrome and retention syndrome and the improved daily QoL after pouch reconstruction was not clear. Regarding the latter, the morphological similarity of the reconstruction might play a critical role in this process.

Conclusion

In summary,TG with jejunal pouch reconstruction for gastric cancer is feasible and safe.It combines the advantages of improved digestive absorption and storage and improved QoL. Based on our results, jejunal pouch reconstruction appears to be a superior surgical approach. However, more randomized controlled clinical studies are essential to verify the benefits of this procedure.

Abbreviations

EJA: Oesophageal-jejunalanastomosis; PNI: Prognostic nutritional index; QoL: Quality of life; RE: Reflux oesophagitis; TG: Total gastrectomy

Acknowledgements

We thank Professors Qun Qian,Qingcong Jiang and Suzhi Liu from the Department of General Surgery of Zhongnan Hospital of Wuhan University for their technical assistance.

Funding

This research was supported by the Fund of the Health and Family Planning Commission of Wuhan Municipality(WX17D05)and the Fund of the Health and Family Planning Commission of Hubei Municipality(WJ2017F015).

Authors' contributions

Study concept and design: JXM and CW; data collection: LHC,DZ and HH; data analysisand interpretation: LHC and DZ; table and figure preparation: DZ and HH; manuscript writing and review: CW and JXM.

Competing interests

The author(s) declare that they have no competing interests.

Author details

[1]Department of Gastrointestinal Surgery, The Central Hospital of the Wuhan, Tongji Medical College, Huazhong University of Science and Technology, Wuhan 430000, People's Republic of China. [2]Department of General Surgery, Zhongnan Hospital of Wuhan University, Wuhan 430014, People's Republic of China. [3]Department of Gastrointestinal Surgery, Hubei Cancer Hospital, Wuhan 430014, People's Republic of China.

References

1. Allum W, Lordick F, Alsina M, Andritsch E, Ba-Ssalamah A, Beishon M, et al. ECCO essential requirements for quality cancer care: oesophageal and gastric cancer. Crit Rev Oncol Hematol. 2018;122:179–93. https://doi.org/10.1016/j.critrevonc.2017.12.019.
2. Lygidakis NJ. Total gastrectomy for gastric carcinoma: a retrospective study of different procedures and assessment of a new technique of gastric reconstruction. Br J Surg. 1981;68:649–55. https://doi.org/10.1002/bjs.1800680913.
3. Chen W, Jiang CQ, Qian Q, Ding Z, Liu ZS. Antiperistaltic side-to-side ileorectal anastomosis is associated with a better short-term fecal continence and quality of life in slow transit constipation patients. Dig Surg. 2015;32:367–74. https://doi.org/10.1159/000437234.
4. Ding X, Yan F, Liang H, Xue Q, Zhang K, Li H, et al. Functional jejunal interposition, a reconstruction procedure, promotes functional outcomes after total gastrectomy. BMC Surg. 2015;15:43. https://doi.org/10.1186/s12893-015-0032-2.
5. Razavi D, Allilaire JF, Smith M, Salimpour A, Verra M, Desclaux B, et al. The effect of fluoxetine on anxiety and depression symptoms in cancer patients. Acta Psychiatr Scand. 1996;94:205–10. https://doi.org/10.1111/j.1600-0447.1996.tb09850.x.
6. Addington-Hall JM, LD MD, Anderson HR. Can the Spitzer Quality of Life Index help to reduce prognostic uncertainty in terminal care? Br J Cancer. 1990;62:695–9. https://doi.org/10.1038/bjc.1990.360.
7. Ahn SH, Jung DH, Son SY, Lee CM, Park DJ, Kim HH. Laparoscopic double-tract proximal gastrectomy for proximal early gastric cancer. Gastric Cancer Off J Int Gastric Cancer Assoc Jpn Gastric Cancer Assoc. 2014;17:562–70. https://doi.org/10.1007/s10120-013-0303-5.
8. Ward MA, Ujiki MB. Creation of a jejunal pouch during laparoscopic total gastrectomy and roux-en-Y esophagojejunostomy. Ann Surg Oncol. 2017;24:184–6. https://doi.org/10.1245/s10434-016-5540-5.
9. Bozzetti F, Bonfanti G, Castellani R, Maffioli L, Rubino A, Diazzi G, et al. Comparing reconstruction with roux-en-Y to a pouch following total gastrectomy. J Am Coll Surg. 1996;183:243–8.

10. Lawrence W Jr. Reservoir construction after total gastrectomy: an instructive case. Ann Surg. 1962;155:191–8. https://doi.org/10.1097/00000658-196200000-00004.
11. Chester JF, Gazet JC. Technique for abdominal radical total gastrectomy. Br J Surg. 1989;76:540. https://doi.org/10.1002/bjs.1800760605.
12. Zhang H, Sun Z, Xu H-M, Shan J-X, Wang S-B, Chen J-Q. Improved quality of life in patients with gastric cancer after esophagogastrostomy reconstruction. World J Gastroent. 2009;15:3183–90.
13. Fuchs KH, Thiede A, Engemann R, Deltz E, Stremme O, Hamelmann H. Reconstruction of the food passage after total gastrectomy: randomized trial. World J Surg. 1995;19:698–705. discussion 705. [Discussion:705–696]
14. Kinoshita A, Onoda H, Imai N, Iwaku A, Oishi M, Fushiya N, et al. Comparison of the prognostic value of inflammation-based prognostic scores in patients with hepatocellular carcinoma. Br J Cancer. 2012;107:988–93. https://doi.org/10.1038/bjc.2012.354.
15. Catarci M, Proposito D, Guadagni S, Carboni M. History of reconstruction after total gastrectomy. J R Coll Surg Edinb. 1997;42:73–81.
16. Westhoff BC, Weston A, Cherian R, Sharma P. Development of Barrett's esophagus six months after total gastrectomy. Am J Gastroenterol. 2004;99:2271–7. https://doi.org/10.1111/j.1572-0241.2004.40249.x.
17. Ojima T, Nakamori M, Nakamura M, Katsuda M, Hayata K, Kato T, et al. Internal hernia after laparoscopic total gastrectomy for gastric cancer. Surg Laparosc Endosc Percutan Tech. 2017;27:470–3. https://doi.org/10.1097/SLE.0000000000000481.
18. Nakagawa M, Kojima K, Inokuchi M, Kato K, Sugita H, Otsuki S, et al. Assessment of serum copper state after gastrectomy with roux-en-Y reconstruction for gastric cancer. Dig Surg. 2015;32:301–5. https://doi.org/10.1159/000431186.
19. Kobayashi I, Ohwada S, Ohya T, Yokomori T, Iesato H, Morishita Y. Jejunal pouch with nerve preservation and interposition after total gastrectomy. Hepato-Gastroenterology. 1998;45:558–62.
20. Gertler R, Rosenberg R, Feith M, Schuster T, Friess H. Pouch vs. no pouch following total gastrectomy: meta-analysis and systematic review. Am J Gastroenterol. 2009;104:2838–51. https://doi.org/10.1038/ajg.2009.456.
21. Nozoe T, Anai H, Sugimachi K. Usefulness of reconstruction with jejunal pouch in total gastrectomy for gastric cancer in early improvement of nutritional condition. Am J Surg. 2001;181:274–8. https://doi.org/10.1016/S0002-9610(01)00554-2.
22. Doussot A, Borraccino B, Rat P, Ortega-Deballon P, Facy O. Construction of a jejunal pouch after total gastrectomy. J Surg Tech Case Rep. 2014;6:37–8. https://doi.org/10.4103/2006-8808.135152.
23. Fujiwara Y, Kusunoki M, Nakagawa K, Tanaka T, Hatada T, Yamamura T. Evaluation of J-pouch reconstruction after total gastrectomy: rho-double tract vs. J-pouch double tract. Dig Surg. 2000;17:475–81. discussion 481. [Discussion:481–72]
24. Miyoshi K, Fuchimoto S, Ohsaki T, Sakata T, Ohtsuka S, Takakura N. Long-term effects of jejunal pouch added to Roux-en-Y reconstruction after total gastrectomy. Gastric Cancer Off J Int Gastric Cancer Assoc Jpn Gastric Cancer Assoc. 2001;4:156–61. https://doi.org/10.1007/s101200100007.
25. Namikawa T, Munekage E, Munekage M, Maeda H, Kitagawa H, Nagata Y, et al. Reconstruction with jejunal pouch after gastrectomy for gastric cancer. Am Surg. 2016;82:510–7.
26. Iivonen MK, Mattila JJ, Nordback IH, Matikainen MJ. Long-term follow-up of patients with jejunal pouch reconstruction after total gastrectomy. A randomized prospective study. Scand J Gastroenterol. 2000;35:679–85. https://doi.org/10.1080/003655200750023327.
27. Bracale U, Marzano E, Nastro P, Barone M, Cuccurullo D, Cutini G, et al. Side-to-side esophagojejunostomy during totally laparoscopic total gastrectomy for malignant disease: a multicenter study. Surg Endosc. 2010;24:2475–9. https://doi.org/10.1007/s00464-010-0988-z.

29

Management of early gastric cancer that meet the indication for radical lymph node dissection following endoscopic resection: a retrospective cohort analysis

Satoru Kikuchi[1*], Shinji Kuroda[1], Masahiko Nishizaki[1], Tetsuya Kagawa[1], Hiromitsu Kanzaki[2], Yoshiro Kawahara[2], Shunsuke Kagawa[1], Takehiro Tanaka[3], Hiroyuki Okada[4] and Toshiyoshi Fujiwara[1]

Abstract

Background: Endoscopic resection (ER) has been widely accepted as the standard treatment for early gastric cancer (EGC). However, in patients considered to have undergone non-curative ER due to their potential risk of lymph node metastasis (LNM), additional gastrectomy is recommended. The aim of the present study was to identify EGC patients after non-curative ER at high risk of LNM.

Methods: A total of 150 patients who had undergone ER for EGC were diagnosed as non-curative ER due to their potential risk of LNM. Clinicopathological data and clinical outcomes were examined retrospectively.

Results: Additional gastrectomy with lymph node dissection was performed in 73 patients, and the remaining 77 patients were followed-up without additional gastrectomy. In patients who underwent additional gastrectomy, 8 patients had local residual tumor, and 8 patients had LNM, which were limited in the peritumoral nodes. Only lymphatic invasion ($p = 0.012$) was a statistically significant factor for LNM. The 5-year overall survival and recurrence-free survival were not significantly different between patients with and without additional gastrectomy.

Conclusion: Additional gastrectomy with lymph node dissection is recommended for patients who were diagnosed as non-curative ER with lymphatic invasion, and minimizing the extent of lymph node dissection may be allowed for these patients.

Keywords: Early gastric cancer, Endoscopic resection, Lymph node metastasis

Background

Gastric cancer is the world's third leading cause of cancer mortality, responsible for 723,000 deaths each year [1]. With advances in diagnostic techniques and the increasing prevalence of screening programs, the percentage of early gastric cancer (EGC) cases is reaching nearly 60% in Japan [2, 3]. Endoscopic resection (ER) including endoscopic mucosal resection (EMR) and endoscopic submucosal dissection (ESD) has been widely accepted as the standard treatment for EGC patients when the risk of lymph node metastasis (LNM) is negligible [4, 5]. However, endoscopic diagnosis of EGC before ER is not always accurate, and some patients are diagnosed as non-curative ER due to the potential risk of LNM histologically after ER [5–7]. In patients diagnosed as non-curative ER, additional gastrectomy with lymph node dissection is generally recommended [7]. However, the LNM rate of patients who have undergone additional gastrectomy after non-curative ER is less than 10% [8–10]. The aim of the present study was to investigate the optimal treatment strategies for non-curative ER patients with a potential risk of LNM based on retrospective analysis in a single institution.

* Correspondence: satorukc@okayama-u.ac.jp
[1]Department of Gastroenterological Surgery, Okayama University Graduate School of Medicine, Dentistry and Pharmaceutical Sciences, 2-5-1 Shikata-cho, Kita-ku, Okayama 700-8558, Japan
Full list of author information is available at the end of the article

Methods

Patients

From January 2004 to August 2013, 707 patients with EGCs treated with ER, including EMR and ESD, at the Endoscopy Center of Okayama University Hospital, Okayama, Japan, were retrospectively studied. A total of 182 patients (25.7%) were subsequently diagnosed as non-curative ER after histological evaluation based on the Japanese gastric cancer treatment guidelines 2010 (version 3) [7] and they were classified into those with a positive hiatal margin (HM) only (n = 32), and those with a potential risk of LNM (n = 150). The clinical records of 150 patients after non-curative ER due to their potential risk of LNM were analyzed retrospectively with regard to clinicopathological findings of ER specimens, additional gastrectomy after ER, histology of surgical specimens, and prognosis.

The formalin-fixed specimens resected by ER were examined histologically using serial sections 2 mm in width according to the Japanese Classification of Gastric Carcinoma [11]. Lymphatic or venous infiltration was evaluated by examination of hematoxylin and eosin (H&E) stained sections. Curability was evaluated based on the histological criteria for curative ER [7]. Non-curative ER was defined as potential risk of LNM or positive lateral resection margin.

For all patients with a potential risk of LNM, additional gastrectomy with lymph node dissection was recommended, but for some patients, strict follow-up was selected due to the surgical risk, other primary cancers and new disorders after gastrectomy. They were divided into two subgroups: patients who underwent additional gastrectomy with lymph node dissection and those who received strict follow-up without gastrectomy.

Surgical specimens were examined according to the recommendations of the Japanese Classification of Gastric Carcinoma [11]. The entire resected stomach area was divided into 5-mm-wide slices, and LNMs were evaluated in the central portion of each lymph node. Local residual tumor was defined as any cancer diagnosed histologically at the ER site.

Statistical analysis

Univariate analysis was performed using Fisher's exact test or the χ^2 test. Variables showing a univariate association ($p < 0.50$) were also subjected to multivariate analysis. Multivariate analysis was performed using logistic regression analysis to identify independent predictors related to LNM and local residual tumor. P values <0.05 were considered statistically significant. Clinical outcomes of patients who had additional gastrectomy and those who underwent strict follow-up were collected and analyzed in April 2017. Overall survival (OS) and recurrence-free survival curves were calculated by the Kaplan-Meier method. Statistical analysis was performed using JMP 11.2 (SAS Institute, Cary, NC, USA).

Results

Seventy-three patients (49.7%) underwent additional gastrectomy (Fig. 1). The remaining 77 patients did not undergo additional gastrectomy by the reason of patient choice, high surgical risk, and other concomitant cancer. The patient's clinical courses are summarized in Fig. 1. The demographics and clinical background characteristics of the 73 patients who underwent additional gastrectomy and the 77 who underwent strict follow-up without gastrectomy are compared in Table 1. The subgroup that underwent additional gastrectomy had a higher percentage of younger patients (68.8 versus 73.4 years; $p < 0.001$), positive lymphatic-vascular involvement (74.0% versus 40.3%; $p < 0.001$) and submucosal deep invasion (76.7% versus 51.9%; $p = 0.002$).

Overall and recurrence-free survival curves are shown in Fig. 2. Among those who underwent additional gastrectomy, the median follow-up time was 4.8 (range 0.5–11.9) years. Two of these patients (2.7%) developed distant metastasis after surgery, and died from gastric cancer. The 5-year overall and recurrence-free survivals were 85.0% and 97.0%, respectively (Fig. 2). Among those who underwent strict follow-up without gastrectomy, the median follow-up time was 4.7 (range 0.2–11.8) years. Three patients (3.9%) developed recurrence (local recurrence in two patients and LNM in one patient), and both of local recurrence patients underwent gastrectomy with lymphadenectomy and are alive without recurrence. The remaining patient who had LNM refused further treatment, and was followed up. The 5-year overall and recurrence-free survivals were 79.4% and 95.3%, respectively (Fig. 2). The 5-year overall and recurrence-free survivals of patients who underwent strict follow-up without gastrectomy were not significantly different from those who underwent gastrectomy.

The median interval between initial ER and additional gastrectomy was 88 (range 21–201) days, and there were no operation-related deaths. In additional gastrectomy specimens, 8 (11.0%) of 73 patients had LNM, which were limited in one or two peritumoral nodes. Primary tumor remained in 8 (11.0%) of 73 patients. Relationships among clinicopathological characteristics, nodal metastasis, and local residual tumor are summarized in Table 2.

On univariate analysis, HM was the only significant factor for local residual tumor ($p = 0.015$). For nodal metastasis, lymphatic invasion was the only significant factor ($p = 0.005$). Moreover, 8 (20.5%) of 39 patients with lymphatic invasion (ly (+)) had lymph node metastasis. On multivariate analysis, HM was the only significant factor for local residual tumor ($p = 0.018$). For LNM, only lymphatic invasion was significant ($p < 0.001$) (Table 2).

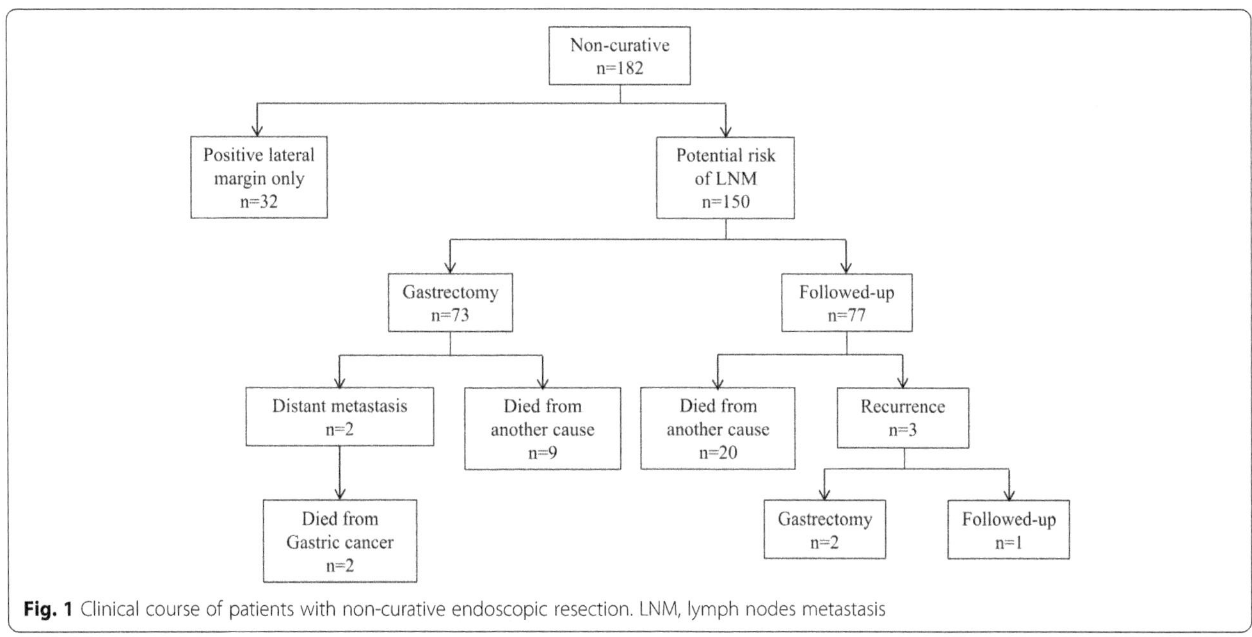

Fig. 1 Clinical course of patients with non-curative endoscopic resection. LNM, lymph nodes metastasis

Discussion

In this retrospective study, 707 EGC patients who were expected to satisfy the criteria for curative ER [7] underwent ER, but, in fact, 25.7% did not. Despite improvements in endoscopic examination, the endoscopic diagnosis of EGC is not always accurate, as several reports have mentioned, and is correct in only 80–90% of cases [12–14]. When patients were diagnosed as non-curative ER based on their potential risk of LNM after pathological examination following ER, additional gastrectomy with lymph node dissection was recommended [7, 15], despite the fact that the incidence of LNM of EGC is rare [9, 10]. Additional gastrectomy with lymph node dissection is necessary for EGC patients with a potential risk of LNM, but most patients without LNM have routinely undergone unnecessary surgery. The conventional gastrectomy with prophylactic lymph node dissection often has acute and chronic complications and reduces the patients' quality of life (QOL). Thus, a specific treatment depending on the individual patient would benefit these patients by allowing them to avoid prophylactic surgery.

Patients diagnosed as non-curative ER were classified into two groups with or without a potential risk of

Table 1 Clinical characteristics of patients diagnosed as non-curative endoscopic resection with a potential risk of LNM

Factors		All (n = 150)	Surgery (n = 73)	Follow-up (n = 77)	p Value
Age		71.2	68.8	73.4	<0.001*
Sex	M:F	128:22	66:7	62:15	0.11
Concomitant disease		22 (14.7%)	9 (12.3%)	13 (16.9%)	0.49
Other cancer		11	5	6	
Hematologic disease		3	2	1	
Cardiovascular disease		3	2	1	
Liver cirrhosis		5	0	5	
Positive lymphatic-vascular involvement		85 (56.7%)	54 (74.0%)	31 (40.3%)	<0.001*
Undifferenciated type		19 (12.7%)	8 (11.0%)	11 (14.3%)	0.63
Deep submucosal invasion (≥ sm2)		96 64.0%)	56 (76.7%)	40 (51.9%)	0.0021*
Minute submucosal cancer (sm1 ≥ 30 mm in size)		9 (6.0%)	4 (5.5%)	5 (6.5%)	1.00
VM positive or unclear		35 (23.3%)	12 (16.4%)	23 (29.9%)	0.056
HM positive or unclear		20 (13.3%)	6 (8.2%)	14 (18.2%)	0.093

The Fisher exact test or the χ2 test was used for the analyses
VM vertical margin, *HM* Hiatal margin, *LNM* lymph node metastasis
Statistical significance defined as $^*p < 0.05$

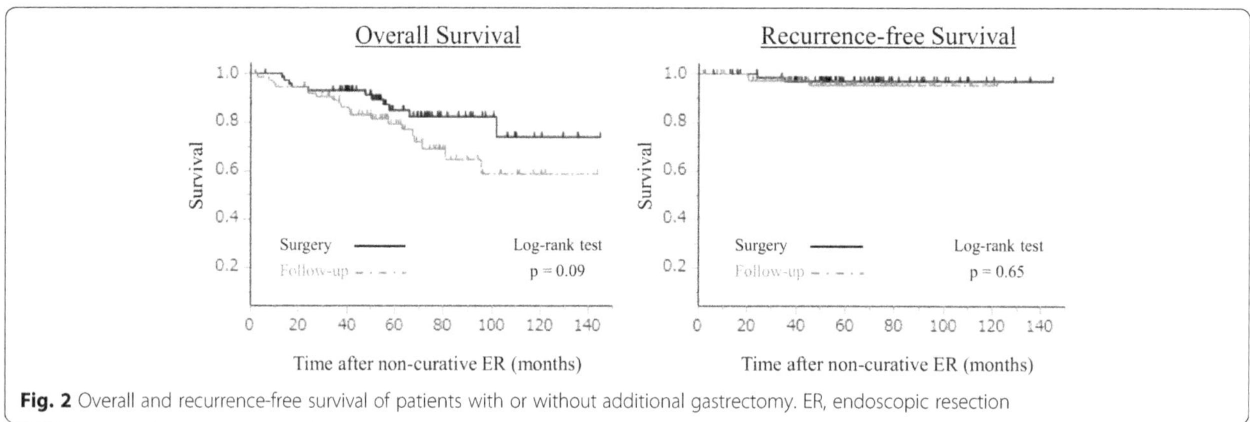

Fig. 2 Overall and recurrence-free survival of patients with or without additional gastrectomy. ER, endoscopic resection

LNM. Non-curative ER with positive HM as the only non-curative factor is generally considered to be an indication for additional local treatment (repeated-ESD or coagulation) or surgery or close observation according to the individual case [9, 16, 17]. However, it is sometimes difficult to achieve an exact diagnosis with ER specimens because of histological modifications that occur with ER [7, 18]. Several articles have reported that none of the patients diagnosed as non-curative ER due only to HM involvement developed LNM [9, 10].

The LNM rate among patients who underwent additional gastrectomy in this study was 11.0%, which was lower than the reported rate of 20% in patients with submucosal invasive cancer [5]. Some lesions with additional gastrectomy in this study had a lower risk of LNM than submucosal invasive cancer overall because they had been treated with curative intent by ER. Similar results have been reported previously, in which less than 10% of patients had LNM in surgical specimens following non-curative ER [19–21].

The 5-year overall and recurrence-free survivals among patients who underwent strict follow-up without gastrectomy were not significantly different from those in patients who underwent gastrectomy. Choi et al. [22] also reported that OS and disease-free survival did not differ significantly between patients treated with additional surgical resection and patients simply followed up after ESD in submucosa-invasive gastric cancer. However, this result should be carefully interpreted, because histological analysis demonstrated that the patients who underwent gastrectomy showed significantly higher lymphatic-vascular involvement and deeper submucosal invasion than those followed up without gastrectomy (Table 1), indicating that the patients with these unfavorable histological findings were more frequently selected for additional gastrectomy. Kawata et al. [20] and Suzuki et al. [21] reported that there

Table 2 Results of univariate and multivariate analysis of pathological findings, remnant tumor, and lymph node metastasis

Factors	Remnant tumor		Univariate *p* Value	Multivariate *p* Value	LNM		Univariatep Value	Multivariate *p* Value
	Presence (*n* = 8)	Absence (*n* = 65)			Presence (*n* = 8)	Absence (*n* = 65)		
Lesion size (mm)	30.3	26.4	0.21	0.35	27.9	26.7	0.81	–
Lymphatic invasion	5 (62.5)	34 (52.3)	0.44	0.31	8 (100)	31 (47.7)	0.005*	<0.001*
Venous invasion	3 (37.5)	20 (30.7)	0.49	0.67	4 (50)	19 (29.2)	0.21	0.05
Undifferenciated type	2 (25)	6 (9.2)	0.21	0.32	1 (12.5)	7 (10.8)	1.00	–
Deep submucosal invasion (≥SM2)	6 (75)	50 (76.9)	0.73	–	7 (87.5)	49 (75.4)	0.67	–
VM Positive or unclear	2 (25)	10 (15.4)	0.39	0.70	1 (12.5)	11 (16.9)	1.00	–
HM Positive or unclear	3 (37.5)	3 (4.6)	0.015*	0.018*	0 (0)	6 (9.2)	1.00	–

Univariate analysis was performed by using the Fisher exact test or the χ^2 test, and multivariate analysis was performed by using logistic regression analysis
Values in parentheses are percentages
VM vertical margin, *HM* hiatal margin
Statistical significance defined as $^*p < 0.05$

was a significant difference in OS between additional surgery and follow-up groups, although disease-specific survival did not differ significantly between the two groups. In patient clinical backgrounds, the follow-up group was significantly older than the additional surgery group, and several patients died of causes other than gastric cancer. Therefore, advanced age or concomitant disease may have contributed to the poor prognosis of the follow-up group. In the current study, all patients in the follow-up group died of causes other than gastric cancer during the study period. This result indicates that strict follow-up instead of additional surgery may be an acceptable management option for certain patients with diagnoses with non-curative ER. Moreover, risk stratification associated with LN or distant metastasis and gastric cancer related death of non-curative ER patients is required for an appropriate treatment strategy.

In this study, 8 of 39 patients (20.5%) with positive lymphatic invasion and 4 of 23 (17.4%) with positive venous invasion had metastasis in regional LNs. Only lymphatic invasion was an independently significant factor of LNM ($p < 0.001$), and there was no LNM in lesions without lymphatic invasion. This result indicates that additional gastrectomy with lymphadenectomy should be performed for lesions with lymphatic invasion. Some similar studies [20, 21] reported that lymphatic invasion was an independent risk factor for LNM in non-curative ER patients. Furthermore, all metastatic nodes were located in the perigastric area close to the primary tumors. This suggests that minimizing the lymphadenectomy and reducing the extent of gastrectomy as additional surgery following non-curative ER may be acceptable. Some articles have reported that function-preserving gastrectomy, such as pylorus-preserving gastrectomy and proximal gastrectomy, improved postoperative QOL, including postoperative symptoms, weight gain, and food intake volume [23–25]. However, inadequate treatment may yield remnant metastatic LNs. In recent years, the validity of sentinel node navigation surgery for EGC was reported by some studies [26, 27]. Though it is unclear whether the sentinel hypothesis is suitable for EGC after ER, function-preserving surgery may be used for patients who have been diagnosed as non-curative ER in the future [28].

The limitations of this study are its retrospective, single-center design, and the differences in the clinicopathological background characteristics of the two groups. A prospective randomized clinical trial (RCT) is needed to establish more appropriate treatment strategies for non-curative ER patients, although it may be difficult to conduct a prospective RCT for ethical reasons.

Conclusion

Additional gastrectomy with lymphadenectomy is strongly recommended for patients with lymphatic invasion among patients diagnosed as non-curative ER due to their potential risk of LNM, and minimizing the extent of lymphadenectomy may be allowed for these patients. However, a RCT is required to establish more appropriate treatment strategies for these patients.

Abbreviations

EGC: Early gastric cancer; EMR: Endoscopic mucosal resection; ER: Endoscopic resection; ESD: Endoscopic submucosal dissection; HM: Hiatal margin; LNM: Lymph node metastasis; OS: Overall survival; QOL: Quality of life; RCT: Randomized clinical trial; VM: Vertical margin

Funding

None.

Acknowledgements

This work was supported by JSPS Grant-in-Aid for Young Scientists B, Grant Number 16 K21185.

Authors' contributions

SKi and MN designed the studies. SKu, TK, TT and HK performed data acquisition. Ski, SKu, MN, TK, HK, YK, Ska, TT, HO and TF performed data analysis and interpretation. Ski and MN prepared the manuscript. SKu, TK, HK, YK, Ska, TT, HO and TF revised paper critically. All authors read and approved the final manuscript.

Competing interests

The authors declare that they have no competing interests.

Author details

[1]Department of Gastroenterological Surgery, Okayama University Graduate School of Medicine, Dentistry and Pharmaceutical Sciences, 2-5-1 Shikata-cho, Kita-ku, Okayama 700-8558, Japan. [2]Department of Endoscopy, Okayama University Hospital, Okayama 700-8558, Japan. [3]Department of Diagnostic Pathology, Okayama University Hospital, Okayama 700-8558, Japan. [4]Department of Gastroenterology and Hepatology, Okayama University Graduate School of Medicine, Dentistry and Pharmaceutical Sciences, Okayama 700-8558, Japan.

References

1. Ferlay J, Soerjomataram I, Ervik M, Dikshit R, Eser S, Mathers C, Rebelo M, Parkin DM, Forman D, Bray F. GLOBOCAN 2012 v1.0, cancer incidence and mortality worldwide. IARC CancerBase No.11. Available: http://globocan.iarc.fr
2. Everett SM, Axon AT. Early gastric cancer in Europe. Gut. 1997;41:142–50.
3. Shimizu S, Tada M, Kawai K. Early gastric cancer: its surveillance and natural course. Endoscopy. 1995;27:27–31.
4. Gotoda T. Endoscopic resection of early gastric cancer. Gastric Cancer. 2007; 10:1–11.
5. Gotoda T, Yanagisawa A, Sasako M, Ono H, Nakanishi Y, Shimoda T, et al. Incidence of lymph node metastasis from early gastric cancer: estimation with a large number of cases at two large centers. Gastric Cancer. 2000;3:219–25.
6. Hirasawa T, Gotoda T, Miyata S, Kato Y, Shimoda T, Taniguchi H, et al. Incidence of lymph node metastasis and the feasibility of endoscopic resection for undifferentiated-type early gastric cancer. Gastric Cancer. 2000;12:148–52.
7. Japanese Gastric Cancer Association. Japanese gastric cancer treatment guidelines 2010 (ver.3). Gastric Cancer. 2011;14:113–23.
8. Nagano H, Ohyama S, Fukunaga T, Seto Y, Fujisaki J, Yamaguchi T, et al. Indications for gastrectomy after incomplete EMR for early gastric cancer. Gastric Cancer. 2005;8:149–54.
9. Oda I, Gotoda T, Sasako M, Sano T, Katai H, Fukagawa T, et al. Treatment strategy after non-curative endoscopic resection of early gastric cancer. Br J Surg. 2008;95:1495–500.

10. Ito H, Inoue H, Ikeda H, Odaka N, Yoshida A, Satodate H, et al. Surgical outcomes and clinicopathological characteristics of patients who underwent potentially noncurative endoscopic resection for gastric cancer: a report of a single-center experience. Gastroenterol Res Pract. 2013;427405
11. Japanese Gastric Cancer Association. Japanese classification of gastric carcinoma– 3rd English edition. Gastric Cancer. 2011;14:101–12.
12. Sano T, Okuyama Y, Kobori O, Shimizu T, Morioka Y. Early gastric cancer. Endoscopic diagnosis of depth of invasion. Dig Dis Sci. 1990;35:1340–4.
13. Seto Y, Shimoyama S, Kitayama J, Mafune K, Kaminishi M, Aikou T, et al. Lymph node metastasis and preoperative diagnosis of depth of invasion in early gastric cancer. Gastric Cancer. 2001;4:34–8.
14. Yanai H, Matsubara Y, Kawano T, Okamoto T, Hirano A, Nakamura Y, et al. Clinical impact of strip biopsy for early gastric cancer. Gastrointest Endosc. 2004;60:771–7.
15. Ryu KW, Choi IJ, Doh YW, Kook MC, Kim CG, Park HJ, et al. Surgical indication for non-curative endoscopic resection in early gastric cancer. Ann of Surg Oncol. 2007;14:3428–34.
16. Lee JH, Kim JH, Kim DH, Jeon TY, Kim DH, Kim GH. Park do Y. Is surgical treatment necessary after non-curative endoscopic resection for early gastric cancer? J of Gastric Cancer. 2010;10:182–7.
17. Jung H, Bae JM, Choi MG, Noh JH, Sohn TS, Kim S. Surgical outcome after incomplete endoscopic submucosal dissection of gastric cancer. Br J Surg. 2011;98:73–8.
18. Gotoda T. A large endoscopic resection by endoscopic submucosal dissection procedure for early gastric cancer. Clin Gastroenterol Hepatol. 2005;3:71–3.
19. Hatta W, Gotoda T, Oyama T, Kawata N, Takahashi A, Yoshifuku Y, et al. Is radical surgery necessary in all patients who do not meet the curative criteria for endoscopic submucosal dissection in early gastric cancer? A multi-center retrospective study in Japan. J Gastroenterol. 2017;52:175–84.
20. Kawata N, Kakushima N, Takizawa K, Tanaka M, Makuuchi R, Tokunaga M, et al. Risk factors for lymph node metastasis and long-term outcomes of patients with early gastric cancer after non-curative endoscopic submucosal dissection. Surg Endosc. 2017;31:1607–16.
21. Suzuki H, Oda I, Abe S, Sekiguchi M, Nonaka S, Yoshinaga S, et al. Clinical outcomes of early gastric cancer patients after noncurative endoscopic submucosal dissection in a large consecutive patient series. Gastric Cancer. 2017; [Epub ahead of print]
22. Choi JY, Jeon SW, Cho KB, Park KS, Kim ES, Park CK, et al. Non-curative endoscopic resection does not always lead to grave outcomes in submucosal invasive early gastric cancer. Surg Endosc. 2015;29:1842–9.
23. Morita S, Katai H, Saka M, Fukagawa T, Sano T, Sasako M. Outcome of pylorus-preserving gastrectomy for early gastric cancer. Br J Surg. 2008;95:1131–5.
24. Nunobe S, Sasako M, Saka M, Fukagawa T, Katai H, Sano T. Symptom evaluation of long-term postoperative outcomes after pylorus-preserving gastrectomy for early gastric cancer. Gastric Cancer. 2007;10:167–72.
25. Ichikawa D, Ueshima Y, Shirono K, Kan K, Shioaki Y, Lee CJ, et al. Esophagogastrostomy reconstruction after limited proximal gastrectomy. Hepato-Gastroenterology. 2001;48:1797–801.
26. Kitagawa Y, Takeuchi H, Takagi Y, Natsugoe S, Terashima M, Murakami N, et al. Sentinel node mapping for gastric cancer: a prospective multicenter trial in Japan. J Clin Oncol. 2013;31:3704–10.
27. Takeuchi H, Kitagawa Y. New sentinel node mapping technologies for early gastric cancer. Ann Surg Oncol. 2013;20:522–32.
28. Mayanagi S, Takeuchi H, Kamiya S, Niihara M, Nakamura R, Takahashi T, et al. Suitability of sentinel node mapping as an index of metastasis in early gastric cancer following endoscopic resection. Ann Surg Oncol. 2014;21:2987–93.

30

Prognostic value of preoperative inflammatory response biomarkers in patients with esophageal cancer who undergo a curative thoracoscopic esophagectomy

Noriyuki Hirahara*, Takeshi Matsubara, Yoko Mizota, Shuichi Ishibashi and Yoshitsugu Tajima

Abstract

Background: Several inflammatory response biomarkers, including lymphocyte-to-monocyte ratio (LMR), neutrophil-to-lymphocyte ratio (NLR), and platelet-to-lymphocyte ratio (PLR) have been reported to predict survival in various cancers. The aim of this study is to evaluate the clinical value of these biomarkers in patients undergoing curative resection for esophageal cancer.

Methods: The LMR, NLR and PLR were calculated in 147 consecutive patients who underwent esophagectomy between January 2006 and February 2015. We examined the prognostic significance of the LMR, NLR, and PLR in both elderly and non-elderly patients. We evaluated the cancer-specific survival (CSS), with the cause of death determined from the case notes or computerized records.

Results: Univariate analyses demonstrated that TNM pStage ($p < 0.0001$), tumor size ($p = 0.0014$), operation time ($p = 0.0209$), low LMR ($p = 0.0008$), and high PLR ($p = 0.0232$) were significant risk factors for poor prognosis. Meanwhile, TNM pStage ($p < 0.0001$) and low LMR ($p = 0.0129$) were found to be independently associated with poor prognosis via multivariate analysis.

In non-elderly patients, univariate analyses demonstrated that TNM pStage ($p < 0.0001$), tumor size ($p = 0.0001$), operation time ($p = 0.0374$), LMR ($p < 0.0001$), and PLR ($p = 0.0189$) were significantly associated with a poorer prognosis. Multivariate analysis demonstrated that TNM pStage ($p = 0.001$) and LMR ($p = 0.0007$) were independent risk factors for a poorer prognosis.

In elderly patients, univariate analysis demonstrated that that TNM pStage ($p = 0.0023$) was the only significant risk factor for a poor prognosis.

Conclusions: LMR was associated with cancer-specific survival (CSS) of esophageal cancer patients after curative esophagectomy. In particular, a low LMR was a significant and independent predictor of poor survival in non-elderly patients. The LMR was convenient, cost effective, and readily available, and could thus act as markers of survival in esophageal cancer.

Keywords: Esophageal cancer, Lymphocyte to monocyte ratio (LMR), Neutrophil to lymphocyte ratio (NLR), Platelet lymphocyte ratio (PLR), Prognostic predictor

* Correspondence: norinorihirahara@yahoo.co.jp
Department of Digestive and General Surgery, Shimane University Faculty of Medicine, 89-1 Enya-cho, Izumo, Shimane 693-8501, Japan

Background

It is now widely recognized that host-related factors, such as performance status, weight loss, smoking, and comorbidity, as well as the biological properties of individual tumors, play an important role in cancer outcomes [1]. Recent studies have shown that preoperative inflammation-based prognostic scores have a significant predictive and prognostic value in various types of cancers [2–4]. A systemic inflammatory response has been reported to be associated with tumor development, apoptosis inhibition, and angiogenesis promotion, thus resulting in tumor progression and metastasis [5, 6]. Furthermore, significant relationships between patient survival and the lymphocyte-to-monocyte ratio (LMR), neutrophil-to-lymphocyte ratio (NLR), and platelet-to-lymphocyte ratio (PLR) have been documented in various cancers [7–9]. However, only a few studies have evaluated the utility of inflammation-based scores for assessing the prognosis of patients with esophageal cancer.

The aim of the present study was to evaluate whether the LMR, NLR, and PLR have prognostic values independent of conventional clinicopathological features in patients undergoing a potentially curative resection for esophageal cancer. Additionally, this study stratified patients into two age groups, elderly patients aged 70 years or older and patients aged under 70 years, because esophageal cancer occurs predominantly in elderly people and age-specific prognostic factors in patients with esophageal cancer have not yet been identified.

Methods

Patients

We retrospectively reviewed a database of medical records from 147 consecutive patients who underwent curative esophagectomy with R0 resection for histologically verified esophageal squamous cell carcinoma between January 2006 and February 2015 at Shimane University Faculty of Medicine. R0 resection was defined as a complete resection without any microscopic resection margin involvement. Video-assisted or thoracoscopic subtotal esophagectomy with three-field lymph node dissection was performed in all patients, followed by laparoscopic gastric surgery with an elevation of the gastric conduit to the neck via the posterior mediastinal or a retrosternal approach with an end-to-end anastomosis of the remnant cervical esophagus and fundus of the gastric conduit. The patients' clinical characteristics, laboratory data, treatment, and pathological data were obtained from medical records. Preoperatively, no patients had clinical signs of infection or other systemic inflammatory conditions. Based on the age distribution of the patients, they were subdivided into two groups in this study: patients <70 years (non-elderly group) and patients ≥70 years (elderly group). We evaluated cancer-specific survival (CSS), with the cause of death determined from case notes or computerized records.

This retrospective study was approved with the ethical board of Shimane University Faculty of Medicine, and was conducted in accordance with the Declaration of Helsinki. Informed consent was obtained from all individual participants included in the study.

Blood sample analysis

Data on preoperative complete blood cell (CBC) counts were retrospectively extracted from patient medical records. Only patients with available preoperative CBC count and blood differential data were included in the study. All white blood cell and differential counts were obtained within 1 week prior to surgery. CBC was measured using ethylenediaminetetraacetic acid-treated blood, and analyzed using an automated hematology analyzer XE-5000 (SYSMEX K1000 hematology analyzer; Medical Electronics, Kobe, Japan). Absolute counts of lymphocytes, monocytes, and platelets were obtained from CBC tests.

LMR, NLR, and PLR evaluations

The LMR was calculated from a routinely performed preoperative blood cell count as the absolute lymphocyte count divided by the absolute monocyte count. White blood cell count data were analyzed in the general routine laboratory of our hospital. The NLR was calculated as a simple ratio between the absolute neutrophil and absolute lymphocyte counts, as provided by the differential white blood cell count. The PLR was calculated from the differential count by dividing the absolute platelet count by the absolute lymphocyte count.

TNM stage

The pathological classification of the primary tumor, degree of lymph node involvement, and presence of organ metastasis were determined according to the TNM classification system [10].

Statistical analysis

Means and standard deviations were calculated, and differences between groups were evaluated using a Student's *t*-test. Differences between categories of each clinicopathological feature were analyzed using a Chi-square (χ^2) test.

We determined the optimal cut-off levels of the LMR, NLR, and PLR by applying receiver operating curve (ROC) analysis. Regarding LMR, the area under curve (AUC) was 0.69 for CSS. A value of 4.0 was chosen as the cut-off level for LMR for CSS as associated with a high sensitivity and specificity for CSS (62.5 and 71.3 %, respectively). Regarding NLR, the AUC was 0.58 for CSS. A value of 1.6 was chosen as the cut-off level for NLR for CSS as associated with a sensitivity and specificity for CSS (57.5 and 66.3 %, respectively). Regarding

PLR, the AUC was 0.65 for CSS. A value of 147 was chosen as the cut-off level for PLR for CSS as associated with a high sensitivity and specificity for CSS (59.6 and 68.4 %, respectively). The patients with LMR, NLR, and PLR greater than these cutoff values were considered to have high LMR, NLR, and PLR, respectively; the remaining patients were considered to have low LMR, low NLR, and low PLR. CSS was calculated using Kaplan–Meier analysis, and differences between the groups were assessed by a log-rank test. Additionally, prognostic factors associated with decreased survival rates were determined using Cox regression analysis.

Univariate analyses were performed to determine which variables were associated with CSS. Variables with a *p*-value <0.05 in univariate analysis were subjected to multivariate logistic regression analysis. The potential prognostic factors for esophageal cancer were as follows: age (<70 vs. ≥70 years); sex (female vs. male); pStage (I, II vs. III); tumor size (<3 cm vs. ≥3 cm); operation time (<600 vs. ≥600 min); intraoperative blood loss (<5 00 mL vs. ≥500 mL); LMR (≥4 vs. <4); NLR (≥1.6 vs. <1.6); PLR (<147 vs. ≥147); weight loss (No vs. Yes: Weight loss was defined as more than 5 % decreasing in the body weight in the last 3 months preceding operation); and serum squamous cell carcinoma (SCC) antigen value (<1.5 vs. ≥1.5). Medical records were retrospectively reviewed to examine these factors.

All statistical analyses were performed using the statistical software JMP (version 11 for Windows; SAS Institute, Cary, NC, USA), and *p*-values <0.05 were considered statistically significant.

Results

Relationships between LMR, NLR, PLR, and clinicopathological features in patients with esophageal cancer

The relationships between LMR, NLR, PLR, and clinicopathological features in 147 patients with esophageal cancer are shown in Table 1.

Significant correlations were observed between the LMR and factors such as lymphocyte count ($p < 0.0001$), monocyte count ($p < 0.0001$), tumor size ($p = 0.014$), tumor depth ($p = 0.0007$), and TNM pStage ($p = 0.0002$). The NLR was significantly correlated with neutrophil count ($p < 0.0001$), lymphocyte count ($p < 0.0001$), and tumor depth ($p = 0.002$). Furthermore, significant correlations were observed between the PLR and lymphocyte count ($p < 0.0001$), platelet count ($p < 0.0001$), and tumor location ($p = 0.042$). It is notable that a low LMR was significantly correlated with more advanced TNM pStage, while the NLR and PLR showed no significant associations with TNM pStage.

Prognostic factors for CSS in overall patients with esophageal cancer

Univariate analyses demonstrated that TNM pStage ($p < 0.0001$), tumor size ($p = 0.0014$), operation time ($p = 0.0209$), low LMR ($p = 0.0008$), and high PLR ($p = 0.0232$) were significant risk factors for poor prognosis (Table 2).

TNM pStage (HR, 4.190; 95 % CI, 2.146–8.562; $p < 0.0001$) and low LMR (HR, 2.372; 95 % CI, 1.198–4.840; $p = 0.0129$) were found to be independently associated with poor prognosis via multivariate analysis (Table 2).

Relationships between LMR, NLR, PLR, and clinicopathological features in non-elderly patients with esophageal cancer

The relationships between LMR, NLR, PLR, and clinicopathological features in non-elderly patients (younger than 70 years) are shown in Table 3. Significant correlations were observed between the LMR and such factors as lymphocyte count ($p < 0.0001$), monocyte count ($p < 0.0001$), tumor location ($p = 0.0169$), tumor size ($p = 0.0309$), tumor depth ($p = 0.0093$), and TNM pStage ($p = 0.0003$). The NLR was significantly correlated with neutrophil count ($p < 0.0001$), lymphocyte count ($p < 0.0001$), tumor size ($p = 0.0452$), tumor depth ($p = 0.0018$), and TNM pStage ($p = 0.0032$). Furthermore, significant correlations were observed between the PLR and lymphocyte count ($p < 0.0001$) as well as platelet count ($p < 0.0001$).

Prognostic factors for CSS in non-elderly patients with esophageal cancer

In non-elderly patients, univariate analyses demonstrated that TNM pStage ($p < 0.0001$), tumor size ($p = 0.0001$), operation time ($p = 0.0374$), LMR ($p < 0.0001$), and PLR ($p = 0.0189$) were significantly associated with a poorer prognosis. Multivariate analysis demonstrated that TNM pStage (HR, 4.009; 95 % CI, 1.731–10.162; $p = 0.001$) and LMR (HR, 4.553; 95 % CI, 1.856–12.516; $p = 0.0007$) were independent risk factors for a poorer prognosis (Table 4).

Relationships between LMR, NLR, PLR, and clinicopathological features in elderly patients with esophageal cancer

The relationships between LMR, NLR, PLR, and clinicopathological features in elderly patients (70 years or older) are shown in Tables 5. Significant correlations were observed between the LMR and such factors as lymphocyte count ($p < 0.0001$), monocyte count ($p = 0.0001$), and serum SCC antigen ($p = 0.0342$). The NLR was significantly correlated with factors such as WBC ($p = 0.0146$), age ($p = 0.012$), lymphocyte count ($p < 0.0001$), and neutrophil count ($p = 0.0009$). Furthermore, significant correlations were observed between the PLR and lymphocyte count ($p < 0.0001$) as well as platelet count ($p = 0.0009$).

Table 1 Relationships between LMR, NLR, PLR and clinicopathologic features of 147 all patients

Characteristics	Total patients	LMR			NLR			PLR		
		<4 (*n* = 64)	≥4 (*n* = 83)	*p* value	1.6< (*n* = 37)	≥1.6 (*n* = 110)	*p* value	147< (*n* = 79)	≥147 (*n* = 68)	*p* value
Age (years)		65.8 ± 7.4	65.7 ± 8.2	0.934	65.4 ± 8.0	65.9 ± 7.9	0.72	66.8 ± 8.1	64.6 ± 7.6	0.097
Gender				0.052			0.163			0.562
Male	132	61	71		31	101		72	60	
Female	15	3	12		6	9		7	8	
WBC		6082.2 ± 2153.2	5844.3 ± 1788.2	0.466	5284.1 ± 1667.3	6171.2 ± 1996.5	0.016	6190.9 ± 1723.0	5665.6 ± 2167.2	0.104
Neutrophil		3944.7 ± 1804.6	3412.8 ± 1470.4	0.051	2491.0 ± 948.3	4032.3 ± 1643.7	<0.0001	3509.3 ± 1300.5	3801.3 ± 1960.9	0.283
Lymphocyte		1322.0 ± 546.4	1942.5 ± 584.5	<0.0001	2187.6 ± 658.6	1499.0 ± 541.8	<0.0001	2029.2 ± 586.3	1257.7 ± 426.2	<0.0001
Monocyte		546.8 ± 211.3	328.7 ± 111.1	<0.0001	379.0 ± 161.3	438.7 ± 203.3	0.1074	418.2 ± 171.3	430.0 ± 220.2	0.714
Platelet		236.6 ± 79.2	226.9 ± 66.2	0.42	231.0 ± 76.9	231.2 ± 70.7	0.987	203.5 ± 49.2	263.2 ± 80.9	<0.0001
Location of tumor				0.09			0.313			0.042
Ce	6	5	1		1	5		0	6	
Ut	8	4	4		0	8		5	3	
Mt	65	29	36		20	45		32	33	
Lt	52	23	29		11	41		31	21	
Ae	16	3	13		5	11		11	5	
Tumor size (mm)		4.9 ± 1.9	3.9 ± 2.7	0.014	3.8 ± 2.8	4.5 ± 2.3	0.134	4.0 ± 2.5	4.8 ± 2.3	0.056
Depth of tumor				0.0007			0.002			0.06
T1a-1b	66	20	46		18	48		40	26	
2	12	2	10		8	4		9	3	
3	56	33	23		8	48		26	30	
4a-4b	13	9	4		3	10		4	9	
Lymph node metastasis				0.2732			0.1532			0.0639
N0	79	30	49		22	57		43	36	
N1	42	19	23		12	30		25	17	
N2	12	8	4		3	9		8	4	
N3	14	7	7		0	14		3	11	
Pathological stage				0.0002			0.1338			0.3497
1a-1b	59	14	45		20	39		36	23	
2a-2b	33	21	12		6	27		16	17	
3a-3c	55	29	26		11	44		27	28	
Operation time (min)		644.8 ± 162.2	663.5 ± 159.2	0.4843	655.9 ± 177.2	655.2 ± 155.0	0.9798	676.5 ± 149.0	630.8 ± 170.2	0.0845
Intraoperative blood loss (ml)		751.8 ± 622.8	581.6 ± 633.4	0.1059	568.8 ± 511.1	684.9 ± 667.8	0.3359	598.5 ± 633.1	722.2 ± 629.7	0.2384
SCC antigen		1.19 ± 1.06	1.12 ± 1.12	0.7208	1.04 ± 1.12	1.19 ± 1.08	0.7643	1.05 ± 0.91	1.27 ± 1.26	0.8858

LMR **lymphocyte to monocyte ratio,** ***NLR*** **neutrophil to lymphocyte ratio,** ***PLR*** **platelet lymphocyte ratio**

Table 2 Prognostic factors for cancer-specific survival in 147 patients with esophageal cancer

Variables	Patients ($n = 147$)	Category or characteristics	Univariate			Multivariate		
			HR	95 % CI	*p* value	HR	95 % CI	*p* value
Gender	15/132	(female/male)	0.942	0.406–2.740	0.9007			
Age	46/101	(70</≥70)	1.427	0.742–2.639	0.2771			
pStage	92/55	(1,2/3)	4.876	2.625–9.420	<0.0001	4.19	2.146–8.562	<0.0001
Tumor size	45/102	(3</≥3)	3.405	1.548–8.981	0.0014	1.433	0.580–4.056	0.4493
Operation time	99/48	(600</≥600)	2.041	1.116–3.741	0.0209	1.425	0.757–2.681	0.2699
Intraoperative blood loss	72/75	(500</≥500)	1.321	0.723–2.463	0.3663			
LMR	83/64	(≥4.0/4.0<)	2.829	1.537–5.378	0.0008	2.372	1.198–4.840	0.0129
NLR	37/110	(≥1.6/1.6<)	1.469	0.753–2.734	0.2494			
PLR	79/68	(147</≥147)	2.013	1.100–3.783	0.0232	1.12	0.611–2.404	0.5999
SCC antigen	109/38	(1.5</≥1.5)	1.3	0.603–2.564	0.4842			

LMR lymphocyte to monocyte ratio, *NLR* neutrophil to lymphocyte ratio, *PLR* platelet lymphocyte ratio, *SCC* squamous cell carcinoma, *HR* hazard ratio, *CI* confidence interval

Prognostic factors for CSS in elderly patients with esophageal cancer

In elderly patients, univariate analysis demonstrated that that TNM pStage ($p = 0.0023$) was the only significant risk factor for a poor prognosis (Table 6).

Postoperative CSS based on LMR, NLR, and PLR in all patients with esophageal cancer

Patients with a low LMR had a significantly poorer prognosis in terms of CSS than those with a high LMR ($p = 0.0006$). In contrast, patients with a high PLR had a significantly poorer prognosis than those with a low PLR ($p = 0.0169$), whereas no significant differences in CSS were observed between patients with a low or high NLR ($p = 0.3214$; Fig. 1a-c).

Postoperative CSS based on LMR, NLR, and PLR in non-elderly patients with esophageal cancer

Patients with a low LMR had a significantly poorer prognosis in terms of CSS than those with a high LMR ($p < 0.0001$). In contrast, patients with a high PLR had a significantly poorer prognosis than those with a low PLR ($p = 0.0172$), whereas no significant differences in CSS were observed between patients with a low or high NLR ($p = 0.3714$; Fig. 2a-c).

Postoperative CSS based on LMR, NLR, and PLR in elderly patients with esophageal cancer

In the elderly group, no significant differences in CSS were observed between patients with either low or high LMR ($p = 0.4700$), NLR ($p = 0.9698$), or PLR ($p = 0.5386$; Fig. 3a-c).

Discussion

Pathological features, including tumor stage, nodal status, and resection margin, are considered important in determining cancer patient survival [11]. However, it is now clear that cancer survival is not solely determined by tumor pathology; indeed, recent studies have shown that preoperative inflammation-based prognostic scores can predict the overall survival of patients with various types of cancers [2–4]. In the present study, we retrospectively analyzed the clinical data of patients undergoing a potentially curative resection for esophageal cancer to determine whether the LMR, NLR, and PLR have prognostic values according to each TNM pStage. The results demonstrated that the LMR can be used as a novel predictor of postoperative CSS in patients with esophageal cancer after curative esophagectomy. Additionally, univariate analyses revealed that a low LMR was a significant risk factor for poor prognosis in stage III patients, whereas no prognostic factor was detected in patients with stage I or II cancer.

Interleukin-6 (IL-6) is a multifunctional inflammatory cytokine that triggers the proliferation and differentiation of a variety of cell types, including immune competent cells and hematopoietic cells. IL-6 induces not only neutrophil proliferation, but also the differentiation of megakaryocytes to platelets, and these events are similar to those underlying the systemic inflammatory response (SIR) [12, 13]. Theoretically, dynamic changes in the SIR resulting from tumor-host interactions are best estimated by directly measuring the serum IL-6 level. However, routine measurement of IL-6 in cancer patients in the clinical setting is expensive and inconvenient. On the other hand, the LMR, NLR, and PLR are based on blood cell components whose levels are regulated by cytokines, most notably, IL-6; these blood cell components proliferate and differentiate immediately after inflammatory cytokine release [14]. Moreover, measurement of the LMR, NLR, and PLR is easy, convenient, and cost-effective and therefore can be performed routinely.

In this study, we examined the prognostic significance of the LMR, NLR, and PLR in both elderly and non-

Table 3 Relationships between LMR, NLR, PLR and clinicopathologic features of 101 nonelderly patients

Characteristics	Total patients	LMR			NLR			PLR		
		<4 (*n* = 43)	≥4 (*n* = 58)	*p* value	1.6< (*n* = 25)	≥1.6 (*n* = 76)	*p* value	147< (*n* = 54)	≥147 (*n* = 47)	*p* value
Age (years)		61.9 ± 5.2	61.6 ± 5.6	0.7778	61.1 ± 5.8	61.9 ± 5.3	0.7249	62.4 ± 5.2	60.8 ± 5.5	0.1294
Gender				0.1283			0.2392			0.1171
Male	91	41	50		21	70		51	40	
Female	10	2	8		4	6		3	7	
WBC		6261.2 ± 2234.8	5951.4 ± 1747.8	0.7819	5654.4 ± 1725.4	6224.3 ± 2028.8	0.2101	6242.2 ± 1660.6	5900.6 ± 287.0	0.3863
Neutrophil		4020.2 ± 1757.4	3506.3 ± 1522.4	0.9402	2645.3 ± 978.7	4080.3 ± 1659.8	<0.0001	3481.2 ± 1252.0	4005.4 ± 1969.1	0.109
Lymphocyte		1352.8 ± 621.1	1964.2 ± 584.6	<0.0001	2362.7 ± 651.4	1487.2 ± 520.4	<0.0001	2068.7 ± 601.1	1284.7 ± 473.7	<0.0001
Monocyte		574.3 ± 223.8	336.1 ± 109.6	<0.0001	395.8 ± 163.2	451.3 ± 215.8	0.2417	438.1 ± 172.2	436.9 ± 238.6	0.9756
Platelet		230.1 ± 76.1	233.0 ± 70.2	0.8422	215.2 ± 64.4	237.2 ± 74.5	0.9051	205.7 ± 47.3	261.7 ± 84.3	<0.0001
Location of tumor				0.0169			0.5489			0.1445
Ce	4	4	0		0	4		0	4	
Ut	4	3	1		0	4		3	1	
Mt	49	23	26		14	35		24	25	
Lt	31	11	20		8	23		19	12	
Ae	13	2	11		3	10		8	5	
Tumor size (mm)		4.9 ± 2.1	3.9 ± 2.8	0.0309	3.4 ± 2.7	4.6 ± 2.5	0.0452	4.0 ± 2.8	4.7 ± 2.2	0.2116
Depth of tumor				0.0093			0.0018			0.0943
T1a-1b	44	12	32		13	31		29	15	
2	6	1	5		5	1		4	2	
3	40	23	17		5	35		17	23	
4a-4b	11	7	4		2	9		4	7	
Lymph node metastasis				0.5691			0.1307			0.3183
N0	56	22	34		18	38		32	24	
N1	28	13	15		6	22		16	12	
N2	6	4	2		1	5		3	3	
N3	11	4	7		0	11		3	8	
Pathological stage				0.0003			0.0032			0.1024
1a-1b	41	9	32		17	24		27	14	
2a-2b	20	15	5		1	19		8	12	
3a-3c	40	19	21		7	33		19	21	
Operation time (min)		617.8 ± 142.7	666.4 ± 148.0	0.101	643.33 ± 151.1	646.5 ± 146.8	0.9246	680.2 ± 147.9	606.0 ± 137.2	0.107
Intraoperative blood loss (ml)		727.9 ± 578.1	538.5 ± 523.1	0.0543	616.4 ± 567.6	620.1 ± 551.2	0.9772	563.0 ± 531.4	683.7 ± 574.5	0.2753
SCC antigen		1.01 ± 0.76	1.20 ± 1.26	0.3828	1.11 ± 1.36	1.11 ± 1.02	0.9667	1.04 ± 0.97	1.20 ± 1.19	0.465

LMR lymphocyte to monocyte ratio, *NLR* neutrophil to lymphocyte ratio, *PLR* platelet lymphocyte ratio

Table 4 Univariate and multivariate analysis of prognostic factors in 101 non-elderly patients with esophageal cancer

Variables	Patients (*n* = 101)	Category or characteristics	Univariate			Multivariate		
			HR	95 % CI	*p* value	HR	95 % CI	*p* value
Gender	10/91	(female/male)	0.608	0.233–20.78	0.388			
pStage	61/40	(1,2/3)	5.022	2.321–11.715	<0.0001	4.009	1.731–10.162	0.001
Tumor size	34/67	(3</≥3)	8.34	2.491–51.782	0.0001	3.115	0.788–20.674	0.1114
Operation time	67/34	(600</≥600)	2.219	1.048–4.752	0.0374	1.109	0.490–2.540	0.803
Intraoperative blood loss	49/52	(500</≥500)	1.53	0.723–3.373	0.2679			
LMR	58/43	(≥4/4<)	5.076	2.259–12.909	<0.0001	4.553	1.856–12.516	0.0007
NLR	25/76	(≥1.6/1.6<)	1.593	0.656–4.750	0.322			
PLR	54/47	(147</≥147)	2.475	1.160–5.592	0.0189	1.163	0.499–2.845	0.5999
SCC antigen	76/25	(1.5</≥1.5)	0.915	0.305–2.244	0.857			

LMR lymphocyte to monocyte ratio, *NLR* neutrophil to lymphocyte ratio, *PLR* platelet lymphocyte ratio, *SCC* squamous cell carcinoma, *HR* hazard ratio, *CI* confidence interval

elderly patients undergoing thoracoscopic esophagectomy for esophageal cancer. Esophageal cancer is the eighth most common cancer and the sixth most common cause of cancer deaths worldwide [15]. It occurs predominantly in elderly people, and the average age at the time of diagnosis continues to rise, with a peak incidence between 70 and 75 years of age [16]. Because age-specific prognostic factors in patients with esophageal cancer have not yet been described, we divided patients into two age groups in order to determine the age-specific prognostic values of the LMR, NLR, and PLR. The reason we chose a cut-off value of 70 years is because "elderly" is typically defined as a patient aged over 70 years in a plurality of studies on elderly patients with esophageal cancer [17–19].

Platelets are a key element linking the processes of hemostasis, inflammation, and tissue repair. Previous studies have shown that proinflammatory mediators stimulate megakaryocyte proliferation and are responsible for platelet production [20, 21]. Consequently, platelet activation causes angiogenic growth factor release as well as platelet adherence to tumor microvessels and extravasation via increased vascular permeability; this process leads to platelet activation [22, 23]. Lymphocytes can cause systemic inflammation by releasing numerous inhibitory immunologic mediators, particularly interleukin-10 and transforming growth factor-ß, which may consequently cause suppression of antitumor immunity via decreased regulatory T cell levels [6]. Accordingly, there is increasing evidence that lymphocytes are essential for antitumor immune reactions owing to several mechanisms, including the ability to enhance tumor cell apoptosis, inhibition of tumor cell proliferation, and promotion of metastasis [24]. Neutrophils are known to not only produce angiogenic cytokines, but have also been shown to generate matrix metalloproteinase-9, which induces an angiogenic state in cancer cells [25].

Based on such inflammatory responses, systemic inflammatory markers such as the LMR, NLR, and PLR have been shown to predict mortality and recurrence in a variety of cancers, but their role in esophageal cancer remains controversial [7, 20, 26].

We revealed that a low LMR in patients with esophageal cancer was significantly correlated with more advanced TNM pStage ($p = 0.0002$), but a low LMR was found to be independently associated with poor prognosis via multivariate analysis (HR, 2.372; $p = 0.0129$), as determined by Kaplan-Meier analysis and a log-rank test ($p = 0.0006$). A definitive explanation for our findings remains speculative. Monocytes are known to promote tumorigenesis and angiogenesis through local immune suppression and stimulation of tumor neovasculogenesis [25]. Moreover, tumor-associated macrophages developing from mononuclear cell lineages have been demonstrated to be able to inhibit cancer progression and spread of metastatic tumors [27, 28]. This could explain why an elevated monocyte count confers poor clinical outcomes in various types of cancers [29]. A poor prognosis was observed in patients with a low LMR in this study, which is reasonable because both lymphopenia and monocytosis induce immune suppression, as mentioned above. Moreover, the results of subgroup analysis revealed that the preoperative LMR was the most significant prognostic factor in non-elderly patients (HR, 4.553; $p = 0.0007$), as determined by Kaplan-Meier analysis and a log-rank test ($p < 0.0001$), but not in elderly patients. The present study may have failed to demonstrate a prognostic significance of the LMR in elderly patients because these patients were more likely to have advanced age-related conditions that cause immune suppression. Further investigations are required to elucidate the precise mechanisms that affect the prognosis of esophageal cancer patients.

Changes in platelet count and platelet function have been identified as part of a paraneoplastic syndrome in

Table 5 Relationships between LMR, NLR, PLR and clinicopathologic features of 46 elderly patients

Characteristics	Total patients	LMR			NLR			PLR		
		<4 ($n = 21$)	≥4 ($n = 25$)	p value	1.6< ($n = 12$)	≥1.6 ($n = 34$)	p value	147< ($n = 25$)	≥147 ($n = 21$)	p value
Age (years)		74.0 ± 3.8	75.4 ± 4.4	0.8781	74.3 ± 3.0	75.0 ± 4.5	0.6094	76.2 ± 4.3	73.1 ± 3.3	0.012
Gender				0.2226			0.453			0.2226
Male	41	20	21		10	31		21	20	
Female	5	1	4		2	3		4	1	
WBC		5715.7 ± 1976.4	5596.0 ± 1891.6	0.835	4512.5 ± 1281.2	6052.4 ± 1946.8	0.0146	6080.0 ± 1881.6	5139.5 ± 1858.8	0.0966
Neutrophil		3790.0 ± 1932.6	3195.8 ± 1346.0	0.2271	2169.4 ± 828.4	3925.1 ± 1626.7	0.0009	3570.0 ± 1424.7	3344.5 ± 1909.4	0.649
Lymphocyte		1258.9 ± 352.0	1892.1 ± 593.0	<0.0001	1822.8 ± 528.1	1525.4 ± 594.0	0.1327	1943.9 ± 555.2	1197.2 ± 294.4	<0.0001
Monocyte		490.2 ± 174.3	311.6 ± 115.0	0.0001	344.1 ± 158.3	410.5 ± 171.8	0.2469	375.1 ± 164.4	414.7 ± 176.4	0.4351
Platelet		250.0 ± 85.7	212.8 ± 54.3	0.0805	263.8 ± 92.6	217.8 ± 60.4	0.0563	198.8 ± 53.8	266.6 ± 74.7	0.0009
Location of tumor				0.6568			0.1274			0.2753
Ce	2	1	1		1	1		0	2	
Ut	4	1	3		0	4		2	2	
Mt	16	6	10		6	10		8	8	
Lt	21	12	9		3	18		12	9	
Ae	3	1	2		2	1		3	0	
Tumor size (mm)		4.9 ± 1.5	3.9 ± 2.5	0.0987	4.6 ± 3.2	4.3 ± 1.7	0.6459	3.9 ± 1.8	4.9 ± 2.4	0.0987
Depth of tumor				0.0716			0.3997			0.2032
T1a-1b	22	8	14		5	17		11	11	
2	6	1	5		3	3		5	1	
3	16	10	6		3	13		9	7	
4a-4b	2	2	0		1	1		0	2	
Lymph node metastasis				0.1229			0.2441			0.0875
N0	23	8	15		4	19		11	12	
N1	14	6	8		6	8		9	5	
N2	6	4	2		2	4		5	1	
N3	3	3	0		0	3		0	3	
Pathological stage				0.0825			0.3939			0.8129
1a-1b	18	5	13		3	15		9	9	
2a-2b	13	6	7		5	8		8	5	
3a-3c	15	10	5		4	11		8	7	
Operation time (min)		700.0 ± 187.8	656.8 ± 185.7	0.4385	682.3 ± 227.3	674.5 ± 172.6	0.9021	668.5 ± 154.0	686.2 ± 221.6	0.7515
Intraoperative blood loss (ml)		800.7 ± 718.7	681.5 ± 840.3	0.3057	469.8 ± 368.3	829.9 ± 866.8	0.1723	675.2 ± 818.5	808.2 ± 746.9	0.2854
SCC antigen		1.56 ± 1.44	0.96 ± 0.68	0.0342	0.90 ± 0.80	1.35 ± 1.21	0.2379	1.07 ± 0.78	1.42 ± 1.43	0.2961

LMR lymphocyte to monocyte ratio, *NLR* neutrophil to lymphocyte ratio, *PLR* platelet lymphocyte ratio

Table 6 Univariate and multivariate analysis of prognostic factors in 46 elderly patients with esophageal cancer

Variables	Patients ($n = 46$)	Category or characteristics	Univariate			Multivariate		
			HR	95 % CI	p value	HR	95 % CI	p value
Gender	5/41	(female/male)	3.114	0.611–56.892	0.201			
pStage	31/15	(1,2/3)	5.22	1.824–16.080	0.0023	5.22	1.824–16.080	0.0023
Tumor size	11/35	(3</≥3)	0.976	0.333–3.529	0.9666			
Operation time	32/14	(600</≥600)	1.761	0.615–4.929	0.2822			
Intraoperative blood loss	23/23	(500</≥500)	0.981	0.349–2.820	0.9707			
LMR	25/21	(≥4/4<)	1.118	0.368–3.175	0.837			
NLR	12/34	(≥1.6/1.6<)	0.853	0.464–1.535	0.718			
PLR	25/21	(147</≥147)	1.3	0.464–3.712	0.616			
SCC antigen	33/13	(1.5</≥1.5)	2.261	0.689–6.565	0.167			

LMR lymphocyte to monocyte ratio, *NLR* neutrophil to lymphocyte ratio, *PLR* platelet lymphocyte ratio, *SCC* squamous cell carcinoma, *HR* hazard ratio, *CI*, confidence interval

many cancers [30], and a high platelet count was found to be closely associated with TNM pStage, metastasis, as well as a high risk of recurrence in many types of cancer [31, 32]. Consequently, the PLR may act as a marker of the balance between host inflammatory and immune responses. However, to the best of our knowledge, the relationship between the PLR and esophageal cancer has not yet been described. We therefore focused on the PLR and CSS in esophageal cancer patients. Although univariate analysis demonstrated that the PLR was a significant risk factor for poorer CSS, as determined by Kaplan-Meier analysis and a log-rank test ($p = 0.0169$), multivariate analysis failed to confirm that the PLR was a significant predictor of CSS. Similarly, in non-elderly patients, univariate analysis demonstrated that the PLR was a significant risk factor for poorer CSS ($p = 0.0172$), but this significance was lost when analysis was confined to elderly patients. Recent studies have demonstrated that termed combination of platelet count and mean platelet volume is a predictor for postoperative survival in esophageal cancer patients [33]. Further studies are necessary to examine the role of these inflammatory biomarkers in various types of cancers.

The NLR has been reported to be highly promising in stratifying the outcome in large cohorts of patients with cancer [34, 35]. The relationship between the NLR and

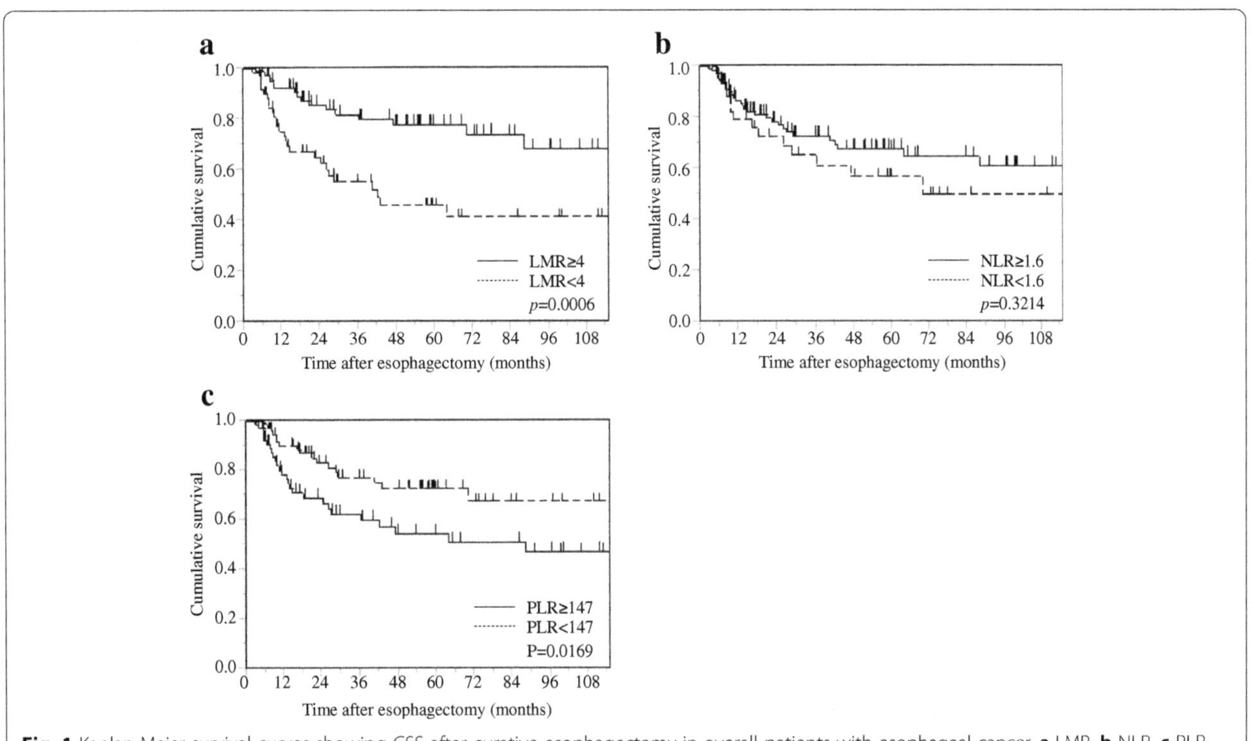

Fig. 1 Kaplan-Meier survival curves showing CSS after curative esophagectomy in overall patients with esophageal cancer. **a** LMR. **b** NLR. **c** PLR

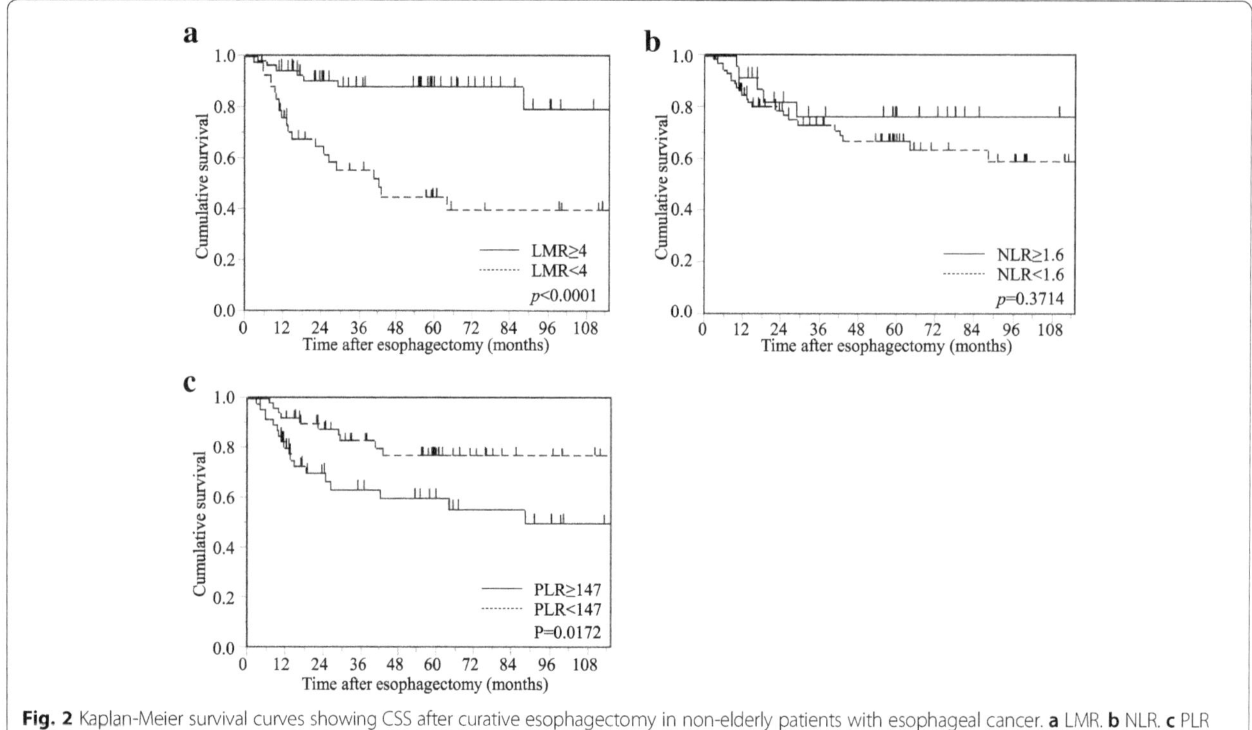

Fig. 2 Kaplan-Meier survival curves showing CSS after curative esophagectomy in non-elderly patients with esophageal cancer. **a** LMR. **b** NLR. **c** PLR

prognosis is probably complex and remains unclear. Recently, many studies have shown that a high NLR may indicate an impaired host immune response to the tumor [36]. In this study, the NLR did not affect the prognosis of esophageal cancer patients following curative resection, which may be due to the small retrospective sample size and short follow-up duration of the study. However, other components of the systemic inflammatory response, including cytokines and chemokines, have proven prognostically important in some studies [37].

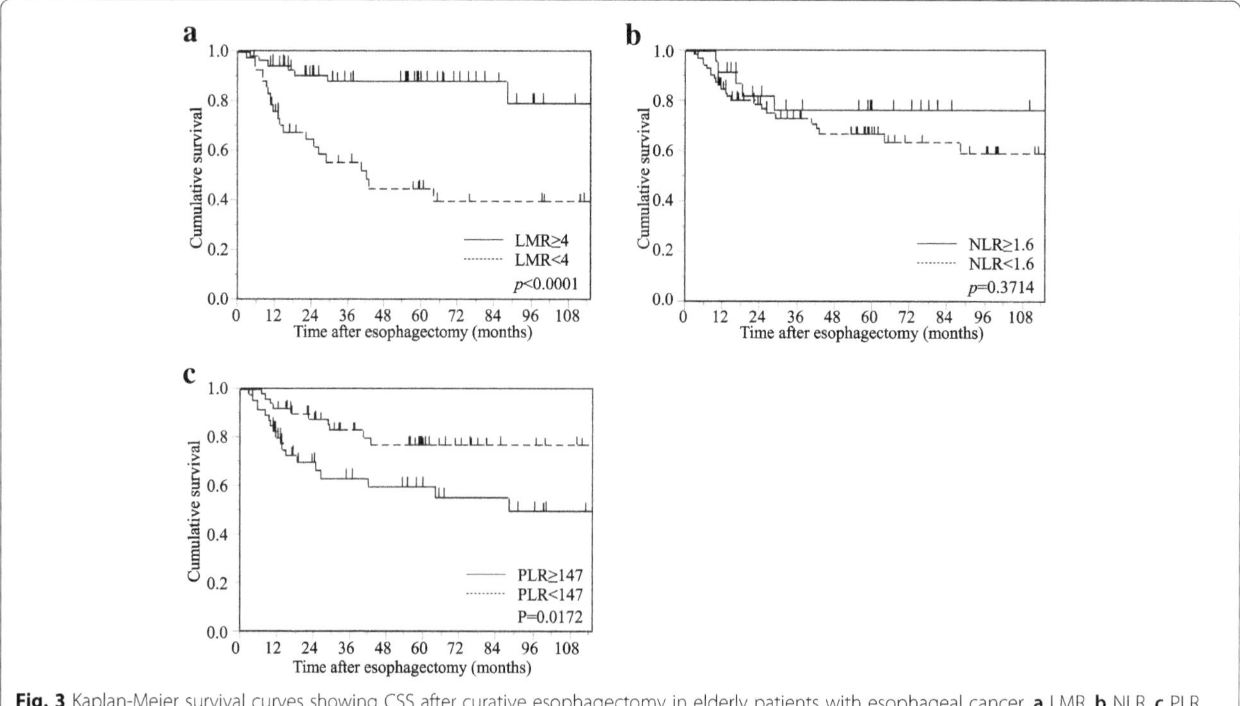

Fig. 3 Kaplan-Meier survival curves showing CSS after curative esophagectomy in elderly patients with esophageal cancer. **a** LMR. **b** NLR. **c** PLR

There were several potential limitations that warrant consideration in our study, which include single-institution retrospective analysis, short follow-up periods, and a small sample size, especially elderly patients. Furthermore, we excluded patients who had received adjuvant chemotherapy and/or radiotherapy, which may have influenced our analysis. Thus, large, prospective, randomized controlled trials are needed to confirm these preliminary results. In addition, the amount of weight loss are well-known prognostic factors for various types of cancers. Minimal weight loss and a good performance status are considered favorable prognostic factors. Needless to say significant weight loss may impact bone marrow function as well as the patient's ability to mount a host-tumor response. But we could not reveal that weight loss were proven to be independent prognostic factors in esophageal cancer, because our study is retrospective analysis, and data about the weight loss are insufficient.

Conclusion

In conclusion, our study demonstrated that the LMR and PLR were associated with CSS of esophageal cancer patients after curative esophagectomy. Moreover, the results of subgroup analysis revealed that the preoperative LMR and PLR were the most significant prognostic factors in non-elderly patients, as determined by Kaplan-Meier analyses and log-rank tests. In particular, a low LMR was a significant and independent predictor of poor survival. In non-elderly patients, a low LMR was also an independent risk factor for a poorer prognosis. The LMR and PLR are convenient, cost effective, and readily available as a part of routine complete blood counts, and could thus act as markers of survival in this malignancy.

Abbreviations

AUC: Area under curve; CBC: Complete blood cell; CSS: Cancer-specific survival; LMR: Lymphocyte to monocyte ratio; NLR: Neutrophil to lymphocyte ratio; PLR: Platelet lymphocyte ratio; ROC: Receiver operating curve; SCC: Squamous cell carcinoma

Acknowledgements

None.

Funding

None.

Authors' contributions

NH was the lead author, and conceived this study. TM, DK, YM, and SI collected data, performed analysis, and drafted the manuscript. YT reviewed paper and technique of surgery. All authors read and approved the final manuscript.

Competing interests

The authors declare that they have no competing interests.

References

1. Roxburgh CS, McMillan DC. Role of systemic inflammatory response in predicting survival in patients with primary operable cancer. Future Oncol. 2010;6:149–63.
2. Porrata LF, Ristow K, Colgan JP, Habermann TM, Witzig TE, Inwards DJ, Ansell SM, Micallef IN, Johnston PB, Nowakowski GS, Thompson C, Markovic SN. Peripheral blood lymphocyte/monocyte ratio at diagnosis and survival in classical Hodgkin's lymphoma. Haematologica. 2012;97:262–9. doi:10.3324/haematol.2011.050138.
3. Szkandera J, Gerger A, Liegl-Atzwanger B, Absenger G, Stotz M, Friesenbichler J, Trajanoski S, Stojakovic T, Eberhard K, Leithner A, Pichler M. The lymphocyte/monocyte ratio predicts poor clinical outcome and improves the predictive accuracy in patients with soft tissue sarcomas. Int J Cancer. 2014;135:362–70. doi:10.1002/ijc.28677.
4. Hirahara N, Matsubara T, Hayashi H, Takai K, Fujii Y, Yajima Y. Impact of inflammation-based prognostic score on survival after curative thoracoscopic esophagectomy for esophageal cancer. Euro J Surg Oncol. 2015;41:1308–15. doi:10.1016/j.ejso.2015.07.008.
5. Dunn GP, Old LJ, Schreiber RD. The immunobiology of cancer immunosurveillance and immunoediting. Immunity. 2004;21:137–48.
6. Hoffmann TK, Dworacki G, Tsukihiro T, Meidenbauer N, Gooding W, Johnson JT, Whiteside TL. Spontaneous apoptosis of circulating T lymphocytes in patients with head and neck cancer and its clinical importance. Clin Cancer Res. 2002;8:2553–62.
7. Deng Q, He B, Liu X, Yue J, Ying H, Pan Y, Sun H, Chen J, Wang F, Gao T, Zhang L, Wang S. Prognostic value of pre-operative inflammatory response biomarkers in gastric cancer patients and the construction of a predictive model. J Transl Med. 2015;13:66. doi:10.1186/s12967-015-0409-0.
8. Li ZM, Huang JJ, Xia Y, Sun J, Huang Y, Wang Y, Zhu YJ, Li YJ, Zhao W, Wei WX, Lin TY, Huang HQ, Jiang WQ. Blood lymphocyte-to-monocyte ratio identifies high-risk patients in diffuse large B-cell lymphoma treated with R-CHOP. PLoS One. 2012;7:e41658. doi:10.1371/journal.pone.0041658.
9. Neofytou K, Smyth EC, Giakoustidis A, Khan AZ, Williams R, Cunningham D, Mudan S. The preoperative lymphocyte-to-monocyte ratio is prognostic of clinical outcomes for patients with liver-only colorectal metastases in the neoadjuvant setting. Ann Surg Oncol. 2015;22:4353–62. doi:10.1245/s10434-015-4481-8.
10. Sobin LH, Gospodarowicz MK, Wittekind C. TNM classification of malignant tumors. 7th ed. Oxford: Wiley-Blackwell; 2010.
11. Liu YP, Ma L, Wang SJ, Chen YN, Wu GX, Han M, Wang XL. Prognostic value of lymph node metastases and lymph node ratio in esophageal squamous cell carcinoma. Eur J Surg Oncol. 2010;36:155–9.
12. Imai T, Koike K, Kubo T, Kikuchi T, Amano Y, Takagi M, Okumura N, Nakahata T. Interleukin-6 supports human megakaryocytic proliferation and differentiation in vitro. Blood. 1991;78:1969–74.
13. Ruscetti FW. Hematologic effects of interleukin-1 and interleukin-6. Curr Opin Hematol. 1994;1:210–5.
14. Ohsugi Y. Recent advances in immunopathophysiology of interleukin-6: an innovative therapeutic drug, tocilizumab (recombinant humanized anti-human interleukin-6 receptor antibody), unveils the mysterious etiology of immune-mediated inflammatory diseases. Biol Pharm Bull. 2007;30:2001–6.
15. Parkin DM, Bray F, Ferlay J, Pisani P. Global cancer statistics, 2002. CA Cancer J Clin. 2005;55:74–108.
16. Yamamoto M, Weber JM, Karl RC, Meredith KL. Minimally invasive surgery for esophageal cancer: review of the literature and institutional experience. Cancer Control. 2013;20:130–7.
17. Ma JY, Wu Z, Wang Y, Zhao YF, Liu LX, Kou YL, Zhou QH. Clinicopathologic characteristics of esophagectomy for esophageal carcinoma in elderly patients. World J Gastroenterol. 2006;12:1296–9.
18. Poon RT, Law SY, Chu KM, Branicki FJ, Wong J. Esophagectomy for carcinoma of the esophagus in the elderly: results of current surgical management. Ann Surg. 1998;227:357–64.
19. Sabel MS, Smith JL, Nava HR, Mollen K, Douglass HO, Gibbs JF. Esophageal resection for carcinoma in patients older than 70 years. Ann Surg Oncol. 2002;9:210–4.
20. Asher V, Lee J, Innamaa A, Bali A. Preoperative platelet lymphocyte ratio as an independent prognostic marker in ovarian cancer. Clin Transl Oncol. 2011;13:499–503. doi:10.1007/s12094-011-0687-9.
21. Cooper ZA, Frederick DT, Juneja VR, Sullivan RJ, Lawrence DP, Piris A, Sharpe AH, Fisher DE, Flaherty KT, Wargo JA. BRAF inhibition is associated with increased clonality in tumor-infiltrating lymphocytes. Oncoimmunology 2013;2:e26615

22. Bergers G, Brekken R, McMahon G, Vu TH, Itoh T, Tamaki K, Tanzawa K, Thorpe P, Itohara S, Werb Z, Hanahan D. Matrix metalloproteinase-9 triggers the angiogenic switch during carcinogenesis. Nat Cell Biol. 2000;2:737–44.
23. Kono SA, Heasley LE, Doebele RC, Camidge DR. Adding to the mix: fibroblast growth factor and platelet-derived growth factor receptor pathways as targets in non-small cell lung cancer. Curr Cancer Drug Targets. 2012;12:107–23.
24. Fridman WH, Pagès F, Sautès-Fridman C, Galon J. The immune contexture in human tumours: impact on clinical outcome. Nat Rev Cancer. 2012;12: 298–306. doi:10.1038/nrc3245.
25. Koh YW, Kang HJ, Park C, Yoon DH, Kim S, Suh C, Go H, Kim JE, Kim CW, Huh J. The ratio of the absolute lymphocyte count to the absolute monocyte count is associated with prognosis in Hodgkin's lymphoma: correlation with tumor-associated macrophages. Oncologist. 2012;17:871–80. doi:10.1634/theoncologist.2012-0034.
26. Ying HQ, Deng QW, He BS, Pan YQ, Wang F, Sun HL, Chen J, Liu X, Wang SK. The prognostic value of preoperative NLR, d-NLR, PLR and LMR for predicting clinical outcome in surgical colorectal cancer patients. Med Oncol. 2014;31:305. doi:10.1007/s12032-014-0305-0.
27. Condeelis J, Pollard JW. Macrophages: obligate partners for tumor cell migration, invasion, and metastasis. Cell. 2006;124:263–6.
28. Pollard JW. Tumour-educated macrophages promote tumour progression and metastasis. Nat Rev Cancer. 2004;4:71–8.
29. Donskov F, von der Maase H. Impact of immune parameters on long-term survival in metastatic renal cell carcinoma. J Clin Oncol. 2006;24:1997–2005.
30. Stone RL, Nick AM, McNeish IA, Balkwill F, Han HD, Bottsford-Miller J, Rupairmoole R, Armaiz-Pena GN, Pecot CV, Coward J, Deavers MT, Vasquez HG, Urbauer D, Landen CN, Hu W, Gershenson H, Matsuo K, Shahzad MM, King ER, Tekedereli I, Ozpolat B, Ahn EH, Bond VK, Wang R, Drew AF, Gushiken F, Lamkin D, Collins K, DeGeest K, Lutgendorf SK, Chiu W, Lopez-Berestein G, Afshar-Kharghan V, Sood AK. Paraneoplastic thrombocytosis in ovarian cancer. N Engl J Med. 2012;366:610–8. doi:10.1056/NEJMoa1110352.
31. Li FX, Wei LJ, Zhang H, Li SX, Liu JT. Signifcance of thrombocytosis in clinicopathologic characteristics of prognosis of gastric cancer. Asian Pac J Cancer Prev. 2014;15:6511–7.
32. Unal D, Eroglu C, Kurtul N, Oguz A, Tasdemir A. Are neutrophil/lymphocyte and platelrt/lymphocyte rates in patients with non-small cell lung cancer associated with treatment response and prognosis? Asian Pac J Cancer Prev. 2013;14:5237–42.
33. Zang F, Chen C, Wang P, Hu X, Gao Y, He J. Combination of platelet count and mean platelet volume (COP-MPV) predicts postoperative prognosis in both resectable early and advanced stage esophageal squamous cell cancer patients. Tumor Biol. doi:10.1007/s13277-015-4774-3
34. Proctor MJ, Morrison DS, Talwar D, Balmer SM, Fletcher CD, O'Reilly DS, Foulis AK, Horgan PG, McMillan DC. A comparison of inflammation-based prognostic scores in patients with cancer. A Glasgow Inflammation Outcome Study. Eur J Cancer. 2011;47:2633–41.
35. Proctor MJ, McMillan DC, Morrison DS, Fletcher CD, Horgan PG, Clarke SJ. A derived neutrophil to lymphocyte ratio predicts survival in patients with cancer. Br J Cancer. 2012;107:695–9.
36. Walsh SR, Cook EJ, Goulder F, Justin TA, Keeling NJ. Neutrophil-lymphocyte ratio as a prognostic factor in colorectal cancer. J Surg Oncol. 2005;91:181–4.
37. Proctor MJ, Horgan PG, Talwar D, Fletcher CD, Morrison DS, McMillan DC. Optimization of the systemic inflammation-based Glasgow prognostic score: a Glasgow Inflammation Outcome Study. Cancer. 2013;119:2325–32.

31

Pylorus drainage procedures in thoracoabdominal esophagectomy – a single-center experience and review of the literature

Stefan Fritz*, Katharina Feilhauer, André Schaudt, Hansjörg Killguss, Eduard Esianu, René Hennig† and Jörg Köninger†

Abstract

Background: Pylorotomy and pyloroplasty in thoracoabdominal esophagectomy are routinely performed in many high-volume centers to prevent delayed gastric emptying (DGE) due to truncal vagotomy. Currently, controversy remains regarding the need for these practices. The present study aimed to determine the value and role of pyloric drainage procedures in esophagectomy with gastric replacement.

Methods: A retrospective review of prospectively collected data was performed for all consecutive patients who underwent thoracoabdominal resection of the esophagus between January 2009 and December 2016 at the Katharinenhospital in Stuttgart, Germany. Clinicopathologic features and surgical outcomes were evaluated with a focus on postoperative nutrition and gastric emptying.

Results: The study group included 170 patients who underwent thoracoabdominal esophageal resection with a gastric conduit using the Ivor Lewis approach. The median age of the patients was 64 years. Most patients were male (81%), and most suffered from adenocarcinoma of the esophagus (75%). The median hospital stay was 20 days, and the 30-day hospital death rate was 2.9%. According to the department standard, pylorotomy, pyloroplasty, or other pyloric drainage procedures were not performed in any of the patients. Overall, 28/170 patients showed clinical signs of DGE (16.5%).

Conclusions: In the literature, the rate of DGE after thoracoabdominal esophagectomy is reported to be approximately 15%, even with the use of pyloric drainage procedures. This rate is comparable to that reported in the present series in which no pyloric drainage procedures were performed. Therefore, we believe that pyloric drainage procedures may be unwarranted in thoracoabdominal esophagectomy. However, future randomized trials are needed to ultimately confirm this supposition.

Keywords: Thoracoabdominal esophagectomy, Pylorotomy, Pyloroplasty, Pylorus drainage, Delayed gastric emptying

* Correspondence: st.fritz@klinikum-stuttgart.de
†Equal contributors
Department of General, Visceral, Thoracic and Transplantation Surgery, Katharinenhospital Stuttgart, Kriegsbergstraße 60, 70174 Stuttgart, Germany

Background

Thoracoabdominal esophagectomy for esophageal cancer has been associated with high rates of morbidity and mortality in the past. Until the 1980s, postoperative in-hospital death rates were reported to range around 30% [1, 2]. Due to significant improvements in surgery, anesthesiology, and intensive care management, a reduction in mortality to less than 10% has been achieved in the last 10–20 years [3–5]. Along with improvements in peri- and postoperative outcomes, surgical techniques have also been evaluated with regard to non-life-threatening postoperative complications and quality of life.

Delayed gastric emptying (DGE) is a frequent functional disorder of the pylorus following esophagectomy with a gastric conduit. Depending on the definition and the surgical technique performed, clinical symptoms during the postoperative course reportedly occur in 10% to 50% of patients [6, 7]. Gastric outlet obstruction results from truncal vagotomy and is thought to be associated with an increased incidence of postoperative complications, including aspiration with subsequent pneumonia and anastomotic leaks. Consequently, DGE is reported to lead to decreased patient satisfaction and a prolonged hospital stay [8–10].

Although gastric tube reconstruction, rather than reconstruction of the entire stomach, has been sufficiently demonstrated to be associated with a significantly reduced risk of DGE [11], superior quality-of-life scores during the first postoperative year, and less reflux esophagitis, controversy surrounds the need for pyloric drainage procedures [9, 12]. Based on historical experience with truncal bilateral vagotomies during peptic ulcer surgery, pyloric drainage procedures were routinely performed in many high-volume centers to prevent DGE. The choice of procedure, including pylorotomy, pyloroplasty, finger fracture, or botulinum toxin injection, mainly depended on the surgeon's preference. Recent series have questioned the benefit of these procedures [13]. Currently, ongoing controversy remains concerning the need for pyloric drainage procedures following esophageal substitution with gastric interposition [8, 14, 15].

Limited data are available on short-term postoperative outcomes regarding DGE following esophagectomy with gastric pull-up. Moreover, most reports are based on series that include patients who underwent surgery in the 1980s and 1990s or even earlier [16–19]. At that time, mortality rates were two- to three-times higher compared to those in more recently published series in high-volume centers. Furthermore, the use of pyloric drainage procedures was based on different surgical schools and not on evidence or randomized clinical trials. In recent years, the rate of laparoscopic esophagectomies has continuously increased. Certainly, pylorus drainage procedures can be performed laparoscopically. However, this technique is relatively sophisticated and may be related to morbidity. Especially for the laparoscopic approach, it is important to be sure whether pylorus drainage procedures will be beneficial compared to no intervention. Therefore, the present study aimed to determine the value and role of pylorus drainage procedures in esophagectomy.

Methods

Patients

All consecutive patients who underwent thoracoabdominal esophagectomy at the Department of General, Visceral and Transplantation Surgery of the Katharinenhospital in Stuttgart, Germany between January 2009 and December 2016 were prospectively evaluated from a database. The study was approved by the institutional review board of the Klinikum Stuttgart and is in compliance with the Declaration of Helsinki. Clinicopathologic features including age, sex, body mass index, tumor location and stage, and nutrition management were assessed. Clinical courses and outcomes were evaluated with a focus on postoperative nutrition and gastric emptying difficulties. Among other variables, the rate of gastric outlet obstruction symptoms, the median postoperative day of return to a normal full diet, and postoperative surgical and non-surgical complications were assessed. Moreover, clinical management of gastric outlet obstruction was investigated with regard to success rates and outcomes.

Preoperative work-up

All patients included in the study had undergone preoperative thin-sliced radiological imaging using computed tomography or magnetic resonance imaging (MRI). All images were accessed and viewed using the PACS online imaging system of the Katharinenhospital in Stuttgart, Germany (GE Healthcare, Barrington, USA). For preoperative staging, all patients underwent endoscopic ultrasonography examination (EUS) to assess tumor size, infiltration depth and enlargement of lymph nodes. All patients were presented at an interdisciplinary tumor board for therapeutic management planning. According to preoperative tumor staging, patients received neoadjuvant chemotherapy or radiochemotherapy as indicated.

Surgical procedure

All study patients except for three underwent open Ivor Lewis thoracoabdominal esophagectomy. In brief, an upper abdominal incision and a right-sided posterolateral thoracotomy were applied for surgical access. The procedure was mainly performed on tumors of the middle- and lower-third of the esophagus. In cases of uncertain resectability or lesions suspected of metastasis in the liver or lung, an exploratory laparotomy and/or thoracotomy was performed before surgical esophageal resection. Patients who did not undergo curative resection were excluded from the study. Only patients with the stomach as the site of esophageal replacement were included in the present study. Patients with colonic or jejunal interposition were excluded. The gastric conduit for esophageal replacement (Fig. 1) was brought up to the thorax using a posterior mediastinal route. Three patients underwent laparoscopic mobilization of the stomach and open thoracotomy for gastric pull-up and anastomosis.

Postoperative management

Patients were routinely transferred to an intensive care unit postoperatively for three days, followed by another three days in an intermediate care unit with cardiopulmonary monitoring. The gastric tube was removed on postoperative day one in all patients regardless of the amount of reflux. On day one, patients were allowed to drink clear liquids ad libitum. Return to regular diet was routinely started on postoperative day four. Abdominal drainages were removed on day two and thoracic drainage according to the amount and quality of fluid production.

Results

Patient characteristics

A total of 170 consecutive patients who underwent thoracoabdominal resection of the esophagus with gastric replacement were included in the study (Table 1). The entire group included 137 men (80.6%) and 33 women (19.4%), with a median age of 64 years (range: 39–87 years). Most of the patients were male (80.6%). The mean body mass index of all patients was 26 kg/m^2 (range: 16.3–41.8 kg/m^2), with body weight ranging from 48 to 131 kg (mean: 78.2 kg).

Most of the patients (128/170) suffered from adenocarcinoma of the esophagus (75.3%). Thirty-six patients suffered from squamous cell carcinoma (21.2%). Three patients had neuroendocrine tumors of the esophagus (1.8%), and one patient suffered from a gastrointestinal stroma tumor (GIST). Two patients underwent surgery for non-neoplastic disease, including a 73-year-old male with peptic stenosis and a 72-year-old patient who suffered from distal scarred stenosis following iatrogenic perforation during endoscopic dilation for achalasia (Table 2).

Excluding arterial hypertension, 51/170 patients (30.0%) had cardiovascular comorbidities such as coronary heart disease with status post cardiac infarction or bypass surgery. According to the American Society of Anesthesiologists (ASA) classification, 108/170 patients were categorized as ASA III (63.5%), and 60 were categorized as ASA II (35.3%).

Table 1 Demographics and comorbidities of the patients ($n = 170$)

Feature		Number	Percent
Age (years)	Median: 64		
	Range: 39–87		
Sex	Male	137	80.6
	Female	33	19.4
Body mass index (kg/m^2)	Mean: 26.7		
	Range: 16.3–41.8		
	≤18.5	7	4.1
	> 18.5 and ≤25.0	73	42.9
	> 25.0 and ≤30.0	65	38.3
	> 30.0 and ≤35.0	17	10.0
	> 35.0	8	4.7
Body weight (kg)	Mean: 78.2		
	Range: 48–131		
Smoking history	Current smoker	66	38.8
	Former smoker	22	13.0
	Never	82	48.2
Alcohol history	Current alcohol abuse	35	20.6
	Former alcohol abuse	12	7.1
	Never	123	72.3
Comorbidity	Cardiovascular (hypertension excluded)	51	30.0
	Pulmonary	27	15.9
	Renal	12	7.1
	Diabetes mellitus	30	17.6
ASA risk classification	I	2	1.2
	II	60	35.3
	III	108	63.5
	IV	0	0

The indication for surgical resection and the histological characteristics and locations of the tumors are listed in Table 2. Most patients (118/170) had lymph node-positive disease (69.4%) and received neoadjuvant chemo- or radiochemotherapy (65.3%).

Surgical resection

All patients underwent thoracoabdominal esophageal resection using the Lewis-Tanner approach as described in the Patients and Methods section. According to the department standard, pyloric drainage procedures such as pylorotomy, pyloroplasty, pylorus buginage or botulinum toxin injection were not applied in any of the patients. The mean operative time was 256 min (range: 117–386 min).

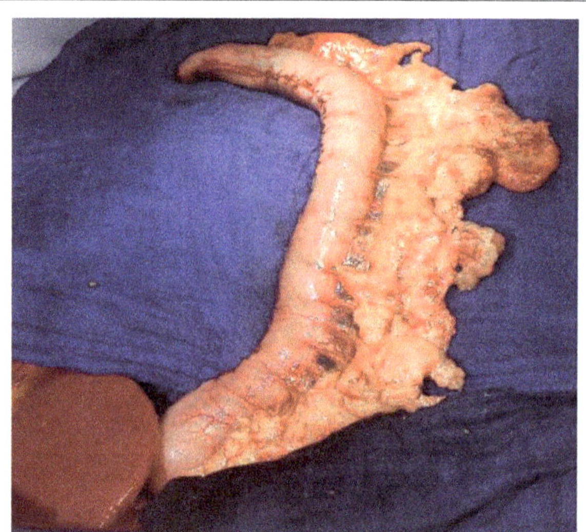

Fig. 1 Gastric conduit for esophageal replacementAll patients received thoracoabdominal esophagectomy with gastric pull-up. The gastric conduit was small, with a diameter of 3–5 cm. None of the patients received any pyloric drainage procedure such as pylorotomy, pyloroplasty, pylorus buginage or botulinum toxin injection.

Postoperative management

In most patients (83%), the nasogastric tube was removed on postoperative day one or two. Clinical signs of gastric outlet obstruction were observed in 28/170 patients (16.5%). DGE was primarily treated conservatively with re-insertion of a gastric tube and prokinetic drugs. In 5 of 170 patients (2.9%), DGE was severe and persistent and required intervention. In these cases, endoscopic dilation of the stenotic region was performed (Table 3). In all five patients, the intervention was successful. The median return to a regular diet was satisfactory at six days postoperatively.

Table 2 Disease-specific and oncological characteristics

Feature		Number	Percent
Histological type of disease	Adenocarcinoma	128	75.2
	Squamous cell carcinoma	36	21.2
	Neuroendocrine tumor (NET)	3	1.8
	Other	3	1.8
Tumor location	Upper-third (0–18 cm)	1	0.6
	Middle-third (19–29 cm)	32	18.8
	Lower-third (30–45 cm)	137	80.6
Clinical T-stage at diagnosis	cT1	5	2.9
	cT2	38	22.4
	cT3	90	52.9
	cT4	35	20.6
	Not determined	2	1.2
Clinical N-stage at diagnosis	cN0	50	29.4
	cN+	118	69.4
	Not determined	2	1.2
Neoadjuvant therapy	Chemo- or radiochemotherapy	111	65.3

Surgical outcomes

The median hospital stay was 20 days (range: 8–112 days), including a mean of six days in the intensive care unit. The 30-day hospital death rate was 2.9%. Postoperative endoscopy was performed in 45.9% of the cases. Implantation of a stent or endosponge was performed in 21.2% of the cases, and endoscopic balloon dilation was applied in 2.9% of the cases. Anastomotic leakage was observed in 24.1% of the cases. However, most leakages (36/41) were sufficiently treated with endoscopic stenting or endosponge therapy (87.8%). Re-operation for anastomotic leakage was required in 7/170 patients (4.1%). Other reasons for re-operation were chylous fistula (2.9%), postoperative bleeding (1.8%), and ischemia of the gastric conduit (1.2%). Overall, surgical re-intervention was required in 18/170 cases (10.6%).

The rates of postoperative non-surgical complications are listed in Table 3. Generally, the most frequent non-surgical complications were pneumonia (27.1%) and pleural effusion (24.7%).

Pathology

Of all 170 resected patients, 168 had an oncological diagnosis (98.8%). One patient suffered from peptic stenosis and another from stenosis following iatrogenic injury during endoscopy. Most patients had histological T3 or T4 tumors (49.7%), 35.8% of the patients had a T1 or T2 tumor, and 14.5% had ypT0 or ypTis tumors. Overall, 50.6% of the patients with an oncological diagnosis had lymph node-positive disease, and 49.4% had lymph node-negative findings on final histopathology.

Discussion

DGE is one of the major causes of severe aspiration pneumonia, which is associated with a poor early postoperative outcome following esophagectomy with gastric replacement [20]. In the past, different surgical techniques, such as pyloromyotomy, pyloroplasty, or pylorus buginage, were implemented to reduce the incidence of gastric outlet obstruction [14].

Currently, the value of these pyloric drainage procedures remains controversial [9]. The potential advantage of these procedures is possible prevention of DGE [21]. Some authors argue that by reducing gastric outlet obstruction, the incidence of aspiration pneumonia may decrease, potentially improving early postoperative outcomes [17]. Others argue that only a minority of patients show signs of DGE. Furthermore, pyloric drainage

Table 3 Operative procedure and postoperative outcomes

Feature		Number	Percent
Operative time (minutes)	Mean: 256		
	Range: 117–386		
Surgical complications	Anastomotic leak	41	24.1
	Surgical site infection	29	17.1
	Delayed gastric emptying (DGE)	28	16.5
	Delayed gastric emptying (DGE) requiring intervention	5	2.9
	Chylothorax	8	4.7
	Postoperative bleeding	8	4.7
Non-surgical complications	Pneumonia	46	27.1
	Pleural effusion	42	24.7
	Cardiovascular complications	11	6.5
	Postoperative delirium	11	6.5
	Renal failure	5	2.9
Postoperative endoscopy	Not required	92	54.1
	Diagnostic endoscopy	78	45.9
	Stenting/endosponge	36	21.2
	Balloon dilation	5	2.9
Surgical re-intervention	Total	18	10.6
	Re-operations for early anastomotic leak	7	4.1
	Ligature of the thoracic duct	5	2.9
	Postoperative bleeding	3	1.8
	Other	3	1.8
Length of hospital stay (days)	Median: 20		
	Range: 8–112		
30-day mortality		5	2.9

procedures may predispose patients to dumping and duodenal reflux, which could impede late postoperative functional outcomes [14, 20, 22, 23].

In 1991, Fok et al. published a prospective randomized study on 200 patients who underwent esophagectomy with gastric replacement [17]. Based on their findings, the authors recommended pyloroplasty for patients in whom the entire stomach was used for reconstruction after esophagectomy. These results are not comparable to those of more recent studies because most centers today do not use the entire stomach for esophageal replacement but only a small conduit of 3–5 cm in diameter [11]. By analyzing 2 RCTs and 5 cohort studies, Akkermann et al. found that the overall rate of DGE was significantly lower in patients who underwent gastric tube reconstruction compared with that in patients who underwent reconstruction using the whole stomach [9].

In 2002, Urschel et al. performed a meta-analysis including nine randomized controlled trials with a total of 553 patients [21]. According to this study, pyloric drainage procedures at the time of esophagectomy reduced the occurrence of early gastric outlet obstruction ($p = 0.046$) but had little effect on mortality, pulmonary complications and late postoperative foregut function.

Although two recent systematic reviews including 827 and 668 patients did not find a benefit of pyloric drainage procedures versus no intervention [9, 15], Arya et al. found a non-significant trend toward fewer anastomotic leaks, fewer pulmonary complications and less gastric stasis when pyloric drainage procedures were performed [8]. However, most studies included in these systematic reviews were performed at a time when the morbidity and mortality rates of esophagectomy were generally much higher compared to today. For example, the study of Akkerman et al. included patients who underwent surgery in the 1980s and 1990s or even earlier [9]. As mentioned above, the postoperative outcomes of these patients are not comparable to those of current studies due to improvements in intensive care and relevant modifications of operative techniques, including minimally invasive approaches.

In a recent randomized clinical trial, Mohajeri et al. found that pyloromyotomy or pylorus buginage could not reduce the incidence of DGE after esophagectomy with gastric pull-up [24]. Moreover, there is evidence that patients who undergo pyloric drainage procedures may suffer from increased biliary reflux and dumping syndrome long term [25, 26]. Wang et al. analyzed 368 patients following esophagectomy with esophageal substitute and found a greater incidence of both of these undesirable outcomes in patients who underwent pyloroplasty [27].

The present study aimed to evaluate surgical outcomes following esophagectomy with gastric replacement with a special focus on gastric outlet obstruction in a large single-center series. In this series, clinical signs of DGE were observed in 16.5% of the cases, and pneumonia was observed in 27.1% of the cases, which is consistent with the current literature. Most authors report a DGE rate ranging around 15% [28, 29], and most centers describe comparable rates of postoperative pneumonia [4]. Since no pyloric drainage procedures were performed in the current study, we can conclude that these procedures are not necessary. Moreover, most of the patients with clinical signs of DGE were successfully treated with conservative therapy. Only a few patients required endoscopic balloon dilation (3.8%), and none of the patients with DGE required reoperation or underwent a so-called rescue pyloroplasty.

In the present series, postoperative endoscopy with exploration of the anastomosis was performed whenever a patient had any obvious clinical signs or unexplained increasing levels of inflammatory parameters in the blood, which explains the relatively high rate of postoperative endoscopies. The reason for this approach is based on our experience that in the case of an anastomotic leak, an early intervention, such as stenting or placement of an endoscopic vacuum sponge, is helpful to prevent a severe and prolonged postoperative course. Some of the patients with anastomotic leakage only showed small leaks without necrosis and mild clinical symptoms, which explains the low rate of re-operation for anastomotic leakage and the relatively low 30-day hospital morbidity of 2.9%.

There are limitations in the present study design. First, this was a single-center observational study without a control group. According to the department standard, none of the patients underwent pyloric drainage procedures. Therefore, the data can only be compared to the existing literature. Still, we believe that our data are clinically relevant since many recent studies refer to historical clinical data of patients who underwent surgery in the 1980s or 1990s. Since this time, not only the surgical procedure but also postoperative intensive care management, including mobilization and nutrition regimens, have changed tremendously.

It has been reported that pyloric drainage procedures are not only ineffective in preventing DGE but also can add relevant morbidity, such as esophageal leakage or stenosis, in the long-term follow-up. For example, Richardson et al. described a patient who developed late pyloroplasty leakage on postoperative day 16 following esophagectomy [30]. Likewise, Antonoff et al. described two major complications directly related to pyloric drainage procedures, accounting for 0.6% of their study collective. One patient was re-explored on the first postoperative day because of bilious drainage from the midline abdominal incision due to a pin-point hole at the pyloromyotomy. Another patient developed a leak at the pyloroplasty site and ultimately died following a complicated postoperative course [25]. Zieren et al. reported one patient who died following insufficient pyloroplasty and another patient who developed a severe stricture secondary to surgical pyloric drainage, accounting for 3.8% of their study group [31]. Although the overall surgical complication rate after pylorus drainage procedures seems to be relatively low, these practices are associated with significant morbidity and even mortality.

In more recent studies, the value of botulinum toxin injection in reducing gastric outlet obstruction was evaluated. In 2016, Fuchs et al. reported a trial in which 14 patients received botulinum toxin injections versus 27 who did not receive injections [32]. In this study, the rate of postoperative pyloric dysfunction was found to be significantly lower in the botulinum toxin group. Moreover, patients who received botulinum toxin injections were discharged earlier (7.4 versus 10.7 days, $p < 0.05$), and no differences were observed regarding anastomotic strictures or leaks. In contrast, Eldaif et al. found that patients receiving botulinum injections exhibited a higher rate of postoperative reflux symptoms and increased use of promotility agents and more frequently required postoperative endoscopic interventions. Therefore, the authors concluded that intrapyloric botulinum toxin injections should not be used as an alternative to standard drainage procedures [33]. Consequently, the value of botulinum toxin injections as an alternative approach to reduce postoperative gastric outlet obstruction remains controversial. More randomized clinical studies with larger samples are required before this method can be generally recommended.

For postoperative DGE therapy, conservative approaches or endoscopic pyloric balloon dilation are safe and effective in most patients [34–36]. For example, Maus et al. performed 89 pylorus balloon dilations after esophagectomy without complications. In this study, the total re-dilation rate for a 30-mm balloon was 20% [37]. In rare cases of endoscopic therapy failures, rescue pyloroplasty has been described to be helpful and well tolerated. For example, Datta et al. reported that rescue pyloroplasty was successful in 9 of 13 cases (69%), leading to decreased rates of nausea, vomiting, bloating, prokinetic use, and total parenteral nutrition dependence [38].

Conclusions

Our current single-center study aimed to evaluate whether pyloric drainage procedures are necessary to achieve an acceptable early postoperative outcome. In the present series, DGE was observed in the early postoperative course in 16.5% of cases. Pneumonia as a potential consequence of gastric outlet obstruction was observed in 27.1% of cases. Both of these values are consistent with the current literature regardless of whether pyloric drainage procedures were applied. Therefore, we propose that pyloric drainage procedures may be unwarranted in thoracoabdominal esophagectomy. In fact, these procedures can be associated with complications that may lead to morbidity or even mortality. To ultimately address the question of whether pylorus drainage procedures are beneficial versus no intervention, future prospective randomized controlled trials are needed.

Abbreviations

ASA: American Society of Anesthesiologists; BMI: Body mass index; DGE: Delayed gastric emptying; EUS: Endoscopic ultrasonography; GIST: Gastrointestinal stroma tumor; MRI: Magnetic resonance imaging; NET: Neuroendocrine tumor

Acknowledgements

The authors would like to thank Annika Brückner for technical assistance and data collection.

Funding

The study was not funded.

Authors' contributions

SF, AS and EE were responsible for data collection. SF, AS and HK analyzed and interpreted the patient data, particularly regarding patient demographics and clinical outcomes. JK and RH were major contributors to the writing of the manuscript. KF and RH contributed significantly by proof-reading the manuscript. All authors read and approved the final manuscript.

Competing interests

The authors declare that they have no competing interests.

References

1. Earlam R, Cunha-Melo JR. Oesophageal squamous cell carcinoma: I. A critical review of surgery. Br J Surg. 1980;67(6):381–90.
2. Muller JM, Erasmi H, Stelzner M, et al. Surgical therapy of oesophageal carcinoma. Br J Surg. 1990;77(8):845–57.
3. Raymond DP, Seder CW, Wright CD, et al. Predictors of major morbidity or mortality after resection for esophageal cancer: a Society of Thoracic Surgeons general thoracic surgery database risk adjustment model. Ann Thorac Surg. 2016;102(1):207–14.
4. Whooley BP, Law S, Murthy SC, et al. Analysis of reduced death and complication rates after esophageal resection. Ann Surg. 2001;233(3):338–44.
5. van Hagen P, Hulshof MC, van Lanschot JJ, et al. Preoperative chemoradiotherapy for esophageal or junctional cancer. N Engl J Med. 2012;366(22):2074–84.
6. Poghosyan T, Gaujoux S, Chirica M, et al. Functional disorders and quality of life after esophagectomy and gastric tube reconstruction for cancer. J Visc Surg. 2011;148(5):e327–35.
7. Chen KN. Managing complications I: leaks, strictures, emptying, reflux, chylothorax. J Thorac Dis. 2014;6(Suppl 3):S355–63.
8. Arya S, Markar SR, Karthikesalingam A, et al. The impact of pyloric drainage on clinical outcome following esophagectomy: a systematic review. Dis Esophagus. 2015;28(4):326–35.
9. Akkerman RD, Haverkamp L, van Hillegersberg R, et al. Surgical techniques to prevent delayed gastric emptying after esophagectomy with gastric interposition: a systematic review. Ann Thorac Surg. 2014; 98(4):1512–9.
10. Martin JT, Federico JA, McKelvey AA, et al. Prevention of delayed gastric emptying after esophagectomy: a single center's experience with botulinum toxin. Ann Thorac Surg. 2009;87(6):1708–13. discussion 1713-4
11. Bemelman WA, Taat CW, Slors JF, et al. Delayed postoperative emptying after esophageal resection is dependent on the size of the gastric substitute. J Am Coll Surg. 1995;180(4):461–4.
12. Beham A, Dango S, Ghadimi BM. Management of delayed complications after esophagectomy. Chirurg. 2015;86(11):1029–33.
13. van der Schaaf M, Johar A, Lagergren P, et al. Surgical prevention of reflux after esophagectomy for cancer. Ann Surg Oncol. 2013;20(11):3655–61.
14. Lanuti M, de Delva PE, Wright CD, et al. Post-esophagectomy gastric outlet obstruction: role of pyloromyotomy and management with endoscopic pyloric dilatation. Eur J Cardiothorac Surg. 2007;31(2):149–53.
15. Gaur P, Swanson SJ. Should we continue to drain the pylorus in patients undergoing an esophagectomy? Dis Esophagus. 2014;27(6):568–73.
16. Cheung HC, Siu KF, Wong JI. Pyloroplasty necessary in esophageal replacement by stomach? A prospective, randomized controlled trial. Surgery. 1987;102(1):19–24.
17. Fok M, Cheng SW, Wong J. Pyloroplasty versus no drainage in gastric replacement of the esophagus. Am J Surg. 1991;162(5):447–52.
18. Manjari R, Padhy AK, Chattopadhyay TK. Emptying of the intrathoracic stomach using three different pylorus drainage procedures–results of a comparative study. Surg Today. 1996;26(8):581–5.
19. Law S, Cheung MC, Fok M, et al. Pyloroplasty and pyloromyotomy in gastric replacement of the esophagus after esophagectomy: a randomized controlled trial. J Am Coll Surg. 1997;184(6):630–6.
20. Lanuti M, DeDelva P, Morse CR, et al. Management of delayed gastric emptying after esophagectomy with endoscopic balloon dilatation of the pylorus. Ann Thorac Surg. 2011;91(4):1019–24.
21. Urschel JD, Blewett CJ, Young JE, et al. Pyloric drainage (pyloroplasty) or no drainage in gastric reconstruction after esophagectomy: a meta-analysis of randomized controlled trials. Dig Surg. 2002;19(3):160–4.
22. Cerfolio RJ, Bryant AS, Canon CL, et al. Is botulinum toxin injection of the pylorus during Ivor Lewis [corrected] esophagogastrectomy the optimal drainage strategy? J Thorac Cardiovasc Surg. 2009;137(3):565–72.
23. Palmes D, Weilinghoff M, Colombo-Benkmann M, et al. Effect of pyloric drainage procedures on gastric passage and bile reflux after esophagectomy with gastric conduit reconstruction. Langenbeck's Arch Surg. 2007;392(2):135–41.
24. Mohajeri G, Tabatabaei SA, Hashemi SM, et al. Comparison of pyloromyotomy, pyloric buginage, and intact pylorus on gastric drainage in gastric pull-up surgery after esophagectomy. J Res Med Sci. 2016;21:33.
25. Antonoff MB, Puri V, Meyers BF, et al. Comparison of pyloric intervention strategies at the time of esophagectomy: is more better? Ann Thorac Surg. 2014;97(6):1950–7. discussion 1657-8
26. Lerut T, Coosemans W, De Leyn P, et al. Gastroplasty: yes or no to gastric drainage procedure. Dis Esophagus. 2001;14(3–4):173–7.
27. Wang LS, Huang MH, Huang BS, et al. Gastric substitution for resectable carcinoma of the esophagus: an analysis of 368 cases. Ann Thorac Surg. 1992;53(2):289–94.
28. Greene CL, DeMeester SR, Worrell SG, et al. Alimentary satisfaction, gastrointestinal symptoms, and quality of life 10 or more years after esophagectomy with gastric pull-up. J Thorac Cardiovasc Surg. 2014;147(3): 909–14.
29. Scarpa M, Valente S, Alfieri R, et al. Systematic review of health-related quality of life after esophagectomy for esophageal cancer. World J Gastroenterol. 2011;17(42):4660–74.

30. Richardson J, Richardson M, Nijjar R. Fistula after pyloroplasty - a novel approach to the management of a leak following oesophagectomy. J Surg Case Rep. 2012;2012(2):9.
31. Zieren HU, Muller JM, Jacobi CA, et al. Should a pyloroplasty be carried out in stomach transposition after subtotal esophagectomy with esophago-gastric anastomosis at the neck? A prospective randomized study. Chirurg. 1995;66(4):319–25.
32. Fuchs HF, Broderick RC, Harnsberger CR, et al. Intraoperative endoscopic Botox injection during Total Esophagectomy prevents the need for Pyloromyotomy or dilatation. J Laparoendosc Adv Surg Tech A. 2016;26(6): 433–8.
33. Eldaif SM, Lee R, Adams KN, et al. Intrapyloric botulinum injection increases postoperative esophagectomy complications. Ann Thorac Surg. 2014;97(6): 1959–64. discussion 1964-5
34. Li B, Zhang JH, Wang C, et al. Delayed gastric emptying after esophagectomy for malignancy. J Laparoendosc Adv Surg Tech A. 2014; 24(5):306–11.
35. Blackmon SH, Correa AM, Wynn B, et al. Propensity-matched analysis of three techniques for intrathoracic esophagogastric anastomosis. Ann Thorac Surg. 2007;83(5):1805–13; discussion 1813.
36. Sutcliffe RP, Forshaw MJ, Tandon R, et al. Anastomotic strictures and delayed gastric emptying after esophagectomy: incidence, risk factors and management. Dis Esophagus. 2008;21(8):712–7.
37. Maus MK, Leers J, Herbold T, et al. Gastric outlet obstruction after Esophagectomy: retrospective analysis of the effectiveness and safety of postoperative endoscopic pyloric dilatation. World J Surg. 2016;40(10): 2405–11.
38. Datta J, Williams NN, Conway RG, et al. Rescue pyloroplasty for refractory delayed gastric emptying following esophagectomy. Surgery. 2014;156(2): 290–7.

32

Robotic vs laparoscopic distal gastrectomy with D2 lymphadenectomy for gastric cancer: a retrospective comparative mono-institutional study

Fabio Cianchi[1*], Giampiero Indennitate[2], Giacomo Trallori[3], Manuela Ortolani[2], Beatrice Paoli[2], Giuseppe Macrì[3], Gabriele Lami[3], Beatrice Mallardi[4], Benedetta Badii[1], Fabio Staderini[1], Etleva Qirici[1], Antonio Taddei[1], Maria Novella Ringressi[1], Luca Messerini[5], Luca Novelli[5], Siro Bagnoli[3], Andrea Bonanomi[3], Caterina Foppa[1], Ileana Skalamera[1], Giulia Fiorenza[1] and Giuliano Perigli[1]

Abstract

Background: Robotic surgery has been developed with the aim of improving surgical quality and overcoming the limitations of conventional laparoscopy in the performance of complex mini-invasive procedures. The present study was designed to compare robotic and laparoscopic distal gastrectomy in the treatment of gastric cancer.

Methods: Between June 2008 and September 2015, 41 laparoscopic and 30 robotic distal gastrectomies were performed by a single surgeon at the same institution. Clinicopathological characteristics of the patients, surgical performance, postoperative morbidity/mortality and pathologic data were prospectively collected and compared between the laparoscopic and robotic groups by the Chi-square test and the Mann-Whitney test, as indicated.

Results: There were no significant differences in patient characteristics between the two groups. Mean tumor size was larger in the laparoscopic than in the robotic patients (5.3 ± 0.5 cm and 3.0 ± 0.4 cm, respectively; $P = 0.02$). However, tumor stage distribution was similar between the two groups. The mean number of dissected lymph nodes was higher in the robotic than in the laparoscopic patients (39.1 ± 3.7 and 30.5 ± 2.0, respectively; $P = 0.02$). The mean operative time was 262.6 ± 8.6 min in the laparoscopic group and 312.6 ± 15.7 min in the robotic group ($P < 0.001$). The incidences of surgery-related and surgery-unrelated complications were similar in the laparoscopic and in the robotic patients. There were no significant differences in short-term clinical outcomes between the two groups.

Conclusions: Within the limitation of a small-sized, non-randomized analysis, our study confirms that robotic distal gastrectomy is a feasible and safe surgical procedure. When compared with conventional laparoscopy, robotic surgery shows evident benefits in the performance of lymphadenectomy with a higher number of retrieved and examined lymph nodes.

Keywords: Gastric cancer, Robotic surgery, Laparoscopy, Lymphadenectomy, Distal gastrectomy

* Correspondence: fabio.cianchi@unifi.it
[1]Department of Surgery and Translational Medicine, Center of Oncological Minimally Invasive Surgery (COMIS), University of Florence, Largo Brambilla 3, 50134 Florence, Italy
Full list of author information is available at the end of the article

Background

Minimally invasive surgery for gastric cancer has evolved rapidly and has increased in popularity during the last two decades mainly in the Far East and for patients with early-stage tumors [1, 2]. A number of non-randomized trials, randomized controlled trials and meta-analyses have confirmed that laparoscopic surgery for gastric cancer can improve short-term results and the patient's quality of life when compared with open surgery [3–7]. Nevertheless, the development of laparoscopic surgery for gastric cancers in the Western world has been slow because most gastric cancers are diagnosed in an advanced stage for which laparoscopic gastrectomy is not yet considered an acceptable alternative to standard open surgery [8, 9]. This skepticism is basically due to the technical complexity of laparoscopic gastrectomy and concerns the feasibility of an oncologically acceptable lymphadenectomy. For these reasons, laparoscopic gastrectomy is considered one of the most difficult operations, requiring a long learning curve of about 40–50 cases [10, 11].

Robotic surgery has been introduced to overcome some of the technical limitations of laparoscopic surgery, such as two-dimensional vision, amplified physiological tremor, restricted range of motion and ergonomic discomfort [12, 13]. Robotic systems include operator-controlled 3-dimensional cameras that ensure steady and effective surgical fields of view with motion scaling and multiple degrees of freedom. It is believed that this technological evolution can assist the surgeon with complex surgical procedures that are required in radical gastrectomy, such as precise lymph node dissection and intracorporeal anastomoses [14].

Several studies have compared the feasibility and efficacy of robotic-assisted gastrectomy to that of laparoscopic-assisted gastrectomy for gastric cancer [15]. Robotic gastrectomy was reported to be associated with less operative blood loss and shorter hospital stay than laparoscopic gastrectomy [16, 17]. However, an overt advantage of robotic surgery in comparison with the laparoscopic technique in the treatment of gastric cancer has not been demonstrated yet.

This study was designed to analyze our early experience with robotic gastric surgery and compare the short-term clinical outcomes after laparoscopic and robotic distal gastrectomy for gastric cancer.

Methods

A total of 41 laparoscopic distal gastrectomies (LDG) for gastric cancer have been performed since June 2008 at the Center of Oncologic Minimally Invasive Surgery (COMIS), University of Florence, Florence, Italy. After the introduction of the daVinci Si surgical system (Intuitive Surgical Inc., Sunnyvale, CA, USA) in April 2014 at our hospital, we have performed 30 robotic distal gastrectomies (RDG) for gastric cancer between June 2014 and September 2015. All of the laparoscopic and robotic procedures were performed by a single surgeon (F.C.) and these cases were his initial experience with robotic gastrectomy.

We prospectively collected and retrospectively compared the clinicopathological characteristics, surgical performance and postoperative outcomes/morbidities between these two groups of patients. All patients underwent diagnostic and preoperative staging work-up according to a standard protocol which includes upper digestive endoscopy with gastric biopsy and computed tomography of the abdomen and chest. Patients with distant metastases, para-aortic lymph node involvement and/or pre- or intraoperative diagnosis of T4 lesions (i.e., local invasion of other organs, including spleen, pancreas or peritoneum), were excluded from the study. All patients had been thoroughly informed about the study and gave their written consent for the investigation in compliance with the Helsinki Declaration and in accordance with the ethical committee of our University Hospital.

The characteristics of patients, such as age, gender, body mass index (BMI) and tumor location, pathological results and surgical outcomes (operative time, blood loss, postoperative morbidity and mortality, time-to-first flatus, time-to-first oral intake and postoperative hospitalization) were collected.

Tumor localization was classified as middle or lower third of the stomach. The extension of lymph node dissection, namely D1 + α/β or D2, was performed according to the lymph node classification of the Japanese Gastric Cancer Association [18]. Tumors were classified according to the 7th edition of the AJCC/TNM tumor staging [19]. They were also classified according to Lauren's histotype, i.e., intestinal, diffuse or mixed.

Surgical technique

Trocar placement and docking the robotic arms

The preoperative procedures of RDG are not different from those of LDG except for the use of robotic ports and articulating robotic instruments. Under general anesthesia, the patient was placed in supine, reverse Trendelenburg position with legs abducted. In the robotic technique, the camera port was inserted by the open method through an umbilical transverse incision with a 12-mm trocar. After establishing pneumoperitoneum, three 8-mm trocars for the robotic arms were inserted: one in the upper right quadrant, one in the lower right quadrant, and one in the upper left quadrant. A final fourth 12-mm trocar was inserted in the lower left quadrant for the assistant. Either a hook or a monopolar shear was held in the first robotic arm located at the patient's left side. A Maryland bipolar forceps and a Cadiere forceps were held in the second and third arms, respectively, at the patient's right side.

The LDG surgical technique includes four trocars (two 12-mm and two 5-mm trocars) that are placed as previously described [20].

Distal gastrectomy

Most of the operative steps during RDG were the same as those during LDG. First, a routine exploration of the abdominal cavity was performed. D1 + α/β or D2 lymphadenectomy and gastric dissection were performed as previously described [20]. A key difference between RDG and LDG is that robotic dissection of lymph nodes was performed with the robotic wristed instruments. Moreover, some procedures, such as operating the stapler, applying hemoclips, inserting and removing surgical gauzes, are performed by the first operator during LDG whereas they are performed by the assistant during RDG.

In both procedures, mechanical intracorporeal either Billroth II or Roux-en-Y gastrojejunal anastomosis was performed. In the last 25 laparoscopic and in all robotic procedures, we reinforced the duodenal stump with a running, barbed suture after the duodenal transaction. The surgical specimen was placed in a polyethylene endobag and pulled out of the peritoneal cavity through the umbilical port which was extended to a length of 4–6 cm.

Statistical analysis

Categorical variables within laparoscopic and robotic groups were compared using Fisher's exact test or the chi-square test. Quantitative variables were summarized by means and SEM or medians and range. Groups were compared using the Mann-Whitney test.

Results

Table 1 shows the clinicopathological characteristics of the patients in the LDG and RDG groups. There were no significant differences in terms of age, sex or BMI. Patients in the LDG group had a larger mean tumor size than those in the RDG group. However, tumor stage distribution was similar between the two groups. Most of the tumors were located in the lower third of the stomach in both groups.

Surgical performance is detailed in Table 2. Robotic procedures showed significantly higher operative times when compared to laparoscopic surgery. No significant difference was found between the two groups in terms of blood loss. More Billroth II reconstructions were performed in the RDG group even if the difference was not statistically significant. No patients required open conversion in either group. No tumor involvement of the proximal or distal margin was found in any patient in either of the two groups. A higher number of lymph nodes was retrieved and examined in the RDG group when compared with the LDG group after D2 dissection (39.1 ± 3.7 vs 30.5 ± 2.0, respectively, $P = 0.02$).

Table 1 Clinicopathological characteristics of patients undergoing laparoscopic and robotic distal gastrectomy

	Laparoscopic group $N = 41$	Robotic group $N = 30$	*P* value
Gender (male/female)	19/22	14/16	NS
Age (year) (median, range)	74 (40–87)	73 (45–86)	NS
BMI (kg/m^2) (median, range)	26.0 (23–30)	27.0 (23–38)	NS
Tumor location			NS
Middle third	17 (41.5 %)	10 (33.3 %)	
Lower third	24 (58.5 %)	20 (66.7 %)	
Lauren classification			NS
Intestinal	19 (46.3)	19 (66.3)	
Diffuse	13 (31.7)	5 (16.7)	
Mixed	9 (22.0)	6 (20.0)	
Tumor size (cm) (mean ± SD)	5.3 ± 0.5	3.0 ± 0.4	$P = 0.02$
Stage distribution			NS
I	15 (36.6)	11 (36.7)	
II	15 (36.6)	10 (33.3)	
III	11 (26.8)	9 (30.0)	

The incidence of postoperative complications (surgery-related and surgery-unrelated), reoperations and mortality rates were similar in the two groups (Table 3). There were two mortalities in the LDG group and one in the RDG group. The cause of the two mortalities in the LDG group included one duodenal stump leakage with peritonitis and sepsis and one case of acute myocardial infarction. The case of duodenal stump leakage occurred before the introduction of the manual reinforcement with a running suture over the duodenal stump closure. One 89-year-old female patient in the RDG group who experienced a postoperative intestinal occlusion received laparotomy but eventually died of a cerebral vascular accident.

No significant differences were found between the two groups in terms of time to diet, bowel function recovery or length of hospital stay (Table 3).

Discussion

The clinical efficacy and advantages of the laparoscopic technique in the treatment of gastric cancer have now been recognized [21]. However, laparoscopic gastric surgery is still considered a technically demanding procedure. In particular, the technical threshold of performing lymph node dissection and intracorporeal suture during laparoscopic gastrectomy remains high and requires a steep learning curve [10, 11]. The robotic platform provides some

Table 2 Comparison of surgical performance between the laparoscopic and the robotic groups

	Laparoscopic group $N = 41$	Robotic group $N = 30$	P value
Type of reconstruction			NS
Billroth II	22 (53.7 %)	21 (70.0 %)	
Rou-en-Y	19 (46.3 %)	9 (30.0 %)	
Lymph node dissection			NS
D1 + α/β	4 (9.8 %)	2 (6.6 %)	
D2	37 (90.2 %)	28 (93.3 %)	
Mean operative time (min) (mean ± SEM)	262.6 ± 8.6	312.6 ± 15.7	<0.001
Blood loss (ml) (mean ± SEM)	118.7 ± 10.7	99.5 ± 7.6	NS
Conversion to open surgery	0	0	NS
Positive resection margin	0	0	NS
No. of retrieved lymph nodes after D2 dissection (mean ± SEM)	30.5 ± 2.0	39.1 ± 3.7	0.02

Table 3 Comparison of short-term clinical outcomes between the laparoscopic and the robotic groups

	Laparoscopic group $N = 41$	Robotic group $N = 30$	P value
Time-to-first flatus (day) (mean ± SD)	3.0 ± 0.3	3.2 ± 0.3	NS
Time-to-first oral feeding (day) (mean ± SD)	5.4 ± 0.5	5.2 ± 0.3	NS
Surgery-related complications (total)	5 (12.1 %)	4 (13.2 %)	NS
Focal pancreatitis	1 (2.4 %)	0	
Duodenal stump leakage	2 (4.9 %)	0	
Intestinal obstruction	0	2 (6.6 %)	
Anastomotic bleeding	1 (2.4 %)	0	
Delayed gastric emptying	1 (2.4 %)	2 (6.6 %)	
Surgery-unrelated complications (total)	3 (7.2 %)	2 (6.6 %)	NS
Urinary tract infections	1 (2.4 %)	0	
Arrhythmia	1 (2.4 %)	0	
Deep venous thrombosis	0	1 (3.3 %)	
Cerebral vascular accident	0	1 (3.3 %)	
Myocardial infarction	1 (2.4 %)	0	
Reoperations	2 (4.9 %)	1 (3.3 %)	NS
Postoperative mortality	2 (4.9 %)	1 (3.3 %)	NS
Hospital length stay (day) (mean ± SD)	8.1 ± 0.5	9.5 ± 1.0	NS

technical improvements, such as improved vision, wristed instrument, tremor filtration system and motion scaling, that enable surgeons to easily perform precise lymphadenectomy and anastomoses. A number of studies have shown the feasibility and safety of robotic gastric surgery but a clear superiority of robotic surgery over laparoscopy has not yet been demonstrated [22–26]. No substantial reduction in time-to-first flatus, time-to-first oral feeding and length of hospital stay has been reported after robotic surgery when compared to laparoscopy. Our early experience in robotic gastrectomy confirms these previously published results: we did not find any significant difference in short-term clinical outcomes between patients in the robotic and those in the laparoscopic group. However, our inability to show robotic surgery to be superior to laparoscopic surgery is not surprising in light of previous studies that have compared laparoscopic with open surgery. In numerous studies, laparoscopic gastrectomy facilitated less blood loss, earlier bowel function recovery and shorter length of stay than open gastrectomy [27]. Thus, conceivably, optimal peri-operative surgical outcomes may have already been achieved with laparoscopic surgery, leaving little room for improvement via robotic surgery.

One crucial step in gastric cancer surgery is lymphadenectomy since the removal of an adequate number of lymph nodes has been shown to improve the accuracy of staging and regional disease control [28]. This procedure is typically considered to be technically difficult to perform in conventional laparoscopic surgery, especially when D2 lymphadenectomy is mandatory [10, 11, 29]. This is mainly due to the use of conventional straight forceps in laparoscopic surgery that do not allow the surgeon to reach deep-seated vessels and areas such as the supra-pancreatic one. Stable exposure and use of wristed instruments with the robotic system may help the surgeon to efficiently perform lymph node dissection in these delicate areas, in particular around the posterior aspect of the common hepatic artery and the splenic vessels [30]. In the present study, we found that robotic surgery can improve the quality of lymphadenectomy in distal gastric resection when compared with conventional laparoscopy. Indeed, the mean number of retrieved lymph nodes in the robotic group was significantly higher than in the laparoscopic group (39.1 vs 30.5, respectively) and, importantly, the mean values in both groups were much higher than the recommended number (i.e., 25) for adequate D2 lymphadenectomy [31]. Importantly, this number was even higher than what we found in a group of matched patients who were operated on by open distal gastrectomy between 2008 and 2012 at our institution [20].

Despite the evident technical advantages offered by the robotic system, recent meta-analyses comparing robotic and laparoscopic gastrectomy have failed to show a significant increase in the number of retrieved lymph nodes in patients operated robotically [15–17, 32]. This may be explained by the fact that the majority of the analyzed studies were carried out in the Far East where patients generally have a low BMI. Recently, Lee et al. [33] have shown that the benefits of a robotic approach were more evident in high versus normal BMI patients when performing distal gastrectomy with D2 lymphadenectomy, particularly in terms of achieving a consistent number of retrieved lymph nodes (>25). The authors concluded that robotic surgery may overcome the technical difficulties due to excessive intra-abdominal fat and thick abdominal walls during laparoscopic lymphadenectomy. Our findings seem to confirm these previously published results: the BMIs of our patients (26.0 and 27.0 kg/m^2 in the laparoscopic and robotic group, respectively) were similar to those of high-BMI patients reported by Lee et al. (26.8 and 26.9 kg/m^2 in the two groups, respectively), thus showing that robotic surgery may offer consistent quality of lymphadenectomy for patients with high BMI. Importantly, the present results were achieved during our very early experience in gastric robotic surgery. This suggests that surgeons with sufficient experience in laparoscopic gastrectomy can rapidly overcome the learning curve for robotic gastrectomy and high-quality surgery is achievable even after a relatively low number of cases [34]. These advantages could be more helpful in Western countries or lower volume centers, where high BMI patients are more common and where there is a lower incidence of gastric cancer, which limits the number of gastric cancer surgeries to be performed through a minimally invasive approach.

All sorts of studies that have been published about robotic gastric surgery, have reported that operative time was prolonged when compared with the laparoscopic approach and our findings are in line with these results [15–17, 32]. There are a number of possible reasons for this: first, robotic surgery is associated with an increased set-up time needed to position the robot before beginning surgery. However, docking times can be shortened after accumulation of greater experience. Secondly, the prolonged time may be due to camera motion interrupting the operative procedure and the unadapted optical system with an absence of a large general view of the operative field which prevents a safe continuous dissection and necessitates slow manipulation. However, longer operation times have never been shown to translate into increased perioperative complications and thus should not discourage surgeons from investigating the novel utility of robotic surgery.

One of the limitations of the present study was the lack of a detailed comparative analysis of cost-effectiveness between robotic and laparoscopic gastric surgery. Robotic gastric surgery undoubtedly has higher costs than laparoscopic surgery as clearly demonstrated by Park et al. [35]. The only way its use can be justified would be through improved patient survival achieved through more efficient surgery. The present study seems to show potentially relevant advantages, such as a higher number of retrieved lymph nodes, that would justify the higher costs of robotic systems. However, a multicenter, randomized study is needed to confirm this clinical benefit and evaluate whether it may effectively translate into improvement of long-term patient survival and quality of life.

Conclusions

Within the limitation of a small-sized, non-randomized analysis, our study confirms that robot-assisted gastrectomy is a feasible and safe surgical procedure. When compared with conventional laparoscopy, robotic surgery shows evident benefits in performing lymphadenectomy with a higher number of retrieved and examined lymph nodes.

Abbreviations

LDG: Laparoscopic distal gastrectomyRDG: Robotic distal gastrectomyBMI: Body mass indexAJCC: American joint committee of cancer

Acknowledgements

Not applicable.

Funding

This study was supported by a grant from the Ente Cassa di Risparmio di Firenze.

Authors' contributions

FC performed all surgical operations and was a major contributor in writing the manuscript. BB, FS, EQ, AT, MNR, CF, IS, GF, and GP were part of the same surgical unit and were involved in patient care, follow-up and acquisition, analysis and interpretation of the data. GI, GT, MO, PB, GM, GL, BM, SB, and AB were part of different endoscopic units from different hospitals in Florence and were involved in the recruitment of patients and significantly contributed to acquisition and critical revision of the data during the entire length of the study period (8 years). LM and LN are pathologists and were involved in drafting the manuscript and revising it critically for important intellectual content. All authors read and approved the final manuscript.

Competing interests

The authors declare that they have no competing interests.

Author details

[1]Department of Surgery and Translational Medicine, Center of Oncological Minimally Invasive Surgery (COMIS), University of Florence, Largo Brambilla 3, 50134 Florence, Italy. [2]IFCA, Florence, Italy. [3]Unit of Gastroenterology, University Hospital Careggi, Florence, Italy. [4]ISPO, Florence, Italy. [5]Department of Experimental and Clinical Medicine, University of Florence, Florence, Italy.

References

1. Kitano S, Shiraishi N, Uyama I, Sugihara K, Tanigawa N, Japanese Laparoscopic Surgery Study Group. A multicenter study on oncologic outcome of laparoscopic gastrectomy for early cancer in Japan. Ann Surg. 2007;245:68–72.
2. Koeda K, Nishizuka S, Wakabayashi G. Minimally invasive surgery for gastric cancer: the future standard of care. World J Surg. 2011;35:1469–77.
3. Huscher CG, Mingoli A, Sgarzini G, Sansonetti A, Di Paola M, Recher A, et al. Laparoscopic versus open subtotal gastrectomy for distal gastric cancer: five-year results of a randomized prospective trial. Ann Surg. 2005;241:232–7.
4. Hayashi H, Ochiai T, Shimada H, Gunji Y. Prospective randomized study of open versus laparoscopy-assisted distal gastrectomy with extraperigastric lymph node dissection for early gastric cancer. Surg Endosc. 2005;19:1172–6.
5. Kim HH, Hyung WJ, Cho GS, Kim MC, Han SU, Kim W, et al. Morbidity and mortality of laparoscopic gastrectomy versus open gastrectomy for gastric cancer: an interim report—a phase III multicenter, prospective, randomized Trial (KLASS Trial). Ann Surg. 2010;251:417–20.
6. Kodera Y, Fujiwara M, Ohashi N, Nakayama G, Koike M, Morita S, et al. Laparoscopic surgery for gastric cancer: a collective review with meta-analysis of randomized trials. J Am Coll Surg. 2010;211:677–86.
7. Ding J, Liao GQ, Liu HL, Tang J. Meta-analysis of laparoscopy-assisted distal gastrectomy with D2 lymph node dissection for gastric cancer. J Surg Oncol. 2012;105:297–303.
8. Strong VE, Devaud N, Karpeh M. The role of laparoscopy for gastric surgery in the West. Gastric Cancer. 2009;12:127–31.
9. Yamamoto M, Rashid OM, Wong J. Surgical management of gastric cancer: the East vs West perspective. J Gastrointest Oncol. 2015;6:79–88.
10. Kim MC, Jung GJ, Kim HH. Learning curve of laparoscopy-assisted distal gastrectomy with systemic lymphadenectomy for early gastric cancer. World J Gastroenterol. 2005;1:7508–11.
11. Jin SH, Kim DY, Kim H, Jeong IH, Kim MW, Cho YK, et al. Multidimensional learning curve in laparoscopy-assisted gastrectomy for early gastric cancer. Surg Endosc. 2007;21:28–33.
12. Lanfranco AR, Castellanos AE, Desai JP, Meyers WC. Robotic surgery: a current perspective. Ann Surg. 2004;239:14–21.
13. Diana M, Marescaux J. Robotic surgery. Br J Surg. 2015;102:15–28.
14. Obama K, Sakai Y. Current status of robotic gastrectomy for gastric cancer. Surg Today. 2016;46:528–34.
15. Hyun MH, Lee CH, Kim HJ, Tong Y, Park SS. Systematic review and meta-analysis of robotic surgery compared with conventional laparoscopic and open resections for gastric carcinoma. Br J Surg. 2013;100:1566–78.
16. Marano A, Choi YY, Hyung WJ, Kim YM, Kim J, Noh SH. Robotic versus Laparoscopic versus Open Gastrectomy: A Meta-Analysis. J Gastric Cancer. 2013;13:136–48.
17. Zong L, Seto Y, Aikou S, Takahashi T. Efficacy evaluation of subtotal and total gastrectomies in robotic surgery for gastric cancer compared with that in open and laparoscopic resections: a meta-analysis. PLoS One. 2014;9:103312.
18. Japanese Gastric Cancer Association. Japanese classification of gastric carcinoma, 2nd English ed. Gastric Cancer. 1998;1:10–24.
19. Edge SB, Byrd DR, Compton CC, Fritz AG, Greene FL, Trotti III A. AJCC cancer staging manual. 7th ed. New York: Springer; 2009.
20. Cianchi F, Qirici E, Trallori G, Macrì G, Indennitate G, Ortolani M, et al. Totally laparoscopic versus open gastrectomy for gastric cancer: a matched cohort study. J Laparoendosc Adv Surg Tech A. 2013;23:117–22.
21. Antonakis PT, Ashrafian H, Isla AM. Laparoscopic gastric surgery for cancer: where do we stand? World J Gastroenterol. 2014;20:14280–91.
22. Huang KH, Lan YT, Fang WL, Chen JH, Lo SS, Li AF, et al. Comparison of the operative outcomes and learning curves between laparoscopic and robotic gastrectomy for gastric cancer. PLoS One. 2014;9:111499.
23. Junfeng Z, Yan S, Bo T, Yingxue H, Dongzhu Z, Yongliang Z, et al. Robotic gastrectomy versus laparoscopic gastrectomy for gastric cancer: comparison of surgical performance and short-term outcomes. Surg Endosc. 2014;28:1779–87.
24. Yoon HM, Kim YW, Lee JH, Ryu KW, Eom BW, Park JY, et al. Robot-assisted total gastrectomy is comparable with laparoscopically assisted total gastrectomy for early gastric cancer. Surg Endosc. 2012;26:1377–81.
25. Hyun MH, Lee CH, Kwon YJ, Cho SI, Jang YJ, Kim DH, et al. Robot versus laparoscopic gastrectomy for cancer by an experienced surgeon: comparisons of surgery, complications, and surgical stress. Ann Surg Oncol. 2013;20:1258–65.
26. Eom BW, Yoon HM, Ryu KW, Lee JH, Cho SJ, Lee JY, et al. Comparison of surgical performance and short-term clinical outcomes between laparoscopic and robotic surgery in distal gastric cancer. Eur J Surg Oncol. 2012;38:57–63.
27. Deng Y, Zhang Y, Guo TK. Laparoscopy-assisted versus open distal gastrectomy for early gastric cancer: A meta-analysis based on seven randomized controlled trials. Surg Oncol. 2015;24:71–7.
28. Coburn NG. Lymph nodes and gastric cancer. J Surg Oncol. 2009;99:199–206.
29. Zou ZH, Zhao LY, Mou TY, Hu YF, Yu J, Liu H, et al. Laparoscopic vs open D2 gastrectomy for locally advanced gastric cancer: a meta-analysis. World J Gastroenterol. 2014;20:16750–64.
30. Kim YW, Reim D, Park JY, Eom BW, Kook MC, Ryu KW, et al. Role of robot-assisted distal gastrectomy compared to laparoscopy-assisted distal gastrectomy in suprapancreatic nodal dissection for gastric cancer. Surg Endosc. 2016;30:1547–52.
31. Verlato G, Roviello F, Marchet A, Giacopuzzi S, Marrelli D, Nitti D, et al. Indexes of surgical quality in gastric cancer surgery: experience of an Italian network. Ann Surg Oncol. 2009;16:594–602.
32. Shen WS, Xi HQ, Chen L, Wei B. A meta-analysis of robotic versus laparoscopic gastrectomy for gastric cancer. Surg Endosc. 2014;28:2795–802.
33. Lee J, Kim YM, Woo Y, Obama K, Noh SH, Hyung WJ. Robotic distal subtotal gastrectomy with D2 lymphadenectomy for gastric cancer patients with high body mass index: comparison with conventional laparoscopic distal subtotal gastrectomy with D2 lymphadenectomy. Surg Endosc. 2015;29:3251–60.
34. Park SS, Kim MC, Park MS, Hyung WJ. Rapid adaptation of robotic gastrectomy for gastric cancer by experienced laparoscopic surgeons. Surg Endosc. 2012;26:60–7.
35. Park JY, Jo MJ, Nam BH, Kim Y, Eom BW, Yoon HM, et al. Surgical stress after robot-assisted distal gastrectomy and its economic implications. Br J Surg. 2012;99:1554–61.

33

Gastric volvulus through Morgagni hernia and intestinal diverticulosis in an adult patient: a case report

Zoya Fatima Rizwan Ladiwala[1], Rija Sheikh[1], Ayesha Ahmed[1], Ibrahim Zahid[1*] and Amjad Siraj Memon[2]

Abstract

Background: Morgagni's hernia (MH) is a rare type of congenital diaphragmatic hernia with limited available literature. Late presentations are infrequent and the ones complicated due to gastric volvulus are even rarer. Another uncommon association of MH is with small bowel diverticulosis. We herein discussed a case of gastric volvulus as the content of MH, and small bowel diverticulosis present in a patient concomitantly.

Case presentation: A 30 year old woman, who presented with a one year history of epigastric burning and indigestion, occasionally associated with pain and vomiting. On clinical examination, no clue to the diagnosis could be ascertained. Her chest and abdominal x-ray indicated an abnormal air-fluid level at right hemithorax, which prompted a Computed Tomography (CT) scan, showing organo-axial gastric volvulus. MH with gastric volvulus was observed during laparotomy and trans-thoracic reduction of the contents was performed, along with repair of the defect. Multiple intestinal diverticuli were also found and the largest diverticulum was excised.

Conclusions: Gastric volvulus through MH is a rare but potentially life-threatening condition. Non-specific symptoms like epigastric pain and vomiting can delay the diagnosis and management, however, advanced imaging techniques like CT scan can speed up this process. After the diagnosis is made, surgical repair should be attempted regardless of symptoms.

Keywords: Diaphragmatic hernia, Morgagni hernia, Gastric volvulus, Diverticulosis, Computed tomography, Laparotomy, Gastrostomy, Gastropexy

Background

Morgagni's hernia (MH) is an uncommon birth defect accounting for about 3% of all congenital diaphragmatic hernias, with substantial morbidity and mortality [1]. It is a result of abdominal contents entering the thoracic cavity through an antero-medial defect of the diaphragm and is usually diagnosed early in life [2]. MH rarely presents with gastric volvulus [3], which is the abnormal torsion of the stomach along its longitudinal or horizontal axis [4]. Another unusual incidence of MH is with small bowel diverticulosis (SBD). SBD is characterized by multiple sac like mucosal out-pouchings through weak points in the intestinal wall [5]. Here we describe a case report where gastric volvulus was herniating through the foramen of Morgagni and the patient had concurrent SBD. To the best of our knowledge such a case has never been reported previously.

* Correspondence: ibrahim_zahid@hotmail.com
[1]Dow University of Health Sciences, Karachi, Pakistan
Full list of author information is available at the end of the article

Case presentation

A 30-year-old female presented with complaints of epigastric burning and indigestion for 1 year, which was occasionally associated with pain and vomiting. On a previous oesophago-gastroduodenoscopy, multiple oesophageal ulcers were noted, located from 30 to 35 cm and the mucosa was seen to be circumferentially hyperaemic. Upon investigation, chest and abdominal X-ray showed abnormal air-fluid level at right hemithorax as shown in Fig. 1. Computed Tomography (CT) scan demonstrated organo-axial gastric volvulus accompanied with right hemi-diaphragm elevation and a slight mediastinal shift to the left, with gastric bubble above the diaphragm (Fig. 2), and sections through the lower chest showed mild bilateral pleural effusion with basal atelectasis of the right

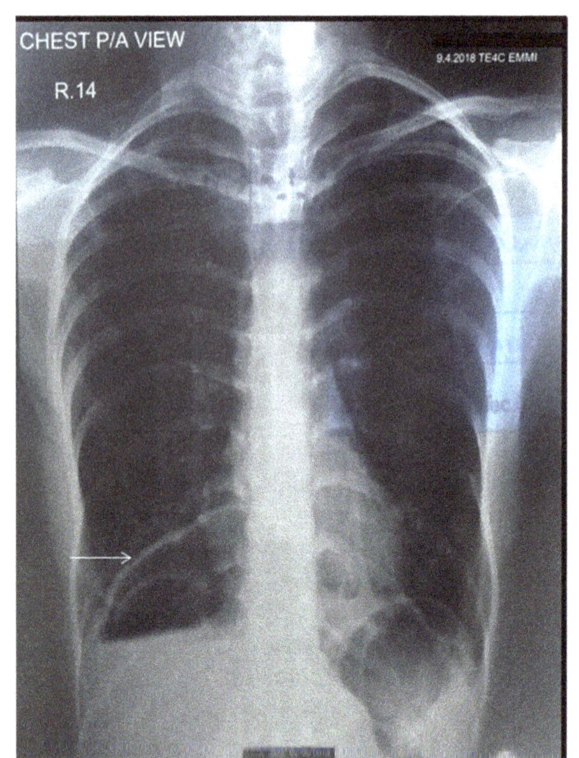

Fig. 1 Plain postero-anterior chest X-ray showing abnormal air fluid level (white arrow) in the right basal hemi-thorax above the diaphragm

lower lobe. The small and large bowel loops were unremarkable and there was no evidence of bowel obstruction.

An elective laparotomy was performed through a midline incision. Stomach was not seen in the abdominal cavity, but pull on the gastrocolic ligament revealed the greater curvature of the stomach through foramen of Morgagni in the right hemi-diaphragm, with the defect measuring 4 × 5 cm (Fig. 3). The hernia was reduced, with excision of the hernial sac and the defect was repaired using a size zero non-absorbable polypropylene suture—no mesh was placed. Since there was a high jejunal repair, a gastrostomy was created which served to secure the stomach in place. Following the reduction of hernia, on further exploration, multiple diverticuli were observed in the small and large intestine (Fig. 4). Interestingly, these were unremarkable on CT scan. Only the largest and most proximal jejunal diverticulum (Fig. 5), which was about 6 cm in size, was resected using a linear stapler as it had a narrow neck. A pelvic drain was placed and the wound was closed in layers using absorbable polyglactin suture. Figure 6 exhibits the normal anatomy and a schematic diagram of this case depicting the presence of gastric volvulus through MH on the right side. The post-operative period was uneventful and the patient was discharged on the 10th post-operative day. The patient was stable and asymptomatic on follow up after one month, and she is doing well as of writing of this report. 'Timeline for Case Report' in Additional file 1 represents the events of this case in a chronologic order.

Discussion and conclusions

MH is the rarest form of congenital diaphragmatic hernia which occurs through a developmental defect as a result of failure of fusion between the sternal and costal portions of the muscle [6]. Usually it occurs on the right side where it contains the omentum, followed by colon and small intestine [7]. Conversely, left-sided hernias commonly bear the stomach as reported by a review done in India [8]. Our case however, presented with a right sided hernia associated with gastric volvulus. These hernias are congenital in origin, but an acquired increase in abdominal pressures such as vomiting or coughing can cause true herniation [8]. MH may present with acute symptoms usually caused by respiratory distress or volvulus of its contents; it can also be detected incidentally with mild generic respiratory/bowel symptoms [8]. It is interesting to note that our case presented with enteric symptoms only, despite having lung abnormalities which were found on the CT scan.

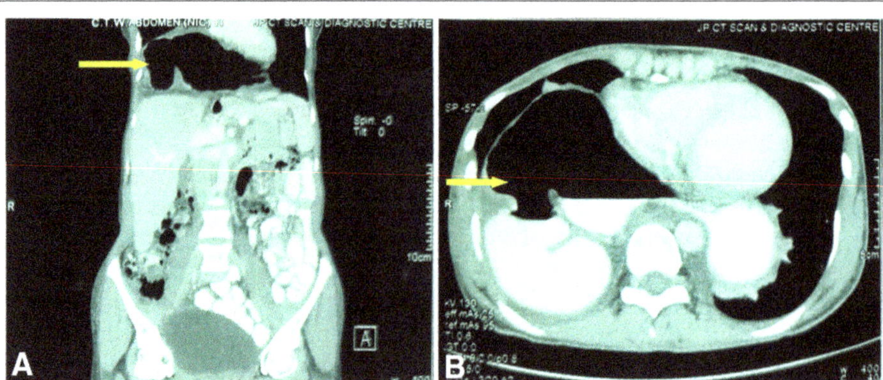

Fig. 2 Preoperative coronal (**a**) and axial (**b**) computed tomography slice showing gastric bubble (yellow arrow) indicating herniation of stomach into the thorax

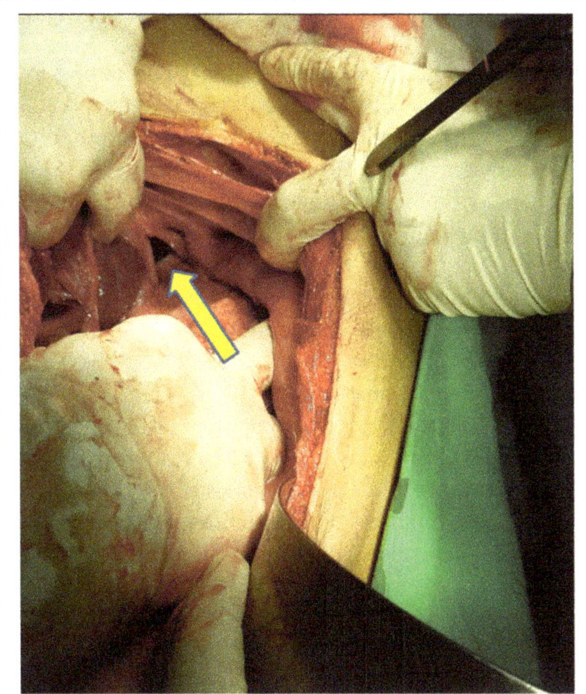

Fig. 3 Intra-operative view of Morgagni's defect (yellow arrow)

Diagnosis of MH is facilitated by chest x-ray, abdominal x-rays, barium studies or ultrasound, but currently CT scan is the diagnostic modality of choice [9]. The scans must include sections through the lower chest as well as the abdomen to determine the extent of the hernia [1]. Treatment is primarily based on surgical repair [9], even if the hernia sac only contains the omentum [10], and trans-abdominal approach with interrupted non-absorbable sutures is widely preferred [9]. Nevertheless, recent advances in thoracoscopic [9] and laparoscopic [3, 9] techniques offer innovative approaches to its management [9]. In fact, laparoscopy has been concluded as the gold standard procedure for uncomplicated MH [11]. In addition to being minimally invasive, it offers better visualization of the surgical field, easy manipulation and accessibility, aesthetic benefit, fewer complications and faster recovery of the patient [10]. Several laparoscopic techniques are being practiced, which include primary closure of the defect with different variety of intra-corporeal sutures, staples or mesh [12], but no single technique has been advocated as ideal. We opted for an open surgical approach due to limitation of resources and required surgical expertise for laparoscopic repair of MH.

Literature revealed very few cases of gastric volvulus into the foramen of Morgagni, with presenting features in most cases being hematemesis, melena, abdominal bloating, and vomiting [10, 13]. Gastric volvulus occurs in conditions which increase the laxity of structures supporting the stomach, such as pyloric stenosis, pyloric hypertrophy or chronic gastric distension [10]. Several predisposing factors, such as hiatal or incisional hernias, eventration of the diaphragm, trauma, surgical injury, gastric ulcers and neoplasms, are found in about half of the patients who present with this disease [3]. Similarly in this case, the CT scan indicated diaphragmatic eventration associated with organo-axial rotation of the herniated stomach. This type of volvulus is more commonly associated with MH than its mesentro-axial counterpart [3]. The definitive treatment of gastric volvulus is gastropexy where the stomach is fixed to the diaphragm and/or anterior abdominal wall either through a laparoscopic or an open abdominal approach [4].

In order to prevent recurrences of gastric volvulus, a temporary gastrostomy may be added to act as a diversion thereby protecting the high jejunal repair and to fix the stomach to the anterior abdominal wall, serving as a gastropexy. The location of gastrostomy tube is essential, as recurrence of volvulus has been reported after gastrostomy, acting as two fixed points of the axis [14]. Literature search revealed that Bhasin endoscopically reduced a chronic gastric volvulus in 10 patients without performing any percutaneous endoscopic gastrostomy placement, but on follow up, 3 cases eventually recurred and required surgical treatment [15]. It emphasizes the significance of adding a gastrostomy tube while managing gastric volvulus. Percutaneous endoscopic gastrostomy has an added advantage for patients who have difficulties with oral intake [16] thus

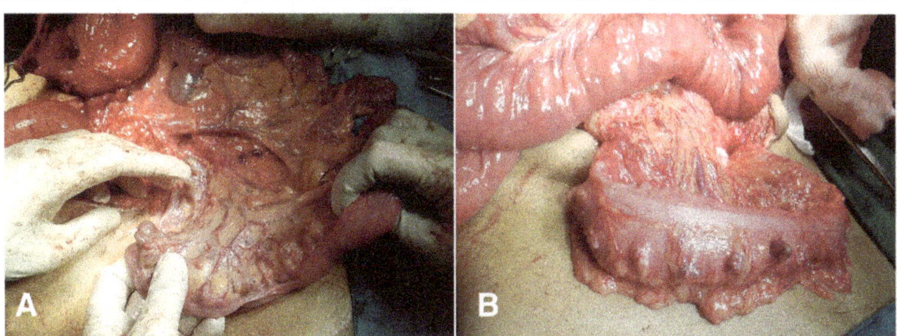

Fig. 4 Intra-operative picture showing small bowel (**a**) and large bowel (**b**) diverticulosis

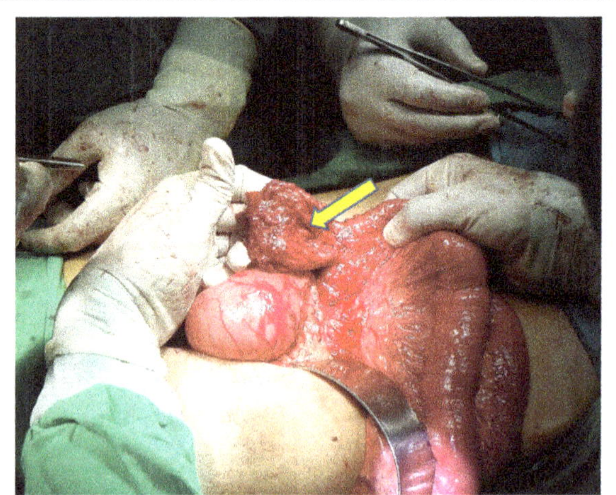

Fig. 5 Intra-operative picture of a large jejunal diverticulum (yellow arrow)

permitting the fixation of the stomach together with provision of enteral nutrition.

SBD occurs due to abnormal peristalsis resulting from motor dysfunction of the gut. It is more frequently confined to the proximal jejunum and distal ileum due to a wider diameter of vasa recta in these segments [5]. Clinically the disease is asymptomatic until it presents with complications which are determined by performing a diagnostic laparoscopy [5]. Complications like perforation, abscess and mechanical obstruction identified on laparoscopy, are managed by an exploratory laparotomy allowing diverticulectomy with resection of the diseased bowel and performing primary anastomosis [17].

In conclusion, MH along with gastric volvulus and small bowel diverticulosis is a rare occurrence, and may not be identified clinically; meticulous analysis of CT scan followed by surgical exploration allows definitive diagnosis. Hernia closure using non-absorbable sutures along with gastropexy and diverticulectomy yields good results with no major sequelae.

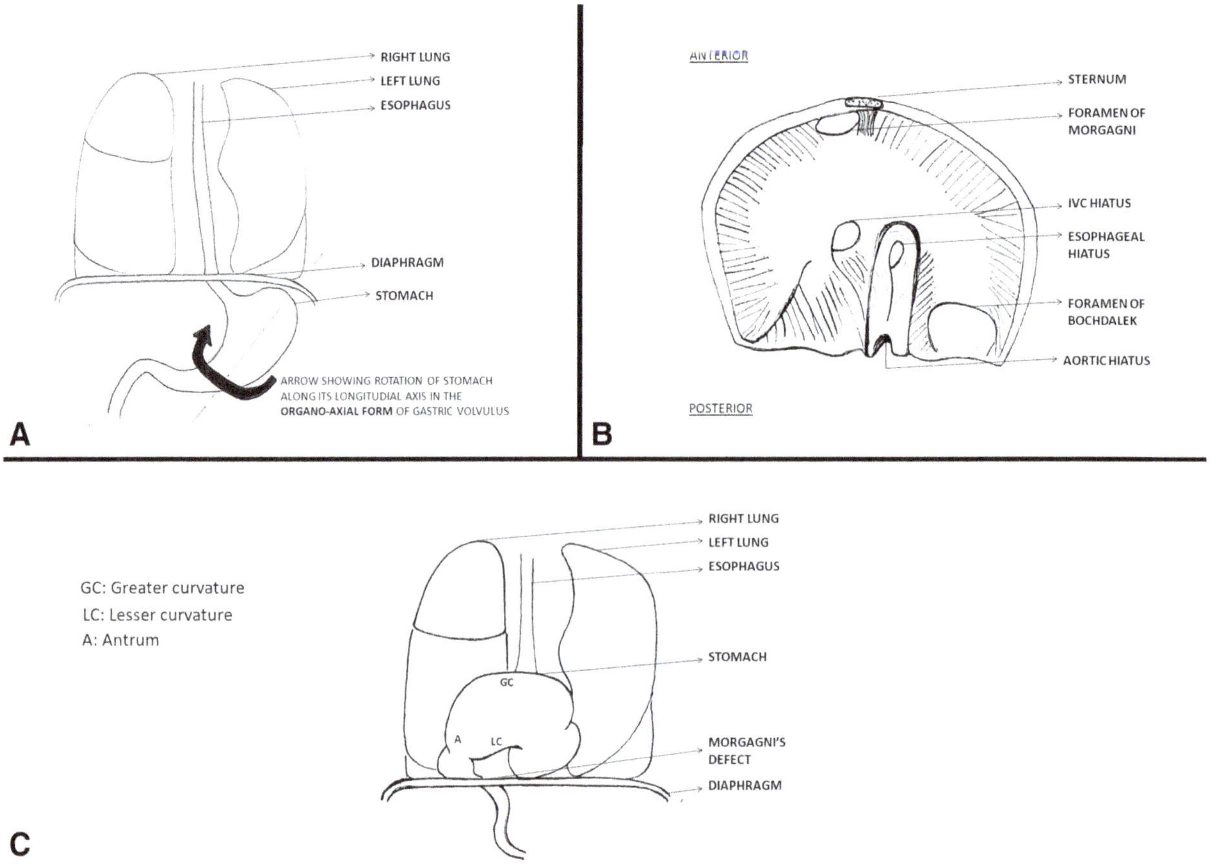

Fig. 6 a Normal anatomic diagram with an arrow showing the axis of rotation of stomach in this case. **b** Axial section of the diaphragm showing the presence of foramen of Morgagni in the right antero-medial part. **c** Anatomical schema of the case showing the greater curvature of stomach being displaced superiorly, after its organo-axial rotation, and the herniating stomach into the thorax through the defect (of Morgagni) in the diaphragm

Abbreviations

CT: Computed Tomography; MH: Morgagni Hernia; SBD: Small Bowel Diverticulosis

Authors' contributions

IZ is the corresponding author, drafted a part of the manuscript, reviewed the report and implemented the suggested changes by the reviewer including the schematic diagram. ZFRL provided the pre-surgical data of the patient, drafted the discussion of the manuscript and finalized the visualization of the anatomical changes. RS and AA accessed the postoperative data, acquired the patient's permission for publication, drafted a part of the manuscript and assisted in making the necessary changes according to reviewers' comments. ASM was the head surgeon for the case; he acquired the patients' data and the intra-operative pictures, revised the manuscript critically for important intellectual content and provided us with the background information. All authors read and approved the final manuscript.

Competing interests

The authors declare that they have no competing interests.

Author details

[1]Dow University of Health Sciences, Karachi, Pakistan. [2]Department of General Surgery, Dow University of Health Sciences, Civil Hospital Karachi, Karachi, Pakistan.

References

1. Park A, Doyle C. Laparoscopic Morgagni hernia repair: how I do it. J Gastrointest Surg. 2014;18(10):1858–62. PubMed PMID: 24898515
2. Federico JA. General Thoracic Surgery. 5. Philadelphia: Lippincott Williams and Wilkins; 2000. Foramen of Morgagni hernia; pp. 647–660.
3. Sonthalia N, Ray S, Khanra D, Saha A, Maitra S, Saha M, et al. Gastric Volvulus Through Morgagni Hernia: An Easily Overlooked Emergency. J Emerg Med. 2013 2013/06/01/;44(6):1092–1096.
4. Rodriguez-Garcia H, Wright A, Yates R. Managing obstructive gastric volvulus: challenges and solutions. Open Access Surgery. 2017;10:15–25.
5. Janevska D, Trajkovska M, Janevski V, Serafimoski V. Small bowel diverticulosis as a cause of ileus: a case report. Pril (Makedon Akad Nauk Umet Odd Med Nauki). 2013;34(1):175–7. PubMed PMID: 23917752. Epub 2013/08/07. eng
6. Court FG, Wemyss-Holden SA, Fitridge R, Maddern GJ. Unusual case of Morgagni hernia associated with malrotation. ANZ J Surg 2003 Sep;73(9): 772–773. PubMed PMID: 12956800.
7. Ambrogi V, Forcella D, Gatti A, Vanni G, Mineo TC. Transthoracic repair of Morgagni's hernia: a 20-year experience from open to video-assisted approach. Surg Endosc 2007 Apr;21(4):587–591. PubMed PMID: 17180292. Epub 2006/12/21. eng.
8. Abraham V, Myla Y, Verghese S, Chandran BS. Morgagni-larrey hernia- a review of 20 cases. The Indian journal of surgery 2012 Oct;74(5):391–395. PubMed PMID: 24082592. Pubmed Central PMCID: PMC3477412. Epub 2013/10/02. eng.
9. Minneci PC, Deans KJ, Kim P, Mathisen DJ. Foramen of Morgagni hernia: changes in diagnosis and treatment. Ann Thorac Surg 2004 Jun;77(6):1956–1959. PubMed PMID: 15172245. Epub 2004/06/03. eng.
10. Coulier B, Broze B. Gastric volvulus through a Morgagni hernia: multidetector computed tomography diagnosis. Emerg Radiol 2008 May; 15(3):197–201. PubMed PMID: 17701234. Epub 2007/08/19. eng.
11. Li S, Liu X, Shen Y, Wang H, Feng M, Tan L. Laparoscopic repair of Morgagni hernia by artificial pericardium patch in an adult obese patient. J Thorac Dis. 2015;7(4):754–7.
12. Shah RS, Sharma PC, Bhandarkar DS. Laparoscopic repair of Morgagni's hernia: an innovative approach. J Indian Assoc Pediatr Surg. 2015;20(2):68–71.
13. Cybulsky I, Himal HS. Gastric volvulus within the foramen of Morgagni. Can Med Assoc J. 1985;133(3):209–10. PubMed PMID: 4016626. Pubmed Central PMCID: PMC1346152. Epub 1985/08/01. eng
14. Golash V. Laparoscopic reduction of acute intrathoracic herniation of colon, omentum and gastric volvulus. Journal of Minimal Access Surgery. 2006;2(2): 76–8.
15. Bhasin DK. Endoscopic management of chronic organoaxial volvulus of the stomach. Am J Gastro. 1990;85(11):1486–8.
16. Baudet JS, Ammengol-Miro JR, Medin C, Accarino AM, Vilaceca J, Malagelada JR. Percutaneous endoscopic gastrostomy as a treatment for chronic gastric volvulus. Endoscopy. 1997;29:147–8.
17. Kassahun WT, Fangmann J, Harms J, Bartels M, Hauss J. Complicated small-bowel diverticulosis: a case report and review of the literature. World J Gastroenterol 2007 Apr 21;13(15):2240–2242. PubMed PMID: 17465510. Pubmed Central PMCID: PMC4146853. Epub 2007/05/01. eng.

34

Safety of expanded criteria for endoscopic resection of early gastric cancer in a Western cohort

Rimantas Bausys[1,2], Augustinas Bausys[1,2*], Kazimieras Maneikis[1], Viktorija Belogorceva[1], Eugenijus Stratilatovas[1,2] and Kestutis Strupas[1,3]

Abstract

Background: Endoscopic resection is widely accepted treatment option for early gastric cancer if tumors meet the standard or expanded indications. However, the safety of expanded criteria is still under investigation. Furthermore, discussion, if any additional treatment is necessary for patients who underwent endoscopic resection but exceeded expanded criteria, is rising. This study aimed to evaluate the safety of extended indications for endoscopic resection of early gastric cancer in a Western cohort. Also, we aimed to analyze the lymph node metastasis rate in tumors which exceeds the extended criteria.

Methods: Two hundred eighteen patients who underwent surgery for early gastric cancer at National Cancer Institute, Vilnius, Lithuania between 2005 and 2015 were identified from a prospective database. Lymph node status was examined in 197 patients who met or exceeded extended indications for endoscopic resection.

Results: Lymph node metastasis was detected in 1.7% of cancers who met extended indications and in 30.2% of cancers who exceeded expanded indications. Lymphovascular invasion and deeper tumor invasion is associated with lymph node metastasis in cancers exceeding expanded indications.

Conclusions: Expanded criteria for endoscopic resection of early gastric cancer in Western settings is not entirely safe because these tumors carry the risk of lymph node metastasis.

Keywords: Early gastric cancer, Endoscopic resection, Expanded indications, Safety, West

Background

Worldwide, the overall incidence of gastric cancer (GC) has steadily declined over the past 50 years, but in some regions (Asia, South America and Eastern Europe) it remained high [1, 2]. Furthermore, the incidence of early gastric cancer (EGC) in these areas is even rising [3]. According to the Japanese classification of gastric cancer, EGC is defined when tumor invasion is confined to the mucosa or submucosa, irrespective of the presence of lymph node metastasis (LNM) [4]. Surgery remains the only potentially curative treatment option for GC, but the extent of surgery for EGC and advanced GC may differ dramatically. Radical gastrectomy with regional lymphadenectomy remains the gold-standard for advanced GC, while endoscopic resection (ER) is sufficient procedure to treat EGC without LNM. According to studies from different regions, the rate of LNM in tumors confined to the mucosa varies between 2.7 and 6.5% and in submucosal tumors between 22.9 and 26.0%. There is a tendency, that rate of LNM in Western countries is higher compared to Asian countries [1]. Since radiological imaging accuracy for LNM detection is insufficient, indications for ER is based on histological tumor characteristics. The absolute indication for ER includes differentiated-type adenocarcinoma without ulcerative findings, of which the depth of invasion is clinically diagnosed as T1a, and the diameter is ≤2 cm [5]. However, only a small part of EGCs fulfill these criteria. The expansion of the standard criteria has been proposed in Japan from clinical observations that too

* Correspondence: abpelikanas@gmail.com
[1]Faculty of Medicine, Vilnius University, Ciurlionio str, 21 Vilnius, Lithuania
[2]Department of Abdominal surgery and Oncology, National Cancer Institute, Vilnius, Lithuania
Full list of author information is available at the end of the article

strict indication leads to unnecessary surgery [6, 7]. From the dataset of 5265 patients who underwent gastrectomy for EGC Gotoda et al. identified four additional groups of tumors, which have very low possibility of LNM when they are not accompanied with lymphovascular infiltration [8, 9]. These criteria are described as expanded indications in Japanese Gastric Cancer guideline: 1) differentiated-type mucosal cancer without ulceration and greater than 2 cm in diameter; 2) differentiated-type mucosal cancer with ulceration and up to 3 cm in diameter; 3) undifferentiated-type mucosal cancer without ulceration and up to 2 cm in diameter and 4) differentiated-type submucosal cancer (SM1, < 500 μm from the muscularis mucosae) up to 3 cm in diameter [5] (Table 1).

However, extending the indications for endoscopic EGC treatment remains controversial because the long-term outcomes of these procedures have not been adequately documented [10].

Also, some authors reported LNM in tumors which fulfill extended criteria [3, 10, 11].

Indications for ER of EGC were established in the Asian population. These findings translation to the Western world may be controversial because two recently published studies identified non-Asian race as an independent risk factor for LNM [12, 13]. Furthermore, it is not clear if any additional treatment is necessary for patients who underwent ER, but histological examination showed that tumor exceeds expanded criteria.

Therefore, our study aimed to evaluate the safety of extended indications for ER of EGC in a Western population. Also, we analyzed the LNM rate in tumors which exceeds the extended criteria.

Methods

Regional ethical committee approval was given before study was conducted. Retrospective analysis of prospectively collected GC database was performed. Between January 2005 and December 2015, a total of 1564 patients underwent curative surgery for gastric cancer at the National Cancer Institute, Vilnius, Lithuania. From this cohort, 218 (13.9%) patients underwent open gastrectomy with a D1 or D2 lymph node dissection for early gastric cancer. They were initially enrolled in this study. The clinicopathological characteristics of these patients were reviewed, and 197 patients with tumors who met or exceeded the extended indications for ER were identified and included to further analysis.

Statistical analysis

All statistical analyses were conducted using the statistical program SPSS 22.0 (SPSS, Chicago, IL, USA). Clinicopathological characteristics were analyzed by the 2-tailed t-test, one-way ANOVA test, Chi-square test or Fisher exact test. Binary logistic regression was performed to identify independent risk factors for lymph node metastasis in the group of patients who exceed the extended indications for endoscopic early gastric cancer treatment. In all statistical analyses, a p-value of < 0.05 was considered to be significant.

Results

Table 2 shows the clinicopathological characteristics of the 218 patients with EGC. 99 (45.4%) patients were diagnosed with intramucosal cancers and 119 (54.6%) with submucosal cancers.

The rate of lymph node metastasis, the presence of lymphovascular invasion and rate of tumors with greater diameter were significantly higher in submucosal cancer group. 21 patients had tumors which met standard indications for ER and they were excluded from further analysis. 58 patients met and 139 patients exceeded the extended indications for endoscopic EGC treatment. Table 3 shows clinicopathological data of these two groups.

Groups were comparable only according to age, retrieved lymph node number, and male: female ratio.

Of 58 cancer who met extended criteria, one (1.7%) had lymph node metastasis in 2 of 22 retrieved lymph nodes. It was not ulcerated, moderately differentiated mucosal cancer with greater than 2 cm diameter (2.2 × 1.8 × 1.5 cm).

LNM was found in 42 (30.2%) of 139 tumors who exceeded the extended criteria. Submucosal tumor invasion (36.2% vs. 11.8%, $p = 0.009$) and presence of lymphovascular invasion (61.3% vs. 21.3%, $p = 0.001$) was revealed as risk factors for LNM at univariate analysis (Table 4).

Binary logistic regression confirmed univariate analysis findings and showed submucosal tumor invasion (OR = 5.57, 95% CI: 1.40–22.08, $p = 0.014$) and lymphovascular

Table 1 The standard and expanded indications for endoscopic resection of early gastric cancer

The absolute indication for endoscopic resection of EGC	The expanded indications for endoscopic resection of EGC
Differentiated-type mucosal adenocarcinoma without ulcerative findings and the diameter is ≤2 cm	1) Differentiated-type mucosal cancer without ulceration and greater than 2 cm in diameter 2) Differentiated-type mucosal cancer with ulceration and up to 3 cm in diameter 3) Undifferentiated-type mucosal cancer without ulceration and up to 2 cm in diameter 4) Differentiated-type submucosal cancer (SM1, < 500 μm from the muscularis mucosae) up to 3 cm in diameter

Table 2 Clinicopathological characteristics of patients with mucosal and submucosal early gastric cancer

	Mucosal tumor invasion ($n = 99$)	Submucosal tumor invasion ($n = 119$)	p value
Age (mean ± SD)	63.5 ± 12.9	67.3 ± 11.6	**0.024**
Gender			
Male	44 (44.4%)	73 (61.3%)	**0.014**
Female	55 (55.6%)	46 (38.7%)	
Histology			
Differentiated	53 (53.5%)	61 (51.3%)	0.786
Undifferentiated	46 (46.5%)	58 (48.7%)	
Lauren classification			
Intestinal	54 (58.7%)	69 (60.5%)	0.902
Mix	8 (8.7%)	11 (9.6%)	
Diffuse	30 (32.6%)	34 (29.8%)	
Lymphanodectomy			
D1	11 (11.1%)	12 (10.1%)	0.828
D2	88 (89.9%)	107 (89.9%)	
No. of retrieved lymph nodes (mean ± SD)	19.4 ± 8.3	20.3 ± 10.7	0.454
Lymph node metastasis			
LNM+	5 (5.1%)	38 (31.9%)	**0.001**
LNM-	94 (94.9%)	81 (68.1%)	
Ulceration			
UL+	30 (30.3%)	48 (40.3%)	0.156
UL-	69 (69.7%)	71 (59.7%)	
Lymphovascular invasion			
LV+	3 (3.0%)	28 (23.5%)	**0.001**
LV-	96 (97.0%)	97 (76.5%)	
Tumor size			
< 2 cm	55 (55.6%)	42 (35.3%)	**0.009**
2–3 cm	25 (25.2%)	40 (33.6%)	
> 3 cm	19 (19.2%)	37 (31.1%)	

All the values in bold shows significance

invasion (OR = 7.13, 95% CI: 2.46–20.64, p = 0.001) as independent prognostic factors for LNM.

Discussion

EGC treatment with traditional gastrectomy and lymphadenectomy leads to excellent oncological outcomes. Several studies reported 5-year overall survival rate of up to 99% [14, 15]. However, compared to ER, surgery has some disadvantages. It is more invasive treatment method, associated with higher costs and reduced quality of life [16].

Avoidance of unnecessary surgery for appropriately selected EGC patients would lead to treatment improvement. Ideal selection of candidates for ER or surgery would consist of reliable preoperative radiological imaging and identification of LNM before choosing an appropriate surgical method for the individual patient. Unfortunately, available methods are not sufficiently accurate. Currently used endoscopic ultrasonography and computed tomography can reach only 50–87% accuracy [3, 17]. Therefore, the indications for ER is based on LNM risk presumption based on a set of histological tumor characteristics. As mentioned in the introduction section, several reasons exist to consider if expanded indications are entirely safe, especially in the Western population. A study published by Jee et al. [3] confirmed this uncertainty when reported 2.8% LNM rate in a cohort of patients who underwent gastrectomy for ECG which met the extended indications for ER. Alike, data from our present study showed 1.7% LNM rate in the similar cohort.

Furthermore, Jee et al. [3] showed the risk of LNM in three of four expanded criteria, but not in differentiated-type mucosal cancer, without ulceration, greater than 2 cm in

Table 3 Clinicopathological characteristics of patients who met and exceeded extended indications for endoscopic early gastric cancer treatment

	Extended indications group (*n* = 58)	Exceeding extended indications group (*n* = 139)	p value
Age (mean ± SD)	65.7 ± 11.3	65.2 ± 12.7	0.438
Gender			
Male	34 (58.6%)	71 (51.1%)	0.352
Female	24 (41.4%)	68 (48.9%)	
Histology			
Differentiated	40 (70.2%)	52 (37.4%)	**0.001**
Undifferentiated	17 (29.8%)	87 (62.6%)	
No. of retrieved lymph nodes (mean ± SD)	20.7 ± 10.8	19.0 ± 7.1	0.212
Tumor invasion			
Mucosal	44 (75.5%)	34 (24.5%)	**0.001**
Submucosal	14 (24.1%)	105 (75.5%)	
Lymph node metastasis			
LNM+	1 (1.7%)	42 (30.2%)	**0.001**
LNM-	57 (98.3%)	97 (69.8%)	
Ulceration			
UL+	8 (13.8%)	70 (50.3%)	**0.001**
UL-	50 (86.2%)	69 (49.7%)	
Lymphovascular invasion			
LV+	0 (0%)	31 (22.3%)	**0.001**
LV-	58 (100%)	108 (77.7%)	
Tumor size			
< 2 cm	34 (58.6%)	41 (29.4%)	**0.001**
2–3 cm	16 (27.6%)	49 (35.3%)	
> 3 cm	8 (13.8%)	49 (35.3%)	

All the values in bold shows significance

diameter. Therefore, authors proposed to consider this indication as safe [3]. In contrast, our study showed that this criterion also carries the risk of LNM. Thus, our result together with previous Jee et al. [3] findings indicates that possibility of LNM exists in every extended criterion.

Two recent studies showed the non-Asian race as a risk factor for LNM in gastric cancer [12, 13]. Our study cohort was very homogenous according to race and ethnicity. All patients were a Caucasian race. Despite, we failed to show a higher rate of LNM in tumors who meet extended criteria compared to the rate reported from similar Asian study [3]. These unexpected findings, together with a fact, that GC incidence in Eastern Europe is significantly higher compared to the rest of Western world, perfectly illustrates heterogenicity of the disease between different regions and different populations. Therefore, multicenter studies with large sample sizes from different racial and ethnical populations are needed to understand the risk of nodal involvement in EGC better. Only new and high-quality evidence will let us establish accurate and reliable clinical practice guidelines for EGC management.

While LNM risk in patients who meets expanded indications for ER is relatively low, patients who exceed these criteria are at high risk. We founded LNM in 30.2% of tumors who exceeded the expanded criteria. Nowadays ER for those tumors is considered as a non-curative treatment. However, some authors discuss that even non-curative ER could lead to satisfactory clinical outcomes. A large multi-center study published by Hatta et al. [18] compared long-term outcomes of patients who underwent either additional radical surgery or only follow-up after non-curative endoscopic resection. Results of the study showed that patients who underwent additional radical surgery had better 3- and 5-year overall survival (OS) and disease-specific survival (DSS) rates. Obviously, it should be declared, that the difference in DSS rates was rather small (99.4% vs.

Table 4 Univariate analysis of risk factors for lymph node metastasis in patients who exceed extended indications for endoscopic early gastric cancer treatment

	LNM- (*n* = 97)	LNM+ (*n* = 42)	p value
Age (mean ± SD)	64.6 ± 12.6	66.4 ± 12.8	0.441
Gender			
Male	53 (54.6%)	18 (42.9%)	0.268
Female	44 (45.4%)	24 (57.1%)	
Histology			
Differentiated	39 (40.2%)	13 (31.0%)	0.344
Undifferentiated	58 (59.8%)	29 (69.0%)	
Lauren classification			
Intestinal	50 (51.6%)	18 (42.9%)	0.553
Mix	11 (11.3%)	7 (16.7%)	
Diffuse	36 (37.1%)	17 (40.4%)	
Tumor invasion			
Mucosal	30 (30.9%)	4 (9.5%)	**0.009**
Submucosal	67 (69.1%)	38 (90.5%)	
Ulceration			
UL+	50 (51.6%)	20 (47.6%)	0.670
UL-	47 (48.4%)	22 (52.4%)	
Lymphovascular invasion			
LV+	12 (12.4%)	19 (45.2%)	**0.001**
LV-	85 (87.6%)	23 (54.8%)	
Tumor size			
< 2 cm	30 (30.9%)	11 (26.2%)	0.319
2–3 cm	31 (32.0%)	19 (45.2%)	
> 3 cm	36 (37.1%)	12 (28.6%)	

All the values in bold shows significance

98.7%) compared to the difference in OS rates (96.7% vs. 84.0%). Also, the rates of recurrence were significantly different, although in both groups they were low - 1.3% and 3.1% in the radical surgery group and the follow-up group, respectively. However, good outcomes in the follow-up group according to DSS and recurrence rates should be treated carefully due to different background characteristics of the study groups. Some major risk factors for LNM (lymphatic invasion or deeper submucosal invasion) were significantly more frequent in the additional radical surgery group [18, 19], and these differences may influence the study results. Furthermore, Suzuki et al. [20] recently published results from the similar study and showed a clear superiority of additional surgery after non-curative ESD compared to follow-up. After propensity score matching analysis, they founded significantly higher rates of 5-year DSS rate (99.0% vs 96.8%) and 5-year OS (91.0% vs. 75.5%) in the additional surgery group [19]. Results of those two studies and a high rate of LNM revealed in our study indicate, that EGC which exceeds expanded criteria for ER should be treated with gastrectomy and appropriate lymphadenectomy.

Some limitations of the present study should be mentioned as well. First, 5 (8.6%) of 58 patients with EGC that met expanded indications for ER underwent D1 lymphadenectomy. Because of limited lymphadenectomy, the risk of LNM in this group could be underestimated. Second, our study sample size was small compared to reports from Asian countries. Only 58 patients were in a group of tumors who met extended criteria for ER. However, lack of reports from Western countries increases the scientific value of our paper. Furthermore, despite the small sample size we managed to reach our study goal and showed the risk of LNM in tumors who meet expanded indications for ER.

Conclusion

Implementation of expanded criteria for endoscopic resection of EGC in a Western setting is not entirely safe because cancers who meet these indications carry the risk of LNM.

EGC who exceeds expanded indications has a high risk of LNM, therefore gastrectomy with lymphadenectomy should remain a standard treatment option.

Acknowledgments

This research received no specific grant from any funding agency in the public, commercial, or not-for-profit sectors.

Authors' contributions

RB, KS, ES and AB were responsible for study concept and design. KM, AB and VB were responsible for data collection and analysis. Manuscript was prepared by AB and KM. RB, VB, ES, KS were major contributors in writing, editing and revising the manuscript. All authors read and approved the final form of manuscript.

Competing interests

The authors declare that they have no competing interests.

Author details

[1]Faculty of Medicine, Vilnius University, Ciurlionio str, 21 Vilnius, Lithuania. [2]Department of Abdominal surgery and Oncology, National Cancer Institute, Vilnius, Lithuania. [3]Vilnius University Hospital Santaros Clinics, Center of Abdominal Surgery, Vilnius, Lithuania.

References

1. Bollschweiler E, Berlth F, Baltin C, Mönig S, Hölscher AH. Treatment of early gastric cancer in the Western world. World J Gastroenterol WJG. 2014;20(19):5672–8.
2. Mickevicius A, Ignatavicius P, Markelis R, Parseliunas A, Butkute D, Kiudelis M, et al. Trends and results in treatment of gastric cancer over last two decades at single east European Centre: a cohort study. BMC Surg. 2014;14:98.
3. Jee YS, Hwang S-H, Rao J, Park DJ, Kim H-H, Lee H-J, et al. Safety of extended endoscopic mucosal resection and endoscopic submucosal dissection following the Japanese gastric Cancer association treatment guidelines. Br J Surg. 2009;96(10):1157–61.

4. Japanese Gastric Cancer Association. Japanese classification of gastric carcinoma: 3rd English edition. Gastric Cancer Off J Int Gastric Cancer Assoc Jpn Gastric Cancer Assoc. 2011;14(2):101–12.
5. Association JGC. Japanese gastric cancer treatment guidelines 2014 (ver. 4). Gastric Cancer. 2017;20(1):1):1–19.
6. Gotoda T. Endoscopic resection of early gastric cancer. Gastric Cancer Off J Int Gastric Cancer Assoc Jpn Gastric Cancer Assoc. 2007;10(1):1–11.
7. Min YW, Min B-H, Lee JH, Kim JJ. Endoscopic treatment for early gastric cancer. World J Gastroenterol WJG. 2014;20(16):4566–73.
8. Gotoda T, Yanagisawa A, Sasako M, Ono H, Nakanishi Y, Shimoda T, et al. Incidence of lymph node metastasis from early gastric cancer: estimation with a large number of cases at two large centers. Gastric Cancer Off J Int Gastric Cancer Assoc Jpn Gastric Cancer Assoc. 2000;3(4):219–25.
9. Hirasawa T, Gotoda T, Miyata S, Kato Y, Shimoda T, Taniguchi H, et al. Incidence of lymph node metastasis and the feasibility of endoscopic resection for undifferentiated-type early gastric cancer. Gastric Cancer Off J Int Gastric Cancer Assoc Jpn Gastric Cancer Assoc. 2009;12(3):148–52.
10. Ishikawa S, Togashi A, Inoue M, Honda S, Nozawa F, Toyama E, et al. Indications for EMR/ESD in cases of early gastric cancer: relationship between histological type, depth of wall invasion, and lymph node metastasis. Gastric Cancer Off J Int Gastric Cancer Assoc Jpn Gastric Cancer Assoc. 2007;10(1):35–8.
11. Nagano H, Ohyama S, Fukunaga T, Hiki N, Seto Y, Yamaguchi T, et al. Two rare cases of node-positive differentiated gastric cancer despite their infiltration to sm1, their small size, and lack of lymphatic invasion into the submucosal layer. Gastric Cancer. 2008;11(1):53–8.
12. Fukuhara S, Yabe M, Montgomery MM, Itagaki S, Brower ST, Karpeh MS. Race/ethnicity is predictive of lymph node status in patients with early gastric cancer. J Gastrointest Surg Off J Soc Surg Aliment Tract. 2014;18(10): 1744–51.
13. Ikoma N, Blum M, Chiang Y-J, Estrella JS, Roy-Chowdhuri S, Fournier K, et al. Race is a risk for lymph node metastasis in patients with gastric Cancer. Ann Surg Oncol. 2017;24(4):960–5.
14. Green PH, O'Toole KM, Slonim D, Wang T, Weg A. Increasing incidence and excellent survival of patients with early gastric cancer: experience in a United States medical center. Am J Med. 1988;85(5):658–61.
15. Huang Q, Zou X. Clinicopathology of early gastric carcinoma: an update for pathologists and gastroenterologists. Gastrointest Tumors. 2017;3(3–4):115–24.
16. Peng LJ, Tian SN, Lu L, Chen H, Ouyang YY, Wu YJ. Outcome of endoscopic submucosal dissection for early gastric cancer of conventional and expanded indications: systematic review and meta-analysis. J Dig Dis. 2015; 16(2):67–74.
17. Polkowski M, Palucki J, Wronska E, Szawlowski A, Nasierowska-Guttmejer A, Butruk E. Endosonography versus helical computed tomography for Locoregional staging of gastric Cancer. Endoscopy. 2004;36(07):617–23.
18. Hatta W, Gotoda T, Oyama T, Kawata N, Takahashi A, Yoshifuku Y, et al. Is radical surgery necessary in all patients who do not meet the curative criteria for endoscopic submucosal dissection in early gastric cancer? A multi-center retrospective study in Japan. J Gastroenterol. 2017;52(2):175–84.
19. Bausys R, Bausys A, Vysniauskaite I, Maneikis K, Klimas D, Luksta M, et al. Risk factors for lymph node metastasis in early gastric cancer patients: report from Eastern Europe country- Lithuania. BMC Surg. 2017;17(1):108.
20. Suzuki S, Gotoda T, Hatta W, Oyama T, Kawata N, Takahashi A, et al. Survival benefit of additional surgery after non-curative endoscopic submucosal dissection for early gastric Cancer: a propensity score matching analysis. Ann Surg Oncol. 2017;24(11):3353–60.

Permissions

All chapters in this book were first published in SURGERY, by BioMed Central; hereby published with permission under the Creative Commons Attribution License or equivalent. Every chapter published in this book has been scrutinized by our experts. Their significance has been extensively debated. The topics covered herein carry significant findings which will fuel the growth of the discipline. They may even be implemented as practical applications or may be referred to as a beginning point for another development.

The contributors of this book come from diverse backgrounds, making this book a truly international effort. This book will bring forth new frontiers with its revolutionizing research information and detailed analysis of the nascent developments around the world.

We would like to thank all the contributing authors for lending their expertise to make the book truly unique. They have played a crucial role in the development of this book. Without their invaluable contributions this book wouldn't have been possible. They have made vital efforts to compile up to date information on the varied aspects of this subject to make this book a valuable addition to the collection of many professionals and students.

This book was conceptualized with the vision of imparting up-to-date information and advanced data in this field. To ensure the same, a matchless editorial board was set up. Every individual on the board went through rigorous rounds of assessment to prove their worth. After which they invested a large part of their time researching and compiling the most relevant data for our readers.

The editorial board has been involved in producing this book since its inception. They have spent rigorous hours researching and exploring the diverse topics which have resulted in the successful publishing of this book. They have passed on their knowledge of decades through this book. To expedite this challenging task, the publisher supported the team at every step. A small team of assistant editors was also appointed to further simplify the editing procedure and attain best results for the readers.

Apart from the editorial board, the designing team has also invested a significant amount of their time in understanding the subject and creating the most relevant covers. They scrutinized every image to scout for the most suitable representation of the subject and create an appropriate cover for the book.

The publishing team has been an ardent support to the editorial, designing and production team. Their endless efforts to recruit the best for this project, has resulted in the accomplishment of this book. They are a veteran in the field of academics and their pool of knowledge is as vast as their experience in printing. Their expertise and guidance has proved useful at every step. Their uncompromising quality standards have made this book an exceptional effort. Their encouragement from time to time has been an inspiration for everyone.

The publisher and the editorial board hope that this book will prove to be a valuable piece of knowledge for researchers, students, practitioners and scholars across the globe.

List of Contributors

Marc Schiesser, Pierre-Alain Clavien and Antonio Nocito
Department of Visceral and Transplantation Surgery, University Hospital Zurich, Raemistrasse 100, 8091 Zurich, Switzerland

Daniel C Steinemann
Department of Visceral and Transplantation Surgery, University Hospital Zurich, Raemistrasse 100, 8091 Zurich, Switzerland
Department of Surgery, Cantonal Hospital Bruderholz, 4104 Bruderholz, Switzerland

Mikito Inokuchi, Keiji Kato, Hirofumi Sugita and Sho Otsuki
Department of Surgical Oncology, Tokyo Medical and Dental University, Tokyo, Japan

Kazuyuki Kojima
Department of Minimally Invasive Surgery, Tokyo Medical and Dental University, Tokyo, Japan

Roberto Cirocchi, Stefano Trastulli, Jacopo Desiderio and Amilcare Parisi
Department of Digestive and Liver Surgery Unit, St Maria Hospital, Terni, Italy

Carlo Boselli, Piero Covarelli, Claudio Renzi, Chiara Listorti and Giuseppe Noya
Department of General and Oncologic Surgery, University of Perugia, Perugia, Italy

Alberto Santoro, Salvatore Guarino and Adriano Redler
Department of Surgical Sciences, "Sapienza" University of Rome, Rome, Italy

Andrea Coratti
Department of General Surgery, Misericordia Hospital, Grosseto, Italy

Villy Våge, Camilla Laukeland and Jan Behme
Department of Surgery, Førde Central Hospital, 6807 Førde, Norway

Vetle Aaberge Sande
Department of Clinical Science, University of Bergen, 5020 Bergen, Norway

Gunnar Mellgren
Department of Clinical Science, University of Bergen, 5020 Bergen, Norway
Hormone Laboratory, Haukeland University Hospital, 5021 Bergen, Norway

John Roger Andersen
Department of Surgery, Førde Central Hospital, 6807 Førde, Norway
Department of Health, Sogn og Fjordane University College, 6803 Førde, Norway

Christina Hackl, Felix C Popp, Volker Benseler, Philipp Renner, Martin Loss, Hans J Schlitt and Marc H Dahlke
Department of Surgery, University Medical Center Regensburg, Regensburg 93042, Germany

Katharina Ehehalt
Department of Anaesthesia, University Medical Center Regensburg, Regensburg, Germany

Lena-Marie Dendl
Department of Radiology, University Medical Center Regensburg, Regensburg, Germany

Jurgen Dolderer and Lukas Prantl
Department of Trauma, Plastic and Hand Surgery, University Medical Center Regensburg, Regensburg, Germany

Thomas Kühnel
Department of Otorhinolaryngology, University Medical Center Regensburg, Regensburg, Germany

Giovanni Aprea, Alfonso Canfora, Antonio Ferronetti, Antonio Giugliano, Francesco Guida, Antonio Braun, Melania Battaglini Ciciriello, Federica Tovecci, Giovanni Mastrobuoni and Bruno Amato
Department of General, Geriatric, Oncologic Surgery and Advanced Technologies, University "Federico II" of Naples, Via Pansini, 5 - 80131 - Naples, Italy

Fabrizio Cardin
Department of Surgical and Gastroenterological Sciences, Padova University Hospital, Italy Via Giustiniani n.2, 35126 Padova, Italy

Junqiang Chen, Jianji Pan, Jiancheng Li and Yu Lin
Department of Radiation Oncology, The Teaching Hospital of Fujian Medical University, Fujian Provincial Cancer Hospital, 91 Maluding, Fuma Road, Fuzhou, Fujian 350014, China

Sangang Wu
Xiamen Cancer Center, Department of Radiation Oncology, the First Affiliated Hospital of Xiamen University, Xiamen 361003, China

Xiongwei Zheng
Departments of Pathology, The Teaching Hospital of Fujian Medical University, Fujian Provincial Cancer Hospital, Fuzhou 350014, China

Kunshou Zhu and Yuanmei Chen
Departments of Surgery, The Teaching Hospital of Fujian Medical University, Fujian Provincial Cancer Hospital, Fuzhou 350014, China

Lianming Liao
Center of Oncology Research, Academy of Integrative Medicine, Fujian University of Traditional Chinese Medicine, Fuzhou 350014, China

Zhongxing Liao
Department of Radiation Oncology, The University of Texas M. D. Anderson Cancer Center, Unit 97, 1515 Holcombe Boulevard, Houston, TX, USA

Wei-Juan Zeng, Lin-Wei Wang, Chun-Wei Peng, Gui-Fang Yang and Yan Li
Departments of Oncology and Pathology, Zhongnan Hospital of Wuhan University, Hubei Key Laboratory of Tumor Biological Behaviors and Hubei Cancer Clinical Study Center, Wuhan 430071, China

Wen-Qin Hu and Shu-Guang Yan
Department of Surgery, Heji Hospital Affiliated to Changzhi Medical College, Changzhi 046000, China

Jian-Ding Li
Department of Medical Imaging, The First Affiliated Hospital of Shanxi Medical University, No 85, South Jiefang Road, Taiyuan City 030001, Shangxi Province, China

Hao-Liang Zhao
Department of General Surgery, Shanxi University Hospital, No 99, Longcheng Street, Taiyuan City 046000, Shangxi Province, China

Noëlle Geubbels, Ingrid Kappers and Arnold W. J. M. van de Laar
Department of Surgery, Slotervaart hospital, Amsterdam, The Netherlands

Tobias S Schiergens, Michael N Thomas and Wolfgang E Thasler
Department of Surgery, University of Munich, Campus Grosshadern, Munich, Germany

Thomas P Hüttl
Department of Surgery, Chirurgische Klinik München-Bogenhausen, Munich, Germany

Yan-Na Wang, Kun-Tang Shen, Jia-Qian Ling, Xiao-Dong Gao, Xue-Fei Wang, Jing Qin, Yi-Hong Sun and Xin-Yu Qin
Department of General Surgery, Zhongshan Hospital of Fudan University, No 180 Fenglin Road, Shanghai 200032, China

Ying-Yong Hou
Department of Pathology, Zhongshan Hospital of Fudan University, No 180 Fenglin Road, Shanghai 200032, China

Duminda Subasinghe
General Surgery, University Surgical Unit, The National Hospital of Sri Lanka, Colombo, Sri Lanka

Chathuranga Tisara Keppetiyagama
Gastrointestinal Surgery, University Surgical Unit, The National Hospital of Sri Lanka, Colombo, Sri Lanka

Dharmabandhu N Samarasekera
University Surgical Unit, The National Hospital of Sri Lanka, 28/1, Ishwari road, Colombo 06 Colombo, Sri Lanka

Marta Guimarães, Pedro Rodrigues, Gil Gonçalves and Mário Nora
Department of General Surgery, Hospital de São Sebastião, Santa Maria da Feira, Portugal

Mariana P Monteiro
Endocrinology Unit of Hospital São Sebastião, Hospital de São Sebastião, Santa Maria da Feira, Portugal
Department of Anatomy, Multidisciplinary Unit for Biomedical Research (UMIB), ICBAS, University of Porto, Porto, Portugal

Bruno Martella, Fabrizio Cardin, Renata Lorenzetti and Carmelo Militello
Department of Molecular Medicine, University of Padua, Italy

Claudio Terranova
Department of Surgical and Gastroenterological Sciences, University of Padua, Italy

Bruno Amato
University of Naples Federico II - Department of General Surgery, Italy

Ming Wang, Jia Xu, Yun Zhang, Lin Tu, Wei-Qing Qiu, Chao-Jie Wang and and Hui Cao
Department of General Surgery, Ren Ji Hospital, School of Medicine, Shanghai Jiao Tong University, Floor 11, Building 7, NO. 1630, Dongfang Road, Shanghai 200127, China.

Yan-Ying Shen and Qiang Liu
Department of Pathology, Ren Ji Hospital, School of Medicine, Shanghai Jiao Tong University, Shanghai, China

IM Luppino, R Spagnuolo, R Marasco and P Doldo
Gastroenterology and Endoscopy Unit, T. Campanella Oncological Foundation, Catanzaro, Italy

B Amato
General Surgery Unit, Dept of General Surgery, Geriatric and Endoscopy, University Federico II, Naples, Italy

A Puzziello, G Orlando, R Gervasi and MA Lerose
Endocrine Surgery Unit, Department of Surgical and Medical Sciences, University Magna Graecia, Catanzaro, Italy

Jingge Yang, Cunchuan Wang, Guo Cao, Wah Yang, Shuqing Yu, Hening Zhai and Yunlong Pan
Department of General Surgery, First Affiliated Hospital of Jinan University, Guangzhou 510630, China

Shinichiro Kobayashi, Kengo Kanetaka, Masahiko Nakayama, Ryo Matsumoto, Mitsuhisa Takatsuki and Susumu Eguchi
Department of Surgery, Nagasaki University Graduate School of Biomedical Sciences, Sakamoto 1-7-1, Nagasaki 8528102, Japan

Yasuhiro Nagata
Department of Surgery, Nagasaki University Graduate School of Biomedical Sciences, Sakamoto 1-7-1, Nagasaki 8528102, Japan
Center for Comprehensive Community Care Education, Nagasaki University Graduate School of Biomedical Sciences, Sakamoto 1-12-4, Nagasaki, Japan

Hong-Xia Ren, Li-Qiong Duan, Xiao-Xia Wu, Bao-Hong Zhao and Yuan-Yuan Jin
Department of Pediatric Surgery, Shanxi Children's Hospital, 13 New People Avenue, Taiyuan 030013, Shanxi, China

Ke Chen, Yu Pan, Bin Zhang, Xian-fa Wang and Xiu-jun Cai
Department of General Surgery, Sir Run Run Shaw Hospital, School of Medicine, Zhejiang University, 3 East Qingchun Road, Hangzhou, Zhejiang Province 310016, China

Hendi Maher
School of Medicine, Zhejiang University, 866 Yuhangtang Road, Hangzhou, Zhejiang Province 310058, China

Shota Kuwabara, Yuma Ebihara, Yoshitsugu Nakanishi, Toshimichi Asano, Takehiro Noji, Yo Kurashima, Soichi Murakami, Toru Nakamura, Takahiro Tsuchikawa, Keisuke Okamura, Toshiaki Shichinohe and Satoshi Hirano
Department of Gastroenterological Surgery II, Hokkaido University Graduate School of Medicine, North 15 West 7, Kita-ku, Sapporo, Hokkaido 0608638, Japan

Wei Wang, Lei Liu, Minxin Shi, Yixin Zhang and Qiang Wang
Department of Surgery, The Affiliated Tumor Hospital of Nantong University, Nantong, Jiangsu Province, China

Min Wei and Qi He
Department of Breast, International Peace Maternity and Child Health Hospital, Shanghai Jiao Tong University, Shanghai, China

Tianlong Ling and Ziang Cao
Department of Thoracic Surgery, Shanghai Renji Hospital Affiliated to Shanghai Jiao Tong University School of Medicine, Shanghai, China

Zhiwei Wang
Department of Breast, International Peace Maternity and Child Health Hospital, Shanghai Jiao Tong University, Shanghai, China
Department of Thoracic Surgery, Shanghai Renji Hospital Affiliated to Shanghai Jiao Tong University School of Medicine, Shanghai, China

Fanny Sellberg, Sofie Possmark and Daniel Berglind
Department of Public Health Sciences, Karolinska Institutet, K9, Social Medicin, SE-171 77 Stockholm, Sweden

Ata Ghaderi
Department of Clinical Neuroscience, Karolinska Institutet, SE-171 77 Stockholm, Sweden

Erik Näslund
Division of Clinical Sciences, Danderyd Hospital, Karolinska Institutet, SE-182 88 Stockholm, Sweden

Mikaela Willmer
Department of Health and Caring Sciences, University of Gävle, SE-801 76 Gävle, Sweden

Per Tynelius
Department of Public Health Sciences, Karolinska Institutet, K9, Social Medicin, SE-171 77 Stockholm, Sweden
Centre for Epidemiology and Community Medicine, Stockholm County Council, Box 45436, SE-104 31 Stockholm, Sweden

Anders Thorell
Department of Clinical Science at Danderyd Hospital, Karolinska Institutet, SE-116 91 Stockholm, Sweden
Department of Surgery, Ersta Hospital, SE-116 91 Stockholm, Sweden

Magnus Sundbom
Department of Surgical Sciences, Uppsala University, SE-751 85 Uppsala, Sweden

Joanna Uddén
Department of Medicine, Karolinska Institutet, SE-141 86 Stockholm, Sweden
Department of Endocrine and Obesity, Capio st Görans Hospital, SE-141 86 Stockholm, Sweden

Eva Szabo
Department of Surgery, Faculty of Medicine and Health, Örebro University, SE-701 85 Örebro, Sweden

Yukinori Yamagata, Kazuyuki Saito, Kosuke Hirano, Yawara Kubota, Ryuji Yoshioka, Takashi Okuyama, Emiko Takeshita, Nobumi Tagaya, Shinichi Sameshima, Tamaki Noie and Masatoshi Oya
Department of Surgery, Dokkyo Medical University Koshigaya Hospital, 2-1-50 Minami-Koshigaya, Koshigaya City, Saitama 343-8555, Japan

Robert Grützmann, Nikolaos Vassos, Aristotelis Perrakis and Roland S Croner
Department of Surgery, University Hospital Erlangen, Krankenhausstrasse 12, 91054 Erlangen, Germany

Alexandros Mekras, Vasileios Kalles and Cem Atamer
Department of Surgery, S. Elisabeth Hospital, Bernkastel/Wittlich, Germany

Veit Krenn
MVZ-Zentrum für Histologie, Zytologie und Molekulare Diagnostik, Trier, Germany

Chien-An Liu
Department of Radiology, Taipei Veterans General Hospital, Taipei City, Taiwan.
School of Medicine, National Yang-Ming University, Taipei City, Taiwan

Chew-Wun Wu, Yi-Ming Shyr and Wen-Liang Fang
Division of General Surgery, Department of Surgery, Taipei Veterans General Hospital, No. 201, Sec 2, Shipai Rd., Beitou District, Taipei City 11217, Taiwan
School of Medicine, National Yang-Ming University, Taipei City, Taiwan

Kuo-Hung Huang
Division of General Surgery, Department of Surgery, Taipei Veterans General Hospital, No. 201, Sec 2, Shipai Rd., Beitou District, Taipei City 11217, Taiwan
School of Medicine, National Yang-Ming University, Taipei City, Taiwan
Institute of Clinical Medicine, School of Medicine, National Yang-Ming University, Taipei City, Taiwan

Ming-Huang Chen
Division of Medical Oncology, Department of Oncology, Taipei Veterans General Hospital, Taipei City, Taiwan

School of Medicine, National Yang-Ming University, Taipei City, Taiwan

Su-Shun Lo
School of Medicine, National Yang-Ming University, Taipei City, Taiwan
National Yang-Ming University Hospital, Yilan City, Taiwan

Anna Fen-Yau Li
Department of Pathology, Taipei Veterans General Hospital, Taipei City, Taiwan
School of Medicine, National Yang-Ming University, Taipei City, Taiwan

Chaoyong Shen, Haining Chen, Yuan Yin, Jiaju Chen, Bo Zhang, Zhixin Chen and Jiaping Chen
Department of Gastrointestinal Surgery, West China Hospital, Sichuan University, Chengdu 610041, Sichuan, China

Luyin Han
Intensive Care Unit, West China Hospital, Sichuan University, Chengdu 610041, China

Wei Chen, Xumian Jiang and Hui Huang
Department of Gastrointestinal Surgery, The Central Hospital of the Wuhan, Tongji Medical College, Huazhong University of Science and Technology, Wuhan 430000, People's Republic of China

Zao Ding
Department of General Surgery, Zhongnan Hospital of Wuhan University, Wuhan 430014, People's Republic of China

Chihua Li
Department of Gastrointestinal Surgery, Hubei Cancer Hospital, Wuhan 430014, People's Republic of China

Satoru Kikuchi, Shinji Kuroda, Masahiko Nishizaki, Tetsuya Kagawa, Shunsuke Kagawa and Toshiyoshi Fujiwara
Department of Gastroenterological Surgery, Okayama University Graduate School of Medicine, Dentistry and Pharmaceutical Sciences, 2-5-1 Shikata-cho, Kita-ku, Okayama 700-8558, Japan

Hiromitsu Kanzaki and Yoshiro Kawahara
Department of Endoscopy, Okayama University Hospital, Okayama 700-8558, Japan

Takehiro Tanaka
Department of Diagnostic Pathology, Okayama University Hospital, Okayama 700-8558, Japan

Hiroyuki Okada
Department of Gastroenterology and Hepatology, Okayama University Graduate School of Medicine, Dentistry and Pharmaceutical Sciences, Okayama 700-8558, Japan

Noriyuki Hirahara, Takeshi Matsubara, Yoko Mizota, Shuichi Ishibashi and Yoshitsugu Tajima
Department of Digestive and General Surgery, Shimane University Faculty of Medicine, 89-1 Enya-cho, Izumo, Shimane 693-8501, Japan

Stefan Fritz, Katharina Feilhauer, André Schaudt, Hansjörg Killguss, Eduard Esianu, René Hennig and Jörg Köninger
Department of General, Visceral, Thoracic and Transplantation Surgery, Katharinenhospital Stuttgart, Kriegsbergstraße 60, 70174 Stuttgart, Germany

Fabio Cianchi, Benedetta Badii, Fabio Staderini, Etleva Qirici, Antonio Taddei, Maria Novella Ringressi, Caterina Foppa, Ileana Skalamera, Giulia Fiorenza and Giuliano Perigli
Department of Surgery and Translational Medicine, Center of Oncological Minimally Invasive Surgery (COMIS), University of Florence, Largo Brambilla 3, 50134 Florence, Italy

Giampiero Indennitate, Manuela Ortolani and Beatrice Paoli
IFCA, Florence, Italy

Giacomo Trallori, Giuseppe Macrì, Gabriele Lami, Siro Bagnoli and Andrea Bonanomi
Unit of Gastroenterology, University Hospital Careggi, Florence, Italy

Beatrice Mallardi
ISPO, Florence, Italy

Luca Messerini and Luca Novelli
Department of Experimental and Clinical Medicine, University of Florence, Florence, Italy

Zoya Fatima Rizwan Ladiwala, Rija Sheikh, Ayesha Ahmed and Ibrahim Zahid
Dow University of Health Sciences, Karachi, Pakistan

Amjad Siraj Memon
Department of General Surgery, Dow University of Health Sciences, Civil Hospital Karachi, Karachi, Pakistan

Kazimieras Maneikis and Viktorija Belogorceva
Faculty of Medicine, Vilnius University, Ciurlionio str, 21 Vilnius, Lithuania

Rimantas Bausys, Augustinas Bausys and Eugenijus Stratilatovas
Faculty of Medicine, Vilnius University, Ciurlionio str, 21 Vilnius, Lithuania
Department of Abdominal surgery and Oncology, National Cancer Institute, Vilnius, Lithuania

Kestutis Strupas
Faculty of Medicine, Vilnius University, Ciurlionio str, 21 Vilnius, Lithuania
Vilnius University Hospital Santaros Clinics, Center of Abdominal Surgery, Vilnius, Lithuania

Index

www.ingramcontent.com/pod-product-compliance
Lightning Source LLC
Chambersburg PA
CBHW061259190326
41458CB00011B/3713

9781632416094